MEG–EEG PRIMER

MEG–EEG PRIMER

SECOND EDITION

Riitta Hari, MD, PhD

Professor Emerita of Systems Neuroscience and Neuroimaging

Department of Art and Media

Aalto University

Espoo, Finland

Aina Puce, PhD

Eleanor Cox Riggs Professor in Social Justice and Ethics

Department of Psychological & Brain Sciences

Indiana University

Bloomington, IN, USA

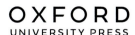

OXFORD

UNIVERSITY PRESS

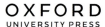

Oxford University Press is a department of the University of Oxford. It furthers
the University's objective of excellence in research, scholarship, and education
by publishing worldwide. Oxford is a registered trade mark of Oxford University
Press in the UK and certain other countries.

Published in the United States of America by Oxford University Press
198 Madison Avenue, New York, NY 10016, United States of America.

Library of Congress Cataloging-in-Publication Data
Names: Hari, Riitta, author. | Puce, Aina, author.
Title: MEG–EEG Primer 2nd Ed./by Riitta Hari and Aina Puce.
Description: New York, NY: Oxford University Press, [2023] |
Includes bibliographical references and index.
Identifiers: LCCN 2016039489 | ISBN 9780197542187 (alk. paper)
Subjects: | MESH: Magnetoencephalography—methods |
Electroencephalography—methods | Brain—physiology | Brain Mapping |
Brain Diseases—diagnosis
Classification: LCC RC386.6.M36 | NLM WL 141.5.M24 | DDC 616.8/047548—dc23
LC record available at https://lccn.loc.gov/2016039489

DOI: 10.1093/med/9780197542187.001.0001

Printed by Integrated Books International, United States of America

CONTENTS

■ SECTION 3

PREFACE TO THE SECOND EDITION

We are delighted by the interest and positive feedback that the first edition of our *Primer* received. We are especially gratified that it has been a useful source for training new students, researchers, and faculty entering the field. Our aims in this second edition remain unchanged: to introduce the basic principles of magnetoencephalography (MEG) and electroencephalography (EEG) as tools to noninvasively study human brain dynamics and to generate an *integrated understanding of the two techniques*.

Over the last 5 years, interest in high-resolution, time-sensitive methods has increased rapidly in the whole human brain-imaging community, requiring us to slightly broaden our scope. We still attempt to provide a solid basis for applying the MEG and EEG methods—including the underlying physics and physiology, instrumentation, recording techniques, data analysis, and interpretation—without comprehensively covering the rapidly expanding literature in this field.

We have made updates to all chapters, especially in Sections 2 and 3. We have expanded text on MEG/EEG sensor types and amplifiers, artifacts, new analysis tools, open data repositories, and novel instrumentation. Due to a new concern, brought about by the COVID-19 pandemic, we now discuss general infection control in all MEG/EEG measurements. Moreover, we now introduce interoception as an interesting emerging research field. We end with a broader chapter on the future of understanding human brain function to stimulate our readers' thinking beyond their own research topics.

We have added some citations to both old and new key literature in the field. Some minor errors have been corrected, and the index has been expanded. The second edition is over 100 pages longer than the original and contains 34 totally new illustrations, with small edits to 36 existing figures. Despite the reorganization, we have tried to keep the *Primer* as close to the original as possible, to serve as the "ABC book" for all researchers interested in immersing themselves into the exciting world of human brain dynamics. Therefore, we recognize that we have omitted important topics and data and have not been able to expand the presentation as much as some of our readers would have liked to (especially regarding anatomy, clinical applications, and some analysis methods). After all, this is a primer that aims to stimulate the reader to search for additional information and hands-on databases and to embark on the never-ending adventure of studying the secrets of the human brain.

We cordially thank our colleagues Synnöve Carlson, Matti Hämäläinen, Veikko Jousmäki, Lauri Parkkonen, Ben Ramsden, Jari Saramäki, Samu Taulu, and Koichi Yokosawa for many helpful discussions on various topics in this book. We also received excellent comments from five anonymous reviewers who were invited by the publisher to read the first edition; we highly appreciate their constructive suggestions. We are especially grateful to two prereaders of our second edition: Juan Avenado (Aalto University, Finland), with his keen eyes, spotted multiple inconsistencies in our text and figures, and Ann-Sophie Barwich (Indiana University, USA) guided us to improve the text flow. We are also greatly indebted to Peter Molfese and Kami Salibayeva for help in proofreading the Primer.

A huge thank you also to Matt Winter and Kami Salibayeva (Social Neuroscience Lab at Indiana University) for assistance with collection and analysis of ExG data for new figures: together we learned to use our new EEG/ExG recording system without on-site technical support during the COVID-19 lockdown! Matt also provided valuable feedback and comments on isolated sections of our chapters. We thank Satu Ilta for drawing and editing most of the new or revised figures of the second edition. We are also immensely grateful again to the digital librarians at Indiana University Libraries for their continued tenacious sourcing of obscure and almost forgotten manuscripts for this second edition.

We thankfully acknowledge Craig Panner from OUP for his enduring patience and humanity. We have appreciated his continued collaboration and facilitation over the years as he shepherded both editions of our *Primer* to the publication stage.

When preparing the first edition, we were privileged to interact with Professor Fernando Lopes da Silva (1935–2019), a pioneer in advocating the importance of combining EEG and MEG methods in the assessment of human brain dynamics. We miss Fernando's kind support and presence but hope that his legacy will live on in new generations of EEGers and MEGers.

Riitta Hari acknowledges funding from Louis Jeantet Foundation and thanks the Department of Art and Media, Aalto University, Finland, for stimulating working environment for an emerita.

Aina Puce expresses her gratitude to both Eleanor Cox Riggs and also the College of Arts and Sciences at Indiana University (Bloomington) for continued support and funding. She also acknowledges her wonderful colleagues and students in the Department of Psychological and Brain Sciences, at Indiana University.

PREFACE TO THE FIRST EDITION

The aim of this primer is to provide an introduction to the basic principles of magneto-encephalography (MEG) and electroencephalography (EEG). MEG and EEG are time-sensitive methods that allow the noninvasive study of human brain activity. We target our message to beginning and intermediate users of MEG/EEG, assuming that most readers will be graduate students or postdoctoral fellows in systems, cognitive, affective, social, or clinical neuroscience, or perhaps faculty looking to move into these areas. We also hope that scientists interested in interdisciplinary research linked to these research fields may find this primer useful.

Even the best tools cannot yield sound results if the principles underlying the recording techniques, the generation of the signals, as well as the fundamentals of the analysis methods are not well understood. In this primer we thus focus on the basic physical and physiological background of MEG and EEG signals and principles of appropriate experimentation, data analysis, and interpretation. Our goal is to provide the reader with useful information on the practical aspects and typical technical problems faced in MEG or EEG recordings. We thus discuss at some length possible sources of artifacts, the procedures to judge the quality of the recording, and the care required in physiological interpretation.

Consequently, we do not exhaustively review the existing MEG and EEG literature but rather give examples of typical signals and refer to previous review papers and textbooks. Whenever possible, we try to point out connections to interesting brain functions and brain-imaging methods to emphasize that the MEG and EEG technologies are not independent of other approaches in neuroscience.

MEG and EEG have often been discussed separately, which has led many researchers to neglect their close relationship. The current neuroscience literature frequently examines results of one or two functional neuroimaging methods in a fairly unbalanced manner. For example, both MEG and EEG papers often cite functional magnetic resonance imaging (fMRI) literature, MEG papers more often cite EEG literature than vice versa, and fMRI papers either largely ignore electrophysiology or may cite scalp or invasive electric potential measurements (electrocorticography or depth electrode measurements) but rarely MEG. To remediate this problem, we try to discuss MEG and EEG in parallel, hoping that the very direct connections between these two methods thereby become clear. At the same time, it is important to develop a common language to facilitate successful interdisciplinary science.

We are indebted to our research teams and colleagues for feedback on the contents of this book, and especially the following individuals who have commented on drafts: Elizabeth

Bendycki, Sara Driskell, Tommi Himberg, Aapo Hyvärinen, Matti Hämäläinen, Veikko Jousmäki, Miika Koskinen, Kaisu Lankinen, Nancy Lundin, Ben Motz, Timo Nurmi, Ben Ramsden, Elina Pihko, Eero Smeds, and Noah Zarr. We thank Satu Ilta for drawing and redrawing the illustrations, and Lotta Hirvenkari for additional assistance in image preparation. We thank Elizabeth da Silva, Mia Illman, Isaiah Innis, Veikko Jousmäki, Anne Mandel, Timo Nurmi, and Lauri Parkkonen for help in the collection of some new MEG/EEG data for illustrations in this primer and Nancy Lundin and John Purcell for modeling the EEG caps and nets in Chapter 6. We acknowledge Matti Hämäläinen and Ben Ramsden for in-depth discussions on the contents of this primer. Finally, we thank the Staff at the Indiana University Libraries, Bloomington, for their determination in sourcing the more difficult-to-access publications.

ABOUT THE AUTHORS

Riitta Hari is a professor emerita of systems neuroscience and neuroimaging at Aalto University, Finland, currently working at the Aalto University's Department of Art and Media. She is an MD PhD who, after her doctoral education at the Department of Physiology, University of Helsinki, Finland, received specialization in clinical neurophysiology at the Helsinki University Central Hospital, where she worked as a clinical neurophysiologist at the Epilepsy Unit of the Department of Neurology and at the Department of Neurosurgery. In 1982, she moved to Helsinki University of Technology (currently Aalto University) where, for over 30 years, she led a multidisciplinary Brain Research Unit. She has published extensively on MEG research in basic and clinical human neuroscience. She was a founding member of a five-member team of Mustekala Ky, which laid the foundation for the MEG-instrument development company Neuromag Oy (currently MEGIN Oy, Helsinki, Finland). Her most recent interests are in the brain basis of human social interaction and in bridging neuroscience and art without privileging either one. She has been financially supported by the Academy of Finland, the European Research Council, the Sigrid Jusélius Foundation, the SalWe Research Program for Mind and Body (by Tekes, the Finnish Funding Agency for Technology and Innovation), the Louis Jeantet Foundation, the Finnish Cultural Foundation, and the Aalto University.

Aina Puce is currently the Eleanor Cox Riggs Professor of Social Ethics and Justice in the Department of Psychological & Brain Sciences at Indiana University, Bloomington, Indiana. She completed her PhD in the Department of Medicine, University of Melbourne, Australia, and then worked as a postdoctoral fellow and then research scientist in the Department of Neurosurgery at the Yale University School of Medicine, New Haven, Connecticut. Her research in face/object perception provided major contributions to invasive electrical brain mapping studies in epilepsy-surgery patients and to fMRI studies in healthy subjects. She has served as the deputy director for the Brain Sciences Institute, Swinburne University in Melbourne, Australia; the director of neuroimaging in the Department of Radiology at the West Virginia University School of Medicine, and the director of the Imaging Research Facility at Indiana University. She has published work on basic and clinical human neuroscience using scalp and intracranial EEG, MEG, and fMRI. Her academic interests are rooted in the brain bases of human nonverbal communication and more recently with art and the brain. She has been heavily involved in international efforts to develop and disseminate best practices in EEG and MEG data acquisition, analysis, and sharing. Her work has been supported by the National Health & Medical Research Council (Australia), the Australia Research Council, the National Institutes for Health (NINDS and NIBIB, USA), West Virginia University, Eleanor Cox Riggs, and the College of Arts and Sciences of Indiana University.

PREAMBLE

In the early 1990s, a 38-year-old man entered the magnetoencephalography (MEG) laboratory of the Brain Research Unit of the Helsinki University of Technology. He had suffered from epileptic seizures since the age of 14. His seizures typically started by convulsions of the side of his face, which then progressed to a full-blown generalized seizure with loss of consciousness. Now his generalized seizures were well controlled with modern antiepileptic drugs, but he was left with a type of "focal epilepsy," consisting of frequent convulsions of his left face but without associated loss of consciousness. These convulsions could occur spontaneously or could be triggered by touching the left side of his mouth or gum: he had a rare type of reflex epilepsy that was touch triggered.

Because of the resistance of the facial convulsions to medication, surgery was planned to remove the brain area, or "epileptic focus," that was giving rise to the convulsions. Typical for patients with focal seizure disorders, he had already gone through an exhaustive set of examinations to identify the epileptic focus; the examinations included multiple scalp electroencephalography (EEG) and videotelemetric recordings, as well as positron emission tomography (PET). Despite this extensive workup, the brain regions responsible for the epileptic seizures had not been identified. The hope was now to put MEG to the task as it is not affected by the skull, which dampens and smears EEG signals. The first whole-scalp-covering MEG device had just been developed in Finland to simultaneously pick up signals from both hemispheres.

During the MEG recording, the patient triggered a seizure by touching his left gum with his tongue. Figure P.1 shows MEG signals recorded over a 20-s interval where, soon after the touch, epileptic spikes, sharp transients, and complex spikes started to appear in the right hemisphere (red trace in panel a), contralateral to the touched gum. The abnormal discharges soon became continuous and spread to the left hemisphere as well (both traces in b), and simultaneously convulsions started in the patient's left cheek. The whole seizure, as determined from the MEG signals, lasted for 14 seconds and then ended abruptly (in both traces in c).

The source analysis of the MEG signals—aiming to attribute the measured signals to particular brain regions—indicated that the epileptic discharges started from the face representation area of the right primary motor cortex and then spread, within 22 ms, to the left hemisphere (see the insert of Figure P.1). This time lag was determined by careful analysis of the time courses of the sources of right- and left-hemisphere spikes, and it agreed with interhemispheric conduction via myelinated fibers of about 1 μm in diameter (Aboitiz

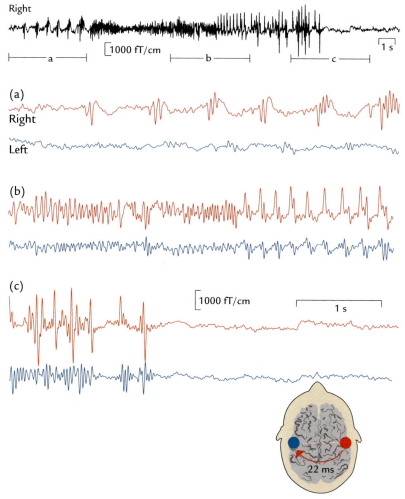

FIGURE P.1. MEG signals in a patient with touch-triggered focal epilepsy. A 20-s trace from one (planar) MEG sensor over the right sensorimotor region is shown at the top of the figure, with calibration bars for signal amplitude and time. The segments a, b, and c indicate times of interest that are magnified in the subsequent traces from homologous right- (red) and left-hemisphere (blue) MEG sensors. (a) Immediately after touch, epileptic spikes appear in the right hemisphere. (b) Abnormal discharges are seen in both hemispheres but are significantly larger on the right. (c) The epileptic discharge ends abruptly in both hemispheres. The schematic axial section of the brain depicts the transfer of the spikes in 22 ms from the right to the left hemisphere. Adapted and reprinted from Forss N, Mäkelä JP, Keränen T, Hari R: Trigeminally triggered epileptic hemifacial convulsions. *Neuroreport* 1995, 6: 918–920. With permission from Wolters Kluwer Health, Inc.

et al., 1992). Thus, the primary epileptic focus had been identified in the right hemisphere with a "mirror" focus in the left hemisphere (Forss et al., 1995).

The quite rare types of epileptic discharges seen in this patient raise several questions: How do MEG and EEG differ from each other? What essential steps do we need to take to record reliable MEG and EEG signals, and how can we be sure that the measured signals arise from the brain and not from some external source or from another part of the body? How do we preprocess, analyze, and model the signals, and how do these results relate to findings obtained by other neuroimaging methods? How do we interpret the results from the neuroscientific and clinical points of view? How can we expect these methods to improve in the future? In this *Primer*, we try to address these questions.

■ REFERENCES

Aboitiz F, Scheibel A, Fisher R, Zaidel E: Fiber composition of the human corpus callosum. *Brain Res* 1992, 598: 143–153.

Forss N, Mäkelä JP, Keränen T, Hari R: Trigeminally triggered epileptic facial convulsions. *Neuroreport* 1995, 6: 918–920.

SECTION 1

CHAPTER 1

INTRODUCTION

When all you have is a hammer, everything looks like a nail.

Abraham Maslow

One of the secrets of cooking is to learn to correct something if you can, and bear with it if you cannot.

Julia Child

Neuronal communication in the brain is associated with minute electrical currents that give rise to both electrical potentials on the scalp (measurable by means of electro-encephalography [EEG]) and magnetic fields outside the head (measurable by means of magnetoencephalography [MEG]). Both MEG and EEG are noninvasive neurophysiolog-ical methods used to study brain dynamics, temporal changes in the activation patterns and sequences. The differences between MEG and EEG mainly reflect differences in the spread of electric potentials and magnetic fields generated by electric currents in the human brain. In this chapter, we give an overall description of the main principles of MEG and EEG, going deeper into details in the following chapters.

■ MEG AND EEG SETUPS

Figure 1.1 illustrates MEG and EEG measuring set-ups. During a conventional MEG re-cording (top panel), the subject is sitting with her head inside a helmet-shaped "dewar" vacuum flask that in this specific supercooled device houses an array of 306 extremely sen-sitive magnetic-field detectors (middle panel, left); the name of this vacuum-insulated flask honors its inventor, James Dewar (1842–1923). To eliminate or dampen external ambient magnetic disturbances, the measurements are performed within a magnetically shielded room. To unravel which part of the brain the MEG signals are coming from, the position of the head with respect to the sensor array must be determined before each session, and it is often—depending on the availability of this option in the applied measurement device—continuously monitored during the recording.

Eye movements and blinks that cause prominent artifacts in the recording are best monitored by means of an electro-oculogram (electrical activity from eye and lid move-ments) or with an infrared camera (as shown in Figure 1.1, top panel), although they can be detected also from the frontal MEG (and EEG) channels. During the recording, the subject must keep her head as still as possible in the relatively tight helmet-shaped

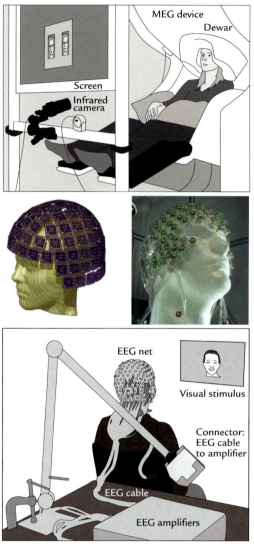

FIGURE 1.1. MEG and EEG recording setups. Schematic MEG layout (top panel) displays subject sitting comfortably with her head placed in a "dewar." In front of her are a back-projection screen for visual stimulus presentation and an infrared camera for monitoring eye movements. EEG setup (bottom panel) shows a subject, with attached EEG sensors, sitting in front of a computer monitor for visual stimulation. EEG amplifiers (to which the electrodes are connected via the thick EEG cable) appear in the foreground. Middle panels show MEG (left) and EEG (right) sensor arrays, respectively.

dewar housing the sensor array. She can speak and moderately move her hands and eyes, although in that case some artifact-suppression methods may be needed. Her facial and bodily actions can be recorded with a video and monitored with response pads, accelerometers, and surface electromyogram (electrical activity from muscles), also including the electro-oculogram. The electrocardiogram (electrical activity from the heart) can also be recorded.

During the EEG recording (Figure 1.1, bottom panel), the subject is more free to move, although head and body movements may cause artifacts and, as with MEG, are in most cases discouraged. The subject wears an EEG cap or elasticized "net," in this case with 256 electrodes, attached to the scalp (middle panel, right). A response pad is on the subject's lap (not seen in the figure), and a monitor to present visual stimuli is located at a distance in front of the subject to minimize electrical interference. As with MEG recordings, other electrical signals from the body—such as the heart and muscles—can also be recorded together with the EEG. To avoid other types of external electrical interference, EEG is preferably measured inside a Faraday cage that dampens power-line artifacts and other electrical noise, although recordings of sufficient quality can also be performed in regular rooms, operating theaters, and even in real-life settings using mobile EEG devices.

EEG can be recorded simultaneously with MEG, provided that the EEG electrodes and wires are nonmagnetic and do not take up too much space to prevent the subject's head from fitting into the MEG helmet.

EEG and MEG signals are closely related. Figure 1.2 shows that a neuronal current (depicted with an arrow) in a local brain area, here representing activation of the auditory cortex to an abrupt sound, generates both MEG (magnetic field, left) and EEG (electric potential, middle) signal distributions. The resulting MEG pattern can be predicted using the "right-hand rule" (as outlined in Figure 1.2, right panel).

Figure 1.2 also shows that the MEG and EEG patterns are at right angles with respect to each other. The electric potential distribution on the scalp is more widespread than the corresponding pattern of the radial component of the magnetic field, here also computed on the scalp, although in practice the MEG signals are recorded about 20 mm above the scalp. This difference in spread between the MEG and EEG patterns arises because the concentrically layered structure of the head with different electrical conductivities for cerebrospinal fluid, skull, and scalp tissues leads to spread, or "smearing" of the electric potentials, but

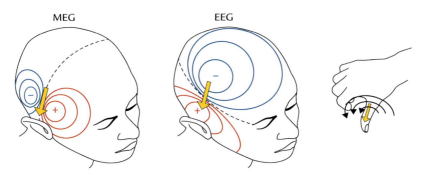

FIGURE 1.2. **Relationship between the site and direction of intracellular current and MEG and EEG signal distributions on the head.** The schematic example depicts isofield lines for MEG (left) and isopotential lines for EEG (center) about 100 ms after a sound that activates the auditory cortex; the elicited net current (dipole) is displayed by the yellow arrow. The MEG and EEG patterns are rotated by 90 degrees with respect to one another. For MEG, positive and negative signs signify magnetic flux leaving and entering the head, respectively. For EEG, positive and negative signs indicate the polarities of the scalp potentials. The broken lines on each field pattern show the respective isofield and isopotential lines where the signal is zero. The MEG pattern can be understood on the basis of the "right-hand rule" that is illustrated in the panel on the right: when the current flows to exit the right thumb, the magnetic field lines curl in the direction of the fingers of the right hand.

TABLE 1.1 Approximate Sizes of Different Magnetic Fields of the Environment and the Body (in units of femtotesla or 10^{-15} tesla = 10^{-15} T)

Magnetic resonance imaging	3,000,000,000,000,000 (= 3 T)
Steady magnetic field of the earth	50,000,000,000
Magnetocardiogram	100,000
Brain's alpha rhythm	1,000
Brain's evoked responses	100
Sensitivity of a magnetometer	3
Noise within a magnetically shielded room	1

does not affect the magnetic field. Its distribution is only altered by the distance between brain sources and the locations from which the MEG signals are recorded.

If we have measured the magnetic field at multiple locations outside the head and/or the potential distribution on the scalp, we can estimate the locations and strengths of the "source currents" giving rise to the measured signals. In other words, the field and potential distributions outside the head can be used to model the likely site of the original current inside the head. This inference of the sources of the measured signals is the so-called *inverse problem*, which is discussed further in Chapters 3 and 10.

In MEG, tiny magnetic fields, in the order of femto- and picotesla (1 fT = 10^{-15} tesla and 1 pT = 10^{-12} tesla), are detected with an array of sensors that are located around the head. As the typical MEG signal is of the order of 100 fT and thus a mere 10^{-8} times the strength of the earth's steady magnetic field, the best-quality MEG recordings are carried out inside special magnetically shielded rooms (see Chapter 5). However, even there, only the most sensitive sensors can pick up the brain's tiny magnetic fields. For approximate sizes of different magnetic fields in the environment and body, see Table 1.1.

The most commonly used sensors are SQUIDs (superconducting quantum interference devices), which do not make direct contact with the head as they are immersed within the large, vacuum-insulated liquid-helium-containing dewar. The magnetic fields emanating from the head induce current flow in the SQUIDs. The circuit associated with the SQUID functions as a flux–voltage amplifier, transforming the magnetic flux sensed by the SQUID to a voltage readable by the electronics. Recent developments using different types of sensor technologies now allow MEG measurements to be made at room temperature (see Chapter 5).

In EEG, electrodes are fixed to the scalp and electric potentials are measured between two electrodes at a time (potential difference is the same as voltage). Scalp EEG signals typically are about 50 to 100 µV (1 µV = 10^{-6} volt) in amplitude, whereas intracranial EEG signals can be an order of magnitude larger. The smaller amplitude of the scalp EEG is the result of the increased distance between the sources in the brain and the electrodes and signal attenuation by the scalp, the skull, and the cerebrospinal fluid. (One very important additional factor is the size of the active area, as the potential decreases considerably faster as a function of distance for small relative to large areas of active tissue, see e.g., Mitzdorf, 1985.) Compare these EEG potentials with the up to 1 million times higher voltages (of 110–240 V) used to power home appliances.

Because of their small size, both MEG and EEG signals must be amplified. They need to be filtered before they are digitized (sampled to discrete values) and subjected to further analysis; we discuss these preprocessing steps in Chapter 8.

■ COMPARISON OF MEG AND EEG

When examining the properties of MEG and EEG signals, it is convenient to assume, as the first approximation, that the head is a sphere where we have only local activations that we model as "current dipoles." In a sphere, the relationships between (neural) currents and the associated magnetic fields and electric potentials are relatively simple, and they serve as good first approximations for the interpretation of real MEG and EEG signals.

To avoid confusion, it is necessary to first make a distinction between different dipoles: a current dipole, an electric dipole, and a magnetic dipole, all shown schematically in Figure 1.3. The *current dipole* (Figure 1.3, top), indicated here as a yellow arrow, is an approximation to describe locally moving charges (i.e., a current concentrated to a point). As we explain in Chapter 3, the current dipole represents the intracellular "primary current" due to net flow of ions within the cell bodies (soma) and projections (dendrites) of the activated neurons.

The current dipole is situated in a conducting medium (a volume conductor), and the primary current is always associated with return currents (or volume currents) that close

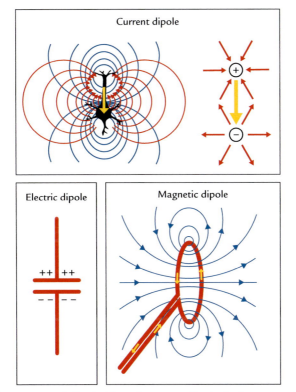

FIGURE 1.3. **Three types of dipole.** Top. A current dipole (yellow arrow) depicted in two different ways. At left, the blue lines show the isopotential lines and the red lines show the paths of the volume (return) currents in a schematic neuron. At right, the volume currents have been replaced by two radially symmetric current distributions: currents (red arrows) entering the positive end of the dipole and currents leaving the negative pole of the current dipole. Bottom left. An electric dipole (a charged capacitor) with no current flow. Bottom right. Magnetic dipole (a current loop) with the associated magnetic field lines (shown in blue); the small yellow arrows indicate the current direction in the loop.

the loop. The currents cannot accumulate in any part of the brain because of small capacitances of the tissues.

In Figure 1.3 (top panel), the volume currents associated with the current dipole are presented as current paths that connect the two ends of the neuron; the left schematic shows these paths as red lines and the right schematic shows an equivalent distribution of two radially symmetric current distributions, one at each end of the activated neuron (red arrows). For the neuron on the left, the blue isopotential lines indicate where in the extracellular space the potential is the same. Current dipoles like these are commonly used as source models for MEG and EEG signals.

Positive and negative static charges, for example, in a charged capacitor, form an *electric dipole* (Figure 1.3, bottom left), which by itself does not generate electric current or a magnetic field. The *magnetic dipole* (Figure 1.3, bottom right) is a current loop that, in the ideal case, does not produce any electric potential, but a very focal magnetic field goes through the loop (e.g., a wire) and returns via the environment, as is shown by the blue field lines. In transcranial magnetic stimulation (TMS; see Chapter 21), the opposite situation occurs: A brief current pulse delivered to a coil will induce a short-lasting strong magnetic field that can be used to focally stimulate the brain.

To understand how MEG and EEG signals are generated, it is useful to examine three types of current dipoles situated in a sphere (Figure 1.4): a radial dipole, a tangential dipole, and a deep source in the middle of the sphere. It is through a combination of these types of currents that we can represent currents of *any* orientation in the sphere, because we can divide any current into tangential and radial components with respect to the sphere's surface. Radial currents are oriented along the radius of the sphere, and tangential currents are orthogonal (at 90°) to them (see the dashed lines depicting two radii in Figure 1.4a). A local current in the middle of the sphere is always radial.

Figure 1.4 illustrates some interesting properties of magnetic fields generated by various local currents in a spherical volume conductor. Note that all current dipoles (arrows) shown in the figure represent the primary (intracellular) currents. First, the radial currents (both the intracellular current represented by the arrow and the associated return currents that are not illustrated in this image) are symmetric with respect to the direction of the

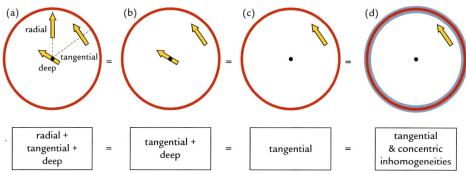

FIGURE 1.4. **MEG in a nutshell.** Panel (a) shows a radial, a tangential, and a deep dipole in a spherical volume conductor. The produced external magnetic field pattern will be identical for this panel and for panels (b)–(d), and even for panel d, where concentric inhomogeneities have been added to the sphere. See text for further explanation. Adapted and reprinted from Hari R, Levänen S, Raij T: Timing of human cortical functions during cognition: role of MEG. *Trends Cogn Sci* 2000, 4: 455–462. With permission from Elsevier.

current dipole and *do not* produce any magnetic field *outside the sphere*. This rather surprising result can be demonstrated formally (see, e.g., Hämäläinen et al., 1993). In contrast to radial dipoles, tangential current dipoles are associated with volume currents that are *not* symmetric with respect to the primary current (and thereby also not with respect to the sphere) and *do* produce a net magnetic field outside the sphere. Note, however, that even in this case the magnetic field outside the sphere can be computed directly from the size (and location) of the primary current, without taking into account the volume currents.

Thus, the magnetic field (MEG signal) produced by the three dipoles in Figure 1.4a is exactly the same as without the radial dipole (Figure 1.4b). Because all dipoles in the center of the sphere are radial, the external field is still the same even without the deep dipole in the center of the volume conductor (Figure 1.4c). In other words, all magnetic fields outside the ideal sphere arise from tangential currents only or from the tangential components of tilted (i.e., not perfectly tangential or radial) currents.

Keep in mind that we are speaking here about a fundamental property of the generation of magnetic fields within a sphere, meaning that it is the current orientation with respect to the sphere that matters, and it is not possible to see magnetic fields produced by the radial currents by any manipulation, such as tilting the orientation of the MEG sensors (outside the sphere) with respect to the dipole orientation.

Another important point is that the external magnetic field remains the same even if the sphere is comprised of concentric shells of different electrical conductivities (Figure 1.4d). Concentric inhomogeneities mean that the conductivity σ (see Chapter 3) is a function of the radius r only: $\sigma(x) = \sigma(r)$, where x is a point in the medium. Here the brain, the cerebrospinal fluid, the skull, and the scalp can be considered to form concentric inhomogeneities.

We can thus say that MEG sees directly into the brain, without distortion from the intervening tissues, and we are left with the notion that—in a sphere that contains only concentric shells of electric inhomogeneities—solely tangential currents (or the tangential components of tilted currents) will contribute to MEG signals measured outside the sphere. Although the real head is not an ideal sphere, these main principles are most useful in understanding the neuronal contributions to the MEG signals.

Figure 1.5 continues these MEG-in-a-nutshell considerations. Panel (a) shows that the magnetic field for two current dipoles of opposite directions at the same place is equal in size but opposite in polarity. Panel (b) demonstrates the linear additivity of the magnetic fields. Panel (c) repeats the message from Figure 1.4 in that radial currents do not produce any magnetic field outside the sphere. As a consequence, one can add to the sphere any number of radial currents as was done in panel (d), where a tangential current was replaced by a current loop running via the origin of the sphere. The formed current loop will produce a magnetic field that is equal to that produced by the tangential current dipole (Ilmoniemi et al., 1985; Hari & Ilmoniemi, 1986). This equivalence has been used to build elegant "dry phantoms" to test the accuracy of MEG localization: a tangential current dipole in a sphere can be replaced with a triangular current loop that passes through the origin of the sphere, without the need to use a wet volume conductor.

For EEG, the situation is different because all of the currents, of different orientations and different depths, contribute to the EEG potentials on the surface of the sphere. Moreover, the electric inhomogeneities (such as the skull and scalp) dampen and smear the potential distribution, resulting in the more widespread pattern for EEG than MEG as was shown in Figure 1.2. For radial currents, the maximum scalp potentials are just above the current location, whereas tangential currents produce potential maxima of different polarities at the two ends of the current dipole. For both MEG and EEG, the distance between the two signal extrema depends on the depth of the tangential current.

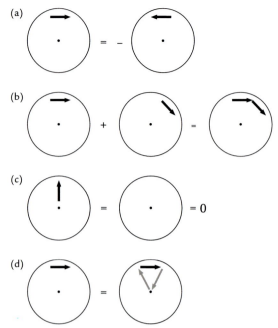

FIGURE 1.5. Schematic presentation of magnetic fields associated with different current-dipole configurations. (a) If the current flow reverses, the polarity of the magnetic field will reverse as well. (b) Superposition principle of magnetic fields. (c) Radial currents do not produce any external magnetic field. (d) Since radial currents do not produce any magnetic field, one can add those to any existing current distributions. Here the gray arrows (that pass the origin of the sphere) have replaced volume currents. See text for further explanation.

An interesting point to note is that, compared with the identical current dipole in an infinitely large homogeneous conductor, the interface between the head and air (or brain and skull) in fact magnifies the potential at the surface by a factor of three (Hari & Katila, 1982). We will fine-tune these general principles about MEG/EEG generation in the following chapters when the anatomy and physiology of the human brain are taken into account.

The main source currents of both MEG and EEG arise in the cortical pyramidal neurons. A pyramidal neuron (see Figures 1.6 and 2.1) consists of a cell body (soma), dendrites that receive input from other cells, and an axon that carries the neuron's impulse to other neurons. Because of their shape (elongated apical dendrites) and alignment perpendicular to the cortical surface, the pyramidal neurons effectively generate intracellular currents perpendicular to the cortical surface. This critical spatial alignment sets the scene for microscopic currents associated with each apical dendrite to collectively sum to (detectable) macroscopic net currents at the cortical surface, so that each pyramidal neuron can be considered to be a tiny current dipole, as shown in Figure 1.6.

Nonpyramidal neurons lack these essential geometric hallmarks and therefore contribute very little to MEG/EEG signals. These geometric proclivities of pyramidal neurons thus yield mainly radial current sources in the convexial cortex (the upper surfaces of the gyri) and tangential currents in the walls of cortical fissures (or sulci); see Figure 1.6.

EEG measures voltage differences between different parts of the scalp and is most sensitive to currents in convexial cortex just under the electrode. In addition to these superficial

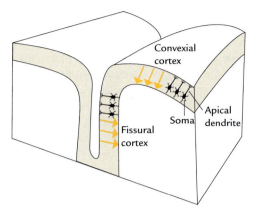

FIGURE 1.6. **Convexial and fissural currents.** Schematic representation of neurons (black) with their main axis oriented perpendicular to the cortical surface. The somas of the neurons are in the deeper layers of cortex, and the current flow following excitation of the apical dendrites can be modeled as intracellular current dipoles pointing from surface to deeper layers (yellow arrows). Note that the current flow may be of the opposite direction, depending on the type of postsynaptic current (excitatory/inhibitory) and the locations of synapses (see Figure 2.1).

radial currents, it can also sense tangential currents and (strong) deep currents. For example, auditory-evoked brainstem responses (Chapter 13) can be picked up far more easily with EEG than with MEG. However, the broad spatial sensitivity of EEG also means that it may be difficult to discern multiple active sources from the recorded signals.

The high sensitivity (and, in the case of a sphere, even selectivity) of MEG to tangential currents means that MEG mainly measures activity occurring in the walls of cortical fissures. This is an advantage, as about two-thirds of the cerebral cortex is located within fissures (including all primary sensory cortices) that are difficult places to reach even with intracranial recordings. Because of MEG's insensitivity to electric inhomogeneities, the inverse solution (computing the most likely generator currents, or the "sources") on the basis of the measured signal patterns is more straightforward for MEG than for EEG. For EEG, additional assumptions are required about the conductivities of different head-tissue layers.

An additional important difference between MEG and EEG is that EEG recordings measure voltage differences (potentials) *between* two recording sites (i.e., between "active" and "reference" electrodes; see Chapter 5), whereas MEG recordings provide information on the magnetic flux or its gradients exactly at the measurement site.

A major advantage of EEG is that it is relatively inexpensive and portable, relative to MEG, and it can be more easily incorporated for simultaneous use with functional magnetic resonance imaging (fMRI), transcranial magnetic stimulation, and transcranial direct current stimulation (Chapter 21).

All methods have their own characteristics that make them appropriate tools for some purposes but not for others. For cutting, for example, scissors are the tool of choice for making tiny paper decorations, whereas a sharp knife would be preferred for slicing an apple into many pieces. Similarly, all functional neuroimaging methods have their own niches. MEG and EEG are optimal and complementary methods to reveal the brain's neurodynamics, the temporal variations of brain activity at a (sub)millisecond time scale. In principle, simultaneous recordings of MEG and EEG provide the most complete direct picture of the ongoing neuronal mass activity in the human brain.

■ STRUCTURE OF THIS PRIMER

After this brief introduction to MEG and EEG, we begin our tour with a concise survey of brain structure and function, which is necessary to place MEG and EEG results into the proper perspective, and we discuss the neural currents underlying MEG and EEG (Chapter 2). We then proceed to the basic physics of electricity, currents, volume conduction, magnetic fields, and superconductivity (Chapter 3). In the last chapter of Section 1, we review briefly the history of EEG and MEG recordings and give an overview of the most common spontaneous and evoked EEG and MEG signals; we also briefly list the advantages and disadvantages of MEG and EEG in the study of human brain function (Chapter 4).

Section 2 deals with the practicalities of acquiring and analyzing data. In Chapters 5 and 6, we discuss instrumentation, including shielding and stimulators, as well as practical aspects of sound MEG/EEG experimentation. Next, in Chapters 7 and 8, we describe data acquisition and preprocessing of signals, and in Chapter 9 we discuss common artifacts and their prevention and elimination. In Chapter 10, we proceed to common methods of data analysis, including signal averaging, some single-trial analysis methods, and source analysis.

In Section 3, in Chapters 11 through 19, we provide examples of various MEG and EEG signals, including spontaneous and stimulus-, task-, and event-related activity, always attempting to discuss MEG and EEG findings side by side. We include discussion on the integration of other bodily signals with recordings of MEG or EEG activity (e.g., skeletal-muscle activity, heart rate, electrical activity of the gut, action monitoring, eye tracking, etc.) to allow a more embodied interpretation of brain function. We also describe simultaneous recordings from two or more individuals ("hyperscanning"). We briefly examine the use of MEG/EEG in various brain disorders in Chapter 20. In Chapter 21, we consider the uses of MEG and EEG together, as well as with other brain imaging methods to study brain function. Finally, we look to the future and special state-of-the-art recording and analysis techniques (Chapter 22). We also try to broaden the reader's view by discussing some challenges in understanding how the human brain works and how MEG and EEG studies with their accurate temporal information could contribute to this very multidisciplinary endeavor.

We hope that after reading this primer you, our reader, independent of your education and training, will be on equal footing with the members of your multidisciplinary MEG/EEG research team as far as the basics of these methods are concerned. Your metaphorical toolbox will then contain—in addition to a hammer for nails—a screwdriver for screws, a wrench for nuts, and whatever other gadgets and gizmos that might be needed.

■ REFERENCES

Hämäläinen M, Hari R, Ilmoniemi RJ, Knuutila JET, Lounasmaa OV: Magnetoencephalography—theory, instrumentation, and applications to noninvasive studies of the working human brain. *Rev Mod Phys* 1993, 65: 413–497.

Hari R, Ilmoniemi RJ: Cerebral magnetic fields. *CRC Crit Rev Biomed Engin* 1986, 14: 93–126.

Hari R, Katila T: Notes on magnetic fields produced by the human brain. In: Malmivuo J, Lekkala J, eds. *Proceedings of the 4th National Meeting on Biophysics and Medical Engineering, Tampere Finland*. Tampere, Finland: Finnish Society for Medical Physics and Medical Engineering, 1982: 49–52.

Ilmoniemi RJ, Hämäläinen MS, Knuutila J: The forward and inverse problems in the spherical model. In Weinberg H, Stroink G, Katila T, eds.: *Biomagnetism: Applications and Theory*. New York: Pergamon, 1985, 278–282.

Mitzdorf U: Current source-density method and application in cat cerebral cortex: investigation of evoked potentials and EEG phenomena. *Physiol Rev* 1985, 65: 37–100.

CHAPTER 2

INSIGHTS INTO THE HUMAN BRAIN

Anatomy is usually right but boring,
physiology is usually wrong but exciting.

SEMIR ZEKI

We know almost everything about the brain,
except how it works.

RODOLFO LLINAS

The aim of MEG and EEG recordings is to obtain new information about human brain function, especially with respect to the millisecond-range neurodynamics in both healthy and diseased brains. Here we review some basic principles of human brain structure and function that may be relevant for the design and interpretation of MEG and EEG recordings.

OVERVIEW OF THE HUMAN BRAIN

Our brains are the product of evolution, individual development (ontogenesis), and culture. Stated briefly, the brain is an organ that predicts the future on the basis of the past, thereby helping the individual survive and perpetuate the species. Genetic information settles the main framework for brain development, but it is the active individual–environment interactions that shape the human brain and mind throughout life. The healthy human brain remains plastic during the entire lifespan, allowing the individual to keep gathering and remembering information, as well as learning new skills.

Different brain regions—which are currently known well even at a microstructural level (Fischl & Sereno, 2018)—are connected to each other, as well as to the sensory and motor periphery, by fibers (axons) that form the brain's white matter. The white color refers to the visual appearance of myelin sheaths that surround a large number of these fibers and allow them to conduct impulses faster than fibers without myelin sheaths.

In newborns and infants, maturation of brain areas can be judged on the basis of myelination (Dehaene-Lambertz & Spelke, 2015). The earliest cortical areas to mature, already before birth, are the primary sensory projection cortices and the visual-motion-sensitive cortical area MT/V5. The maturation of the corpus callosum, the superhighway of information transfer between the hemispheres, continues up to early adulthood (Tanaka-Arakawa et al., 2015). Follow-up studies with different structural magnetic resonance imaging (MRI) methods indicate that brain development beyond infancy is associated with thinning of different cortical regions in a specific order (Gogtay et al., 2004). Whereas myelinization was originally quantified by staining of postmortem histological samples, today special MRI sequences allow noninvasive estimation of myelin content (Glasser & Van Essen, 2011).

■ HOW TO OBTAIN INFORMATION ABOUT BRAIN FUNCTION

Historically, brain injuries and the accompanying sensorimotor and cognitive deficits have been informative regarding the putative functional roles of specific brain regions, and quintessential information related to brain–behavior relationships has been obtained from animal neurophysiology. Most recently, the emergence of various neuroimaging methods has allowed noninvasive studies of the structure and function of the human brain in living individuals, in contrast to the previous focus on postmortem studies of brain structure.

We can now use fMRI, positron emission tomography (PET), scalp EEG, intracranial EEG, MEG, and near-infrared spectroscopy (NIRS) for recordings of brain activity. The information obtained by these methods can be merged with data from brain stimulation methods (which may perturb or stimulate certain brain areas), such as transcranial magnetic stimulation (TMS), transcranial direct current stimulation (tDCS), intracranial electric brain stimulation, or even focused transcranial ultrasonic stimulation (see Chapter 21).

Many neuroimaging publications depict beautifully colored "blobs" of brain activity related to various stimuli and tasks. However, we must remember that only lesions can be localized, not functions. Similarly, as the lack of electricity after a broken fuse does not mean that the fuse generates the electricity, a behavioral symptom after a brain lesion (or transient suppression of activity by direct electrical stimulation of the cortex or by TMS) may not have anything to do with the real function of that brain area. Local lesions may also sever the connections between brain regions so that the behavioral manifestations may arise from other parts of the brain. Consider, for example, the famous case of Phineas Gage, in whom a rather restricted brain lesion in the prefrontal cortex resulted in dramatic deficits in affect and cognition, likely because the lesion also interrupted the brain's widespread interareal connections, thus causing symptoms that cannot be explained by the lesion site only (Van Horn et al., 2012).

Information about cognitive functions can be obtained at various temporal and spatial scales. In addition to brain measurements, it is always important to carefully describe the behavioral phenomena of interest and their changes during task modifications. Without sufficient characterization of behavioral phenomena, especially motor behavior and its context, appropriate interpretation of neural activity may be compromised. In certain experiments, it may be useful to also record other signals of interest (e.g., heart rate, pupil dilation, etc.) to relate changes in the subject's physiological state and to specifically examine brain function connected to interoception (see Chapter 16).

■ TIMING IN HUMAN BEHAVIOR

Accurate timing is important for many brain processes devoted to perception, action, and cognition. The relevant time scales vary from tens of microseconds (e.g., in directional hearing) to tens and hundreds of milliseconds (e.g., in cortical processing of sensory information) to seconds and minutes. Table 2.1 gives rough estimates of temporal scales of human behavior and some neuronal events.

Although millisecond timing is needed, for example, for dancing to a fast salsa rhythm, multisensory asynchrony—such as the time lag between voice and visual mouth

TABLE 2.1 Temporal scales of human behavior and neural activity

• Auditory localization	50 μs
• Auditory click separation	1 ms
• Action potential	1–3 ms
• One cycle of gamma-range oscillation	25 ms
• One cycle of beta-range oscillation	50 ms
• One cycle of alpha-range oscillation	100 ms
• Reaction time	150–300 ms
• Multisensory asynchrony	100–250 ms
• Attentional blink	500 ms
• Preparation for motor action	500–2000 ms

Note: ms = milliseconds; μs = microseconds.

movements in a movie—can be tolerated for surprisingly long time spans of up to 100 to 250 ms (see Chapter 16).

The relevant time windows of signal processing in the brain seem to be hierarchically organized and supported by spatially different networks, so that the shortest time windows (associated with the most rapid processing) occur in brain areas closest to sensory projection cortices and the longest time windows in nonsensory brain regions. This organizational principle has been demonstrated from seconds to tens of seconds using fMRI (Hasson et al., 2008) and from milliseconds to hundreds of milliseconds with MEG; the MEG data further indicate that multiple time windows can exist within the same brain area (Hari et al., 2010).

In general, slower brain rhythms can modulate faster ones, as "nested oscillations" (Hyafil et al., 2015). For example, during speech perception, specific integration windows exist for consonants (20–50 ms) and syllables (200–300 ms) (Boemio et al., 2005), as well as for phrases (up to 2 s) (Bourguignon et al., 2013). In several brain disorders, such as Parkinson's disease, temporal sequencing of action may slow down (see Chapter 20). MEG/EEG have just the right temporal sensitivity for monitoring these rapid changes.

■ FUNCTIONAL STRUCTURE OF THE HUMAN CEREBRAL CORTEX

The human cerebral cortex, a 3- to 4-mm thick layer on the brain surface and the main target of MEG and EEG studies, is only about 1.5% of body weight, but consumes about 15% of total blood flow (the whole brain uses about 20%). Lamination of pyramidal neurons differs between neocortex and allocortex: Neocortex that comprises 90% of total cortical area has six layers and allocortex, including the hippocampus and the olfactory cortex located in the mesial temporal lobes, has only three or four layers.

In trying to understand how the brain works, keep in mind both the functional generality of the cerebral cortex as a whole and variability from area to another. Functional generality suggests the existence of some kind of fundamental operations that are connected to the vertical (along the main orientation of cortical pyramidal cells) organization of the cortex. In contrast, the diversity of "cytoarchitectonic" areas (differing, e.g., in cell size, shape and connectivity) may result from different afferent projection systems and efferent target structures (that is, connections between different brain areas, as well as between the brain and the world).

In the human brain, the cortical surface is heavily folded, which allows more cortex to be fitted into the cranial space. Gyrification (formation of the cortical folds) starts prenatally and is probably not only caused by brain size but also by the tension exerted by the fiber tracts connecting different brain areas (Dubois et al., 2008; Zilles et al., 2013; Dehaene-Lambertz & Spelke, 2015). The area of unfolded human cerebral cortex is about 2000 to 2200 cm^2, of which about two-thirds—on average 1400 cm^2—are within sulcal walls, forming so-called fissural cortex.

At a submillimeter scale, microelectrode recordings have demonstrated a characteristic columnar structure perpendicular to the cortical surface, with columns of about 0.5 mm in diameter where neurons have similar preferences to stimulus properties, especially sharing receptive fields for sensory input. These columns consist of about 50–300 minicolumns, each with about 100 neurons. Here the pioneering work was done in the somatosensory cortex by Vernon Mountcastle (1957, 1997) and in the visual cortex by Nobel laureates David Hubel and Torsten Wiesel (Hubel & Wiesel, 1962). A similar columnar organization has been found also for the prefrontal cortex (Goldman & Schwartz, 1982).

The cortex has macroscopic organizational maps ("feature maps"), the most well known of which are the retinotopic map of the visual cortex, the tonotopic map of the auditory cortex, and the somatotopic maps of the primary somatosensory and motor cortices. In the retinotopic map, two neighboring regions in the visual field will be mapped to neighboring areas in the visual cortex, with separate maps of, for example, the upper and lower and the left and right visual fields. The cortex also has regions sensitive to certain complex stimulus features, such as faces, houses, and body parts. The feature maps allow for effective local computations, but at the same time they are also parts of extended functional brain networks. For example, distributed patterns of brain activity in widely spread brain areas (rather than "grandmother cells" specific for, e.g., seeing a certain person) are observed after presentation of certain object categories (Ishai et al., 1999; Haxby et al., 2001).

The feature maps have characteristic *magnification* factors that weigh the density of receptors corresponding to highly sensitive parts of the body or visual field. For example, the cortical magnification factor, computed in vision as millimeters of cortical area devoted to a given visual angle, can be as much as 10 times larger for the foveal relative to more eccentric areas of the visual field (Daniel & Whitteridge, 1961). This relationship is expected as the fovea has the highest density of day-light-sensitive photoreceptors. Similarly, in the sensorimotor cortical map, the lips, face, and digits are overrepresented as far as their body areas are concerned but in proportion to the receptor and actuator density in each respective body part. Signs of such topographic maps were already observed in the early 1900s by, for example, Victor Horsley (1857–1916), Fedor Krause (1857–1937), and Otfrid Foerster (1878–1941), and the maps were later summarized as a cartoon-like "homunculus" (Penfield & Boldrey, 1937) that demonstrates the relative proportions of cortical areas devoted to different body parts (for a review, see Feindel et al., 2009). The "classic" homunculus that we know today appeared in its final form years later (Penfield & Rasmussen, 1957, pp. 214–215).

The statistical features of the environment have shaped the cortical representations during phylogeny and ontogeny, but it is our active involvement that finally fine-tunes the feature maps. So, the brain retains some important aspects of neuroplasticity throughout life. For example, only the active use and not just holding of a tool (e.g., a rake to collect food pellets from the table) effectively fuses the tool to the body schema in the monkey cortex (Iriki, 2006). Indeed, many scientists, among them Rodolfo Llinas (2002) and György Buzsáki (2019), have argued that our brains evolved for action, and that neuroscience's focus on perception and representations has skewed our thinking.

■ CEREBELLUM

Studies of the cerebral cortex have dominated cognitive, social, and systems neuroscience in the twentieth century. More recently, given the focus on brain networks, cerebellum's importance has been highlighted in the complex brain–behavior relationship. The Cinderella of the brain now wears her missing glass slipper!

Despite the considerably smaller size of the cerebellum compared with the cerebrum, the cerebellar cortex contains about 3.6 times more neurons than the cerebral cortex (Herculano-Houzel, 2010). The size ratio between cerebellum and cerebrum is larger in humans and great apes than in other primates—potentially related to the importance of the cerebellum for advanced sensorimotor skills and cognition (Barton & Venditti, 2014). In the human cerebellum, partially segregated regions exist for motor, cognitive/language, and emotional functions, with preferential connections to motor, cognitive/language, and limbic regions of the cerebrum (Buckner, 2013; D'Angelo, 2018; Schmahmann et al., 2019).

Three features differentiate cerebellum very clearly from the other parts of the brain: (1) characteristic "cauliflower" anatomy, with tightly spaced cortical grooves forming thin folia that resemble the bellows of an accordion; (2) canonical configuration of neuronal circuits, with inhibition as the main operational principle; and (3) predominance of feedforward connections, unlike in other parts of the brain.

The cerebellar cortex has only three layers. The lowest layer contains granule cells, the middle layer the GABA-ergic Purkinje cells, and the top layer the dendritic trees of the Purkinje cells as well as inhibitory interneurons (stellate and basket cells) that synapse onto Purkinje cells. Purkinje cells (discovered by the Czech physiologist Jan Evangelista Purkyně in 1839) have characteristic bushy dendritic trees and up to 200,000 synapses.

The highly stereotypical neural circuitry of the cerebellar cortex comprises two main inputs to the Purkinje cells: strong input arrives via the climbing fibers from the inferior olive nucleus and weaker input via the parallel fibers (axons of the granule cells). The granule cells themselves receive excitatory sensory input (visual, auditory, tactile, proprioceptive) via mossy fibers. Animal neurophysiological and more recently human TMS studies (Fernandez et al., 2018) have indicated that efferent impulses from cerebellar Purkinje cells can inhibit the primary motor cortex, thereby fine-tuning ongoing movements.

The cerebellum is involved in multiple tasks, from motor coordination, accurate timing (including balance and gait), and motor learning to various sensory and cognitive processes that are relevant to behavior. Cerebellum's medial part, the spinocerebellum, fine-tunes body and limb movements and displays clear functional topography for somatosensory input, with the foot representation at the dorsal aspect. The lateral parts, called cerebrocerebellum (or neocerebellum), receive input only from the cerebral cortex. The anterior lobe of the cerebellum is connected with sensorimotor cerebral cortex, supporting motor execution, whereas the posterior lobe has been linked with motor planning, action prediction, and internal models. Lesions in these cerebellar regions can result in motor deficits, such as erratic movements, ataxic gait and hand movements, dysarthria, difficulties in producing rapid alternating movements with hands or feet, and "dysmetria" in pointing tasks and even in thought (Schmahmann, 1998).

The lateral and posterior regions of the cerebellum support cognitive functions, including working memory, as is evident from lesions in these areas that can impair language and attention. Posterior cerebellum, particularly the vermis, is critical for emotional and affective experiences, and it is therefore sometimes called the "limbic cerebellum" (Schmahmann et al., 2019).

Given this rich functional tapestry of cerebellar function, recording and visualizing human cerebellar activity is attracting increasing interest. In Chapter 22 we discuss findings of the few available human intracranial recordings and examine the extent noninvasive MEG and EEG recordings have detected cerebellar activity.

■ COMMUNICATION BETWEEN BRAIN AREAS

Thalamocortical Connections

Information from all senses—with the exception of olfaction—reaches the cerebral cortex via the thalamus, which functions as a relay station that regulates and controls traffic from the periphery to the cortex. The thalamus is a sensory gate from the world to the brain, but it also receives *about 10 times more afferents from the cortex than from the periphery*. Accordingly, the input from modality-specific thalamic nuclei to the cortex forms only 1% of all the input the cortex receives (Braitenberg, 1974). We thus come to the conclusion that the local cortical activity very much depends on what goes on in other parts of the cortex. In a way, the cortex is ruminating on its own output.

Although much of the processing of the healthy brain is only loosely related to sensory input, external stimulation is vital for normal brain function. In total isolation, such as during sensory deprivation (when a person is lying in the dark in a water pool with all sounds dampened), thoughts start to become muddled, and it is difficult to maintain and develop a particular thought; moreover, hallucinations can occur (Vernon, 1966).

Thalamic and thalamocortical communication likely have strong links to the emergence of awareness of different events and objects. The "global neuronal workspace" hypothesis, although not unanimously accepted today (Koch et al., 2016), suggests that a percept can become conscious only if the stimulus-related activation is amplified in sensory brain regions, if synchrony appears between far-away brain areas, and if the network comprising prefrontal and parietal areas is "ignited," i.e., activated rapidly (Dehaene & Changeux, 2011; Dehaene et al., 2017).

Intrabrain Connectivity

Different brain areas are connected with a multitude of fibers of different diameters, some of them myelinated and some unmyelinated. Axons are actually quite poor conductors of electricity: an electric pulse applied to one end of a copper wire will reach the other end 10^7 times faster than it would do in an axon. In myelinated axons, the *conduction velocity* (CV) is directly proportional to fiber diameter, and in nonmyelinated axons it is proportional to the square root of the fiber diameter (Kuffler et al., 1984). The diameters of axons in the central nervous system vary from 0.1 to 10 μm, and the CVs are maximally 100 m/s in the thick myelinated fibers, typically 40 to 60 m/s in peripheral nerves, and only 0.5 m/s in unmyelinated fibers. For reference, 60 m/s is slightly below the top speed of a Formula One racecar and thus is pretty fast, although it is far below the speed of light at which electric and magnetic fields spread.

Note that, in myelinated axons, action potentials (APs) "jump" from one short gap in the myelin sheath to the next, and this *saltatory conduction* considerably speeds up AP propagation. The gaps in the myelin are called nodes of Ranvier, and they are separated by about 0.2–2 mm, depending on the fiber.

Interestingly, all mammals seem to have similar neuronal density of about 10^5 neurons/mm^2 across all brain areas; the only exception is the primary visual cortex (V1) where neuronal packaging is doubled. Thus, the cortex of one cerebral hemisphere—about 1000 cm^2 in area—contains about 10^{10} pyramidal cells. The corpus callosum, the main information highway between the hemispheres, consists of 100 to 200 million ($1–2 \times 10^8$) fibers, meaning that callosal fibers can connect about 1% of cortical pyramidal cells (see Ringo et al., 1994).

Because axonal bundles are comprised of fibers of different diameters, considerable jitter arises in timing: neural volleys that start at the same time at one end of the bundle arrive at the other end at very different times. In the corpus callosum, the wide spectrum of fiber diameters predicts interhemispheric delays of 4 to 300 ms (Aboitiz et al., 1992).

One may think that such a wide variability of interhemispheric transmission times is disadvantageous to ongoing brain processes. However, such dispersion might also have benefits as it maintains flexibility in the system: the jitter prevents the excessive "neurons that fire together wire together" phenomenon that means that strong synchrony in firing will fuse neurons functionally, leading to dedifferentiation of the system (Hari et al., 2010).

Although speed is desirable in brain function, speeding up signal transfer by increasing fiber size is not an option because doubling the diameters of callosal axons to speed up interhemispheric conduction would result in a 50% increase in brain size, which would be a huge metabolic burden and the end of normal deliveries of babies (Ringo et al., 1994).

Although the cross-sectional area of the corpus callosum is linearly related to the total cortical surface, the distribution of axon diameters remains largely the same independent of brain size (Ringo et al., 1994). Interestingly and surprisingly, however, the signal transfer has been optimized so that independently of mammalian brain size—varying from shrews and mice to humans and whales—the shortest interhemispheric time lags are less than 5 ms (Wang et al., 2008). This optimization has been realized by inclusion of a few very large-diameter fibers that keep the delays short enough even in big brains; importantly, the fiber diameters in the thickest-diameter tail of the fiber distribution scale with brain size (Wang et al., 2008).

The thickest fibers guarantee rapid signaling over long distances whereas the unmyelinated fibers, although conducting slowly and therefore showing much temporal jitter over longer distances, are important to secure dense and widespread connectivity. Overall, the distribution of fiber sizes and their varying targets may contribute to the instantiation of different cortical rhythms (Buzsáki, 2011), an idea we examine further in Chapter 11.

■ ELECTRIC SIGNALING IN NEURONS

Information is transmitted along the neurons to other neurons in the form of APs that then trigger, via synapses, postsynaptic potentials (PSPs) in the next neuron. Only when the total amount of excitation from excitatory postsynaptic potentials (EPSPs) exceeds a certain threshold will an AP be triggered in the next neuron. The PSPs can also be inhibitory (i.e., inhibitory postsynaptic potentials [IPSPs]), whereby the likelihood of APs in the next neurons will be lowered.

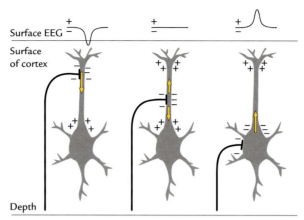

FIGURE 2.1. Surface potentials and currents associated with synaptic activation of a pyramidal neuron aligned perpendicular to the cortical surface. Three pyramidal cells receive excitatory synaptic input via thalamocortical afferents to different parts of the neuron (and at different depths of the cortex), which thereby results in different intracellular current flow (yellow arrows) and consequently in different EEG signals on the surface. We assume here that the reference electrode is far away from these neurons. In practice, of course, detectable EEG signals would require many more neurons to be active. This toy example shows how polarities of scalp potentials may arise.

We have already mentioned that pyramidal neurons in the cerebral cortex are the main sources of both MEG and EEG signals (for the possibility to record signals from the cerebellum, see above). Figure 2.1 shows that, depending on the site of the afferent fibers (that in this figure are excitatory only), the current direction can be either toward the deep or the superficial layers of the cortex. Synaptic inputs due to EPSPs and IPSPs at the same location on a neuron would result in intracellular currents of opposite direction.

In the cerebral cortex, most excitatory synapses are clustered on the apical dendrites, whereas the inhibitory synapses concentrate on the soma and basal dendrites of the pyramidal cells, and these spatial distributions of synapses critically affect the net currents giving rise to the MEG/EEG signals. However, neither MEG nor EEG, nor intracranial EEG measured directly from the cortical surface, can distinguish between currents that result from EPSPs or IPSPs, because the net current visible by MEG/EEG results from a summation of postsynaptic currents occurring in any depth of the cortex at a given time.

Glial cells are known to monitor and adjust potassium concentration in the extracellular space. Their role for brain signaling is still poorly understood, but they respond to sensory stimulation with current flow that can be at least equal to that in neighboring neurons with which they are in contact with (Schummers et al., 2008). Recent work emphasizes the dynamical nature of the interaction between glia and neurons, including trophic and metabolic support (Poskanzer & Molofsky, 2018). Glial cells have been suggested to contribute to low-frequency (< 1 Hz) EEG phenomena by amplifying or modifying the source currents (Galambos & Juhasz, 1997); we discuss such slow MEG and EEG signals in Chapters 11 and 12. In turtle cerebellum, where influential animal neurophysiology related to MEG signal generation has been performed, glial cells contribute to MEG signals produced during spreading depression—a likely neuronal mechanism for a migrainous aura (Okada et al., 1987).

Membrane Potentials

Resting neurons have a stable membrane potential so that their inside is about 60 mV more negative than their outside (range from –40 to –80 mV). This potential difference is actively maintained by means of energy-consuming ion-transport mechanisms. APs and PSPs are distortions of this stable membrane potential.

Figure 2.2 (top panel) shows schematically that, in a resting neuron, sodium (Na^+) and chloride (Cl^-) are more abundant outside the cell, and potassium (K^+) is more abundant inside the cell. Intracellular concentrations of Na^+, K^+, and Cl^- are about 20, 140, and 20 mmol/liter, respectively, and the extracellular concentrations are about 140, 5, and 120 mmol/liter. Membrane "pumps," consisting of ion transporter proteins within the cell membrane (itself a 10-nm-thick bilayer of phospholipids), transport ions against their concentration gradients using chemical energy (in the form of adenosine triphosphate, ATP). At the same time, the ions can leak in the direction of their concentration gradients through "ion channels" that are proteins sitting in the membrane, with ion-specific pores in the middle. In a resting neuron, the permeability is much larger for potassium than sodium, which is beneficial for the membrane potential as the cell interior becomes more negative with respect to the outside when the positive potassium ions diffuse along their concentration gradient out of the cell, without being replaced by inward flow of positive sodium ions.

The relationship between the ion concentrations inside and outside the membrane determines the membrane potential as expressed by the Goldman equation, shown in Figure 2.2 (top panel). Basically, the resting membrane potential is larger (the inside of the cell is more negative) as positive ions increase and negative ions decrease outside the cell and as positive ions decrease and negative ions increase inside the cell. Note that the net concentrations of the ions stay roughly the same all the time, whereas the permeabilities of the ions change during APs and PSPs.

The ion channels can be opened by transmitter molecules that bind to structures of the ion channels themselves (as happens in the postsynaptic membrane) or by voltage changes (as happens in the axonal membrane when an AP propagates). In addition to these transmitter- and voltage-gated openings, some ion channels can be opened by mechanical force or by light.

Currents related to the relatively slow PSPs rather than to fast APs are considered to be the main generators of both MEG and EEG signals. It is thus important to examine these two phenomena in a little more detail.

Action Potentials

An AP is a pulse of about 100 mV in amplitude that travels, or "propagates," along the axon with constant speed and without losing its strength. The AP is thus an all-or-none phenomenon (Figure 2.2, middle panel). For example, even if a stimulus affecting a peripheral receptor increases in strength, the AP amplitudes remain the same, but the firing rate increases in the afferent fibers.

An AP is initiated when the neuron depolarizes in the axon hillock to the level of firing threshold, typically between –55 and –40 mV. (Interestingly, APs can be triggered also by local depolarization, caused by, e.g., electrical stimulation or mechanical force, in different parts of the axon. Remember that time when your elbow hit the corner of the table and you felt tingling in the hand all the way down to the fingers?)

An AP propagates (moves along the fiber) because the permeability of sodium and potassium ions changes in the voltage-sensitive channels as a result of the approaching AP. The

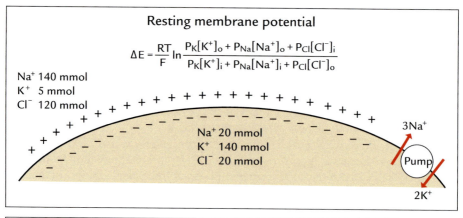

Resting membrane potential

$$\Delta E = \frac{RT}{F} \ln \frac{P_K[K^+]_o + P_{Na}[Na^+]_o + P_{Cl}[Cl^-]_i}{P_K[K^+]_i + P_{Na}[Na^+]_i + P_{Cl}[Cl^-]_o}$$

Na⁺ 140 mmol
K⁺ 5 mmol
Cl⁻ 120 mmol

Na⁺ 20 mmol
K⁺ 140 mmol
Cl⁻ 20 mmol

3Na⁺

Pump

2K⁺

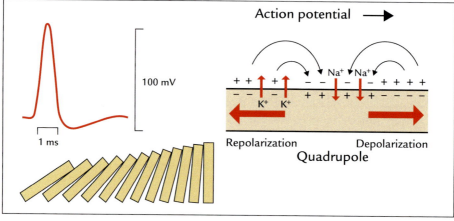

Action potential →

100 mV

1 ms

Na⁺ Na⁺

K⁺ K⁺

Repolarization

Depolarization

Quadrupole

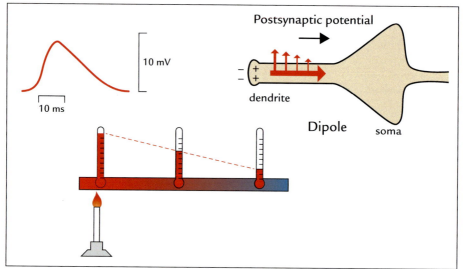

Postsynaptic potential

10 mV

10 ms

dendrite

Dipole

soma

FIGURE 2.2. Schematic representations of the resting membrane potential, action potential, and postsynaptic potential. Top: The resting membrane potential is maintained via an active Na⁺/K⁺ pump, which at each round moves 3 Na⁺ ions out of the cell and 2 K⁺ ions into the cell (at right). Cl⁻ ions follow the Na⁺ ions. The effect of intra- and extracellular K⁺, Na⁺, and Cl⁻ ion concentrations (indicated by [brackets] and by the subscripts i and o, respectively)

propagation thus does not need extra energy, but the process is very similar to the way a row of standing dominoes starts to fall one after another immediately after the first domino has been knocked down (Figure 2.2, middle panel). Instead, energy is needed for picking the dominoes back up and for repairing the membrane potential after the AP has passed.

An AP lasts for 1 to 2 ms and comprises a depolarization and a slightly longer repolarization phase. The leading and trailing edges are associated with intracellular current dipoles of opposite directions, so that the current configuration forms a quadrupole of two close-by dipoles with opposing polarities, as is shown schematically in Figure 2.2, middle panel. (Another common quadrupole is a current loop shown in Figure 1.3, bottom right panel.)

Repolarization progresses in the same direction as depolarization, so that after a few milliseconds the membrane potential is at the resting level again. Importantly, the dipole moments—the intracellular current multiplied by the length constant of the membrane (see Figure 3.4)—are of the same size for the leading and trailing edges of the AP, and the distance between the dipoles can be estimated from the conduction velocity of the fiber. For example, for a peripheral neuron with a conduction velocity of 50 m/s and AP duration of 1 ms, the distance would be 5 cm. In the much more slowly conducting fibers in the brain, the distances between the two opposite dipoles are much shorter.

Because the magnetic field generated by a quadrupolar source diminishes more rapidly as a function of distance than that produced by a PSP (a dipolar source; see next section) and because the duration of an AP is only 1–5% of that of the PSP, *PSPs but not APs* are the main contributors to both MEG and EEG signals.

It is interesting to note that in cardiac muscle, the Ca^{2+}-dependent APs last about 100 times longer (for 100–200 ms) and the repolarization progresses in a direction *opposite* to the depolarization front, thereby effectively preventing the normal heart from going into potentially life-threatening tachycardia.

Postsynaptic Potentials

The dendrites and the soma typically have thousands of synaptic connections from other neurons. When transmitter molecules bind to the receptors on the postsynaptic membrane, they modify the configuration of the receptor molecules, and consequently ion channels will open through the membrane. At typical levels of the resting membrane potential, increased

---

FIGURE 2.2. Continued

on the membrane potential is expressed by the Goldman equation, which appears at the top of the figure. Here, ΔE is the change of the membrane potential, and P_K, P_{Na}, and P_{Cl} represent the permeabilities of the K^+, Na^+, and Cl^- ions, respectively (in units of siemens = coulomb per second per volt of potential; $S = C \times s^{-1} \times V^{-1}$). R = the ideal gas constant (joule/K/mol; here K refers to kelvin units of temperature), T = temperature (K), F = Faraday's constant (coulomb/mol). Middle: The generation of an action potential results in propagating depolarization and a return to baseline by repolarization. The action potential (red trace on the left) lasts only 1 to 2 ms and includes a negative undershoot (hyperpolarization) before the resting membrane potential is re-established. The propagating action potential can be likened to a row of falling dominoes as illustrated. Bottom: Unlike the all-or-none action potential, the postsynaptic potential is graded and is presented here as moving from the apical dendrite towards the soma (triangular shape) of a pyramidal neuron. It spreads along the membrane passively (electrotonically); this spread is analogous to conduction of heat along a metal rod and simultaneous loss of the heat to the surrounding medium, as illustrated.

permeability to Na$^+$ and K$^+$ will lead to *depolarization* and thus to EPSPs, whereas increased permeability to Cl$^-$ ions will result in *hyperpolarization* and thus to IPSPs. Glutamate is a common excitatory neurotransmitter and gamma-aminobutyric acid a common inhibitory neurotransmitter in the cortex. Some transmitter molecules (e.g., acetylcholine) can affect postsynaptic function without opening ion channels; instead they bind to membrane receptors and instigate conformational changes of receptors in the postsynaptic cell, thereby eliciting intracellular "second messenger" biochemical cascades.

Importantly, PSPs do not propagate but rather spread electrotonically, resembling the way heat spreads along a metal rod that is warmed at one end (see Figure 2.2, bottom panel). EPSPs typically last for 10 to 30 ms and IPSPs up to 80 to 100 ms, and both are about 10 mV in amplitude. However, the exact duration of the PSP depends on the synaptic transmitter. For example, the EPSPs associated with feed-forward AMPA (α-amino-3-hydroxy-5-methyl-4-isoxazolepropionic acid) signaling are fast, decaying in less than 30 ms, whereas the EPSPs associated with re-entrant (feedback) NMDA (N-methyl-D-aspartate) based signaling can last over 100 ms. Inhibition also has two very different time scales depending on the transmitter: the fast GABA$_A$-based IPSPs last less than 30 ms, whereas the GABA$_B$-based IPSPs can last even a couple of hundred milliseconds (Gerstner et al., 2004).

The primary current caused by synaptic activity (shown by the intracellular arrow in Figure 2.2) flows inside neurons because the high-resistance cell membranes restrict and channel current flow. However, a small part of the intracellular primary current leaks continuously out of the cell (upward-directed arrows in Figure 2.2, bottom panel), and these returning volume currents close the current path in the extracellular space. Consequently, the intracellular primary current decreases as a function of distance from the synapse along the membrane (see Figure 3.4 and the related discussion in the next chapter).

Excitatory and inhibitory neurotransmitters can each engage more than one receptor type, and many neuropharmacological agents can modulate specific receptor (and synaptic) function differentially. Hence, medical and recreational drug usage must be considered when interpreting MEG and EEG signals. Anesthetic agents can affect excitatory and inhibitory connections differently, which has major implications for comparing earlier studies of electrophysiological data recorded from anesthetized animals with those of awake, behaving human subjects (Chapter 11).

■ REFERENCES

Aboitiz F, Scheibel A, Fisher R, Zaidel E: Fiber composition of the human corpus callosum. *Brain Res* 1992, 598: 143–153.

Barton RA, Venditti C: Rapid evolution of the cerebellum in humans and other great apes. *Curr Biol* 2014, 24: 2440–2444.

Boemio A, Fromm S, Braun A, Poeppel D: Hierarchical and asymmetric temporal sensitivity in human auditory cortices. *Nat Neurosci* 2005, 8: 389–395.

Bourguignon M, De Tiège X, Op de Beeck M, Ligot N, Paquier P, Van Bogaert P, Goldman S, Hari R, Jousmäki V: The pace of prosodic phrasing couples the reader's voice to the listener's cortex. *Hum Brain Mapp* 2013, 34: 314–326.

Braitenberg V: Thoughts on the cerebral cortex. *J Theor Biol* 1974, 46: 421–447.

Buckner RL: The cerebellum and cognitive function: 25 years of insight from anatomy and neuroimaging. *Neuron* 2013, 80: 807–815.

Buzsáki G: *Rhythms of the Brain*. New York: Oxford University Press, 2011.

Buzsáki G: *The Brain From Inside Out*. New York: Oxford University Press, 2019.

D'Angelo E: Physiology of the cerebellum. In: Manto M, Huisman TAGM, eds., *Handbook of Clinical Neurology*, Vol. 154 (3rd series), *The Cerebellum: From Embryology to Diagnostic Investigations* (2018, 85–108). Oxford, UK.

Daniel P, Whitteridge D: The representation of the visual field on the cerebral cortex in monkeys. *J Physiol* 1961, 159: 203–221.

Dehaene S, Changeux JP: Experimental and theoretical approaches to conscious processing. *Neuron* 2011, 70: 200–227.

Dehaene S, Lau H, Kouider S: What is consciousness, and could machines have it? *Science* 2017, 358: 486–492.

Dehaene-Lambertz G, Spelke ES: The infancy of the human brain. *Neuron* 2015, 88: 93–109.

Dubois J, Benders M, Cachia A, Lazeyras F, Ha-Vinh Leuchter R, Sizonenko SV, Borradori-Tolsa C, Mangin JF, Huppi PS: Mapping the early cortical folding process in the preterm newborn brain. *Cereb Cortex* 2008, 18: 1444–1454.

Feindel W, Leblanc R, de Almeida AN: Epilepsy surgery: historical highlights 1909–2009. *Epilepsia* 2009, 50 (Suppl 3): 131–151.

Fernandez L, Major BP, Teo WP, Byrne LK, Enticott PG: Assessing cerebellar brain inhibition (CBI) via transcranial magnetic stimulation (TMS): a systematic review. *Neurosci Biobehav Rev* 2018, 86: 176–206.

Fischl B, Sereno MI: Microstructural parcellation of the human brain. *NeuroImage* 2018, 182: 219–231.

Galambos R, Juhasz G: The contribution of glial cells to spontaneous and evoked potentials. *Int J Psychophysiol* 1997, 26: 229–236.

Gerstner W, Kistler WM, Naud R, Paninski L: *Neuronal Dynamics. From Single Neurons to Networks and Models of Cognition.* Cambridge: Cambridge University Press, 2004. Online book. https://neuronald ynamics.epfl.ch/online/index.html

Glasser MF, Van Essen DC: Mapping human cortical areas in vivo based on myelin content as revealed by T1- and T2-weighted MRI. *J Neurosci* 2011, 31: 11597–11616.

Gogtay N, Giedd JN, Lusk L, Hayashi KM, Greenstein D, Vaituzis AC, Nugent TF 3rd, Herman DH, Clasen LS, Toga AW, Rapoport JL, Thompson PM: Dynamic mapping of human cortical development during childhood through early adulthood. *Proc Natl Acad Sci U S A* 2004, 101: 8174–8179.

Goldman P, Schwartz M: Interdigitation of contralateral and ipsilateral columnar projections to frontal association cortex in primates. *Science* 1982, 216: 755–757.

Hari R, Parkkonen L, Nangini C: The brain in time: insights from neuromagnetic recordings. *Ann N Y Acad Sci* 2010, 1191: 89–109.

Hasson U, Yang E, Vallines I, Heeger D, Rubin N: A hierarchy of temporal receptive windows in human cortex. *J Neurosci* 2008, 28: 2539–2550.

Haxby JV, Gobbini MI, Furey ML, Ishai A, Schouten JL, Pietrini P: Distributed and overlapping representations of faces and objects in ventral temporal cortex. *Science* 2001, 293: 2425–2430.

Herculano-Houzel S: Coordinated scaling of cortical and cerebellar numbers of neurons. *Front Neuroanat* 2010, 4: 12.

Hubel DH, Wiesel TN: Receptive fields, binocular interaction, and functional architecture in the cat's visual cortex. *J Physiol* 1962, 160: 106–154.

Hyafil A, Giraud AL, Fontolan L, Gutkin B: Neural cross-frequency coupling: connecting architectures, mechanisms, and functions. *Trends Neurosci* 2015, 38: 725–740.

Iriki A: The neural origins and implications of imitation, mirror neurons and tool use. *Curr Opin Neurobiol* 2006, 16: 660–667.

Ishai A, Ungerleider LG, Martin A, Schouten JL, Haxby JV: Distributed representation of objects in the human ventral visual pathway. *Proc Natl Acad Sci U S A* 1999, 96: 9379–9384.

Koch C, Massimini M, Boly M, Tononi G: Neural correlates of consciousness: progress and problems. *Nat Rev Neurosci* 2016, 17: 307–321.

Kuffler SW, Nicholls JG, Martin AR: *From Neuron to Brain*, 2nd ed. Sunderland, MA: Sinauer Associates, 1984.

Llinas RR: *I of the Vortex: From Neurons to Self.* Cambridge, MA: Bradford Book, The MIT Press, 2002.

Mountcastle VB: Modality and topographic properties of single neurons of cat's somatic sensory cortex. *J Neurophysiol* 1957, 20: 408–434.

Mountcastle VB: The columnar organization of the neocortex. *Brain* 1997, 120: 701–722.

Okada Y, Lauritzen M, Nicholson C: MEG source models and physiology. *Phys Med Biol* 1987, 32: 43–51.

Penfield W, Boldrey E: Somatic motor and sensory representation in the cerebral cortex of man as studied by electrical stimulation. *Brain* 1937, 60: 389–443.

Penfield W, Rasmussen T: *The Cerebral Cortex of Man. A Clinical Study of Localization of Function.* New York: Macmillan Company, 1957.

Poskanzer KE, Molofsky AV: Dynamism of an astrocyte in vivo: perspectives on identity and function. *Annu Rev Physiol* 2018, 80: 143–157.

Ringo J, Doty R, Demeter S, Simard P: Time is of the essence: a conjecture that hemispheric specialization arises from interhemispheric conduction delay. *Cereb Cortex* 1994, 4: 331–343.

Schmahmann JD: Dysmetria of thought: clinical consequences of cerebellar dysfunction on cognition and affect. *Trends Cogn Sci* 1998, 2: 362–371.

Schmahmann JD, Guell X, Stoodley CJ, Halko MA: The theory and neuroscience of cerebellar cognition. *Annu Rev Neurosci* 2019, 42: 337–364.

Schummers J, Yu H, Sur M: Tuned responses of astrocytes and their influence on hemodynamic signals in the visual cortex. *Science* 2008, 320: 1638–1643.

Tanaka-Arakawa MM, Matsui M, Tanaka C, Uematsu A, Uda S, Miura K, Sakai T, Noguchi K: Developmental changes in the corpus callosum from infancy to early adulthood: a structural magnetic resonance imaging study. *PLoS One* 2015, 10: e0118760.

Van Horn JD, Irimia A, Torgerson CM, Chambers MC, Kikinis R, Toga AW: Mapping connectivity damage in the case of Phineas Gage. *PLoS One* 2012, 7: e37454.

Vernon J: *Inside the Black Room: Studies of Sensory Deprivation.* New York: Penguin Books, 1966.

Wang SS, Shultz JR, Burish MJ, Harrison KH, Hof PR, Towns LC, Wagers MW, Wyatt KD: Functional trade-offs in white matter axonal scaling. *J Neurosci* 2008, 28: 4047–4056.

Zilles K, Palomero-Gallagher N, Amunts K: Development of cortical folding during evolution and ontogeny. *Trends Neurosci* 2013, 36: 275–284.

CHAPTER 3

BASIC PHYSICS AND PHYSIOLOGY OF MEG AND EEG

That theory is worthless. It isn't even wrong!

WOLFGANG PAULI

Experience without theory is blind, but theory without experience is mere intellectual play.

IMMANUEL KANT

■ AN OVERVIEW OF MEG AND EEG SIGNAL GENERATION

This chapter outlines the general principles of physics and physiology underlying MEG and EEG signals. Our aim is to provide information that forms the basis of understanding what MEG and EEG measure and how these methods differ from each other, where the signals arise, and how one can reconstruct the neuronal sources.

Briefly, MEG and EEG signals are thought to be generated as follows:

1. The concerted action of neuronal populations in the brain is associated with synchronous postsynaptic currents that generate very weak $(100–500\ \mathrm{fT})$ magnetic fields outside the head and tiny electric potentials $(1–100\ \mu\mathrm{V})$ on the scalp.
2. The magnetic fields are typically recorded with ultrasensitive SQUID sensors (resulting in MEG signals), and the electric potentials are measured via electrodes (sometimes also referred to as sensors) placed on the scalp (resulting in EEG signals). The MEG and EEG data collected from respective sensors are referred as being in "sensor space."
3. The time courses of both MEG and EEG signals are recorded with millisecond temporal resolution and they display the evolution of brain activity in time. Thus the signals can be related to rapidly changing behavior and processing of information in the brain.
4. By inferring the generator currents in the brain using source modeling based on the measured signals and some physiological constraints, we can estimate where the activations giving rise to the signals have taken place. When sources of MEG and EEG data have been identified, the data are referred to as being in "source space."

■ CHARGES AND ELECTRIC CURRENT

Movements of charges form the electric currents that give rise to both EEG and MEG signals. Hence, it is important to understand the physical relationships between currents and associated electric and magnetic fields, as well as the forces that they exert on their surrounds.

Charges, as such, exist as a property of some materials, in a similar way to which mass is a property of a material. Charges can be either positive or negative. In school physics classes, the generation of charges is classically demonstrated by rubbing a Plexiglas rod with a dry cloth, which results in either attraction or repulsion of other materials because of the built-up electric charges on the rod. For example, when brought close to head, the charged rod makes the hair stand on end. The Ancient Greeks used amber to demonstrate the same phenomenon, and, indeed, the Greek word for amber, *elektron*, resulted in the word *electron* that we currently use to describe a single unit charge, or −e, which is the negative charge of an electron. In other words, charges are "packaged," or quantized, as multiples of −e. Note that a proton, which has a mass 2,000 times that of an electron, has a charge of equal amount (but of opposite polarity) to that of a single electron.

Charges affect nearby charges. *Like* charges (i.e., positive to positive, or negative to negative) repel one another, whereas *Unlike* charges (i.e., positive to negative) attract each other because electric fields exert a force on the nearby charges (Figure 3.1). The direction of the force points radially (inward or outward) along the lines from a single charge, and the magnitude of the force is inversely proportional to the square of the distance between the charges—a relationship that we know today as Coulomb's law.

In electric wires as well as in nerves, negatively charged electrons are the real carriers of charge, and their movement is referred to as *current*. Somewhat paradoxically, the electrons move in the opposite direction to that of electric current that, according to the convention originally proposed by Benjamin Franklin, is the direction of the movement of positive charges.

In a simple electric circuit where a battery is connected, for example to a lamp, the current flows from the positive pole of the battery through the circuit and through the lamp's filament to the negative pole of the battery. Electrons themselves in a wire move very slowly, only 0.1 mm/s, although electric and magnetic fields spread through conductive media at the speed of light. Note that although the body contains positively and negatively charged ions, for example sodium, potassium, and chloride for neuronal signaling, these ions do not travel as current carriers for long distances.

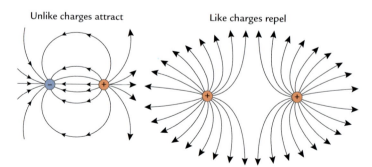

FIGURE 3.1. **Unlike charges attract and like charges repel.** Two unlike charges (on left) attract and two like charges (on right) repel each other. The lines depict the direction of force.

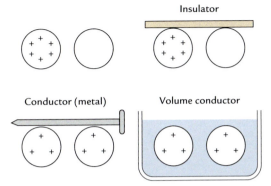

FIGURE 3.2. Charges and their behavior in the presence of insulators and conductors. Top left: One (positively) charged and one uncharged sphere isolated from one another do not change their charged states. Top right: The spheres connected with an insulator do not change their charged states. Bottom left: Connection of the spheres with a conducting metal balances the charges between the spheres. Bottom right: Charge is also balanced when the spheres are immersed in a volume conductor, here a saline bath. Figure stimulated by http://slideplayer.com/slide/4119423/slide 8.

If the charges are in a conducting medium, for example a saline solution (a volume conductor that we discuss later in this chapter) or are connected with a conducting material, such as metal or saline as in Figure 3.2 (bottom panels), the charges start to move (like charges away from each other and unlike changes toward each other to stabilize the potential difference) and thus form an electric current flow. In contrast, the charges will not change their states if they are isolated or connected via an insulator (Figure 3.2 top panels).

The International System of Units (SI) unit of charge is the coulomb (C), which is defined as the amount of charge flowing in 1 s through a wire carrying a current of 1 ampere (A). In these units, the charge of one electron is really tiny: $e = 1.6 \times 10^{-19}$ C.

Also, at the typical frequencies of MEG and EEG signals (< 1 kHz), the magnetic fields elicited by synaptic currents do not induce electric fields, in contrast to the propagation of high-frequency radio waves, for example, where the electric and magnetic fields alternate continuously.

Next we present simple equations needed to understand the evolution of electromagnetic fields and the physics behind the principles of source modeling. In a realistic biological situation, as well as in a metallic conductor, each charge is associated with an electric field, **E**, that exerts a force, **F**, affecting nearby charges by putting them into motion (thereby producing current **J**). **F** is directly proportional to both the electric field, **E**, and the size of the charge, **q**, that **E** is affecting. Stated formally, $\mathbf{F} = \mathbf{E} \times \mathbf{q}$.

An important *superposition principle* holds for both the electric field, **E**, and magnetic field, **B**, stating that fields produced by several charges/currents are linear sums of fields generated by each single charge/current.

■ OHM'S AND KIRCHOFF'S LAWS

In 1827, German physicist George Ohm described a simple relationship between voltage, resistance, and current in a wire. The now-famous Ohm's law states that the current, **I**, is directly proportional to the voltage, *V*, and inversely proportional to resistance, *R*. In other words, $I = V/R$.

In neurons, the primary current $\mathbf{J_p}$ can be thought of as the intracellular current that flows through the neurons themselves, and the returning current (which flows passively outside the cell back to the synaptic area) is equal to the conductivity σ of the medium and the electric field **E**, which acts as a driving force. Thus $\mathbf{J_{return}} = \sigma\mathbf{E}$.

Then Ohm's law for total current, can be written as follows:

$$\mathbf{J_{total}} = \mathbf{J_p} + \mathbf{J_{return}} = \mathbf{J_p} + \sigma\mathbf{E}$$

Each material has a characteristic conductivity, which is a measure that expresses how well a material can *conduct* current over a certain distance; conductivity of a material is expressed in SI units of siemens (Ω^{-1}) per meter = $\Omega^{-1}\,m^{-1}$. Resistivity, **ρ**, is the inverse of conductivity and is a measure of the material's impediment to the flow of current as a function of distance. Consequently, the resistance of an object will be determined by how much of the resistive material it contains: the resistance of a wire made of a certain material depends on both the wire's diameter and length. The SI unit for resistivity is Ω m. For example, a good *conductor*, such as copper, has low resistivity and high conductivity, whereas a good *insulator*, such as rubber, has high resistivity and low conductivity.

When the current encounters a border between two tissue compartments, its distribution will be directly related to the conductivities of the respective tissues. The total current will still be the same (as stated by Kirchoff's law) because of the conservation of charge. Similarly, a river that branches into tributaries of different sizes results in more water flowing through the larger than the smaller branches (analogous to paths with "lower resistance" versus "higher resistance"). Still, the total water that flows in the main river will be equal to the sum of water flowing in all of its branches.

In living tissues, some currents can be *nonohmic*, which means that they do not follow Ohm's law. For example, the transmembrane currents related to the propagation of APs are nonohmic, as they do not follow the conductivity structure of the medium but instead pass through the open ion channels in the membrane (see Figure 2.2).

■ RELATIONSHIP BETWEEN CURRENT AND MAGNETIC FIELD

Quite central for our present-day understanding of the relationship between electricity and magnetism was the observation by the Danish scientist Hans Christian Ørsted in 1820 that electric current flowing in a wire can turn the needle of a nearby compass. Ørsted concluded that the compass was affected because the electric current generated a magnetic field. Modern-day MEG recordings utilize this very same principle: MEG detectors sense the magnetic field elicited by currents flowing in the brain as if the detectors were tiny compasses.

Soon after Ørsted, in the 1820s, André Ampère, Jean B. Biot, and Felix Savart observed that two wires that carry electrical currents could exert a mutual force on one another. The reason is that current in each wire generates a magnetic field, **B**, related to the current by Biot-Savart law, so that the exerted force is directly proportional to the currents in the two wires and inversely proportional to their distance (this relationship is known as Ampère's force law).

In this context remember that permanent magnets consist of magnetized material. The oldest note relating to permanent magnets comes from about 2600 BC when a magnetic stone, likely containing magnetite (Fe_3O_4), was unearthed in China. The first magnetic compasses were invented around 900 BC and then had an enormous impact on navigation, trade, and the spread of culture. But it took well over a millennium before the electromagnetic forces underlying the function of compasses began to be understood.

In 1831, Michael Faraday observed that by moving a permanent magnet it is possible to induce an electrical current into a wire nearby, a phenomenon known as electromagnetic induction. In fact, the earliest recordings of biomagnetic fields from the human heart (in 1963) and brain (in 1968) were made with induction-coil magnetometers that, for improving sensitivity, contained a high number of turns (see Chapter 4). Many contemporaries scoffed at Faraday's theoretical ideas on electromagnetic induction, but finally James C. Maxwell (1831–1879) developed the now-famous and extremely influential "Maxwell equations," which describe the very fundamental relationships between electric charges, electric currents, and electric and magnetic fields. These equations, first presented in 1864 before the Royal Society of London, are central to our modern-day understanding of electromagnetism, as well as to a plethora of technical developments in modern society.

The Maxwell equations also form the basis of solutions to the forward and inverse problems that we apply to model neural sources of the measured MEG and EEG signals (see Chapter 10). Because of the rather low frequencies of most MEG/EEG signals, the time derivatives of the Maxwell equations can be omitted and the equations thereby much simplified to quasistatic form (Hämäläinen et al., 1993).

SUPERCONDUCTIVITY

MEG is most frequently recorded with superconducting SQUIDs, and thus the phenomenon of superconductivity may be of interest to our readers. Close to absolute zero temperature, defined as 0 K (kelvin), equal to –273 °C (celsius) and –460 °F (fahrenheit), some materials lose their resistance and become *superconducting*. This total loss of resistance means that current inserted into a superconducting loop would flow there forever (or as long as the loop remains superconducting), because the nonresistive loop does not lose energy.

In 1913, the Dutch physicist Kamerlingh Onnes received the Nobel Prize in physics for demonstrating superconductivity in mercury. Five years earlier he had been able to liquify helium at the temperature of 4.2 K, and he soon started to study properties of metals at such low temperatures. He observed that close to the temperature at which helium becomes a liquid, the resistance of mercury rapidly dropped, by a factor of 10^{10}. He also demonstrated—by using a compass needle as the indicator—that current was still flowing the next day in the superconducting mercury thread!

When temperature decreases, resistance decreases in *all* conductors, but only some materials become superconducting, meaning that when the so-called critical temperature is reached, the resistance drops directly to zero. For niobium, a chemical element commonly used in SQUID sensors and pickup loops (see Chapter 5), the critical temperature is 9.2 K.

It is interesting to note that Lord Kelvin (1824–1907)—who devised the temperature scale where absolute zero equals 0 K or –273.15 °C—had predicted that close to absolute zero the resistance would *increase* (and not decrease, or even vanish) as he expected the current carriers, the electrons, to freeze at such low temperatures. Had Kelvin devised an experiment in the laboratory, he might have come to another conclusion.

An actual theory of superconductivity had to wait until 1956 when Bardeen, Cooper, and Schrieffer published their BCS theory of superconductivity (the abbreviation derives from the first letters of the discoverers' names). According to the BCS theory, credited with a Nobel Prize in physics in 1972, the current in a superconductor flows in the form of electron pairs, called Cooper pairs. Although negatively charged electrons usually repel each other, in the superconducting state they form interacting and synchronous pairs even if separated by hundreds of atoms. Consequently, the elementary charge in superconductors is $-2e$ instead of $-e$ as seen in metals at room temperatures.

In normal environmental temperatures, the resistance of metals to current (producing waste heat) results from imperfections, such as impurities, in the structure of the material (or crystalline lattice) through which the electrons otherwise very freely move and from (thermal) vibrations of the lattice. These resistive properties disappear in the superconducting state.

Superconductivity can exist in many materials, both pure metals and different alloys, but some metals, such as copper, gold, and silver, never become superconducting. For practical applications (such as superconducting magnets needing large solenoids, coils of wire for current to flow, or high-temperature SQUIDs used for future MEG recordings), the material has to be such that it can be easily shaped to the form of wire, which is not true for all superconducting alloys.

Note also that today MEG signals can be recorded using state-of-the art "room- temperature" technology with special sensor types, including optically pumped magnetometers (OPMs)—an exciting development that we discuss in Chapter 5. At the time of writing, OPM-based MEG recordings must be performed in a shielded room, similar to MEG measurements using SQUID devices.

■ INVERSE PROBLEM

Hermann von Helmholtz, working 150 years ago, is credited as the first person to have formally considered and elaborated on the electrophysiological inverse problem. He showed that the same surface potential can rise in a volume conductor from an infinite number of source-current configurations (electromotive forces, "elektromotorische Kräfte"), meaning that the sources cannot be retrieved uniquely from the known surface potential (Helmholtz, 1853). In other words, the inverse problem does not have a unique solution. The reason is that it is always possible to add other currents to the primary current distribution that are magnetically silent, electrically silent, or both.

Figure 3.3 shows such silent sources in a sphere. While a tangential dipole (panel a) produces both MEG and EEG signals, a radial current or a current in the middle of a sphere is magnetically silent but produces an electric potential (panels b and c) as we have already discussed. Somewhat surprising is the situation of equally distributed radial current dipoles (panel d) that result in no magnetic or electric signals. Here one has to remember that nonzero EEG signals occur only when the two measurement electrodes (the "active" and "reference" electrode) are sitting at different potentials, and we here assume both electrodes to be on the surface of the sphere. On the other hand, a current loop (a magnetic dipole) is electrically silent but produces a magnetic field (panel e). Because of this multitude of potentially silent sources, the inverse problem in its general, nonconstrained form does not have a unique solution.

However, the uniqueness of the inverse problem has colored the entire source modeling discussion far too much, both for MEG and EEG. Careful analysis using *physiologically plausible constraints* can produce reliable interpretations that can be compared with converging evidence from several assessment techniques. Indeed, to this end, the MEG and EEG data can provide a good reality check for other functional neuroimaging methods, such as fMRI, and vice versa, although one must remember that different methods (e.g., those based on neurophysiology versus hemodynamics) will highlight different aspects of neural activity and may not necessarily be directly comparable.

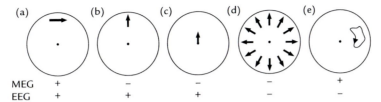

	(a)	(b)	(c)	(d)	(e)
MEG	+	−	−	−	+
EEG	+	+	+	−	−

FIGURE 3.3. **Magnetically or electrically silent sources.** A schematic presentation of a number of sources that can be visible or silent in MEG, EEG, or both. (a) A tangential source is seen (+) by both MEG and EEG. (b) A radial source is seen by EEG (+) and not MEG (−). (c) A source in the middle of the sphere is always radial and (if strong enough) is seen by EEG but not by MEG. (d) A set of radial sources that are evenly distributed across the sphere will produce no MEG nor EEG signals. (e) A current loop will produce an MEG signal but no EEG signal.

■ SOURCE CURRENTS

Primary Current

By finding the primary current **J**, we can locate the neural sources of MEG and EEG signals. $\mathbf{J}(\mathbf{r})$ at a location **r** denotes how much current has flowed across a unit area, for example the cross-sectional area of a current-carrying wire, and this current is measured in units of amperes per square meter (A/m^2).

As we showed in Figure 2.2, small fractions of the intracellular primary current leak out of the cell all the time. Therefore, the intracellular current flow, and thereby also the effectiveness of a single synapse in the apical dendrite on the neuronal firing, depends on the relative resistances across the membrane (r_m) and along the internal space (r_i). This relationship, the so-called length constant (also known as the space constant), λ, of the neuronal membrane is expressed formally as $\lambda = \sqrt{(r_m/r_i)}$ with the units of cm, that is, $\sqrt{(\Omega cm/\Omega cm^{-1})}$. Because r_m decreases in proportion to the surrounding membrane (fiber circumference $2\pi r$) and r_i in proportion to the cross-sectional area (πr^2), it is evident that λ depends on fiber size: λ increases proportional to the square root of fiber diameter, which directly increases **Q** (dipole moment) in large cells, even though the current would be the same. In addition to this λ-based bias favoring larger fibers, larger cells have more surface area and therefore more possibilities to receive synaptic input so that their intracellular net current will be larger than that in small cells.

In a cortical neuron, λ is typically 0.1 to 0.2 mm. From a distance, the current association with a PSP looks like a tiny current dipole (see Figure 2.2) oriented along the dendrite, with strength (or dipole moment) $\mathbf{Q} = \mathbf{J}\lambda$ (Figure 3.4).

A short length constant means that distant synapses are quite ineffective in influencing the firing of the postsynaptic cell. Thus, as long as only the passive electrotonic conduction is considered, a synapse close to the soma can be equivalent to many at more distant sites. However, the real situation may be much more complex, with a nonlinear input–output transformation due to active properties of the dendrites (Johnston et al., 1996; Major et al., 2013). For example, mechanisms exist to make distal synapses more effective, as Ca^{2+}-influx-related dendritic spikes can actually propagate, similar to APs, in some neurons from apical dendrites to the soma (Larkum et al., 1999; Major et al., 2013). Moreover, the diversity of dendritic morphology and channel distribution affects dendritic dynamics (Häusser et al., 2000). How such variability—which may even depend on the brain area under study—influences the generation of MEG and EEG signals remains unknown.

One additional factor affecting the dipole moment, **Q**, is the dependence of λ on input duration: λ is shorter for brief relative to longer input pulses, and it depends on background activity that can thus affect the "electrotonic distance" of the synapse (Figure 3.4). For example, at zero background activity, both synchronized and nonsynchronized inputs were approximately equally effective in triggering APs from the neuron, whereas with background activity at 6 Hz, the synchronous activity was four times more effective (Bernander et al., 1991). Note that these changes in λ may enlarge the measured MEG signals considerably, although the original "battery" current (across the membrane at the site of the synapse) would remain the same. Thus the neuron functionally "shrinks" and "expands" depending on the amount of input it receives: the fewer synapses are active, the longer the length constant is and the more effective a single synapse is in affecting the soma.

In summary, neurophysiological MEG and EEG signals are biased to large neurons and to signals in thick large dendrites. Note that microelectrode recordings from cortex similarly have a preference for larger neurons. Consequently, MEG and EEG signals may reflect partially different phenomena than fMRI that may be more sensitive to information transferred via the dense, but slowly conducting, thin fibers (Hari & Parkkonen, 2015). This idea is supported by the considerably longer interareal delays observed in fMRI than EEG recordings. For example, the signals appear to travel from auditory to motor cortex in 600 ms according to fMRI recordings, but in 250 ms when examined in MEG recordings (Lin et al., 2013). Similarly, during visuospatial mental imagery, latencies between activations of dorsolateral prefrontal cortex and primary motor cortex were of the order

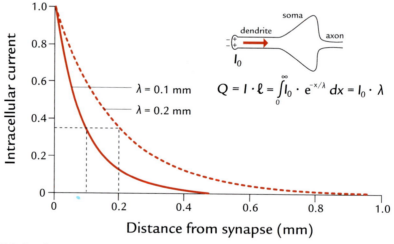

FIGURE 3.4. Electrotonic (passive) spread of current along the neuron. A synapse assumed to be at the left end of the apical dendrite of a pyramidal cell (insert on the top right) will cause an intracellular current that leaks through the membrane (as was also indicated in the lowest panel in Figure 2.2). The length constant λ indicates the distance along which the initial intracellular current, I_0, has decayed to 37% of its original value. Two decay curves are shown for differing values of λ. The equation states that the dipole moment equals the product of current strength and current length (*l*).

of 2.5 s (Formisano et al, 2002)—a surprisingly long delay compared with any activation sequences observed with MEG or EEG.

Layers, Open Fields, and Closed Fields

Both the geometry of single cells and that of neuronal populations determine the resulting potential distributions. When a layer of current dipoles is activated, the curvature of the surface has an effect on the potential distribution: the potential decreases over the convexity but increases in the concavity due to summation of the effects of the single dipoles. As already proposed by Lorente de Nó in 1947, an axial geometry of cells (such as in pyramidal cells) and an alignment of such cells would result in open fields, similar to those caused by single-current dipoles, whereas radial geometry (such as in stellate cells) or radial clustering of axially oriented cells would lead to closed fields, as is shown in Figure 3.5 for "open" and "closed" fields. The cerebral cortex has mainly open distributions, whereas some subcortical nuclei have closed ones (Lorente de Nó, 1947). The hippocampus, which occupies less than 1% of the cortical surface, is an interesting structure in this context as it is well layered, thus producing strong potentials locally, but as it is curved, it can be difficult to detect its potentials at a distance. Intracranial recordings from electrodes placed within or close to the hippocampus in human subjects do, however, show large local potentials (Halgren et al., 1980; McCarthy & Wood, 1987).

Despite the internal complexity of the tissues of the head, the cortical currents of different strengths and directions—when viewed from a distance—sum up to form net currents that produce measurable extracranial magnetic fields and electric scalp potentials.

The magnetic field of a single current dipole decreases with distance as $1/r^2$, more slowly than the $1/r^3$-dependent field of a current quadrupole (e.g., two opposite current dipoles some distance apart associated with an AP, or a current loop) (Hämäläinen et al., 1993). Therefore, far away from the source, the dipolar elements dominate the visible distribution.

The potential generated by a dipole layer decreases in proportion to $1/r$. As a special case, a layer of infinite length would produce a potential that does not decrease as a function

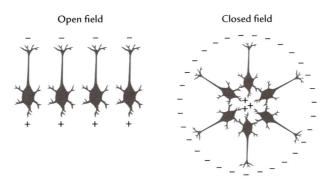

Open field   **Closed field**

FIGURE 3.5. **Open and closed fields.** Polarized (activated) pyramidal cells aligned side-by-side will produce an open field whose potential and magnetic field can be seen at a distance (left panel). If the same elements are in a random order, or are radially symmetric (right panel), they will form a closed field that cannot be seen with MEG nor EEG; instead, a locally sited electrode must be inserted very close to the cluster to be able to record the potential.

of distance at all. The different sizes of dipole layers likely contribute to the variable results on attenuation of EEG potentials from the cortex to the scalp.

Intracortical Cancellation

Synaptic events occur at different depths of the cortex. Because of this misalignment of neurons and because some synapses are excitatory and some inhibitory, producing currents of opposite directions, cancellation of intracortical currents is inevitable. In the neocortex, the pyramidal neurons may have a common orientation, but their somas are at different depths of the cortex. Even when brief stimuli have been applied, the currents in the cortex show temporal asynchrony, which further contributes to the "disappearance" of cortical currents before MEG or EEG can capture any sign of them. It is difficult to estimate how much cancellation takes place. However, the bias of the net current dipole moment toward large fibers, as well as the effect of synchrony on the total signal (see Chapter 10), suggest that we probably have to be satisfied if 0.1–1% of the cortical currents leave any traces on our MEG/EEG recordings. In the very convoluted cerebellar cortex, particularly strong cancellation is expected because of the closely spaced cortical folds.

Volume Conduction

Because of its high content of salt water, the human body acts as a passive *volume conductor*, a medium in which any current can flow. On the other hand, a vacuum, or even atmospheric air, does not qualify as a volume conductor. Volume conduction is a passive spread of current according to the resistivity of the medium, and therefore both the conductivity pattern and the shape of the volume conductor affect the current distribution that is governed by Ohm's and Kirchoff's laws, as already discussed.

Volume conduction explains why electrical activity from the heart (i.e., the electrocardiogram) can be recorded not just from electrodes on the chest but also from a pair of electrodes placed between a hand and a foot, although both locations are far away from the heart. For the same reason, EEG activity can also be reliably recorded from any structures on the human head, such as the earlobes, or the brainstem potentials generated deep in the brainstem can be picked up by electrodes fixed to the scalp.

The electric potential differences caused by a local current source occur at the same time in different parts of the body since the electric field generated by the source spreads with the speed of light (3×10^8 m/s). Therefore, many electric signals can be measured far away from the site of origin at different parts of the body, although the signals have not been transmitted there via nerves, muscles or other special pathways.

We have already mentioned the volume currents that close the current paths initiated by "batteries" in the synapses, resulting in intracellular primary currents and return (volume) currents in the surrounding extracellular volume. We have also mentioned that we can compute the direction and size of the magnetic fields outside the head directly from the primary currents, without taking into account the effects of the volume currents. Because *all* currents elicit magnetic fields, ignoring the volume currents may sound really strange. However, we can neglect the volume currents only in certain geometries of volume conductors, namely in ideal spheres (as well as in infinite half spaces that have been used much in theoretical computations of cardiac biomagnetic fields but that are not that useful for understanding the generation of MEG signals).

Figure 3.6 shows another type of volume conductor geometry, a *cylinder* filled with saline. Let us assume that we will measure the AP volley in a giant axon placed in (a) a very

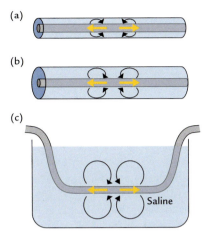

FIGURE 3.6. **Cylinder geometry.** Three examples of volume conductors: (a) a very thin cylinder, (b) a wider cylinder, and (c) a large saline bath. See text for explanation.

tight cylinder just surrounding the axon, (b) a wider cylinder, or (c) a large saline path. Because the volume currents in (a) have to return very close to the primary currents, their magnetic fields largely cancel those of the primary current and the resulting signal will be negligible outside the volume conductor. In the wider cylinder, the volume currents can spread to a wider area and the AP signal can be detected. The best estimate of the magnetic field elicited by the original AP currents is obtained when the nerve is immersed in the large saline path where the effects of the volume currents on the external magnetic field start to disappear.

So we come to the conclusion that removing the borders of the volume conductor close to the primary current will increase the magnetic field measured outside. This idea has been tested in measurements of magnetocardiographic (MCG) signals produced by the heart: when the subject was immersed in a bath of saline, the MCG signal increased in amplitude approximately by a factor of $\sqrt{2}$, varying on the measurement site, relative to when the subject was lying on a bed surrounded by air (Varpula et al., 1985). This example nicely illustrates the effects of volume currents and how they are modified depending on the shape and size of the volume conductor.

Spherical Head Model

We have already stated that a sphere that can be successfully used as the model of the human head is a very special volume conductor, because we do not need to take into account the effects of volume currents while computing the magnitudes of the MEG signals measured outside the sphere. To repeat the logic: First, for radial currents, the vanishing of volume currents can be shown formally by Ampère's law (Hämäläinen et al., 1993). An intuitive understanding can be obtained by considering the equivalent presentation of the volume currents (red lines in Figure 1.3, top panel, left) as two radially symmetric charge clusters (Figure 1.3, top panel, right). These closed radially symmetric charges do not produce any magnetic field outside the sphere. Second, the volume currents of tangential dipoles can be replaced (as was shown in Figure 1.5d) by two equally long current paths that connect the tangential dipole to the origin of the sphere as the produced magnetic field is the same as can be intuitively understood (because radial currents do not produce any magnetic field) and mathematically demonstrated. Thus we can compute the MEG signals produced by any tangential currents by considering only the primary current.

Altogether, in the spherically symmetric volume conductor, only *tangential* primary currents produce a magnetic field outside the sphere. By "production" we mean that (i) the direction of the external magnetic field (or flux) is determined by the right-hand rule (see Figure 1.2) from the direction of the primary current and that (ii) the strength of the magnetic signal can be calculated directly from the primary current without taking into account any other currents, such as the return (volume) currents.

In other words, if the conductor is spherically symmetric, the magnetic field outside can be obtained without explicit reference to the volume currents. Even though the tangential field components are *affected* by the volume currents in a spherically symmetric conductor, they can be computed without knowing the conductivity profile as long as it is concentric, only depending on the radius $\sigma = \sigma(r)$ (Hari & Ilmoniemi, 1986).

For EEG signals, the potential distribution directly reflects the polarities of the volume currents at each location and is strongly affected by the underlying tissue conductivities.

■ SOME GENERAL POINTS ABOUT SOURCE LOCALIZATION

MEG and EEG recordings aim to provide valuable information about the time courses of various brain activations. However, it is also useful to know where in the brain the signals of interest are generated. This information is obtained by source modeling. In general, identification of the neural sources is more straightforward for MEG than EEG recordings. The main reason is MEG's selectivity only to a part of the total current (i.e., fissural currents) and the lack of smearing by the skull, as discussed earlier. Therefore, MEG has perhaps led the way in source modeling approaches. Many MEG-developed source modeling methods have been subsequently adopted for EEG analyses (see Chapter 10).

One important aspect of source localization is its accuracy and *spatial resolution*. In the literature, the concepts of accuracy, precision, and resolution are often intermixed. Figure 3.7 aims to clarify the difference between accuracy and precision: if one stimulates the subject's thumb and finds a source in the hand region of the somatosensory cortex, the *accuracy* of source identification is good. If the same test is repeated and all sources cluster to a small, but different, area of the brain, the *precision* of the method is still good. Note, however, that a good precision (replicability of the test) does not imply that the results are correct, as the estimated sources can cluster tightly to an area (here to the foot area) that is not generating the measured signals. Such a mislocalization could result from a systematic error, for example a mistake or inaccuracy in coordinate transformation.

Spatial *resolution* can be used to discern how well two sources (e.g., the representations of two fingers in the somatosensory cortex) can be separated. Thus spatial resolution can be good even though the accuracy of the method would be poor (but good precision is still needed).

In most cases, both spatial accuracy and spatial resolution are worse for MEG and EEG relative to fMRI, whose resolution is typically in the millimeter range and coregistration errors are small because the functional images can be directly superimposed on the structural images. Importantly, the spatial resolution of MEG and EEG, in contrast to fMRI, depends strongly on the location, number, and configuration of current sources, as well as

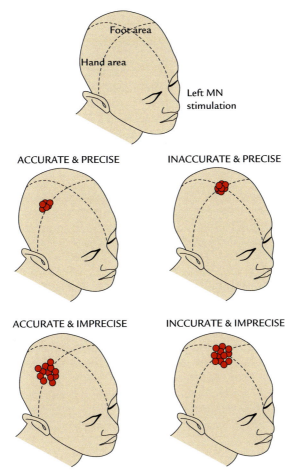

FIGURE 3.7. Accuracy versus precision. A schematic illustration of the differences between accuracy and precision of source localization. After left median-nerve (MN) stimulation, activation is expected in the right-hemisphere hand region of the primary somatosensory cortex. The foot area is shown at the top of the head. See text for further explanation.

on the sensor configuration. That said, the signal-to-noise ratio affects the spatial resolution of all brain-imaging methods, including fMRI and MEG/EEG. At best, the spatial resolution of MEG (related to the differentiation of two nonsimultaneous sources) is on the order of millimeters or even better, for example in differentiating activations elicited by somatosensory stimulation of different digits.

Denser spatial sampling of the magnetic field, or of the potential distribution, will to a certain extent benefit the spatial accuracy of finding the generators of the signals. Hence, MEG arrays of over 300 sensors are now widely available, and 128- and 256-channel EEG recordings are used frequently in basic research. Typically, 32-channel EEG recordings still remain the standard in clinical examinations where the main target is the analysis of the time courses (such as epileptic discharges), frequencies (such as slowing), and morphology (such as the K-complex of sleep) of spontaneous activity for which it is enough to infer the approximate generator sites.

■ REFERENCES

Bernander O, Douglas R, Martin K, Koch C: Synaptic background activity influences spatiotemporal integration in single pyramidal cells. *Proc Natl Acad Sci U S A* 1991, 88: 11569–11573.

Formisano E, Linden DE, Di Salle F, Trojano L, Esposito F, Sack AT, Grossi D, Zanella FE, Goebel R: Tracking the mind's image in the brain I: time-resolved fMRI during visuospatial mental imagery. *Neuron* 2002, 35: 185–194.

Halgren E, Squires NK, Wilson CL, Rohrbaugh JW, Babb TL, Crandall PH: Endogenous potentials generated in the human hippocampal formation and amygdala by infrequent events. *Science* 1980, 210: 803–805.

Hämäläinen M, Hari R, Ilmoniemi RJ, Knuutila JET, Lounasmaa OV: Magnetoencephalography—theory, instrumentation, and applications to noninvasive studies of the working human brain. *Rev Mod Phys* 1993, 65: 413–497.

Hari R, Ilmoniemi RJ: Cerebral magnetic fields. *CRC Crit Rev Biomed Eng* 1986, 14: 93–126.

Hari R, Parkkonen L: The brain timewise: how timing shapes and supports brain function. *Philos Trans R Soc Lond B Biol Sci* 2015, 370: 20140170.

Häusser M, Spruston N, Stuart GJ: Diversity and dynamics of dendritic signaling. *Science* 2000, 290: 739–744.

Helmholtz H: Ueber einige Gesetze der Vertheilung elektrischer Ströme in körperlichen Leitern, mit Anwendung auf die thierisch-elektrischen Versuche. *Ann Phys Chem* 1853, 89: 211–233 & 353–377.

Johnston D, Magee JC, Colbert CM, Cristie BR: Active properties of neuronal dendrites. *Annu Rev Neurosci* 1996, 19: 165–186.

Larkum ME, Zhu JJ, Sakmann B: A new cellular mechanism for coupling inputs arriving at different cortical layers. *Nature* 1999, 398: 338–341.

Lin FH, Witzel T, Raij T, Ahveninen J, Tsai KW, Chu YH, Chang WT, Nummenmaa A, Polimeni JR, Kuo WJ, Hsieh JC, Rosen BR, Belliveau JW: fMRI hemodynamics accurately reflects neuronal timing in the human brain measured by MEG. *NeuroImage* 2013, 78: 372–384.

Lorente de Nó R: Analysis of the distribution of the action currents of nerve in volume conductors. *Stud Rockefeller Inst Med Res Repr* 1947, 132: 384–477.

Major G, Larkum ME, Schiller J: Active properties of neocortical pyramidal neuron dendrites. *Annu Rev Neurosci* 2013, 36: 1–24.

McCarthy G, Wood CC: Intracranial recordings of endogenous ERPs in humans. *EEG Clin Neurophysiol Suppl* 1987, 39: 331–337.

Varpula T, Katila T, Poutanen T, Seppänen M: In vivo study of the effect of the secondary currents on the MCG. In: Weinberg H, Stroink G, Katila T, eds. *Biomagnetism: Applications and Theory.* New York: Pergamon Press, 1985: 180–185.

CHAPTER 4

AN OVERVIEW OF EEG AND MEG

Try to learn something about everything and everything about something.

THOMAS HUXLEY

The older I get the more wisdom I find in the ancient rule of taking first things first. A process which often reduces the most complex human problem to a manageable proportion.

DWIGHT D. EISENHOWER

■ HISTORICAL ASPECTS

MEG and EEG have rather different historical trajectories. EEG has from its earliest beginnings in the 1930s been used as a tool of clinical diagnostics. The widespread clinical use of EEG began by visual inspection of spontaneous EEG activity in patients suffering from various psychiatric or neurological disorders, particularly epilepsy. To this day, this qualitative "eyeballing" or visual pattern recognition remains the main method for reporting on spontaneous, nonaveraged EEG traces in the clinical environment (but machine-learning-based methods may soon change or complement this procedure; see Chapter 14). Although evoked responses had been observed in animals and intracranial human recordings, it was Dawson in 1947 who pioneered a technique by which a sensory stimulus triggered an oscilloscope whose display had a persistence that allowed superimposed individual epochs of human EEG to be visualized (Dawson, 1947). This new method allowed human EEG activity time-locked to the stimulus to be seen clearly for the first time.

For MEG, the evolution of applications has been the opposite of EEG: the first recordings were made in physics and other research laboratories, and only recently, with the advent of whole-scalp-covering devices, MEG has been adopted to clinical use. Moreover, the early MEG evoked-response recordings required averaging of a high number of single trials, and it took some time before low-noise MEG equipment became available to allow single-trial analyses.

■ EARLY EEG RECORDINGS

Richard Caton is generally credited to have been the first to record electrical activity from the brain. He made invasive recordings directly from the cortex of rabbits, cats, and monkeys, and he reported on his findings on "surface negativity" during sensory activation at a meeting of the British Medical Association in Edinburgh in 1875 (Caton, 1875). At that time, his measurement device was a recently invented reflecting galvanometer attached to a small mirror: the brain currents displaced galvanometer coils, and the mirror reflected a spot of light on a wall to produce large and discernable movements. This clever amplifier was sensitive to currents that were of the order of microamperes (μA). Several of his contemporaries, such as Ernst von Fleischl-Marxow from Vienna and Adolph Beck from Krakow, also recorded electric activity from animal brains at around this time, but their findings were reported a number of years later, in 1890. Among the other early players was Vasili Danilevsky from Ukraine, who in 1891 reported results of his thesis work carried out 15 years earlier. This earlier work confirmed Caton's findings regarding spontaneous and evoked activity, and it also demonstrated auditory evoked potentials. For a review of the early history of EEG, see Brazier (1988).

Thus, before the first use of noninvasive human EEG, which we discuss next, many important EEG phenomena were already known from animal experiments. For example, visual, somatosensory, and auditory evoked potentials had already been recorded invasively in single trials. Two different frequency bands of EEG had been observed, corresponding to the alpha and beta bands that Berger later identified in humans (see below). The EEG arousal reaction and the effects of sleep, anesthesia, and death had been reported as well. Moreover, pathological epileptic potentials and focal delta activity had also been observed.

Noninvasive human EEG began to progress significantly following a series of 14 now-classical scientific reports (all with the same title, "Über das Elektroenkephalogramm des Menschen") published by Hans Berger, a psychiatrist in Jena, Germany, in 1929–1938 (for an English translation of the entire set of reports, see Berger & Gloor, 1969). Berger used platinum wires, zinc-plated steel needles, and large plate electrodes, connected to a "Siemens double-coil galvanometer." He recorded the output onto photographic paper and was able to demonstrate, in a recording between one electrode located over the frontal scalp and the other over the occipital scalp, a large and persistent 10-Hz rhythm that he named "alpha." The alpha rhythm was affected by eye opening, painful stimuli, loud noises, and mental effort. Berger studied many brain-injured individuals and epileptic patients, and he started to use EEG as a clinical tool. A compelling insight into Berger's life can be found in Millett (2001).

Berger's first EEG recording was made from a patient with an intact scalp, but an underlying skull defect that created a "window into the brain" without dampening the potentials, and thus EEG signals were clearly discernible. After this initial success, Berger was able to record EEG from healthy subjects, son Klaus and daughter Ilse, whose scalp and skull were intact (Coenen & Zayachkivska, 2013). He systematically investigated factors that altered the EEG, including effects of sleep and anesthesia.

Lord Adrian, a British neuroscientist and Nobel laureate from 1932, became interested in EEG activity in the early 1930s. His experimental approach was more scientifically driven than that of Berger. Adrian and his colleague Matthews observed that alpha oscillations (which they respectfully called "the Berger rhythm") appeared when the cortex had little to do, and they hence proposed, for the first time, an *idling* hypothesis for brain rhythms (Adrian & Matthews, 1934). *Idling* means that a system that is not working is "kept warm" so that it can quickly reach full capacity whenever the need arises. They also noted that alpha-rhythm-like oscillations and reactivity could be seen in nonhuman subjects, and Adrian challenged his colleagues in the Cambridge Physiological Society to tell the difference between potential recordings showing reactive 10-Hz oscillations from the eye of a water-beetle and from the brain of a human subject; see Figure 4.1 (Adrian & Matthews, 1934).

Adrian and Matthews (1934) disagreed with Berger in one aspect: whereas Berger thought that the whole cortex produced alpha-like brain rhythms, Adrian and Matthews consistently showed the alpha to arise in posterior parts of the brain, likely in the visual cortex, as it disappeared when the eyes were opened in light but appeared when the eyes were open but the visual field was homogeneous or the room was dark.

Lord Adrian (1944) understood the problems of recording scalp EEG, stating that "With present methods the skull and the scalp are too much in the way, and we need some new physical method to read through them. . . . In these days we may look with some confidence to the physicists to produce such an instrument, for it is just the sort of thing they can do." With the benefit of twenty-first-century hindsight, we can say that this was a prophetic statement for the development of technologies such as MEG, as well as the dramatically improved analysis methods of both MEG and EEG. However, it would be many years before MEG would be developed because of the technical limitations of the day.

The next important developments of EEG were the emergence of multichannel recordings, first with pen and ink recorders and then in the late 1980s with computer-based paperless recording systems. At the same time, new amplifiers were developed to be more sensitive and to tolerate higher input impedances (see Chapter 5) that made them more resilient to various artifacts and better suited for intracranial recordings. Important additions to clinical EEG were telemetry and videotelemetry to mainly monitor epileptic patients (Chapter 20).

A real leap in EEG applications occurred in the 1960s and 1970s when the first computers became routinely available and made it possible to average EEG signals time-locked to various sensory stimuli, thereby significantly increasing the signal-to-noise ratio. Thus recordings of evoked potentials, as well as of event- and movement-related potentials, started to gain interest (see Chapters 12–19). Another important technical advance was the attempt to plot EEG topographies, pioneered by Mary Brazier at Massachusetts General Hospital, in Boston, in the late 1940s for certain EEG transients (Brazier, 1949) and in the

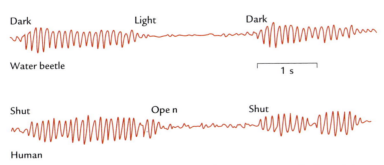

FIGURE 4.1. **Alpha activity recorded by Lord Adrian.** Top trace depicts alpha-range oscillations recorded from a water beetle eye during darkness and light. The bottom trace shows human EEG alpha activity when the subject had the eyes shut versus open. Adapted and reprinted from Adrian ED, Matthews BH: The interpretation of potential waves in the cortex. *J Physiol* 1934, 81: 440–471. With permission from Oxford University Press.

late 1960s, also as a function of time, by Paris-located neuroscientists Nicole Lesèvre and Antoine Remond (Joseph et al., 1969; Remond et al., 1969).

■ EARLY MEG RECORDINGS

Since all electric currents are accompanied by magnetic fields, it was reasonable to expect that brain currents would also produce magnetic fields. However, considerable technical difficulties were encountered in recording of these tiny magnetic fields of the order of only 10 to 100 fT.

In principle, the measurement of magnetic fields is straightforward. If we put a wire loop into a *changing* magnetic field, a current will be induced into the loop. Consequently, we can measure a voltage difference between the ends of the wire forming the loop. The sensitivity of the device can be increased by replacing the single loop with a coil with many turns of wire, as the induced current will increase linearly as a function of the number of turns, as well as with the area of the coil. The sensitivity of this induction-coil magnetometer can be further increased by inserting a high-permeability core inside the coil, so as to increase the magnetic-field density within the coil.

Biomagnetic measurements started with this kind of induction-coil magnetometer when Baule and McFee in 1963, for the first time ever, measured the magnetic field changes associated with the cardiac cycle at room temperature! Their magnetometer contained 2 million turns of copper wire turned around a ferrite core. When they placed one such solenoid over the chest and had an oppositely wound "reference" coil on the side of the subject, the magnetocardiogram, very similar in waveform and timing to the electrocardiogram, could be picked up. However, at that time, averaging with respect to a simultaneously recorded electrocardiogram was necessary to improve the signal-to-noise ratio and thereby observe the small magnetocardiogram signals.

A similar induction-coil magnetometer, again with 2 million turns of copper wire, was used by David Cohen from the Massachusetts Institute of Technology in the first measurements of the human brain's magnetic field, again at room temperature. To pick up the magnetic counterpart of the Berger's alpha rhythm and to improve the signal-to-noise ratio as much as possible, Cohen recorded EEG as a time-reference signal and averaged up to 9,000 epochs of the magnetic signal phase-locked to EEG oscillations (Cohen, 1968). Thus the first MEG had been recorded, some 40 years after the first human EEG recording.

The sensitivity of MEG recordings improved drastically with the invention of superconducting tunneling (Josephson, 1962) that brought the physics Nobel Prize to Brian Josephson in 1973. It then became possible to fabricate SQUIDs, the ultrasensitive detectors of the magnetic field (Silver & Zimmerman, 1965). In the early 1970s, SQUIDs already provided adequate sensitivity for the detection of the brain's spontaneous MEG activity without signal averaging or use of EEG as a time-reference signal (Cohen, 1972).

Little by little, the noise characteristics of SQUIDs were improved so that the SQUID noise is at present close to physically achievable limits. Different types of flux transformer configurations have been applied, and multichannel neuromagnetometers started to emerge in the 1980s. Despite the early concerns about disturbing cross-talk between the channels, it became possible to build multichannel devices; the first whole-scalp-covering neuromagnetometer with 122 sensors became functional in 1992 (Ahonen et al., 1993), followed by systems with over 300 channels at the end of the decade. These whole-scalp-covering devices became quintessential for both clinical applications and studies of cognitive functions beyond simple sensory stimulation, as they produced more reliable neural activation patterns than were possible to obtain with single-channel devices used in sequential measurements from one location at a time, with no guarantee that the subject's state, or head position, stayed stable between the measurements.

Despite these advances, the progress of MEG development has been rather slow compared with fMRI, where the blood-oxygen-level-dependent (BOLD) response was discovered only in 1990 (Ogawa et al., 1990); one reason for the rapid rise of fMRI's popularity was the possibility to make the measurements with the magnets already available in many hospitals for structural imaging. In 2021, about 210–220 laboratories worldwide were equipped with whole-scalp MEG devices.

Over the past three decades, important progress has taken place in the data analysis of both MEG and EEG signals, and we cover some of these developments later in this book.

■ TYPES OF EEG AND MEG SIGNALS

Brain Rhythms

Two well-known and widely applied brain rhythms are the alpha rhythm at the back of the brain and the mu rhythm in the Rolandic areas (sensorimotor cortex around the central sulcus). Figure 4.2 shows the different distribution of alpha and mu across the scalp in an EEG recording, and Figure 4.3 shows spectra of alpha and mu rhythms in a MEG recording. Alpha is strongest when the subjects have their eyes closed, and mu is strongest when the subjects are relaxed and still.

The mu rhythm was described for the first time in Marseille in 1952 by Henri Gastaut, who noted its characteristic arc-like shape (*rythme rolandique en arceau*) and also its reactivity with respect to executed motor actions (Gastaut, 1952); hence *mu* for "motor." The arch-like shape of the mu rhythm indicates that it has at least two frequency components, one around 10 Hz and another around 20 Hz (Hari, 2006), as is also evident in

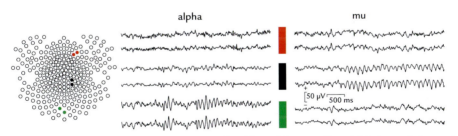

FIGURE 4.2. **EEG alpha and mu rhythms in healthy subjects.** Left: A 256-channel electrode array identifies two right frontal (red circles), central (black circles), and posterior (green circles) scalp electrodes. Middle: EEG displayed from six electrodes at the anterior, central, and posterior scalp shows a clear alpha rhythm that waxes and wanes over the posterior scalp (green electrodes, bottom traces) but is not visible in the other electrodes. In this subject, the sinusoidal rhythm peaks at around 10 Hz. Right: EEG in another healthy subject displayed from the same six electrodes. The central sites over the sensorimotor scalp (black electrodes, middle traces) show a clear mu rhythm that waxes and wanes and is not visible at the anterior and posterior sensors. The signals are low-pass filtered at 45 Hz. The average reference configuration is used to display these data. Calibration bars depict amplitude in μV and time in milliseconds. Data recorded in the Social Neuroscience Laboratory, Indiana University, USA.

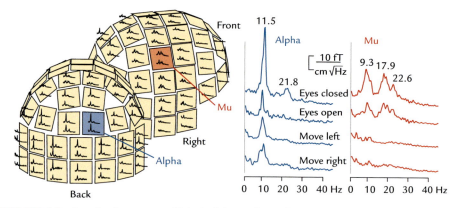

FIGURE 4.3. Amplitude spectra of MEG alpha and mu rhythms. Left: A 122-channel sensor array shown from two viewing angles (back and right). On each sensor unit, spectra are displayed from two orthogonal planar gradiometers. Alpha rhythm (blue) is strongest in the posterior MEG sensors, with a peak at 11.5 Hz, and mu rhythm (red) is strongest in sensors over the sensorimotor cortex. Right: Magnified amplitude spectra from the left panel. Alpha rhythm is greatly diminished by opening of the eyes, and mu rhythm is abolished during unilateral hand movements. Adapted and reprinted from Hari R, Salmelin R: Human cortical oscillations: a view through the skull. *Trends Neurosci* 1997, 20: 44–49. With permission from Elsevier.

Figure 4.3. It is important to note that these two components need not have a harmonic relationship.

When EEG rhythms were increasingly used in clinical studies in the 1930s and 1940s (Collura, 1993; Kennett, 2012), they were typically characterized in terms of their dominant frequency. The same frequency ranges are still in use today (Schomer & Lopes da Silva, 2018; see also Hari et al., 2018, and Pernet et al., 2018, 2020), even though slight variations occur between labs as to what constitutes the precise upper and lower limits in each case. These commonly studied EEG/MEG frequency bands (and when they were first described) are listed in Table 4.1. (For high-frequency oscillatory responses at about 600 Hz, see Chapters 11 and 17).

Importantly, it is not enough just to name the frequency band and, for example, refer to all ~10-Hz oscillations as "alpha." Unfortunately, such inaccurate language has produced some serious confusion in the literature, hampering efforts of investigators who are performing meta-analyses. We thus recommend that *both* the frequency *and* the site of the rhythm always be indicated. The reactivity of different brain rhythms is of interest in many studies and can be quantified by computing their amplitude envelopes and monitoring their changes. The main frequencies can be obtained from the peaks of power spectra, and the width of the spectral peak provides information about the consistency of the frequency; a broader peak indicates fluctuations around the main frequency, for example, because of drowsiness.

Evoked and Event-Related Responses

Besides spontaneous brain activity, rhythmic or not, both MEG and EEG can show time-locked (evoked) responses to various sensory stimuli. These quite small and noisy signals are typically visualized and characterized by increasing the signal-to-noise ratio by averaging

TABLE 4.1 EEG and MEG frequency bands

BAND	FIRST DESCRIBED
ISO: < 0.2 Hz	Nina Aladjalova, 1957
Delta: < 3.5 Hz	Grey Walter, 1936
Theta: 4–7.5 Hz	Grey Walter, 1936
Alpha: 8–13 Hz	Hans Berger, 1929
Beta: 14–30 [or 40] Hz	Hans Berger, 1929
Gamma: > 30 [or 40] Hz	Herbert Jasper & Howard Andrews, 1938

Note: ISO = infra-slow oscillations.
Aladjalova NA: Infra-slow rhythmic oscillations of the steady potential of the cerebral cortex. *Nature* 1957, 179: 957–959.
Berger H: Über das Elektroenkephalogramm des Menschen. *Arch Psychiat Nervenkr* 1929, 87: 527–570.
Jasper H, Andrews H: Electroencephalography III. Normal differentiation of occipital and precentral regions in man. *Arch Neurol Psychiatry* 1938, 39: 96–115.
Walter WG: The location of cerebral tumors by electroencephalography. *Lancet* 1936, 2: 305–308.

tens or even hundreds of single responses. These "evoked responses" have been examined in all sensory modalities with a plethora of stimuli. In MEG, the evoked responses are typically referred to as evoked fields and in EEG as evoked potentials.

The earliest evoked responses can occur within milliseconds from stimulus onset (e.g., auditory-evoked responses from the brainstem) and continue for several hundreds of milliseconds after the stimulus. Quite sustained potentials and fields can be recorded during the presentation of stimuli of longer durations or during tasks involving aspects of motor planning and other cognitive operations.

It is also possible to average signals with respect to some behavioral events, such as reaction times, eye movements, utterances of a words, or voluntary movements. The obtained "event-related responses" can be informative about integrative brain processes, such as attention, memory, and prediction of forthcoming events.

In Chapters 12 through 19, we discuss the features of both evoked and event-related responses from the earliest input to the cortex to later processing and show how the experimental setup (including stimulus repetition rate, filtering of the signals, etc.) strongly affects the kind of responses we are able to see.

▪ ADVANTAGES AND DISADVANTAGES OF MEG AND EEG

We consider MEG and EEG as two sides of the same coin; both are tools that provide complementary information about brain function. Below we summarize some advantages and disadvantages of both methods; some of these issues have been previously elaborated (Hari et al., 2000).

Advantages

1. MEG/EEG are noninvasive and safe for all subjects. Thus it is possible to repeatedly test even infants in a less intimidating environment than an MRI scanner. EEG recordings can also be performed in the operating room or intensive care unit.
2. MEG/EEG's excellent temporal resolution extends to the submillisecond range.
3. MEG/EEG measures direct and instantaneous neural activation. The signals arise mainly from postsynaptic currents, in contrast to fMRI, which measures slow hemodynamic effects associated with neural activity. DC recordings of sustained and infra-slow signals are possible with MEG and with special EEG electrodes.
4. Source modeling of MEG/EEG signals yields information about putative locations and strengths of active neuronal populations. The results can be integrated with structural MRI and fMRI data, expressed in the same 3D space.
5. Some MEG/EEG signals are clearly visible without group-level or individual statistical analyses. Hence, valid conclusions for clinical diagnostics (e.g., in epileptic disorders) can be drawn from single-subject data.
6. Neural activity can be analyzed and visualized without performing subtractions between experimental conditions. This is an important distinction relative to PET and fMRI studies, as we will see in subsequent chapters.
7. MEG signal sources can be modeled without reference to the structure and relative conductivities of the tissues of the head.
8. Compared with EEG, one crucial advantage of MEG is that the signals are recorded without any reference sensor.

Disadvantages

1. Current MEG/EEG recordings using standard methods require subjects to keep their heads and bodies still during the recording. Note, however, that the use of portable EEG instrumentation is rapidly increasing.
2. MEG recordings of children and uncooperative subjects may be especially demanding. Major epileptic seizures fill both MEG and EEG records with muscle artifacts that can prevent reasonable interpretation of the data.
3. External sources of interference can be a problem for MEG/EEG. Currently MEG must be recorded in a magnetically silent (shielded) room—an expensive part of an MEG installation. Some investigators prefer to perform also EEG recordings in shielded rooms, although environmental interference is less of a problem for EEG.
4. The inverse problem in source modeling does not have a unique solution. This nonuniqueness has been noted as the main disadvantage of MEG/EEG. Successful source identification depends on source configuration, which is typically not known in advance. However, interpreting the data with plausible anatomical and physiological constraints produces useful and often spatially accurate information.
5. MEG/EEG requires an understanding of the underlying physics and physiology. We argue that this applies equally to the competent use of any brain-research method.
6. Signal biases are different for MEG and EEG. In MEG, deep and radial currents receive considerably smaller weight than superficial and tangential currents. In EEG, all these currents contribute to recorded signals, but they are harder to identify because of the larger number of sources and the effect of differences in tissue conductivities. When used together, MEG and EEG can thus complement each other.

7. Signals from deep brain structures can be difficult to sample with MEG/EEG. MEG, in particular, can have difficulty picking up deep sources in the thalamus, amygdala, hippocampus, and cerebellum, although signals have been reported from these structures.

8. Cancellation of opposing currents, either intracortically or in neighboring cortical areas, can be considerable, thereby concealing large proportions of brain activity from both MEG and EEG.

■ REFERENCES

Adrian ED, Matthews BH: The interpretation of potential waves in the cortex. *J Physiol* 1934, 81: 440–471.

Adrian ED: Brain rhythms. *Nature* 1944, 153: 360–362.

Ahonen AI, Hämäläinen MS, Kajola MJ, Knuutila JET, Laine PP, Lounasmaa OV, Parkkonen LT, Simola JT, Tesche CD: 122-channel SQUID instrument for investigating the magnetic signals from the human brain. *Phys Scripta* 1993, T49: 198–205.

Baule G, McFee R: Detection of the magnetic field of the heart. *Am Heart J* 1963, 66: 95–96.

Berger H, Gloor P: *On the Electroencephalogram of Man: The Fourteen Original Reports on the Human Electroencephalogram.* Translated and edited by Pierre Gloor. Amsterdam: Elsevier, 1969.

Brazier MAB: The electrical fields at the surface of the head during sleep. *Electroenceph Clin Neurophysiol* 1949, 1: 195–204.

Brazier MAB: *A History of Neurophysiology in the 19th Century.* New York: Raven Press, 1988.

Caton R: The electric currents of the brain. *Br Med J* 1875, 2: 278.

Coenen A, Zayachkivska O: Adolf Beck: a pioneer in electroencephalography in between Richard Caton and Hans Berger. *Adv Cogn Psychol* 2013, 9: 216–221.

Cohen D: Magnetoencephalography: evidence of magnetic fields produced by alpha-rhythm currents. *Science* 1968, 161: 784–786.

Cohen D: Magnetoencephalography: detection of the brain's electrical activity with a superconducting magnetometer. *Science* 1972, 175: 664–666.

Collura TF: History and evolution of electroencephalographic instruments and techniques. *J Clin Neurophysiol* 1993, 10: 476–504.

Dawson GD: Cerebral responses to electrical stimulation of peripheral nerve in man. *J Neurol Neurosurg Psychiat* 1947, 10: 134–140.

Gastaut H: Etude électrocorticographique de la réactivité des rythmes rolandiques. [Electrocorticographic study of the reactivity of Rolandic rhythms]. *Revues Neurologiques (Paris)* 1952, 87: 176–182.

Hari R, Levänen S, Raij T: Timing of human cortical functions during cognition: role of MEG. *Trends Cogn Sci* 2000, 4: 455–462.

Hari R: Action–perception connection and the cortical mu rhythm. *Prog Brain Res* 2006, 159: 253–260.

Hari R, Baillet S, Barnes G, Burgess R, Forss N, Gross J, Hämäläinen M, Jensen O, Kakigi R, Mauguière F, Nakasato N, Puce A, Romani GL, Schnitzler A, Taulu S: IFCN-endorsed practical guidelines for clinical magnetoencephalography (MEG). *Clin Neurophysiol* 2018, 129: 1720–1747.

Joseph JP, Remond A, Rieger H, Lesevre N: The alpha average: II. Quantitative study and the proposition of a theoretical model. *Electroencephalogr Clin Neurophysiol* 1969, 26: 350–360.

Josephson BD: Possible new effects in superconductive tunneling. *Phys Lett* 1962, 1: 251–253.

Kennett R: Modern electroencephalography. *J Neurol* 2012, 259: 783–789.

Millett D: Hans Berger: from psychic energy to the EEG. *Perspect Biol Med* 2001, 44: 522–542.

Ogawa S, Lee TM, Kay AR & Tank DW: Brain magnetic resonance imaging with contrast dependent on blood oxygenation. *Proc Natl Acad Sci USA* 1990, 87: 9868–9872.

Pernet P, Garrido M, Gramfort A, Maurits N, Michel C, Pang E, Salmelin R, Schoffelen JM, Valdes-Sosa PA, Puce A: Best practices in data analysis and sharing in neuroimaging using MEEG. 2018. White paper https://osf.io/a8dhx/

Pernet C, Garrido MI, Gramfort A, Maurits N, Michel CM, Pang E, Salmelin R, Schoffelen JM, Valdés-Sosa PA, Puce A: Issues and recommendations from the OHBM COBIDAS MEEG committee for reproducible EEG and MEG research. *Nat Neurosci* 2020, 23: 1473–1483.

Remond A, Lesevre N, Joseph JP, Rieger H, Lairy GC: The alpha average: I. Methodology and description. *Electroencephalogr Clin Neurophysiol* 1969, 26: 245–265.

Schomer DL, Lopes da Silva FH, eds. *Niedermeyer's Electroencephalography: Basic Principles, Clinical Applications, and Related Fields*, 7th ed. New York: Oxford University Press, 2018.

Silver AH, Zimmerman JE: Quantum transitions and loss in multiply connected superconductors *Phys Rev Lett* 1965, 15: 888–891.

SECTION 2

CHAPTER 5

INSTRUMENTATION FOR EEG AND MEG

Learn to cook brown rice with a little salt and butter or olive oil. Learn to boil noodles properly or sauté onions right. Once you get those basics down, you'll be all good and feel more confident.

DAMARIS PHILLIPS

The first rule of any technology used in a business is that automation applied to an efficient operation will magnify the efficiency. The second is that automation applied to an inefficient operation will magnify the inefficiency.

BILL GATES

In this chapter, we discuss the instrumentation needed for EEG and MEG recordings. We describe "wet" and "dry" EEG (and ExG and intracranial) electrodes, MEG sensors, and the respective amplifiers (including active and passive recording systems for EEG), as well as shielding against external artifacts; here ExG refers to other electrical signals from the body. We discuss portable EEG systems and on-scalp MEG (mainly by means of optically pumped magnetometers [OPMs]).

■ EEG INSTRUMENTATION

EEG is recorded as voltages—that is potential differences—between two (sets of) electrodes. Electrodes convey the signals to amplifiers that produce the required augmentation of the EEG. Over the years, advances in technology have produced a large number of options for recording EEG. In general, the measurement systems can be grouped into a 2×2 matrix according to the electrode and amplifier types. EEG electrodes can be either passive or active, and EEG amplifiers can have either passive or active references. Passive EEG electrodes are simple conductive sensors that connect the scalp to remote EEG amplifiers, whereas active electrodes have some preprocessing (amplification) circuitry on the electrode assembly itself. Passive EEG amplifiers only take in signals from the subject, whereas active EEG amplifiers can inject current into the scalp (see section on EEG amplifiers). So, we can have passive electrodes with passive amplifiers (traditional systems), active electrodes with passive amplifiers, passive electrodes with active amplifiers, and active electrodes with active amplifiers. The choice of instrumentation will vary by laboratory setup.

Users with shielded recording rooms may be more likely to select passive electrode systems with passive amplifiers, as they are working in a low-noise environment. On the other hand, users working in regular rooms near sources of electrical interference may benefit from active electrodes combined with active amplification.

Electrodes

General

Traditional (passive) EEG scalp electrodes have been circular metal plates that, when coupled to a conductive medium, provide a bridge between the scalp and the EEG amplifier. Modern EEG electrodes can vary widely, but different electrode types have been optimized for particular EEG amplifier designs. Wet electrodes make contact with the scalp via a conductive medium, for example, a gel or solution, whereas dry electrodes require none. Irrespective of what type of EEG electrode/amplifier combination is available, the goal is to obtain the best possible signal-to-noise ratio for the EEG signal. Thus the input *impedance* (frequency-dependent resistance to current flow) of the amplifier itself must be very high relative to the impedance of the EEG electrodes, which is an important consideration in EEG amplifier design (see the next section). Moreover, the contact between the electrode and the scalp should be maximized.

When a metal comes into contact with an electrolyte solution, charges can accumulate at the metal–solution interface and result in voltage differences across this interface. Ag/AgCl is less prone to this polarization and thus suffers least from polarization-related drifts that can contaminate recordings of slow potentials (Figure 5.1). Because of these desirable properties, the most commonly used wet EEG electrodes are made of silver and silver chloride (Ag/AgCl) (Figure 5.2).

Originally, when fewer EEG electrodes were used, experimenters coated silver electrodes with thin silver-chloride layers by immersing them into an acidic solution (HCl or KCl) and passed current through an electrical circuit consisting of the electrodes and a resistor attached to a metal wire. The coated Ag/AgCl electrodes had a nice purplish-gray color (Figure 5.2, electrode 4). The problem with this kind of Ag/AgCl layer was, however, that it wore down easily and thus had to be renewed frequently. Therefore, manufacturers today prepare the electrodes by "sintering," a process whereby a homogeneous mixture of finely powdered silver and silver chloride in a specific ratio is compacted under high pressure to form the (sintered) Ag/AgCl electrode (Figure 5.2, most electrodes).

Ag/AgCl electrodes have three favorable properties (Cooper et al., 1974; Tallgren et al., 2005). First, they accurately reproduce extremely slowly changing inputs, as can be seen from Figure 5.1, where two square-wave pulses (shown at the top two traces for voltage and current) have been passed through electrodes made from different metals (traces 3–8): whereas Ag/AgCl electrodes (trace 3) reliably repeat the original signal waveform, electrodes made of platinum, and especially of silver, gold, copper, and stainless steel (traces 4–8), react mainly to the onsets and offsets of slow signals because of their short time constants (Cooper et al., 1974). Second, in addition to low polarization potentials, the Ag/AgCl electrodes generally tend to have low drifts and low noise. Third, they are nonreactive with biological tissue. It is important to note that all electrodes used in a recording should be made from the same material. However, if this is not possible (e.g., in intracranial EEG [iEEG] recordings), materials with as similar recording characteristics as possible (according to polarization, noise, and drift characteristics) should be selected.

Figure 5.2 shows different electrodes used for recording of EEG and other biosignals. EEG electrodes may be purchased as individual leads (for EEG systems with few channels;

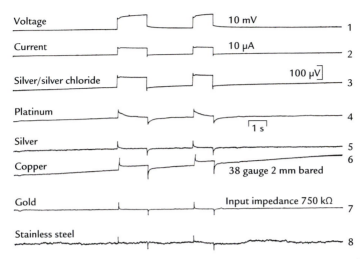

FIGURE 5.1. Different electrode materials and their response to square-wave inputs. Two square-wave pulses (traces 1 and 2; 10 mV voltage and 10 μA current steps) have been passed through electrodes made from different metals (traces 3–8; the 100-μV calibration bar applies to them all; amplifier input impedance is indicated). Of all tested metals, the silver/silver chloride electrode reproduces the signal most accurately. Note that silver, gold, and stainless steel, because of their short time constants, respond only to the transient parts of the input. A 1-s calibration bar is displayed. Reprinted from Cooper R, Osselton JW, Shaw JC: EEG Technology, 2nd ed. London, UK: Butterworth & Co., 1974: 27. ©1980 Elsevier

see Figure 5.2, electrode types 2, 4, 5), or they can be embedded in washable caps or meshes/nets comprising more EEG electrodes (e.g., up to 256; see Figure 5.2, electrode types 1, 3, 9, 10). Such caps and nets can be very convenient for placing the electrodes quickly—often in less than 20 min. Special caps have been designed for newborn and even preterm infants; for a didactic video demonstration of performing neonatal EEG recordings, see Stjerna et al. (2012). Portable EEG systems often have electrodes embedded in headsets that are designed to fit snugly on the head. In some systems, the electrode positions are fixed, in others they can be varied, and in some others the user can select the desired fixed electrode configuration during manufacturing. Portable EEG systems span the consumer–research–clinical markets and currently offer a wide number of channels, ranging from 1 to 256. These systems also offer very different types of electrodes, wet or dry, as we discuss below.

Wet Electrodes

Wet electrodes require some sort of conductive medium to eliminate air gaps between the skin and the electrode itself, thereby lowering the skin–electrode impedance and recording optimal signals (see subsequent section on EEG amplifiers and additional considerations for subject preparation in Chapter 7). Typical input impedances of wet electrodes are between 2 and 10 kOhm, compatible with the input impedances of the associated EEG amplifiers (see next section).

The Ag/AgCl EEG scalp electrodes can be sited within a cloth cap (see Figure 5.2, electrode types 3 and 9), or individual electrodes can be placed on the scalp using an adhesive (typically collodion) (Figure 5.2, electrode type 4), applying thick conductive paste that

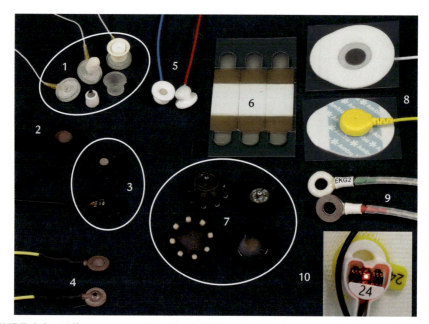

FIGURE 5.2. Different types of Ag/AgCl EEG and ExG electrodes (to be used for EOG, EMG, ECG, etc.). Some electrode groups are encircled for clarity. All electrodes, except 7, are wet, and all, except 3 and 10, are passive. (1) Electrodes for EEG nets. The intact electrode appears at the right of the triplet. The middle disk shows the dry sponge surrounding the electrode after the housing has been removed. In the left disk, the electrode/sponge assembly has been detached from the housing. (2) A general-purpose ExG electrode (includes EEG use) that can be attached to the skin with medical adhesive tape or under an elastic strap. (3) A pair of active EEG electrodes showing both sides of the assembly. Pre-amplifier circuitry is sited in the top of electrode housing that can be inserted into specialized mounts on a cloth EEG cap. The bottom of the assembly is the point of contact with the scalp. (4) Classic collodion cup electrodes. To attach the cup to the scalp, collodion medical adhesive is placed on the flat perimeter of the electrode disk and the surrounding scalp. The cup can then be filled with electrode gel via a syringe/blunted needle. These electrodes are often used for long-term monitoring. (5) General purpose ExG electrodes that can be attached to the skin with medical adhesive tape. (6) Adhesive disposable ExG strip electrodes with 2 separate pre-gelled contacts (brownish squares) and a central (white) adhesive area. The electrodes can be connected to cabling via crocodile/alligator clips. (7) Dry electrodes. Left side shows the top and bottom of a spider/finger EEG electrode made of a composite conductive material with sintered Ag/AgCl tips that make contact with the skin and bypass the hair. Right side displays a smooth disk electrode applicable to non-hairy skin. These electrodes have press studs on their tops and can be easily attached to the headset electrode holder. (8) Pre-gelled disposable ECG electrodes that can also be used for other recording types, e.g., surface EMG. (9) EEG/ExG ceramic donuts (with shielded cables) for simultaneous use with transcranial magnetic stimulation or fMRI, designed to dissipate heat. (10) Active electrode close-up (identical to 3) during impedance measurement procedure. The color of the LED signals the quality of contact (within a certain acceptable range of impedances). (Social Neuroscience Laboratory, Indiana University, USA.)

also adheres to the scalp, or placing electrodes under a set of elastic straps on the head (Figure 5.2, electrode types 2 and 5). These electrode application systems may not work well for subjects with very curly hair. In these cases, special "hair-clip" style Ag/AgCl electrodes can be applied to the scalp after the hair has been braided into "cornrows" (Etienne et al., 2020).

An alternative sintered Ag/AgCl electrode system consists of a flexible "net" of electrodes linked by connecting wires. These electrodes make contact with the scalp via sponges soaked in an electrolyte solution, typically KCl (see Figure 5.2, electrode type 1, and Figure 5.7 right). These electrodes typically have impedances of about 50 kOhm, which is an order of magnitude higher than impedances for the electrodes described above, but comparable to iEEG electrodes. The physiological amplifiers that are designed to work with the higher-impedance net Ag/AgCl or iEEG electrodes will themselves have much higher input impedances than those used with regular wet sintered Ag/AgCl electrodes.

Dry Electrodes

Impedances are much higher for dry than wet electrodes, so that dry-electrode EEG systems must be specially designed to ensure high-fidelity recordings. Thus these amplifiers typically must have much higher input impedances to accommodate dry EEG electrodes. Dry electrodes are desirable for portable (untethered) EEG systems as they require little maintenance and are quick to place. One additional benefit of dry electrodes is that they are not prone to the signal degradation that occurs with wet electrodes when impedances increase due to drying out during prolonged recordings.

Dry electrodes can consist of metallic or nonmetallic conductive materials, and they either make, or do not make, a direct contact with the skin (Grimnes & Martinsen, 2015; Di Flumeri et al., 2019; Shad et al., 2020). Contact electrodes sit directly on the skin and record potentials directly. These electrodes come in a variety of shapes, often being spiky or spider-like with legs or "fingers" designed to make contact with the scalp and bypass the hair (Figure 5.2, electrode type 7, left) (Krachunov & Casson, 2016; Velcescu et al., 2019). A press-stud is present on the top of the electrode so that it can be attached to the EEG headset. Construction materials vary, but often the coating on the electrode is sintered Ag/AgCl. These electrodes can be 3D printed (Debener et al., 2015; Krachunov & Casson, 2016; Velcescu et al., 2019); they typically have high impedances and thus need to be used with amplifiers that in turn have very high input impedances.

Noncontact capacitive electrodes typically consist of a sandwich of materials comprising a conductive plate on the skin (e.g., Ag/AgCl), an insulator, and an additional conductive plate that connects to the EEG preamplifier. Hence, the EEG signal is sensed via capacitive coupling with the skin (Matsuo et al., 1973; Grimnes & Martinsen, 2015). No skin preparation is necessary. However, these electrodes are prone to movement artifacts.

Hybrid or "Semi-Dry" Electrode Configurations

Hybrid electrodes consist of a conductive solid-gel that is composed of a stable base mixed with various moisture-absorbing substances. Some examples of solid-gel mixtures are sodium chloride, calcium chloride dihydrate, glycerol, and pure water (Di Flumeri et al., 2019) or carboxymethylcellulose, calcium chloride, glycerol, and pure water (Toyama et al., 2012). The solid-gel electrodes make direct contact with the scalp and are held in place in electrode sockets that are mounted in a head cap. The electrodes must be hydrated before use by immersion in a saline solution for a few minutes, and they give stable recordings for up to 8 hours (Di Flumeri et al., 2019).

An alternative "semi-dry" electrode is constructed from a superporous hydrogel that slowly releases small amounts of conductive liquid, such as saline, to the scalp (Mota et al., 2013; Li et al., 2021). An important property of a superporous material is the ability to absorb aqueous fluids up to a few hundred times its own weight (Grimnes & Martinsen, 2015), meaning that these types of EEG electrode could theoretically show long-term recording stability. The most recent semi-dry electrode design (Li et al., 2021) consists of a polyacrylamide/polyvinyl alcohol mix that has been polymerized into an electrode cavity. Saline can be "charged" into the material over just a few seconds, allowing the superporous material to swell and absorb the fluid. When the charged electrode is in contact with the scalp, it slowly releases saline to the scalp because of gravity and capillary forces. Importantly, the "charging and discharging" rates of these semi-dry electrodes can be adjusted by changing the design and fabrication (Li et al., 2021). The exciting development of new dry and semi-dry EEG electrode designs will no doubt continue with the emergence of new materials.

Special Electrodes

ELECTRODES FOR INVASIVE RECORDINGS

Intracranial EEG electrodes require surgical placement under general anesthesia and may stay in situ for several weeks during presurgical evaluation for epilepsy or chronically for deep-brain stimulation, which places extra constraints on electrode materials.

Electrocorticography (ECoG) electrodes are typically made from surgical stainless steel or platinum and are embedded in a flexible nonconductive medium, such as silicone. ECoG electrode arrays typically have intercontact distances of 5 or 10 mm and come in a variety of configurations, such as larger "grids" of 8 × 8 electrodes for example, or smaller "strips," such as 1 × 10 or 2 × 8 electrodes—the latter can be straight, curved, or even T-shaped. ECoG arrays are sited subdurally on the brain's gyral surfaces and require a craniotomy.

Stereoencephalography EEG (or SEEG) electrodes are multicontact depth probes made from platinum, typically around 1 mm in diameter, with contacts usually separated by 5–10 mm. Typical numbers of contacts vary from 4 to 12. An SEEG probe is inserted stereotactically into a burr hole in the skull via a rigid guiding stylette and is aimed at a particular target (e.g., hippocampus, amygdala [for epilepsy surgery], or structures in the basal ganglia [for deep-brain stimulation]). Accurate siting is accomplished by matching "fiducial" markers (see Chapter 7) on the patient's head and on their structural MRI (magnetic resonance imaging). (Earlier versions of this procedure required a metal stereotactic frame to literally be bolted to the subject's head, but today frameless stereotaxy, guided by structural MRI, is the common standard.) Some depth probes come with additional fine wires at their distal end, allowing multiunit activity to be sampled from the surrounding tissue.

Thin-needle electrodes, typically made of stainless steel, are sometimes used for acute clinical EEG recordings, for example in comatose patients, by inserting them into the skin. Despite their small size, they do not provide better spatial resolution if they are placed at the same locations as the scalp electrodes. Moreover, their impedance is much higher than that of the surface electrodes, which makes them more prone to artifacts and loss of signal amplitude and quality.

Nasopharyngeal, nasoethmoidal, and sphenoidal electrodes have been used for sampling epileptic activity extracranially from the orbitofrontal and mesial temporal lobes (Morris & Lüders, 1985; Quesney & Gloor, 1987). *Nasopharyngeal electrodes* (Gastaut, 1948; Roubicek & Hill, 1948) are flexible insulated wires with an Ag/AgCl tip. They are inserted through the nostrils down the nasal passage to rest against the nasopharynx. Positioning needs expertise and, despite topical anesthetic gel, is uncomfortable for the patient, who may cough during electrode insertion if the probe is pushed too far. These electrodes are extremely prone to artifacts, but they can detect epileptic discharges that may not be seen in conventional scalp recordings.

Nasoethmoidal electrodes (Lehtinen & Bergström, 1970) are less prone to artifacts and consist of flexible Teflon-coated silver wires with a 1.5- to 2-mm diameter and a rounded tip. They are sited via the nasal passage into the ethmoid sinuses to ideally rest under the cribriform plate of the ethmoid bone. After insertion, electrode locations can be checked by X-ray.

Sphenoidal electrodes, first used in 1949, were steel needles (Christodoulou, 1967). Now, they are insulated silver wires that are inserted by the clinician under local anesthetic by puncturing the skin just below the zygomatic arch on the face and targeting a rigid removable stylette containing the electrode toward the foramen ovale. These electrodes are less prone to artifacts than nasopharyngeal electrodes but require a semi-invasive insertion that is uncomfortable for the patient.

ELECTRODES FOR PORTABLE DEVICES AND BRAIN–COMPUTER INTERFACES

Unique low-density EEG electrode arrays have been developed more recently for use mainly with portable EEG systems and scalp-EEG-based brain–computer interfaces (BCIs). A number of these were developed around the outer human ear, targeted initially to pick up activity from temporal lobes to auditory inputs for BCIs (see Figure 5.3). For example, a C-shaped 10-electrode array or "cEEGrid" is placed on the scalp encircling the earlobe, with wet Ag/AgCI electrodes that can be worn for up to 7 hours (Debener et al., 2015; Mirkovic et al., 2016). Other systems embed the EEG electrodes and also auditory stimulation devices into a personalizable earpiece. Some examples include (1) a 4-channel "EarEEG" system (including a reference electrode) initially developed with wet electrodes (Kidmose et al., 2013), but which now comes with dry electrodes made from titanium coated with iridium-oxide (Kappel et al., 2019); (2) the "EARtrode" system made from silicone rubber and conductive carbon fibers that has a custom-fitted earpiece and ergonomic behind-the-earlobe piece with altogether four EEG channels (Valentin et al., 2021); (3) a flexible, foldable, fractal-like mesh design made from gold (Au) for placement on the outer structures of the ear and the mastoid. The active, reference, and ground electrodes are on a stretchable interconnected structure, aimed for comfortable long-term use for a continuous 2-week period (Norton et al., 2015).

Expertise is needed to obtain good-quality brain signals with all these portable EEG systems. One major concern noted in an extensive meta-analysis of 250 studies on BCIs was that only a small percentage of studies reported if electromyogram (EMG) and electrooculogram (EOG) artifacts had been handled (Fatourechi et al., 2007). This is a worrying problem that needs to be addressed.

A number of commercial whole-scalp, low-density systems have headsets with fixed electrodes that either require the addition of conductive solution/gel or use sponges soaked in conductive solution; these systems can yield good-quality data when used with EEG expertise (e.g., Mullen et al., 2013; Hashemi et al., 2016).

ExG Electrodes

The same electrode application logic used for EEG also applies to measurement of "ExGs," that is, other electrical signals from the body, such as muscle activity (surface EMG), eye movements and blinks (EOG), heart activity (electrocardiogram, EKG or ECG), and activity from the gut (electrogastrogram, EGG). ExG signals are typically measured using wet electrodes, which often are disposable adhesive pre-gelled Ag/AgCI electrodes housed on a press-stud designed to attach to an electrode cable (Figure 5.2, electrode 8). Alternatively,

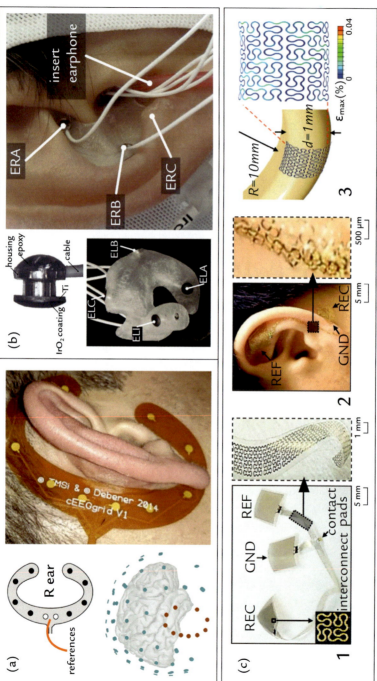

FIGURE 5.3. Some types of EEG electrodes that sit around and in the human ear. (a) Right-ear "cEEGrid", C-shaped assembly. Top left: The schematic shows positions for electrodes (black circles) and 2 reference electrodes (white circles). Bottom left: Electrode positions (red dots) in a 3D anatomical space with corresponding 10–10 electrode positions (blue dots) relative to a lateral view of a brain. Right: The right cEEGrid in situ. (Reproduced with permission from Debener S, Emkes R, De Vos M, Bleichner M: Unobtrusive ambulatory EEG using a smartphone and flexible printed electrodes around the ear. *Sci Rep* 2015, 5: 16743 and from Mirkovic B, Bleichner MG, DeVos M, Debener S: Target speaker detection with concealed EEG around the ear. *Front Neurosci 2016* 10: 349).

single Ag/AgCl disks (similar to those used in EEG) can also be used, but these must be gelled before they are applied to the skin and secured in place with medical adhesive tape.

For some specific ExG applications, very specialized electrodes have been developed. In clinical neurophysiological diagnostics of myopathies and peripheral neurogenic lesions, single motor units and abnormal muscle activity related to damaged innervation are assessed with concentric (coaxial) stainless steel needle electrodes inserted into the muscle; the electrode records potential differences between the tip of the active needle inside and the outside surface of the electrode. With a (tungsten) needle inserted into a peripheral nerve, microneurographic recordings (Zotterman, 1939) can pick up impulses from single nerve fibers (Vallbo, 2018).

Concentric ring electrodes can be applied for noninvasive recordings from the body's surface to improve the spatial specificity of the measured signal prior to sampling. Here two (bipolar) or three (tripolar) rings can mitigate some of the blurring effects that are caused by different conductivities within the volume conductor (the body; see Chapter 3), as for example in recordings of the EGG [electrical activity of the gut]; see Chapter 16). If the center and third rings are short-circuited (connected directly to each other) and activity is recorded between them and the second ring, the spatial derivative (or Laplacian) of the surface potential can be recorded, and artifacts arising far from the electrode, such as the ECG, are suppressed.

Electrodes for Ultra-Slow EEG Signals

One important point needs to be made about EEG electrodes that are stable during recordings of infra-slow or ultra-slow (< 1 Hz or as low as 0.1 Hz) EEG activity, known as full-band EEG recording (fbEEG). As already noted, electrodes can exhibit polarization potentials and other instabilities, and such slow potential drifts can contaminate the recording. To minimize this problem, an insulated wet Ag/AgCl electrode has been designed specifically for these recordings (Vanhatalo et al., 2005; Figure 5.4, top panel) to be used with special "DC-coupled" amplifiers (see next section).

FIGURE 5.3. **Continued**

(b) The "EarEEG" system. Top left: A magnified photograph of a titanium EEG electrode with iridium dioxide coating. Bottom left image shows the entire customized left-sided earpiece with embedded 6 EEG electrodes, of which 4 are visible with their respective electrode labels (ELA, ELB, ELC and ELI, the latter sitting in the ear canal itself). Right: The EarEEG system in situ in right ear, depicting 3 external-ear electrodes (ERA, ERB, and ERC). The 3 ear-canal electrodes and an additional ear insert with sound stimulator cannot be seen in this image. (Reproduced with permission from Kappel SL, Rank ML, Toft HO, Andersen M, Kidmose P: Dry-contact electrode ear-EEG. *IEEE Trans Biomed Eng* 2019, 66: 150–158). (c) Flexible, foldable Peano pattern gold electrode for placement on the ear lobe. Panel 1: The 3 electrodes (RECording, REFerence and GrouND) and 'interconnect' cabling; the inset shows the 2D cabling pattern. Panel 2: The electrodes and interconnect cables in situ on the left ear in one example layout; the inset shows a magnified version of the interconnect cable on the ear. Panel 3: A Finite Element Model showing maximum strains in 2 dimensions across the Peano pattern for a particular size and shape of the ear's helix. (Reproduced with permission from Norton JJS, Lee DS, Lee JW, Lee W, Kwon O, Won P, Jung S-Y, Cheng H, Jeong J-W, Akce A, Umunna S, Na I, Kwon YH, Wang X-Q, Liu Z, Paik U, Huang Y, Bretl T, Yeo W-H, Rogers JA: Soft, curved electrode systems capable of integration on the auricle as a persistent brain-computer interface. *Proc Natl Acad Sci U S A* 2015, 112: 3920–3925).

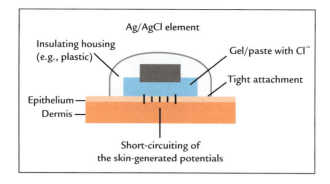

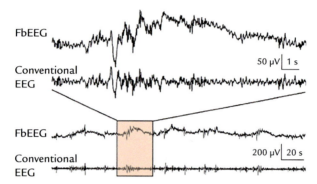

FIGURE 5.4. Full-band EEG recording. Top: Electrode requirements for a stable electrode–skin interface for infra-slow or ultra-slow recordings. A plastic cover insulates the Ag/AgCl electrode and fits so snugly on the skin that it prevents drying of the conductive gel. Skin potentials are short-circuited by scratching or puncturing the epithelium prior to applying the electrode. Bottom: Examples of slow potential shifts recorded during sleep. The traces show the "DC-coupled" full-band (Fb) EEG recording (third trace) and the conventional EEG recording with high-pass filtering at 0.5 Hz (fourth trace). The first and second traces show magnified sections of the same signals shown in the peach-colored square in the lower traces. The slow potentials are clearly visible in the "DC recordings" depicted in the first and third traces, but they have disappeared completely in the EEG recording applying conventional HP filtering (second and fourth traces). DC recordings are discussed in the next section on EEG Amplifiers. Adapted and reprinted from Vanhatalo S, Voipio J, Kaila K: Full-band EEG (FbEEG): an emerging standard in electroencephalography. *Clin Neurophysiol* 2005, 116: 1–8. With permission from Elsevier.

EEG Amplifiers

General

EEG signals are typically amplified at two steps. At the initial analog preamplification stage, some filtering already takes place, before an additional (final) stage of amplification by a power amplifier; the pre- and power amplifiers are connected in series. It is good design practice to augment the tiny EEG signals as close as possible to the subject because a strong, amplified signal is less susceptible to noise during data transfer and digitization. Such avoidance of additional noise and artifacts is particularly important for recordings performed in noisy conditions, as is the case with ambulatory EEG. Often in commercial nonportable

EEG systems, however, both amplification stages take place in the EEG recording device itself, with *passive electrodes* providing only a physical connection to EEG amplifiers. *Active electrodes* will have a preamplifier housed on the electrode itself (Figure 5.2, electrodes 3 and 10), allowing the signal to be amplified before additional noise taints it on the way to the main (remote) EEG amplifier.

Differential Amplifiers and Common-Mode Rejection

EEG recording devices comprise a set of *differential amplifiers* to which the electrodes are connected (Figure 5.5, top panel). As its name suggests, the differential amplifier amplifies the *difference* between the signals at the two inputs (Figure 5.5), and the differential gain indicates how much the signal will be amplified. An important feature of the differential amplifier is the considerable suppression of *common-mode signals* that are the same at both inputs (see Figure 5.5, middle traces). Examples of unwanted common-mode signals are power-line noise and noise arising from a cardiac or a nerve stimulator in another part of the body.

A good amplifier should reject, or strongly suppress, all common-mode signals and amplify only the signals of interest. Thus a measure of interest is the amplifier's common-mode rejection ratio (CMRR), which is the ratio between the differential gain (how much the difference between the inputs is amplified) and the common-mode gain (how much the common signal in both inputs is amplified). CMRR is expressed in decibels as follows:

$$CMRR = 20 \log_{10} [(\text{gain for difference signal})/(\text{gain for common-mode signal})]$$

Note that the gain for common-mode signals is much smaller than the gain for difference signals between the amplifier inputs. Consequently, present-day commercial EEG amplifiers have very high CMRRs, for example, 100 dB or even greater for some portable EEG systems, which means that input differences (our signals of interest) are amplified

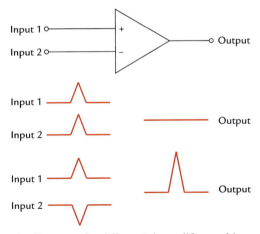

FIGURE 5.5. Schematic diagram of a differential amplifier and its outputs. Top: A differential amplifier has two inputs (one of which inverts the signal) and one amplified output; the ground and the gain-adjusting feedback circuits are not shown. Middle: When identical signals occur at both inputs of the differential amplifier, the output will be zero. If the signals differ, the output reflects at each moment of time the difference between the two. Bottom: If the input signals are equal in size but opposite in polarity, the output will be two times the original signal size (multiplied by the gain of the amplifier).

five orders of magnitude more than the common-mode signals. An amplifier with such a high CMRR effectively reduces electrical power-line noise (50 or 60 Hz depending on the country) *provided* that the electrode impedances are approximately equal for the pair of electrodes connected to the amplifier's inputs.

EFFECT OF AMPLIFIER INPUT IMPEDANCE ON CMRR

As already stated, the input impedance of the amplifier should be many orders of magnitude higher than the electrode–skin impedance so that the amplifier remains as insensitive as possible to small changes in electrode contact. If electrode impedances are too high, the signals may not be amplified as much as the gain of the amplifier would let us predict.

In the following example, we illustrate how EEG recordings can be affected by electrode impedances. If the impedances of a pair of EEG electrodes at an amplifier's inputs are 10 kΩ and the amplifier's input impedance is 1 MΩ (megaohm), then a 100-μV input signal will be measured as 99 μV, resulting in a measurement error (signal drop) of 1%. This error is proportional to the ratio of electrode impedances relative to the input impedance of the amplifier. In contrast, with electrode impedances of 25 kΩ and an amplifier input impedance of 250 MΩ, the corresponding error would be negligible, only 0.01%. The highest input impedances of the present-day portable EEG amplifiers are already on the order of teraohms (10^{12} ohms) (e.g., Chi et al., 2011).

To maximize the CMRR of the amplifier, *impedances should be comparable across electrodes*. In typical EEG recordings, one electrode is the reference—a common input to all EEG amplifiers. Experimenters often take much care in applying the reference electrode, which may result in lower impedance for the reference electrode relative to the other electrodes. A large difference can produce an impedance mismatch, which compromises the CMRR and thereby affects the quality of the EEG recording by weighting the signals toward the voltage occurring at the reference electrode.

MAXIMIZING CMRR: GROUNDING AND SPECIAL FEEDBACK CIRCUITS

A ground electrode, also fixed to the subject, stabilizes any potential difference between the subject and the EEG preamplifier and decreases noise in the EEG recordings. In principle, the location of the ground electrode can be freely chosen, but in commercially available EEG caps or nets the location is typically fixed. On some occasions, different types of ground electrodes may need to be used to minimize noise and artifacts in EEG recordings. For example, during electrical median-nerve stimulation at the wrist, a ring-shaped ground electrode proximal to the stimulation site can effectively decrease the stimulus artifact in the recorded EEG signals (see Chapter 15).

Another way in which noise in the signal can be reduced comes from a special reference configuration, called the "driven right leg" (DRL) circuit, used commercially to reduce power-line noise in electrophysiological signals, including the EEG. The DRL circuit was initially developed for ECG, and it applied the common-mode voltage back to the subject through a low-resistance path from the ECG amplifier's common input, further minimizing common-mode voltages (Winter & Webster, 1983; Acharya, 2011).

An extended variant of the DRL also adds common-mode sensing (CMS) to the mix. In this design, the usual reference and ground electrodes are replaced by two electrodes that act together in a feedback loop. The DRL electrode is placed (ideally) at a distance to the (EEG) recording electrodes, whereas the CMS electrode sits (ideally) in the center of the recording electrodes. The two electrodes form inputs to a differential amplifier that feeds back residual common-mode voltages to the subject and stabilize the potential differences between the subject and the EEG amplifier. Some portable EEG systems have adopted this configuration, but one wonders about how effective this can be, given that all electrodes, including the DRL, are typically located on the face and scalp.

Needless to say, there are electrical safety considerations with these "active" DRL and CMS reference configurations. In physiological amplifiers, these circuits are designed with current limited to 50 microamperes to ensure the electrical safety of the subject and to meet the existing international electrical safety standards.

DC-Coupled EEG Amplifiers

Ultra-slow EEG fluctuations (Aladjalova, 1957) can be recorded only when the amplifiers have very long time constants or are "DC coupled." Note, however, that such recordings are prone to various artifacts arising from movements, electrode polarization, and more. Amplifiers can slowly drift during the recording session, and thus specific technical procedures are necessary to reliably discern brain-originated ultra-slow fluctuations. As already noted in the previous section, special insulated electrodes (Vanhatalo et al., 2005) can allow reliable recordings of slow activity that is not seen in conventional (clinical) EEG recordings with filter settings of 0.5 (or 0.3) to 70 Hz (Figure 5.4, bottom panel). (Filtering is discussed in Chapter 8.) DC-coupled EEG recordings are optimally conducted inside a Faraday cage (or, if carried out with simultaneous MEG, of course within a magnetically shielded room).

EEG Amplifiers for Simultaneous Use With Other Neuroimaging Techniques

For EEG systems used in combination with functional MRI (fMRI) studies, special designs are needed to record reliable signals and minimize the large artifacts caused by MRI-scanner pulses. Special care must be paid to electrode and cable composition as changing gradient fields and radio-frequency pulses may heat the EEG electrodes and cables and potentially cause focal burns to the subject (Pascual-Leone et al., 1990; Laufs et al., 2008). Importantly, EEG cables should not form loops into which the MRI-scanner pulses could induce currents. Given these important safety issues, all EEG devices and electrodes/cabling used within an MRI scanner must be MRI compatible.

Combined transcranial magnetic stimulation (TMS) and EEG studies should use only special TMS-compatible EEG electrodes (Figure 5.2, electrode 9) and amplifiers designed to withstand heating. Although this is not a safety issue, large artifacts arising from TMS pulses can seriously distort the EEG recording, and thus the EEG amplifiers were typically configured not to record signals for the duration of the TMS pulse. (A similar procedure has been used in pain studies when electrical dental pulp stimulation produced large artifacts in the EEG recordings because of the high stimulation voltages that had to be used due to the high, about 2–4 MΩ, impedance of dental enamel.) As we discuss later, it is important that the large artifacts do not saturate the amplifiers or the analog–digital conversion (i.e., reach the limits of their dynamic range).

To summarize, the requirements for a good EEG amplifier are low noise, high input impedance (at least hundreds of MΩ), and high (~100 dB) CMRR. The impedances of EEG electrodes must be comparable across sites and remain, for the entire duration of the recording, within the optimal ranges set by manufacturer's standards.

Standard Electrode Positions

Traditionally, EEG electrodes have been placed in (approximate) standard positions using the International 10–20 system (Jasper, 1958; Klem et al., 1999), which is presented schematically in Figure 5.6 (left). This system has 21 electrodes at locations that are determined by the percentage distances between designated cranial landmarks on the head. The electrodes are referred to with labels comprising an uppercase letter that refers to scalp position (F = frontal, T = temporal, P = parietal, C = central, and O = occipital) and a number that further identifies the electrode's location on the scalp. Odd numbers identify left-hemisphere electrodes and even numbers right-hemisphere electrodes; the letter z electrodes run along the sagittal midline. Additional electrode placements can be on the earlobes (A1 and A2) or mastoids (M1 and M2). Electrode positions are separated by 10% and 20% distances on lines running between cranial landmarks known as the nasion and inion and the preauricular points close to each ear. The nasion is the clear facial indentation just above the bridge of the nose between the eyes, the inion is the most prominent part of the occipital protuberance, and the preauricular points are the indentations in the zygomatic bone just in front of the tragus, in front of the ear canal (see Figure 7.2 for this landmark and a layout of the coordinate system). The vertex (electrode Cz) is in the middle (50%) of the direct line connecting the nasion and inion; it is often useful to define, at the same time, the 50% point of the line connecting the two preauricular points so that the head midline is confirmed. Pinpointing the vertex also aids in finding the other electrode positions.

Figures 5.6 (middle) and 5.7 (left) depict the denser 10–10 system (Chatrian et al., 1985) with a total of 81 electrodes; the interelectrode distances are based on 10% fractions of the nasion–inion and interauricular lines. This system uses a similar lettering and numbering system to the 10–20 system, but because of the larger number of electrodes, the labels had to be expanded, and the nomenclature is not always the most logical one. For example, electrodes P7 and P8 of the 10–10 system denote posterior and inferior electrode sites over the temporal rather than parietal scalp, and their corresponding electrodes in the 10–20 system are T5 and T6. Despite these minor inconsistencies in nomenclature, the 10–10 system is the most widely used one in cloth-cap-housed electrode arrays used in research laboratories.

A further expansion for the high-density EEG electrode system uses even smaller distances to include electrodes that were 5% of the two lines on the head (10–5 system), allowing for a total of over 300 electrodes to be sited (Oostenveld & Praamstra, 2001). However, this system did not really become popular for a number of reasons. First, applying over 300 electrodes takes a lot of time, even when the electrodes are embedded in a cap, as the conductive gel must typically be applied under each electrode. Second, while a large number of electrodes is desirable for identification of neural sources, these electrodes are not equidistant across the entire scalp. In a geodesic array (see schematic in Figure 5.6, right, and electrodes in situ in Figure 5.7, right), the electrodes are spaced with even distances across the head (Tucker, 1993). Importantly, geodesic recording systems sample EEG from the lower face and neck as well, which may offer additional advantages for identification of the generators of the measured signals.

Although skulls and brains vary considerably, X-ray imaging (Homan et al., 1987) of 12 healthy subjects showed a reasonable concordance of electrode locations of the international 10–20 system in relation to the underlying brain anatomy. EEG electrode locations have also been evaluated relative to the Montreal Neurological Institute coordinates, and the electrode locations of the 10–20 and 10–10 systems are often used to designate sites for TMS stimulation as well as sensors of near infrared imaging systems (Herwig et al., 2003; Jurcak et al., 2007). Electrode positions from both the 10–10 and 10–20 systems have been compared using median distances of each geodesic EEG sensor to the closest 10–10 or 10–20 electrode site (Luu & Ferree, 2005). The most recent attempts to determine EEG electrode locations are based on 3D digitization. We cover these approaches in a subsequent section while describing how we can locate the MEG sensor array and the EEG electrodes relative to the head.

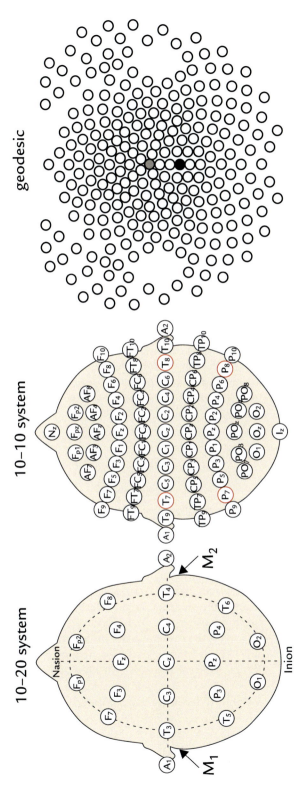

10–20 system

10–10 system

geodesic

FIGURE 5.6. EEG-electrode positions. Left: The International 10–20 system of EEG electrode placement and labeling. The vertical and horizontal broken lines denote the nasion–inion and interauricular lines, respectively. The circular broken line identifies a circumference around the head that encompasses the outer ring of electrodes. The positions of the mastoid electrodes (M1 and M2) are also indicated. For specific electrode distances, see the main text. Middle: The International 10–10 system of EEG electrode placement. Additional electrodes are included at the nasion (Nz) and inion (Iz), between the 10–20 sites themselves and in additional rows that are designated PO (parieto-occipital), TP (temporoparietal), CP (centroparietal), FC (frontocentral), FT (frontotemporal), and AF (anterofrontal). Right: A geodesic electrode array. A 256-channel EEG electrode net covers the scalp, face, and neck. Electrodes are spaced at even distances from each other, although in this 2D representation the spacing does not appear to be equal. (See Figure 5.7 right image of a subject wearing the cap.) The reference electrode is sited at the vertex (in the center of the array; gray circle), and the ground is on the centroparietal midline, behind the reference (black circle). Geodesic electrode arrays also have 64- and 128-electrode versions.

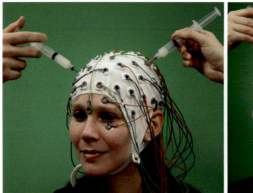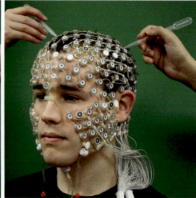

FIGURE 5.7. **EEG-electrode preparation prior to a recording.** Left: A cap embedding 10–10 system with sintered Ag/AgCl electrodes. Additional single electrodes record EOG activity above, below and to the left and right of the left eye. After the cap is sited, gel is added to each electrode using a syringe with a blunted needle. The blunted needle allows the hair to be moved out from under the electrode and to produce mild abrasion of the skin, thereby decreasing electrode–skin impedance. These caps typically require electrode impedances of 2 to 10 kΩ as they are used with EEG amplifiers that have relatively low input impedances. Right: A 256-channel geodesic net with sintered Ag/AgCl electrodes buffered by sponges soaked in KCl solution. After the cap is sited, hair can be moved out from under the sponges using a plastic pipette. KCl solution in the pipette can also be introduced under the sponge if needed. These electrodes typically have impedances around 50 to 70 kΩ (similar to intracranial electrodes) and are appropriate for use with EEG amplifiers that have high input impedances. (Social Neuroscience Laboratory, Indiana University, USA.)

Reference Electrode Configurations

General

Ideally, the reference electrode should be totally neutral and not contribute neural activity to the measurement. However, due to effects of volume conduction, *there is not a single place in the body that would be totally electrically silent* and serve as an inactive reference site for EEG (Nunez, 1981). Because EEG records potential differences between two electrodes, both locations should be taken into account in the analysis and interpretation of the measured signals.

Reference electrodes are typically sited in places that are assumed to be far from the putative activity of interest, and traditionally popular places for reference electrodes have been earlobes, mastoids, and the nose. Notably, these electrodes are not inactive, and the balanced noncephalic reference that has been used in the past is also not inactive (Stephenson & Gibbs, 1951; Lehtonen & Koivikko, 1971). This latter reference configuration requires two electrodes—one on the C7 spinous process and the other near the right sternoclavicular junction—connected via an adjustable resistor so that cardiac artifact can be minimized in the EEG recording. Each subject has a slightly different cardiac dipole (a vector illustrating the main activation direction of the cardiac muscle; see Figure 9.16), as the heart will sit in a slightly different position and orientation in the chest and be of slightly different geometry in each individual; moreover, the heart position changes depending on the position of the person (sitting, lying) and on the phase of respiration. Hence, the resistor setting needs to be adjusted separately for each individual prior to commencing the recording.

The nose reference has been very informative in some special cases. For example, for long-latency, auditory-evoked potentials generated in the supratemporal auditory cortex (Chapter 13), the nose tip is located just at the zero-potential line (Vaughan & Ritter, 1970). Many visual evoked potentials (see Chapter 14) have been recorded with a nose reference (see, e.g., Bentin et al., 1996) as it is far away from the visual cortex. However, a nose reference cannot be recommended in general as, in addition not being inactive, it picks up artifacts from the eyes (movements and blinks) and facial muscles (Chapter 9), and it therefore easily spreads these artifacts to all EEG derivations.

What constitutes a good reference electrode at the time of data acquisition may not be the best reference electrode for data analysis. In many modern EEG caps/nets, the site of the reference electrode is fixed. A reference electrode on an earlobe or the vertex usually works well because it is at a distance from the eyes and facial muscles, which typically can introduce a significant proportion of artifacts into the EEG. Whenever there is flexibility in choosing the (data-acquisition) reference electrode, thought should be given to where the most interesting neural sources for the particular experiment might be located and what the putative data processing plan is. If, for example, the plan is to digitally "re-reference" the data (i.e., to compute with respect to another reference location), then any *single* electrode at a stable place that is not too heavily contaminated by muscular, ocular, or other artifacts can act as a reference in the array of EEG electrodes. In this sense, the stable bony vertex is a much better reference site than the mobile and more artifact-prone nose tip. However, the signals generated close to the vertex would be difficult to see by visual inspection because they would not differ much from signals picked up by the reference electrode located at the vertex.

Whatever the choice for the reference site at data acquisition, one really should use just a *single* reference electrode. For example, *the previously commonly used physically linked-earlobe or physically linked-mastoid electrode configurations should be abandoned.* This type of arrangement was popular in the past because it was thought to give a more balanced (neutral) reference than either earlobe or mastoid alone. However, identification of hemispheric dominance may be hampered because one cannot tell how much each earlobe/mastoid has contributed to the reference signal, which may lead to false lateralization of EEG signals in healthy subjects (Katznelson, 1981; Pivik et al., 1993), as well as in patients with brain lesions (Rodin, 1990). Even if linked-reference electrodes would be used in some rare cases, it is important *not* to combine electrodes *before* the preamplification stage because a low-resistance current path between the two reference sites (which may have clearly different impedances) may distort the potential distribution. There is no way to recover from these distortions once the data have been acquired, resulting in ambiguities in understanding the sources of the signals (see Yao et al., 2019, for a detailed discussion on the issues related to this reference configuration). If the data need to be examined with respect to a linked-mastoid or linked-earlobe reference, for example to compare with past literature, then the recorded signals (and averaged responses) can easily be digitally re-referenced off-line. Recent best-practice EEG guidelines also reinforce this critical issue regarding physically linked earlobes/mastoids (Pernet et al., 2020).

Effect of Reference Electrode Site on the Measured Potential Distribution

The shape of the EEG waveforms may vary strongly depending on where the reference electrode is located, although the corresponding spatial scalp voltage topographies stay the same (Nunez, 1981; Michel et al., 2004; Murray et al., 2008). Figure 5.8 depicts this important issue schematically: depending on the site of the reference electrode, both the "coloring" of the maps and the signal waveforms change so that the lowest amplitudes occur closest to the reference electrode. However, the contours of the spatial distribution remain

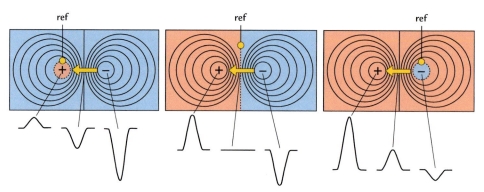

FIGURE 5.8. Schematic illustration of the effect of reference electrode on the potential distribution associated with a tangential current dipole (yellow arrow). The colors indicate positive (pink) and negative (blue) potentials. As the site of the reference electrode (filled yellow circle) changes, its relative potential also changes. Therefore, the border between areas of positive and negative potentials changes, whereas the shape of the topographic distribution remains the same irrespective of reference location. The polarities and amplitudes of responses recorded from three different locations (bottom row) also clearly depend on the reference location.

the same independent of the site of the reference electrode. To use a geographical analogue, the varying terrain of the Swiss Alps will remain the same terrain irrespective of where hikers are standing, although the very same mountain can be either above or below them depending on their respective vantage points.

Figure 5.9 shows the effect of a reference electrode on real EEG responses to visually presented face stimuli; the responses were originally recorded with a vertex reference and then re-referenced computationally with respect to the nasion, linked mastoids, and an average reference. For the vertex reference (Cz; top left) the traces in the middle of the head and for the nasion reference (Nz; top right) traces at frontal sites at the top of the figure show the smallest amplitudes. For a linked-mastoid reference (M1 + M2; bottom left), the responses are suppressed, compared with the other references, over the posterior temporal scalp, and polarity reversals occur between the posterior scalp and anterior scalp/forehead/lower face. The average reference (bottom right; see subsequent discussion) shows maximum amplitudes at the posterior scalp (for the displayed visual activity), with polarity reversals between the posterior scalp and anterior scalp/forehead upper/lower face.

Figure 5.10 shows the corresponding topographical voltage distributions for the same data set, consistent with the schematic in Figure 5.8, with the shapes of the distributions remaining the same (as is evident from the identical patterns of isopotential lines), although the color display changes depending on the site of the reference. Hence, among others, the amplitudes of response peaks at isolated electrode sites (which are typically used for statistical testing) will vary depending on the reference.

When the same reference electrode is used for all derivations, the recordings are often called "monopolar," which is somewhat of a misnomer because EEG always measures potential differences between two locations and thus the recordings are always "bipolar." In clinical EEG jargon, monopolar derivations can also refer to recordings where left-hemisphere electrodes are referenced to the left earlobe and right-hemisphere electrodes to the right earlobe (see Figure 5.11, left). In clinical bipolar recordings, signals are measured between two neighboring electrodes in different standardized configurations.

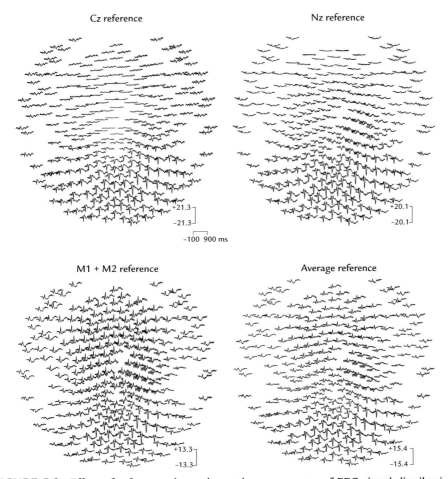

FIGURE 5.9. **Effect of reference electrode on the appearance of EEG signal distribution.** Averaged responses to visual stimuli of a healthy subject. The data were collected with a 256-channel geodesic net with respect to the vertex, Cz (top left), and then digitally re-referenced with respect to nasion, Nz (top right), linked mastoids, M1 + M2 (bottom left), and an average (bottom right) reference. In each plot, the lower face/forehead is at the top and the occipital scalp and neck at the bottom. The small blank oval areas on the left and right sides correspond to discontinuities in the cap for the subject's ears. Time scale (at center) shows a 1000 ms epoch with a 100 ms prestimulus period. Note the minor differences in amplitude scales of the respective plots. In the average-reference data (bottom right), the visual responses show a clear maximum at the right posterior scalp, which is also seen as smaller signals of opposite polarity on the diagonal in the left anterior scalp. Rhythmic periodic activity is seen over the right sensorimotor scalp in the second half of the epoch. Data with vertex reference (top left) also show prominent signals on the right posterior scalp, with diminishing amplitudes at electrode locations closer to the vertex. The Nz-referenced data (top right) show a clear maximum of visual responses at the posterior scalp, particularly in the right hemisphere, and rhythmic activity over the right sensorimotor scalp. Data referenced to the linked mastoids (bottom left) show prominent responses at the right posterior scalp, but the amplitudes diminish at the electrode locations that are more distant from the midline and closer to the mastoids. Rhythmic activity occurs in the second half of the epoch over the right sensorimotor scalp. Data recorded in the Social Neuroscience Laboratory, Indiana University, USA.

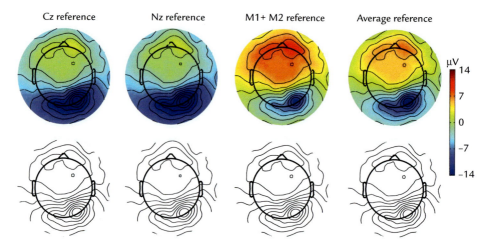

FIGURE 5.10. **Effects of reference electrode on EEG scalp topography.** Topographic scalp-voltage maps of data from Figure 5.9. Maps in the top row show response amplitudes, with colors depending on the site of the reference electrode. The bottom row displays the same maps without colors, demonstrating that the scalp topography (as indicated by the patterns of the isopotential lines) remains unaltered independently of the reference electrode.

Figure 5.11 (right) shows the commonly used "double-banana" montage, which is a set of bilateral longitudinal parasagittal derivations. The aim of using these widely applied montages is to facilitate visualizing the sites that generate epileptic spikes and other abnormalities by searching for "phase reversals" between different derivations to pinpoint the likely source area, as is shown schematically in Figure 5.12.

These kinds of tricks, with separate derivations at the data acquisition phase, add no extra value today as multichannel recordings are available, and all desired montages can be computed offline from data that have been collected with a single (and preferentially stable) reference electrode. Thereby, the recording time can be reduced in many cases (although one often needs to collect data as long as possible to capture a representative sample of epileptiform signals or other abnormalities).

Re-Referencing Relative to an Average Reference

Many decades ago, the *average reference* (AR) was advocated as the proper reference, emerging from ECG studies and implemented in hardware at the analog data acquisition stage (Goldman, 1950; Offner, 1950) or in software at the digital data processing stage (Lehmann & Skrandies, 1980). The assumption underlying AR is that the sum of all measured activity at a given point in time is equal to zero. For example, in a sphere at any given moment in time the voltages around its surface sum to zero. More specifically, the integral of the potential difference over the surface of a sphere that contains only concentric inhomogeneities is zero, and thus the summed potentials of evenly spaced electrodes across the entire surface would be null as well (Bertrand et al., 1985).

While an ideal spherical volume conductor and even distribution of electrodes certainly predicts that the AR would be zero, in practice these conditions are never exactly met because EEG measurements are not sampled from all parts of the head. This shortcoming was a particularly important consideration in the early days when low-density EEG recordings were the norm in both the clinic and the research laboratories (see, e.g., Goldman, 1950;

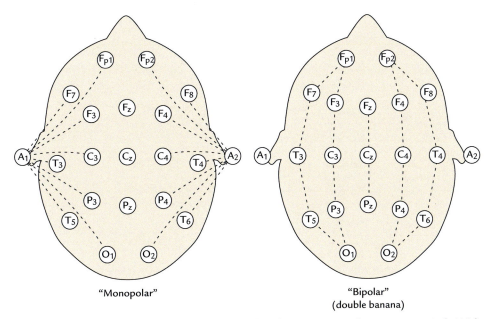

FIGURE 5.11. Examples of "monopolar" and "bipolar" EEG recording montages. Left: With the monopolar montage (set of electrode derivations), multiple EEG channels are recorded with respect to a common reference electrode—in this case, with respect to the left earlobe for left-scalp electrodes and with respect to the right earlobe for the right-scalp electrodes. Right: A common clinical bipolar "double banana" (right) montage records between pairs of electrodes that are located on parasagittal arrays.

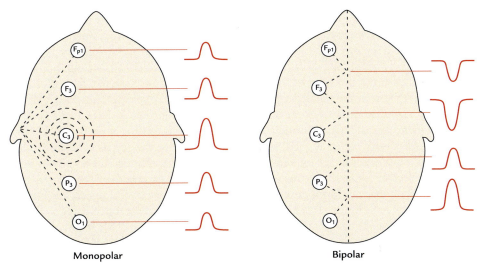

FIGURE 5.12. Phase reversals in EEG recordings. A putative EEG abnormality is located under scalp electrode C3, producing a strong potential change that is seen differently in the monopolar and bipolar derivations. Left: In the monopolar recording, the signal has the same polarity in all derivations, but it is largest at C3. Right: In the bipolar montage, the signal polarity reverses between recording channels containing electrode C3.

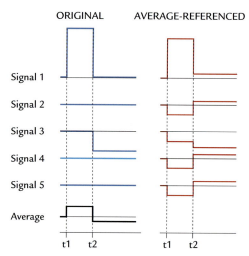

FIGURE 5.13. Schematic illustration of the effect of the average reference. Left: A simulation of two features (Signal 1 and Signal 3) that occurred at times t1 and t2 and were recorded by five "EEG channels" referenced to a single electrode. No changes were visible in Signals 2, 4, and 5. The bottom trace depicts the average of all five original signals. Right: The same signal features represented with respect to the average reference. While the amplitude gradient is similar overall, all five electrode sites now show signal changes both at the t1–t2 interval and after t2, meaning that the original local responses have spread as "ghosts" to all derivations, changing even the waveforms of the original signals.

Offner, 1950). From one perspective, the AR at a single point in time is as good as any other reference because the shape of the potential distribution remains the same regardless of the reference (as already indicated in Figure 5.8). However, in cases where we do not have a *full and equally spaced coverage of the whole sphere (head)*, the level of the AR will vary as a function of time, thereby potentially distorting the waveforms and affecting data interpretation.

Figure 5.13 shows this issue schematically. Assume that we have five derivations, all recorded with the same reference electrode. A large potential shift happens at electrode 1 at time t1 and a smaller one at electrode 3 at time t2. All other derivations have totally flat outputs (and in this toy example the original reference electrode is sitting at zero). The AR level (the left bottom trace in Figure 5.13) is then subtracted from the signals of all electrodes. The result is suppression of the original Signal 1 during t1–t2, although the amplitude with respect to the other signals has remained the same. When at time t2 the AR level changed, we have, as far as the waveforms are concerned, lost a sense of the local signals and instead generated "ghost activations". These are not only changes in the general reference level (as in Figure 5.8) but also changes that vary as a function of time because of the temporally varying baseline level due to fluctuation of the AR potential. Due to the loss of local signals and the ghost activations, the average reference was criticized in the early days (Desmedt et al., 1990), and the criticism continues to the present day (Yao et al., 2019).

The *spatial coverage* and *equidistance* are the most important factors for the behavior of the AR, rather than the number of electrodes per se. The larger the number of electrodes that sample the surface of the head, the more likely it is that the sum of the potentials is zero. Therefore, it is fair to say that these problems with the AR are, in general, the smallest with geodesic electrode configurations that cover large areas of the head. Accordingly, AR configurations have been reported to perform adequately in data sets using 128 or more electrodes (Srinivasan et al., 1998; Nunez & Srinivasan, 2006).

Multiple methods have been used to calculate the AR. For example, the potentials at the original (single) reference electrode are also reconstructed, or spherical splines are generated so that potentials recorded with more sparse electrode coverage would (theoretically) be better approximated (Ferree, 2006). AR calculation may vary across equipment manufacturers and software developers.

After these considerations, it may sound strange and confusing that some source localization software prefers the data to be expressed with respect to the AR (Michel et al., 2004; Litvak et al., 2011; Scherg et al., 2012). For source analysis, however, the aforementioned problems of the AR do not matter because sources are always identified on the basis of the shape, rather than the zero-potential/zero-field lines of the spatial distributions of the signals. However, the temporal waveforms of the signals may be distorted, as we have illustrated in Figure 5.13.

A particular issue for analysis is that the AR will artificially inflate various measures of coherence between signals recorded at different sites around the scalp (Chapter 10), so that in these cases—as well as when examining response waveforms—a single reference site should be used (Fein et al., 1988; Guevara et al., 2005; Srinivasan et al., 2007). Some investigators have advocated the use of an "infinity reference," particularly for measuring coherence between scalp signals (Marzetti et al., 2007). This approach requires source analysis because the infinity reference is reconstructed by first solving the forward problem (see Chapter 10) and then re-expressing the EEG data with respect to a point located at infinity relative to the brain and electrodes (known as a reference electrode standardization technique, REST; Yao, 2001). Although this synthetic reference has its own problems related to calculation errors, it has previously been advocated as a reasonable reference to use (Nunez, 2010). Recently, more sophisticated versions of AR and REST have been proposed (Hu et al., 2018, 2019; Yao et al., 2019), but they are not yet widely used in practice.

Evaluating the data with respect to a number of different reference sites may be both interesting and didactic, especially when the results of the current study need to be compared with previous literature where variable reference configurations have been used. Indeed, when publishing new studies, it might be useful to other investigators in the field if the data were included with respect to another reference derivation as this would better link the older and newer studies (Rossi et al., 2014). Of course, presenting the data in source space would eliminate the need for all these manipulations.

■ MEG INSTRUMENTATION

SQUIDs and SQUID Electronics

The most sensitive MEG sensors at present are superconducting quantum interference devices (SQUIDs), which are made of superconducting material. The brain's weak magnetic fields induce currents in the pickup coil coupled to a SQUID, which together with its electronics functions as a flux–voltage transformer.

Figure 5.14 (left) schematically depicts the SQUID and the associated pickup and input coils. The pickup coil (also called a flux transformer, which can be of different shapes; see Figure 5.15) literally picks up the external magnetic field (B_{ext}), which induces a current into it. The current then flows also in the input coil, and thereby its associated magnetic field ($B_{coupled}$; the red circles) is sensed by the nearby SQUID.

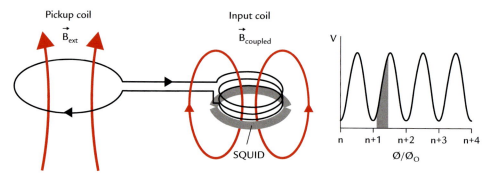

FIGURE 5.14. Schematic of a SQUID circuit. Left: External magnetic field, B_{ext}, induces into the pickup coil (on the left) a current that flows also in the input coil that is located adjacent to the SQUID (on the right). The current in the input coil generates a magnetic field $B_{coupled}$ in the SQUID. Adapted and reprinted from Hari R, Salmelin R: Human cortical oscillations: a neuromagnetic view through the skull. *Trends Neurosci* 1997, 20: 44–49. With permission from Elsevier. Right: The voltage, V, in the SQUID is a periodic function of the number (n) of magnetic flux quanta (Φ/Φ_0). The SQUID is maintained in its optimal working area (shaded with gray) by means of a feedback circuit.

The SQUID itself consists of a superconducting loop interrupted by one or two "weak links," or Josephson junctions (illustrated by the discontinuities in the gray loop), formed by insulation of only a few atoms in width. Magnetic flux Φ threading such a superconducting loop will be quantized, in other words, divided into small packages called magnetic-flux quanta Φ_0 (Figure 5.14, right). The size of each quantum is $\Phi_0 = h/(2e) \approx 2.068 \times 10^{-15}$ Wb, where h is Planck's constant, and e is electron charge; Wb stands for *weber*, which is the unit of magnetic flux (1 Wb = 1 T m^2; in other words, 1 tesla equals the magnetic flux density of 1 weber per 1 square meter). Note that in the flux quanta we see $2e$ as the unit current carrier in a superconductor as was indicated in our discussion in Chapter 3 for Cooper pairs.

The magnetic flux detected by the pickup coil equals the magnetic flux multiplied by the area of the loop. Thus it is possible to increase the sensitivity of the device by increasing the number of turns in the input coil and pickup coil or by increasing the area of the pickup coil; increasing the area will, however, decrease the spatial selectivity of the measurement as signals are collected from a larger area.

The SQUID sensors of the MEG system need to be kept permanently within a working range (marked by the gray band in Figure 5.14, right) by means of a feedback (bias) current so that the voltage over the SQUID becomes a periodic function of the magnetic flux threading the SQUID loop (Figure 5.14, right).

Sometimes magnetic material is accidentally brought close to the SQUID, which in MEG jargon "gets a flux trap" and needs to be reset by transiently heating the sensor(s) above the critical temperature of superconductivity T_c. Localized heating can be performed by applying an electric pulse online, thereby instantaneously recovering the affected sensor or by boiling off the liquid helium of the dewar to warm up all sensors (which would be a whole-day operation). In modern SQUID-MEG devices, flux traps are no more a problem.

SQUID outputs typically show strong low-frequency noise (also called pink or $1/f$ noise, where f is the frequency of the signal). Such $1/f$ noise is a common property of a large variety of physical and biological systems. In a SQUID, the $1/f$ noise typically starts to rise at frequencies lower than 1 Hz, depending on the properties of the SQUID.

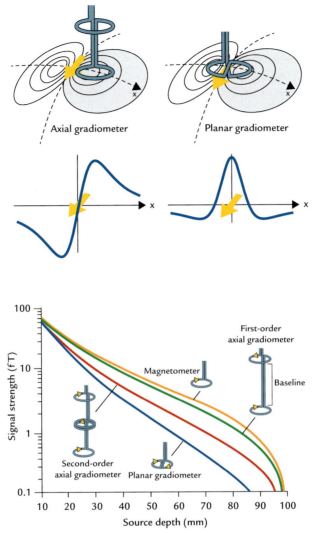

FIGURE 5.15. Effect of different flux transformers on measured signal patterns and strengths. Top: Axial (left) and planar (right) gradiometers pick up the largest signals at different locations of the dipolar field pattern produced by a current dipole (yellow arrow): for an axial gradiometer, the maximum signals are obtained at the two extrema of the dipolar field pattern and for a planar gradiometer just over the source where the gradient is steepest. Adapted and reprinted from Hari R: On brain's magnetic responses to sensory stimuli. *J Clin Neurophysiol* 1991, 8: 157–169. With permission from Wolters Kluwer Health, Inc. Middle: Signal strength plotted along a line above the source, perpendicular to the direction of the current dipole for an axial gradiometer (left) and a planar gradiometer (right). Bottom: The strength of the measured signal (in fT; note the logarithmic scale) as a function of source depth in a sphere with 100-mm radius for different types of flux transformer. The magnetometer will detect the largest signals and the planar gradiometer the smallest signals for sources at all depths. Adapted and reprinted from Hari R, Joutsiniemi S-L, Sarvas J: Spatial resolution of neuromagnetic records: theoretical calculations in a spherical model. *Electroencephalogr Clin Neurophysiol* 1988, 71: 64–72. With permission from Elsevier.

SQUIDs fabricated from niobium are functional when they are immersed in liquid helium at the temperature of 4 kelvin (K) because niobium's critical temperature T_c for superconductivity is 9.2 K. At such a low temperature, the thermal noise is low, and the signal-to-noise ratio of the SQUID good.

The thermal noise generated by the body is at its lowest about $0.1\,f\,T/\sqrt{Hz}$, which forms the lower limit of desirable SQUID sensitivity; the theoretical physical limit is thought to be about $0.5\,f\,T/\sqrt{Hz}$. The noise figures of SQUIDs have rapidly improved from the tens of $f\,T/\sqrt{Hz}$ in the early 1980s to 2 to $4\,f\,T/\sqrt{Hz}$ in the present-day multi-SQUID arrays.

The traditional whole-scalp SQUID-based MEG devices consumed significant amounts of liquid helium (about 80 l/week), but fortunately today, SQUID systems tend to include helium recycling units that capture the escaping helium vapor, liquefy it, and then recirculate it back to the device (Wang et al., 2016), thereby allowing the SQUID-based MEG system to be used continuously during the day and recycling operations to occur overnight. Importantly, this type of internal zero-loss helium recycling has become common practice in commercial MEG systems. If the helium gas is not collected, it is lost forever from the earth—a serious sustainability concern that is also relevant to MRI scanners.

Flux Transformers and Their Configuration

The magnetic field associated with brain currents is first picked up with a flux transformer (i.e., a pickup coil) that may be wound into different shapes, as is illustrated in the bottom panel of Figure 5.15. A *magnetometer* is just a simple loop that picks up the magnetic flux and pattern closest to the real flux but is also very sensitive to various artifacts. *Gradiometers*, on the other hand, comprise two or more loops that are wired in an opposite sense. Such configurations function like differential amplifiers, being sensitive to the *difference* of magnetic flux entering the two (or more loops). They thus see nearby signals but reject those that come from a distance at about the same intensity to both coils. In other words, gradiometric flux transformers are "nearsighted" and less sensitive to distant disturbances.

In axial gradiometers, the coils are along the same axis; Figure 5.15 (bottom) shows both first-order and second-order axial gradiometers, and even third-order axial gradiometers have been used in neuromagnetic recordings. The higher the gradiometer order, the less sensitive the device is to distant homogeneous fields (artifacts) but the more it also dampens the real brain signals of interest. Here one important parameter is the *baseline* of the gradiometer (shown in Figure 5.15, bottom, for the first-order axial gradiometer), that is, the distance between its coils. Typical baselines used in axial gradiometers range from 4 to 14 cm; the gradiometers with the longest baselines record almost the same signals as magnetometers (without significant dampening of the signal by the compensation coil).

With any axial gradiometer (as well as with a magnetometer), the measured field extrema are on the two sides of a local source (see Figure 5.15, left top and middle). The deeper the source within the sphere, the farther apart are the field extrema. Typical distances between the extrema are around 8 cm, depending on the depth of the source and the distance of the sensors from the scalp.

Planar gradiometers (two coils wound up in opposite sense and located on the same plane) pick up the largest signal above the source (Figure 5.15, right top and middle). Thus the best first guess of the generator location is just below the largest signal of the planar gradiometer.

The lowest panel of Figure 5.15 shows that the strength of the measured signals depends on the geometry of the applied flux transformer. The largest signals, even from deep sources, are detected with the magnetometer and the smallest with the planar gradiometer; however, the magnetometer is also extremely sensitive to various noise sources, as it does not have any compensation coil. None of these flux transformers can see a signal from the middle of the sphere, as such sources do not produce any magnetic field outside the sphere, as stated previously (see Figure 1.5).

Large MEG arrays have been constructed using various types of flux transformers, chosen on the basis of various optimization constraints, such as saving space (a problem with long-baseline axial gradiometers) or having all flux transformers as similar as possible (most easily controlled in chip fabrication). Each flux transformer type can be described by its "lead field," that is, how it couples to local source currents. The lead fields can be used in source modeling (see Chapter 10) to take into account different sensor types in a given MEG system. Virtual MEG signals can be computed to compare results between two different MEG systems in signal space.

Toward On-Scalp MEG

Over the years, a number of commercially available SQUID-based MEG devices have come to market with ever-increasing numbers of sensors. The distance between MEG sensors and brain is critical for obtaining an optimum signal-to-noise ratio; thus, some MEG dewars have been built to accommodate the much smaller heads of infants and children. Because the dewar housing the SQUIDs has to be heavily insulated to reduce the evaporation of liquid helium, the sensors of all multichannel SQUID devices are located at least 2 cm above the scalp. Such a distance hampers the detection of the fine details of the field pattern (see Figure 10.11) and hence the discrimination of the underlying brain currents. Thus, it would be optimal if the sensors hugged and resided on the scalp of any individual. For many years, such "on-scalp" sensors have been developed by the MEG community, and they include high-T_c SQUIDs and optically pumped magnetometers (OPMs).

High-T_c SQUIDs

The high-T_c SQUIDs (Faley et al., 2017) function at the temperature of liquid nitrogen (at –196 °C (77 K) and need less insulation than SQUIDs operating at –269 °C (4 K). Because of their higher operating temperature, the high-T_c SQUIDs have more thermal noise than the low-T_c SQUIDs. This is a crucial issue since the considerably higher noise can abolish the benefits of on-scalp sensors. Moreover, some difficulties have arisen in forming the superconducting alloys into solid structures to efficiently fabricate multichannel high-T_c SQUID devices, and therefore the progress in this technology as far as MEG applications are concerned has been slow.

Optically Pumped Magnetometers

Multiple teams have been developing OPMs, and the OPM-based MEG technology is expanding rapidly (Boto et al., 2017, 2018; Iivanainen et al., 2017, 2020; Borna et al., 2020). There are several variants of OPMs. The simplest and most popular OPM (see Figure 5.16) consists of a laser, photodiode, field modulation coils, and a small vapor cell, typically containing rubidium-87 and buffer gas, warmed to 120–180 °C. The laser pumps (align) the spins of the rubidium atoms such that at zero magnetic field the rubidium gas becomes practically transparent, but at non-zero field will absorb the laser light. The changes in the transparency of the vapor cell can be measured (as changes of the incident laser light to them) by the photodiode.

Individual compact OPMs (used as single MEG sensors) can be fabricated and fitted to a wearable, customized sensor array. At the time of writing, a commercial 49-channel OPM

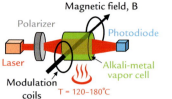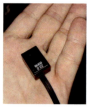

FIGURE 5.16. Left: Schematic of the essential elements of an OPM magnetometer. The laser light travels across the vapor cell from left to right, aligning atomic spins in the alkali vapor. An external magnetic field, B, from the brain (pointing towards the page), affects the absorption of the laser light, and this change can be sensed by a photodiode. Right: A "second-generation" OPM sensor resting on a palm. It is physically smaller than the original OPMs. The center of the vapor cell i.e., the field-sensitive volume, is located 6.5 mm from the (housing) facet to be placed against the head surface. The sensor (housing) covers a scalp area of approximately 12 x 17 mm². Both parts of this figure courtesy of Lauri Parkkonen (Aalto University, Finland).

array had just appeared (Hill et al., 2020), and a 432-channel whole-scalp system had been developed (Pratt et al., 2021). Moreover, the designs of the newer generation of sensors are rapidly decreasing in size, at present resembling 2×4 Lego bricks (see Brookes et al., 2022 and Figure 5.16, right panel).

As OPMs do not need cryogenic cooling, the operating costs of an MEG facility are considerably lowered. Some problems of the current OPMs include (1) higher (by a factor of three or more) noise level than that of SQUIDs; (2) the dependence of the calibration on the ambient magnetic field so that the measurements have to be carried out at very low absolute magnetic field (not only low variability of the field as for SQUIDs), meaning that the remnant magnetic field in a magnetically shielded room has to be compensated to avoid saturation of the sensors or nonlinear changes in their calibration; (3) crosstalk between sensors; and (4) the limitation of the bandwidth to frequencies below about 150 Hz.

Since the OPM arrays are less fixed than SQUID MEG helmets, some additional noise can arise from co-registration errors between individual OPM sensor positions on the subject's head and orientations with respect to the subject's MRI. However, co-registration tests using a printed reference helmet with 85 OPM slots and laser scanning of the sensor locations and orientations demonstrated rotational errors of only 0.23° and translational errors of 0.76 mm (Cao et al., 2021; see Chapter 7).

■ SHIELDING

The strength of the earth's steady magnetic field is about 0.5×10^{-4} T, with irregular fluctuations of about 10 to 20 pT/m. Thus if a SQUID were to be quickly moved for a distance of 5 mm, it would sense a field change of 50 to 100 fT, which is clearly in the range of a typical brain signal. Therefore, MEG measurements are typically made within magnetically shielded rooms, which dampen the environmental magnetic fluctuations. Still, biomagnetic measurements have been performed also without magnetic shielding using higher-order gradiometers where the flux transformers suppress external artifacts. However, the price that is paid is that the brain signals are suppressed as well. Moreover, it is always better to prevent artifacts—for example, performing both the MEG and the EEG measurements in an environment devoid of noise sources—rather than trying to correct or eliminate them in postprocessing.

The main external magnetic artifacts arise from moving vehicles, power lines, and radio transmission. A typical magnetically shielded room used for SQUID-based MEG measurements comprises several layers of aluminum and mu metal that are sandwiched in the wall of the chamber. The shielding factors can be up to 110 dB above 1 Hz and about 45 dB below 1 Hz (e.g., Kelhä et al., 1982). The mu metal that is used for ferromagnetic shielding is an alloy of nickel and iron with very high permeability, which means that environmental magnetic fields tend to spread along the mu-metal layers in the walls of a magnetically shielded room. Aluminum, on the other hand, shields by eddy currents that are induced into the aluminum layer by changing magnetic fields and thus are effective only at frequencies above 50 Hz. A combination of both mu metal and aluminum provides good shielding at the most commonly studied MEG frequencies from DC to 100 Hz.

Some (passive) magnetically shielded rooms are combined with active shielding, which requires the external magnetic field to be continuously monitored with fluxgate magnetometers outside the shielded room (external active shielding) or with some of the magnetometers of the MEG system (internal active shielding). Detected external fields are then compensated, or "fed back," by producing magnetic fields of opposite polarities by activating large Helmholtz coils that surround the room (external active shielding) or are inside the magnetically shielded room (internal active shielding). However, the active shielding is not without problems, as resonances can easily arise, and the compensation may lag the external magnetic fields by about 100 ms.

Cheaper, lightweight magnetically shielded rooms with just a single shell of interleaved mu metal and aluminum layers are currently available as well. In these rooms, the aluminum shielding begins at 1 Hz due to the excellent galvanic coupling between the aluminum plates (gold or tin coating), and the passive shield is combined with active shielding. The space and foundation requirements are less demanding compared with traditional magnetically shielded rooms. Such rooms are especially intended for clinical use, but they also provide sufficient attenuation of external magnetic disturbances for both spontaneous and evoked MEG signals recorded in basic research (Taulu et al., 2014). The performance of these rooms benefits from advanced artifact elimination procedures, such as signal-space separation (see Chapter 9).

Light person-size cylindrical magnetic shields have been constructed and recommended especially for OPM–MEG recordings (He et al., 2019; Borna et al., 2020): the subject lies within the bore of a long cylindrical shield, very much like in an MRI scanner. The advantages of this setup include the more economic price and light weight, but the shield is sensitive to vibrations. Moreover, sensory stimulation is as complicated as in fMRI, limiting various tasks, especially interaction with other persons. Further technological progress is to be expected in this direction.

OPM-based MEG recordings must also be conducted in a magnetically shielded room. Since OPMs—unlike SQUIDs—require a very low absolute magnetic field, the remnant DC field in a typical shielded room must be compensated for. The compensation can be static or dynamic: the compensation coils are driven by a constant DC current such that either the residual field is nulled at the beginning of the MEG measurement or the coil currents are continuously adjusted to keep the field nulled even if the residual field drifts, as happens, for example, when the subject moves during the measurement. In both cases, the compensating fields are generated by large coils placed on both sides of the subject inside the MEG shielded room (Holmes et al., 2018; Iivanainen et al., 2019; Jodko-Władzinska et al., 2020).

EEG recordings are ideally performed in an electrically shielded environment that can be formed by surrounding the room or chamber with a mesh of conducting material. This "Faraday cage" protects its inside from external high-frequency electromagnetic disturbances, as stray currents will run along the well-conducting and well-grounded mesh. However, EEG can be recorded even in hospital intensive-care units, as well as in urban environments while subjects walk on the street. In all cases, however, EEG leads, cables, and amplifiers (and the subject) should be sited as far away from other sources of electrical equipment as possible. Some EEG systems have "active" shielding in the EEG electrodes, so that noise is reduced via feedback to input amplifiers; these systems may be better suited to these high-noise environments.

MEG recordings are often accompanied with simultaneous multichannel EEG recordings to provide a complementary view of the brain function, and in those cases a magnetically shielded room also provides an excellent environment for EEG recordings. To avoid artifacts in MEG, the EEG electrodes have to be totally nonmagnetic. For example, whereas Ag/AgCl electrodes are MEG compatible, gold-plated electrodes are not due to magnetic nickel layers below the gold surface.

■ OTHER WAYS TO MAINTAIN A NOISE-FREE ENVIRONMENT

Most magnetic noise prevention methods aim for the best possible recording environments and include proper design of cabling, stimulators, and other equipment so that they are not magnetic and do not bring radio-frequency or other noise into the magnetically shielded room.

Vibration of the floor and walls of the magnetically shielded room can also produce fluctuations that may even resemble oscillatory brain activity but can usually be differentiated in source space, as the artifacts appear to occur at areas too superficial to be of cerebral origin. Vibrations can arise from beyond the laboratory, for example, from an elevator in the building or from cars, trams, and trains. All these source vibrations may produce large artifacts in MEG recordings.

Additional unwanted magnetic signals can arise from the subjects themselves as they push a response button or move to get more comfortable. These movements can cause vibration in the gantry or table and even elicit tactile-evoked responses via body parts that were not purposefully stimulated (Hari & Imada, 1999).

Fluorescent lighting should be turned off during EEG recordings and not be used in magnetically shielded rooms. Instead, DC-powered lights or fiber-optic video projection systems (that deliver stimuli) can provide good noise-free alternatives for ambient lighting. To prevent perturbations in the EEG signals due to capacitances of a moving human body and in the MEG signals due to vibration of the device, experimenters should avoid moving near the subject during the recording.

Compared with the fMRI environment, the MEG/EEG environment (within a magnetically shielded room) is typically acoustically very quiet. The MEG and EEG systems do not make any sounds when in operation. A magnetically shielded room needs to have several feedthroughs through the walls of the room, and hence the acoustic noise produced by some stimulators even outside the shielded room may need to be masked. Moreover, the experimenters outside the chamber must remember to be silent during the measurement. If the EEG recording is performed in a nonshielded environment, white-noise generators might be installed in various locations around the laboratory to muffle and eliminate acoustic noise external to the lab.

◼ REFERENCES

Acharya V: Improving common-mode rejection using the right-leg drive amplifier (Texas Instruments application report. 2011, SBAA188 July 2011. https://www.ti.com/lit/an/sbaa188/sbaa188.pdf

Aladjalova NA: Infra-slow rhythmic oscillations of the steady potential of the cerebral cortex. *Nature* 1957, 179: 957–959.

Bentin S, Allison T, Puce A, Perez A, McCarthy G: Electrophysiological studies of face perception in humans. *J Cogn Neurosci* 1996, 8: 551–565.

Bertrand O, Perrin F, Pernier J: A theoretical justification of the average reference in topographic evoked potential studies. *Electroencephalogr Clin Neurophysiol* 1985, 62: 462–464.

Borna A, Carter TR, Colombo AP, Jau Y-Y, McKay J, Weisend M, Taulu S, Stephen JM, Schwindt PDD: Non-invasive functional-brain-imaging with an OPM-based magnetoencephalography system. *PLoS One* 2020, 15: e0227684.

Boto E, Meyer SS, Shah V, Alem O, Knappe S, Kruger P, Fromhold TM, Lim M, Glover PM, Morris PG, Bowtell R, Barnes GR, Brookes MJ: A new generation of magnetoencephalography: room temperature measurements using optically-pumped magnetometers. *NeuroImage* 2017, 149: 404–414.

Boto E, Holmes N, Leggett J, Roberts G, Shah V, Meyer SS, Munoz LD, Mullinger KJ, Tierney TM, Bestmann S, Barnes GR, Bowtell R, Brookes MJ: Moving magnetoencephalography towards real-world applications with a wearable system. *Nature* 2018, 555: 657–661.

Brookes MJ, Leggett J, Rea M, Hill RM, Holmes N, Boto E, Bowtell R: Magnetoencephalography with optically pumped magnetometers (OPM-MEG): the next generation of functional neuroimaging. *Trends Neurosci* 2022, 45: 621–634.

Cao F, An N, Xu W, Wang W, Yang Y, Xiang M, Gao Y, Ning X: Co-registration comparison of on-scalp magnetoencephalography and magnetic resonance imaging. *Front Neurosci* 2021, 15: 706785.

Chatrian GE, Lettich E, Nelson PL: Ten percent electrode system for topographic studies of spontaneous and evoked EEG activity. *Am J EEG Technol* 1985, 25: 83–92.

Chi YM, Maier C, Cauwenberghs G: Ultra-high input impedance, low noise integrated amplifier for noncontact biopotential sensing. *IEEE J Emer Sel Topics Circuits Systems* 2011, 1: 526–535.

Christodoulou G: Sphenoidal electrodes. Their significance in diagnosing temporal lobe epileptogenic foci. *Acta Neurol Scand* 1967, 43: 587–593.

Cooper R, Osselton J, Shaw J: *EEG Technology*, 2nd ed. London: Butterworth & Company, 1974.

Debener S, Emkes R, De Vos M, Bleichner M: Unobtrusive ambulatory EEG using a smartphone and flexible printed electrodes around the ear. *Sci Rep* 2015, 5: 16743.

Desmedt JE, Chalklin V, Tomberg C: Emulation of somatosensory evoked potential (SEP) components with the 3-shell head model and the problem of "ghost potential fields" when using an average reference in brain mapping. *Electroencephalogr Clin Neurophysiol* 1990, 77: 243–258.

Di Flumeri G, Aricò P, Borghini G, Sciaraffa N, Di Florio A, Babiloni F: The dry revolution: evaluation of three different EEG dry electrode types in terms of signal spectral features, mental states classification and usability. *Sensors (Basel)* 2019, 19: 1365.

Etienne A, Laroia T, Weigle H, Afelin A, Kelly SK, Krishnan A, Grover P: Novel electrodes for reliable EEG recordings on coarse and curly hair. *Annu Int Conf IEEE Eng Med Biol Soc* 2020, 2020: 6151–6154.

Faley MI, Dammers J, Maslennikov YV, Schneiderman JF, Winkler D, Koshelets VP, Shah NJ, Dunin-Borkowski RE: High-T$_c$ SQUID biomagnetometers. *Supercond Sci Technol* 2017, 30: 083001.

Fatourechi M, Bashashati A, Ward RK, Birch GE: EMG and EOG artifacts in brain computer interface systems: a survey. *Clin Neurophysiol* 2007, 118: 480–494.

Fein G, Raz J, Brown FF, Merrin EL: Common reference coherence data are confounded by power and phase effects. *Electroencephalogr Clin Neurophysiol* 1988, 69: 581–584.

Ferree TC: Spherical splines and average referencing in scalp electroencephalography. *Brain Topogr* 2006, 19: 43–52.

Gastaut H: Présentation d'une electrode pharyngée bipolaire. *Rev Neurol (Paris)* 1948, 80: 623–624.

Goldman D: The clinical use of the "average" reference electrode in monopolar recording. *Electroencephalogr Clin Neurophysiol* 1950, 2: 209–212.

Grimnes S, Martinsen ØG: *Bioimpedance and Bioelectricity Basics*, 3rd ed. Amsterdam: Elsevier, 2015: Chapter 7, Electrodes, 179–254.

Guevara R, Velazquez JL, Nenadovic V, Wennberg R, Senjanovic G, Dominguez LG: Phase synchronization measurements using electroencephalographic recordings: what can we really say about neuronal synchrony? *Neuroinformatics* 2005, 3: 301–314.

Hari R, Imada T: Ipsilateral movement-evoked fields reconsidered. *NeuroImage* 1999, 10: 582–588.

Hashemi A, Pino LJ, Moffat G, Mathewson K, Aimone C, Bennett PJ, Schmidt LA, Sekuler AB: Characterizing population EEG dynamics throughout adulthood. *eNeuro* 2016, 3: ENEURO.0275-16.2016.

He K, Wan S, Sheng J, Liu D, Wang C, Li D, Qin L, Luo S, Qin J, Gao J-H: A high-performance compact magnetic shield for optically pumped magnetometer-based magnetoencephalography. *Rev Sci Instr* 2019, 90: 064102.

Herwig U, Satrapi P, Schonfeldt-Lecuona C: Using the International 10–20 EEG system for positioning of transcranial magnetic stimulation. *Brain Topogr* 2003, 16: 95–99.

Hill RM, Boto E, Rea M, Holmes N, Leggett J, Coles LA, Papastavrou M, Everton SK, Hunt BAE, Sims D, Osborne J, Shah V, Bowtell R, Brookes MJ: Multi-channel whole-head OPM-MEG: helmet design and a comparison with a conventional system. *NeuroImage* 2020, 219: 116995.

Holmes N, Leggett J, Boto E, Roberts G, Hill RM, Tierney TM, Shah V, Barnes GR, Brookes MJ, Bowtell R: A bi-planar coil system for nulling background magnetic fields in scalp mounted magnetoencephalography. *NeuroImage* 2018, 181: 760–774.

Homan RW, Herman J, Purdy P: Cerebral location of international 10–20 system electrode placement. *Electroencephalogr Clin Neurophysiol* 1987, 66: 376–382.

Hu S, Yao D, Valdés-Sosa PA: Unified Bayesian estimator of EEG reference at infinity: rREST (regularized reference electrode standardization technique). *Front Neurosci* 2018, 12: 297.

Hu S, Yao D, Bringas-Vega ML, Qin Y, Valdés-Sosa PA: The statistics of EEG unipolar references: derivations and properties. *Brain Topogr* 2019, 32: 696–703.

Iivanainen J, Stenroos M, Parkkonen L: Measuring MEG closer to the brain: performance of on-scalp sensor arrays. *NeuroImage* 2017, 147: 542–553.

Iivanainen J, Zetter R, Gron M, Hakkarainen K, Parkkonen L: On-scalp MEG system utilizing an actively shielded array of optically-pumped magnetometers. *NeuroImage* 2019, 194: 244–258.

Iivanainen J, Zetter R, Parkkonen L: Potential of on-scalp MEG: Robust detection of human visual gamma-band responses. *Hum Brain Mapp* 2020, 41: 150–161.

Jasper H: The ten–twenty electrode system of the International Federation. *Electroencephalogr Clin Neurophysiol* 1958, 10: 371–375.

Jodko-Władzínska A, Wildner K, Pałko T, Władzínski M: Compensation system for biomagnetic measurements with optically pumped magnetometers inside a magnetically shielded room. *Sensors* 2020, 20: 4563.

Jurcak V, Tsuzuki D, Dan I: 10/20, 10/10, and 10/5 systems revisited: their validity as relative head-surface-based positioning systems. *NeuroImage* 2007, 34: 1600–1611.

Kappel SL, Rank ML, Toft HO, Andersen M, Kidmose P: Dry-contact electrode ear-EEG. *IEEE Trans Biomed Eng* 2019, 66: 150–158.

Katznelson RD: EEG recording, electrode placement, and aspects of generator localization. In: Nunez P, ed. *Electric Fields of the Brain. The Neurophysics of EEG*. New York: Oxford University Press, 1981: 176–213.

Kelhä VO, Pukki JM, Peltonen RS, Penttinen AJ, Ilmoniemi RJ, Heino JJ: Design, construction, and performance of a large volume magnetic shield. *IEEE Trans Magn* 1982, 18: 260–270.

Kidmose P, Looney D, Ungstrup M, Rank M, Mandic D: A study of evoked potentials from ear-EEG. *IEEE Trans Biomed Eng* 2013, 60: 2824–2830.

Klem GH, Lüders HO, Jasper HH, Elger C: The ten-twenty electrode system of the International Federation. The International Federation of Clinical Neurophysiology. *Electroencephalogr Clin Neurophysiol Suppl* 1999, 52: 3–6.

Krachunov S, Casson AJ: 3D printed dry EEG electrodes. *Sensors (Basel)* 2016, 16: 1635.

Laufs H, Daunizeau J, Carmichael DW, Kleinschmidt A: Recent advances in recording electrophysiological data simultaneously with magnetic resonance imaging. *NeuroImage* 2008, 40: 515–528.

Lehmann D, Skrandies W: Reference-free identification of components of checkerboard-evoked multi-channel potential fields. *Electroencephalogr Clin Neurophysiol* 1980, 48: 609–621.

Lehtinen LO, Bergström L: Naso-ethmoidal electrode for recording the electrical activity of the inferior surface of the frontal lobe. *Electroencephalogr Clin Neurophysiol* 1970, 29: 303–305.

Lehtonen JB, Koivikko MJ: The use of non-cephalic reference electrode in recording cerebral evoked potentials in man. *Electroencephalogr Clin Neurophysiol* 1971, 31: 154–156.

Li G, Wang S, Li M, Duan YY: Towards real-life EEG applications: Novel superporous hydrogel-based semi-dry EEG electrodes enabling automatically "charge–discharge" electrolyte. *J Neural Eng* 2021, 18: 046016.

Litvak V, Mattout J, Kiebel S, Phillips C, Henson R, Kilner J, Barnes G, Oostenveld R, Daunizeau J, Flandin G, Penny W, Friston K: EEG and MEG data analysis in SPM8. *Comput Intell Neurosci* 2011, 2011: 852961.

Luu P, Ferree, T: *Technical Note*: Determination of the HydroCel Geodesic Sensor Nets' Average Electrode Positions and Their 10–10 International Equivalents. Eugene, OR: Electrical Geodesics, 2005.

Marzetti L, Nolte G, Perrucci MG, Romani GL, Del Gratta C: The use of standardized infinity reference in EEG coherency studies. *NeuroImage* 2007, 36: 48–63.

Matsuo T, Iinuma K, Esashi M: A barium-titanate-ceramics capacitative-type EEG electrode. *IEEE Trans Biomed Eng* 1973, 20: 299–300.

Michel CM, Murray MM, Lantz G, Gonzalez S, Spinelli L, Grave de Peralta R: EEG source imaging. *Clin Neurophysiol* 2004, 115: 2195–2222.

Mirkovic B, Bleichner MG, DeVos M, Debener S: Target speaker detection with concealed EEG around the ear. *Front Neurosci* 2016, 10: 349.

Morris HH 3rd, Lüders H: Electrodes. *Electroencephalogr Clin Neurophysiol Suppl* 1985, 37: 3–26.

Mota AR, Duarte L, Rodrigues D, Martins AC, Machado AV, Vaz F, Fiedler P, Haueisen J, Nobrega JM, Fonseca C: Development of a quasi-dry electrode for EEG recording. *Sens Actuators A* 2013, 199: 310–317.

Mullen T, Kothe C, Chi YM, Ojeda A, Kerth T, Makeig S, Cauwenberghs G, Jung T-P: Real-time modeling and 3D visualization of source dynamics and connectivity using wearable EEG. *Annu Int Conf IEEE Eng Med Biol Soc* 2013, 2013: 2184–2187.

Murray MM, Brunet D, Michel CM: Topographic ERP analyses: a step-by-step tutorial review. *Brain Topogr* 2008, 20: 249–264.

Norton JJS, Lee DS, Lee JW, Lee W, Kwon O, Won P, Jung S-Y, Cheng H, Jeong J-W, Akce A, Umunna S, Na I, Kwon YH, Wang X-Q, Liu Z, Paik U, Huang Y, Bretl T, Yeo W-H, Rogers JA: Soft, curved electrode systems capable of integration on the auricle as a persistent brain-computer interface. *Proc Natl Acad Sci U S A* 2015, 112: 3920–3925.

Nunez PL: *Electric Fields of the Brain: The Neurophysics of EEG*. New York: Oxford University Press, 1981.

Nunez PL, Srinivasan R: *Electric Fields of the Brain: The Neurophysics of EEG*, 2nd ed. Oxford: Oxford University Press, 2006.

Nunez PL: REST: a good idea but not the gold standard. *Clin Neurophysiol* 2010, 121: 2177–2180.

Offner FF: The EEG as potential mapping: the value of the average monopolar reference. *Electroencephalogr Clin Neurophysiol* 1950, 2: 213–214.

Oostenveld R, Praamstra P: The five percent electrode system for high-resolution EEG and ERP measurements. *Clin Neurophysiol* 2001, 112: 713–719.

Pascual-Leone A, Dhuna A, Roth BJ, Cohen L, Hallett M: Risk of burns during rapid-rate magnetic stimulation in presence of electrodes. *Lancet* 1990, 336: 1195–1196.

Pernet C, Garrido MI, Gramfort A, Maurits N, Michel CM, Pang E, Salmelin R, Schoffelen JM, Valdés-Sosa PA, Puce A: Issues and recommendations from the OHBM COBIDAS MEEG Committee for Reproducible EEG and MEG Research. *Nat Neurosci* 2020, 23: 1473–1483.

Pivik RT, Broughton RJ, Coppola R, Davidson RJ, Fox N, Nuwer MR: Guidelines for the recording and quantitative analysis of electroencephalographic activity in research contexts. *Psychophysiology* 1993, 30: 547–558.

Pratt EJ, Ledbeter M, Jiminez-Martinez R, Shapiro B, Solon A, Iwata GZ, Garber S, Gormley J, Decker D, Delgadillo D, Dellis AT, Phillips J, Sundar G, Leung J, Coyne J, McKinley M, Lopez G, Homan S, Marsh L, ... Alford JK: Kernel Flux: a whole-head 432-magnetometer optically-pumped magnetoencephalography (OP-MEG) system for brain activity imaging during natural human experiences. *Proc SPIE 11700, Optical and Quantum Sensing and Precision Metrology* 2021, 1170032.

Quesney LF, Gloor P: Special extracranial electrodes. In: Wieser HG, Elger CE, eds. *Presurgical Evaluation of Epileptics.* Berlin: Springer, 1987: 162–176.

Rodin E: Is a linked ears reference adequate for topographic EEG analysis? *Electroencephalogr Clin Neurophysiol* 1990, 76: 373–375.

Rossi A, Parada FJ, Kolchinsky A, Puce A: Neural correlates of apparent motion perception of impoverished facial stimuli: a comparison of ERP and ERSP activity. *NeuroImage* 2014, 98: 442–459.

Roubicek J, Hill D: Electroencephalography with pharyngeal electrodes. *Brain* 1948, 71: 77–87.

Scherg M, Ille N, Weckesser D, Ebert A, Ostendorf A, Boppel T, Schubert S, Larsson PG, Henning O, Bast T: Fast evaluation of interictal spikes in long-term EEG by hyper-clustering. *Epilepsia* 2012, 53: 1196–1204.

Shad EHT, Molinas M, Ytterdal T: Impedance and noise of passive and active dry EEG electrodes: a review. *IEEE Sensors J* 2020, 20: 14565–14577.

Srinivasan R, Tucker DM, Murias M: Estimating the spatial Nyquist of the human EEG. *Behav Res Meth Ins C* 1998, 30: 8–19.

Srinivasan R, Winter WR, Ding J, Nunez PL: EEG and MEG coherence: measures of functional connectivity at distinct spatial scales of neocortical dynamics. *J Neurosci Methods* 2007, 166: 41–52.

Stephenson WA, Gibbs FA: A balanced non-cephalic reference electrode. *Electroencephalogr Clin Neurophysiol* 1951, 3: 237–240.

Stjerna S, Voipio J, Metsäranta M, Kaila K, Vanhatalo S: Preterm EEG: a multimodal neurophysiological protocol. *J Vis Exp* 2012, 60: 3774.

Tallgren P, Vanhatalo S, Kaila K, Voipio J: Evaluation of commercially available electrodes and gels for recording of slow EEG potentials. *Clin Neurophysiol* 2005, 116: 799–806.

Taulu S, Simola J, Nenonen J, Parkkonen L: Novel noise reduction methods. In: Supek S, Aine C, eds. *Magnetoencephalography: From Signals to Dynamic Cortical Networks.* Berlin: Springer-Verlag, 2014: 35–72.

Toyama S, Takano K, Kansaku K: A non-adhesive solid-gel electrode for a non-invasive brain-machine interface. *Front Neurol* 2012, 3: 114.

Tucker DM: Spatial sampling of head electrical fields: the Geodesic Sensor Net. *Electroencephalogr Clin Neurophysiol* 1993, 87: 154–163.

Valentin O, Viallet G, Delnavaz A, Cretot-Richert G, Ducharme MI, Monsarat-Chanon H, Voix J: Custom-fitted in- and around-the-ear sensors for unobtrusive and on-the-Go EEG acquisitions: development and validation. *Sensors (Basel)* 2021, 21: 2953.

Vallbo ÅB: Microneurography: how it started and how it works. *J Neurophysiol* 2018, 120: 1415–1427.

Vanhatalo S, Voipio J, Kaila K: Full-band EEG (FbEEG): an emerging standard in electroencephalography. *Clin Neurophysiol* 2005, 116: 1–8.

Vaughan HG Jr, Ritter W: The sources of auditory evoked responses recorded from the human scalp. *Electroencephalogr Clin Neurophysiol* 1970, 28: 360–367.

Velcescu A, Lindley A, Cursio C, Krachunov S, Beach C, Brown CA, Jones AKP, Casson AJ: Flexible 3D-printed EEG electrodes. *Sensors (Basel)* 2019, 19: 1650.

Wang C, Sun L, Lichtenwalter B, Zerkle B, Okada Y: Compact, ultra-low vibration, closed-cycle helium recycler for uninterrupted operation of MEG with SQUID magnetometers. *Cryogenics* 2016, 76: 16–22.

Winter BB, Webster JG: Driven-right-leg circuit design. *IEEE Trans Biomed Eng* 1983, 30: 62–66.

Yao D: A method to standardize a reference of scalp EEG recordings to a point at infinity. *Physiol Meas* 2001, 22: 693–711.

Yao D, Qin Y, Hu S, Dong L, Bringas-Vega M, Valdés Sosa PA: Which reference should we use for EEG and ERP practice? *Brain Topogr* 2019, 32: 530–549.

Zotterman Y: Touch, pain and tickling: an electro-physiological investigation on cutaneous sensory nerves. *J Physiol* 1939, 95: 1–28.

CHAPTER 6

DEVICES FOR SENSORY STIMULATION AND BEHAVIORAL MONITORING

Any sufficiently advanced technology is indistinguishable from magic.

ARTHUR C. CLARKE

The most important tool of the theoretical physicist is his wastebasket.

ALBERT EINSTEIN

B rain research can often move forward by the creation of a clever experimental setup or by the invention of new stimulation devices or data-analysis methods. The MEG environment, in particular, is very challenging for various sensory stimulators because any moving magnetic or magnetized materials near the subject will cause serious artifacts. Special care thus has been taken to develop nonmagnetic stimulators (Jousmäki, 2021), response pads, and monitoring devices. Most MEG monitoring and stimulation equipment can be readily used in the MRI environment but not necessarily vice versa. Although some stimulation settings described below are not in common use today, it is important to understand them so that new results can be compared with older findings.

■ STIMULATORS

Auditory Stimulators

During MEG recordings, different approaches can be taken to deliver sounds to the subject: (a) sound transformers positioned near the subject and connected with short tubing with an ear insert to the subject, (b) loudspeakers kept outside the magnetically shielded room, with the sounds transferred to the subject through large-diameter tubing where the spectral content of the sound is balanced with specific sound-processing software or hardware, and (c) a free-field loudspeaker placed on the inside wall of the magnetically shielded room.

In EEG recordings, sound delivery is more straightforward: one can use loudspeakers placed in suitable locations in the laboratory, or one can use shielded headsets or ear inserts if they can be fitted without affecting the electrodes. Headsets without adequate shielding can produce stimulus artifacts in the EEG recording. For example, the envelopes of speech stimuli, occurring in theta-range frequencies, can mix with the oscillatory brain activity.

Similarly, sound transformers too close to the subject can induce low-amplitude artifacts in MEG recordings. While they may not be seen in the raw MEG signals, they may nevertheless bias the results, for example when correlations are computed between the MEG signals and the acoustic input. A free-field loudspeaker can elicit echoes in the magnetically shielded room. Although these echoes are heavily dampened in the presence of the subject, they can disturb accurate measurements of the sound onset times and durations when the subject is not present in the shielded room.

In any MEG/EEG laboratory, it is important to have on hand devices for accurate measurements of sound loudness, frequency, and duration, as well as the delay from trigger to stimulus onset. If loudspeakers are being used, the acoustic characteristics of the testing room, in addition to the loudspeaker characteristics, should be ascertained as the dimensions and material of the space can all impact how sounds are transmitted, and some frequencies may be augmented relative to others.

A calibrated artificial ear can be used for measurements of the frequency response (and transfer function) of the whole sound-delivery system. In any studies focusing on auditory processing itself, set-ups should be available for measuring the subject's hearing thresholds at multiple frequencies. Delivered stimulus intensities will then be expressed in dB HL (decibels above hearing level) rather than in dB SPL (decibels of sound pressure level). SPL is defined with respect to a reference sound pressure of 2×10^{-5} Pa = 20 μPa. Here Pa refers to *pascal*, which is an unit of pressure according to the International System of Units so that 1 pascal is the pressure that exerts a force of 1 newton (N) perpendicularly upon an area of 1 square meter ($1 \text{ Pa} = 1 \text{ N/m}^2$). Note that different standard scales (e.g., A, B, and C) of sound-level meters are used for measurements of the loudness of environmental sounds; the most commonly used dBA scale has a frequency weighting resembling the human ear and thus approximates how humans would hear the measured environmental sounds.

Visual Stimulators

The traditional visual stimulator for presenting still pictures in EEG and MEG studies was a projector with a rapid shutter that produced instantaneous stimulus delivery. Thereafter, various screens, such as cathode-ray tubes and monitors and video projectors, were used; some of these latter devices can have approximately 20 to 30 ms lags or rise times, which may have a significant effect on the latencies of evoked responses. In the MEG environment, visual stimuli are often presented on a back-projection screen, so that all magnetic parts of the stimulation system can be kept outside the shielded room (see the set-up in Figure 1.1).

It is important to have a photocell-equipped device to accurately measure stimulus timing, especially the onset and rise time of the stimulus on the screen, relative to the timing of the stimulus onset in the stimulus-delivery software. Attention should be paid to the study design to avoid abrupt luminance changes on the screen for stimulus onsets. For example, it is better to set the background display between the stimuli to the mean overall luminance of the stimulus sequence rather than flash bright stimuli from a dark background.

Here, as well as with stimuli of all sensory modalities, experience in measuring the stimulus properties will soon pay for itself as one learns to notice that some unexpected stimulation properties may explain unusual behavior of the brain responses. Such unexpected features may arise from the stimuli themselves or from the stimulus delivery system.

Projectors of different types—based on, for example, liquid crystal display or digital light processing (DLP)—can provide different luminance levels, and thus the results obtained in different laboratories with even the same stimuli may not be comparable. In some projectors the onsets of different colors may differ, and timing may not be precise enough. DLP-based projectors are less likely to have these kinds of timing and luminance problems. Moreover, they present the whole frame at once, and thus the timing is the same on any location of the screen.

The distance of stimuli from the subject's eyes and the two-dimensional size of the image needs to be measured as they affect brain responses (see the visual-angle calculation in Chapter 14). Similarly, other stimulus properties, such as the overall stimulus luminance, contrast, and spatial frequency, should be quantified, for example using image-processing software during stimulus creation. Color stimuli produce additional challenges for stimulus standardization, as the levels of red, blue, green, and grayscale components of the stimulus need to be measured separately.

Movies that are becoming more popular as visual stimuli can trigger clear phase-locking of MEG/EEG signals, resulting in steady-state responses that match the frame rate of the video stimulus (Lankinen et al., 2014).

Somatosensory Stimulators

Various types of somatosensory stimulators preferentially activate different skin receptors. The hairy and nonhairy (glabrous) skin largely differ with respect to predominant receptor type and sensitivity. Receptors activated by touch, pressure, and vibration are connected to the central nervous system via thick myelinated (and thus fast-conducting, about 40–100 m/s) Aα and Aβ fibers. In contrast, receptors sensing temperature, pain (via free nerve endings), and itch are transmitted via slowly conducting, thin myelinated Aδ fibers (2–30 m/s) and unmyelinated C fibers (0.5–2 m/s).

Of the mechanoreceptors, rapidly adapting Pacinian corpuscles sense high-frequency vibration from 150 to 300 Hz and react transiently to stimulus onsets and offsets, whereas slowly adapting Merkel's disks can display sustained responses to skin indentation. Both of these receptors can be activated in MEG/EEG studies. Moreover, the rapidly adapting hair-follicle receptors on the hairy skin can be stimulated by air puffs.

The most common way to activate the dorsal column–lemniscal system is to use *electrical stimulators* to deliver brief electric pulses (typically 0.1–0.2 ms duration) to the skin over a peripheral nerve (such as median or ulnar nerve at the wrist). Note that longer pulses, of the order of 1 ms, will directly activate the muscle underneath. While dependent on intensity, stimulation rates up to 10 Hz can be tolerated well by subjects. At frequencies greater than 20 Hz, the muscle activated via nerve stimulation does not have time to relax and therefore will be tetanically contracted, which can be painful. Textbooks of clinical neurophysiology can be consulted for the appropriate stimulation sites of various nerves. The most commonly used sites in somatosensory-evoked response recordings are the median nerve (on the thumb side) and the ulnar nerve (on the little-finger side) at the wrist, the posterior tibial nerve on the outside lower ankle, and the peroneal nerve on the foot dorsum distal to the ankle.

Constant-voltage stimulators have been used for peripheral nerve stimulation in the past, but it is best to use constant-current stimulators whose current outputs are constant irrespective of electrode–skin impedance. One typically specifies electrical stimuli in terms of the applied current (e.g., 4 mA) and additionally describes whether the intensity has exceeded the sensory or motor threshold and by how much (e.g., "two times the sensory threshold").

Different types of stimulation electrodes can be used to deliver electrical stimuli to the subject. Ring electrodes encircling one or two fingers can be used to stimulate sensory nerves. Two-pad electrodes (with felt pads moistened in saline) placed on the skin overlying a peripheral nerve with Velcro tape are typically used for stimulation of mixed nerves, such as median and ulnar nerves (in the upper limbs) and peroneal and tibial nerves (in the lower limbs). The pad-related skin indentation helps the stimulus to reach the nerve and therefore works better than plate electrodes that are fixed on the skin. Stimulus artifacts associated with electrical pulses can be decreased by encircling the limb, just proximal to the stimulation site, with a wet ground electrode. Electrical stimulation of the face can be problematic because of the very close proximity of stimulating electrodes to recording sensors.

To reduce artifacts in MEG recordings, it is important to minimize any current loops in the stimulation wires and within the stimulation electrode itself as such loops act as magnetic dipoles (see Figure 1.3, bottom right) and thereby produce strong magnetic artifacts. Twisting the stimulation wires tightly together may help considerably.

Air puff stimuli applied to the skin selectively activate hair receptors (Gardner & Costanzo, 1980), with little or no effect on deeper tissues. The stimuli consist of well-directed pulses of pressurized air that can be delivered with very short rise times, on the order of 1 ms.

Pneumatic tactile stimulators are commonly used, with plastic balloon diaphragms fixed to the tips of fingers and driven by pulses of compressed air. The balloons do have a delay in increasing and decreasing their size, and thus the maximum stimulation frequencies are limited to about 20 Hz.

A simple *vibrotactile stimulator* can be built from a thick tube connected to a loudspeaker; the subject is then asked to keep her or his hand(s) on the tube. A balloon at the end of the tube will work nicely as well (Jousmäki & Hari, 1999). Such vibrotactile stimulators can activate Pacinian corpuscles (at 150–300 Hz). Piezoelectric buzzers also produce vibratory stimuli of different frequencies, but with concomitant sounds that have to be masked (e.g., with white noise), and, importantly, their effects on brain activity must be separately controlled for. A recent MEG-compatible somatosensory stimulator uses commercial Braille devices controlled by an Arduino board. Up to five separate devices, one on each finger, can be used simultaneously (Sun & Okada, 2019).

A *manually operated brush stimulator* (Jousmäki et al., 2007; Jousmäki, 2021) is comprised of a bundle of optical fibers, half of them sending and the other half receiving light (see Figure 6.1, left panel). When the brush is brought close to the skin (at a distance that can be adjusted by the experimenter), a trigger pulse will be delivered, and this nonmagnetic device can thus be used to stimulate any part of the body by either the subjects themselves or an experimenter (Hesse et al., 2010). The bundles can be also designed to resemble von Frey hairs, with different weights, and can be used to produce very light touch with accurate timing. The original von Frey hairs are sets of filaments of calibrated rigidity, developed by Maximilian von Frey in 1896 for the assessment of light touch (for a review, see Lambert et al., 2009). When the filament is pushed against the skin, it bends and thereafter does not increase the force to the skin.

Figure 6.1 (middle) depicts the results of brush stimulation of the left hand and lip: two averaged responses (see Chapter 12) show a clear and reproducible pattern with respect to the onset of brush touch (which occurs at time zero). The earliest deflection to hand stimuli peaks at 28 ms and is followed by several distinct deflections. For stimulation of the lower lip, the response waveform is very similar, but the corresponding deflections peak 6 to 10 ms earlier. After data analysis with source modeling (see Chapter 10), activation (modeled

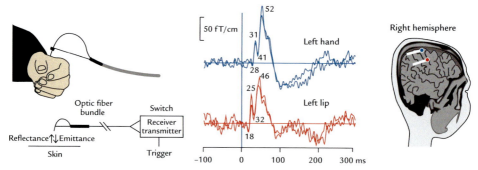

FIGURE 6.1. Fiber-optic brush stimulator. Left: Placement of the device for stimulation of the dorsum of the left hand in the region innervated by the radial nerve (upper part of figure). Diagram of the components of the stimulator (lower part of figure). Stimulation is delivered via manual movement of the bundle of optical fibers. Half of the fibers are sending and the other half are receiving light. When the bundle comes close enough to the skin, the transmitted light is reflected from the skin and transmitted to elicit a trigger pulse that will be used as timing signal for the MEG data-acquisition system. The triggering distance from the skin can be adjusted. Middle: Averaged somatosensory responses to brush stimulation (at time zero) of the left hand and left lip, with traces from two identical experiments superimposed. Passband 0.1–145 Hz. The peak latencies of successive deflections of the response are indicated (in ms). Right: The generator areas of the main (40–55-ms) deflections are superimposed on a parasagittal anatomical MRI slice. Blue and red circles denote current-dipole sources for hand and lip stimulation, respectively, and the white lines indicate the tails of the dipoles. Adapted and reprinted from Jousmäki V, Nishitani N, Hari R: A brush stimulator for functional brain imaging. *Clin Neurophysiol* 2007, 118: 2620–2624. With permission from Elsevier.

as current dipoles) is evident in the left hand and face areas of the primary somatosensory cortex (Figure 6.1, right).

Stimulators for Inducing Acute Pain

Information about noxious stimuli affecting the body is transmitted via myelinated Aδ and unmyelinated C fibers. In pain research, these fibers could be easily stimulated by, for example, strong electrical pulses or by pressure, but the problem is that such stimulation is not selective for pain, and the concomitant activation of tactile fibers will mask the nociceptive responses at the cortical level. Therefore, other types of stimulation have been developed. For example, the thermal pain that can be produced by laser stimuli does not (usually) activate tactile fibers.

Several types of lasers, for example, carbon dioxide (CO_2) and thulium, have been used for studies of acute pain. Whenever laser stimuli are used in the laboratory, both the subject and the experimenter must wear protective glasses (see Figure 6.2). Different lasers have different penetration depths into the tissue, and some can be extremely hazardous. To prevent discomfort and potential burns, the laser stimulator is systematically moved over the area of skin (as demonstrated by the experimenter holding the laser stimulator in Figure 6.2). Drawing an outline of the skin area to be stimulated or even including a drawn grid on skin might be helpful for this purpose. In the figure, the red spot on the skin

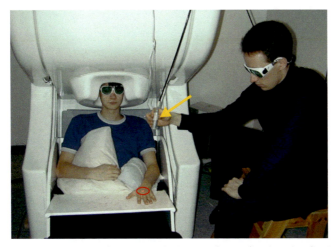

FIGURE 6.2. **Setup for noxious laser stimulation.** A thermal pain stimulus is delivered via a thulium laser to the dorsum of the subject's left hand. The experimenter moves the stimulator probe (indicated by yellow arrow) around a small area over the skin (here highlighted, for visualization purposes only, by the red circle), so as to avoid focal burns to the subject's hand. The red spot on the subject's hand is a guiding light identifying the stimulation site as the laser light itself is invisible. For safety reasons, both the subject and experimenter wear protective glasses. (Setup at the MEG Core, Aalto University, Finland.)

(encircled in red) is a light guide signaling to the experimenter where the invisible laser pulses are being targeted.

An infrared CO_2 laser can stimulate pain afferents, but the types of activated fibers depend on the skin area stimulated (Pertovaara et al., 1984). Progressively increasing stimulus intensity will first cause a sense of warmth, then heat, and finally sharp pain (as a sign of Aδ-fiber activation) or a sensation of dull pain (as the sign of C-fiber activation).

Typical durations for CO_2 laser stimuli (with wavelength of 10.6 microns) are 10 to 70 ms, obtained by interrupting a continuous laser output by a shutter. The now much more commonly used thulium laser (wavelength 2 microns) works in a pulsed mode, and a typical stimulus duration is 1 ms. We discuss responses to thulium-laser stimulation in Chapter 15.

Another possible way to deliver accurately-timed pain stimuli in MEG/EEG studies is by a contact-heat stimulator that allows temperature rises as fast as 70 °C/s, but this procedure requires sophisticated artifact suppression (Gopalakrishnan et al., 2013).

Passive-Movement Stimulators

Well-controlled passive movements of limbs, fingers, and toes provide a means to track proprioceptive afferents to the cortex. The movements can be produced manually so that the experimenter moves the body part (Figure 6.3, left) or automatically with special devices, such as pneumatic artificial muscles (PAMs). PAMs are elastic actuator tubes that shorten when the air pressure increases inside them (Piitulainen et al., 2015). Passive movements are elicited when the subjects rest their finger, toe, hand, or foot on the stimulator (Figure 6.3, right).

One disadvantage common to all passive-movement stimulators is that they simultaneously also activate tactile afferents to a degree that is difficult to judge from the signals themselves and that cannot be totally eliminated by using topical anesthesia.

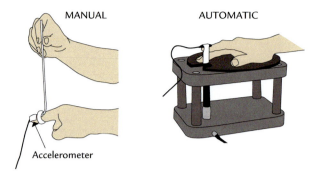

MANUAL　　　　　　　　AUTOMATIC

Accelerometer

FIGURE 6.3. **Two types of passive movement stimulator.** Left: Schematic of a (manual) hand-held passive-movement stimulator consisting of an aluminum stick that the experimenter moves up and down to move the subject's finger; an accelerometer is attached to the subject's finger to monitor the movements. Adapted and reprinted from Piitulainen H, Bourguignon M, De Tiège X, Hari R, Jousmäki V: Cortico-kinematic coherence during active and passive finger movements. *Neuroscience* 2013, 238: 361–370. With permission from Elsevier. Right: A schematic of an automatic stimulator, based on artificial or "pneumatic muscles" that are driven by compressed air. The subject rests the right index finger on the stimulator that will cause the finger to move up and down. An accelerometer is again connected to the finger. Drawn from a photo provided by Harri Piitulainen, Aalto University, Finland. The device has been described in detail in Piitulainen H, Bourguignon M, Hari R, Jousmäki V: MEG-compatible pneumatic device to elicit passive finger and toe movements. *Neuroimage* 2015, 112: 310–317.

Olfactory and Gustatory Stimulators

Studies of smell (olfaction) and taste (gustation) pose particular challenges for the construction of stimulators that are compatible with EEG and MEG. Whereas accurately timed visual, auditory, and tactile stimuli can be delivered quite easily, well-defined smell and taste stimuli require complex stimulation equipment. Chemosensory stimuli must be delivered to the subject as sharply timed boluses that do not contaminate the brain responses by concomitant somatosensory stimulation and that can be washed out quickly from both the stimulus delivery system and the subject's sensory receptors.

Olfaction

Olfactory threshold, discrimination, and smell identification can be tested behaviorally using, for example, "Sniffin'-Sticks" that contain multiple validated odorants (Hummel et al., 1997, 2007). In these kits, desired liquid odorants (or odorant dissolved in propylene glycol) have been filled in felt-tip pen-like objects, from which the odors emerge when the experimenter removes the cap and places the tip of the pen in front of the subject's nostrils. Given that these stimuli lack precise timing, they are not the first choice for EEG or MEG studies as then only changes in spontaneous brain activity could be analyzed.

In stimulus-locked recordings of olfaction-related brain responses, the stimuli should be directed through the nostrils toward the olfactory mucosa at the roof of the nasal cavity. Pure olfactory stimuli should only stimulate olfactory receptors, which is why the use of single-odorant boluses is discouraged because such abrupt single stimuli would additionally activate tactile receptors (due to the local pressure change) and thermal receptors (due to the local temperature change). If the trigeminal nerve innervating the nasal mucosa was inadvertently stimulated, the olfactory brain responses would be contaminated by a somatosensory component, thereby confounding data interpretation. Therefore, the most commonly used olfactometers in EEG/MEG recordings deliver the stimulus as a bolus embedded in a continuous humidified (relative humidity ~80%), constant airflow (6–8 l/min) at body temperature (35–37° C), which avoids inadvertent thermal and mechanical stimulation of the nasal mucosa (Kobal & Plattig, 1978; Evans et al., 1993; Hummel & Kobal, 1999; Lötsch & Hummel, 2006). A pulsed odor (rise time 20 ms and duration 200 ms) is typically embedded into the odorless airstream via a fast valve in a control circuit that includes a vacuum line (Hummel & Kobal, 1999; Lötsch & Hummel, 2006). The continuous airflow is delivered from the olfactometer to the nostril(s) via a long Teflon tube. Stimuli can be presented either asynchronously with respect to breathing in subjects who have been taught to breathe only via mouth (Kobal, 1985; Kettenmann et al., 1996) or synchronized to the inhalation phase of the respiratory cycle (Tonoike et al., 1998).

Figure 6.4 displays a schematic of the main components of a recent olfactometer design (Gotow et al., 2019). This device can also deliver a transient odorant within a background odor, which adds to the complexity of the device but increases the ecological validity of the stimuli. The long tubing and the humidification system require careful disinfection against pathogens that might threaten the subject's health.

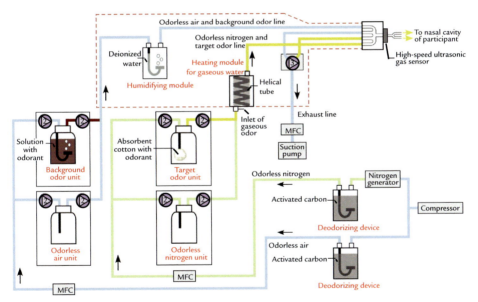

FIGURE 6.4. The main components of an olfactometer that allows presentation of a transient odorant stimulus either on a continuous stream of air or within a background odor. The basic device (with constant airstream) comprises separate units for the target odorant, stream of odorless air (figure middle, light green lines), as well as modules for heating and humidification of the airstream (figure top, box enclosed by broken line). Deodorizing devices clean the air after stimulus presentation. The basic unit can be extended by adding another unit that provides a background odor into which the target odorant can be inserted (left side of figure, blue lines). MFC refers to mass flow controller, and two-way and three-way solenoid valves are indicated with corresponding numbers. Modified and printed by permission from Gotow N, Hoshi A, Kobayakawa T: Expanded olfactometer for measuring reaction time to a target odor during background odor presentation. *Heliyon* 2019, 5: e01254.

One annoying side effect of even partial trigeminal stimulation is reflexive blinking, which is difficult to suppress and shows large intersubject variability. The very long inter-stimulus intervals (e.g., 40 s) necessary to avoid adaptation of the olfactory receptors of the nasal mucosa further accentuate the problem as subjects are easily alerted by each stimulus and thus blink as a part of an automatic orientation reaction. Therefore, monitoring eye-related artifacts with an EOG is a must. Blinks are especially easily triggered by some gases, such as carbon dioxide (used for pain studies) and hydrogen sulfide. With the latter gas, an additional problem is the escape of the unpleasant odor to the test chamber and the whole laboratory. Therefore, both must have efficient ventilation so that any stray odorant can be promptly removed from the research space.

It should also be noted that acoustic stimulation from the sounds of valve opening and closure in the olfactometer may produce auditory evoked responses and thus confound the responses of interest; auditory white-noise masking may thus be necessary during the experiment.

A set of older guidelines exists for collecting and reporting of chemosensory (olfactory) event-related potentials (Evans et al., 1993).

Gustation

Experimental stimulation of taste receptors requires administration of the stimulus directly to the tongue, typically as a liquid bolus consisting of a tasteless carrier mixed with the flavorant of interest. Subjects are not permitted to swallow the stimuli, and thus the liquid stimulus and associated saliva has to be removed from the mouth. A carefully designed gustometer allows for the controlled delivery of a bolus of gustatory liquid, a washout solution, and associated suction and drainage mechanisms that remove the excess liquid from the subject's mouth. The gustometer assembly on the tongue can also include an electrode system for simultaneously measuring tongue potentials (e.g., Feldman et al., 2003).

Figure 6.5 shows a schematic of a gustometer as well as close-ups of the mouthpiece in situ. This device has moving metallic parts close to the subject, and thus design of gustometers that are MEG friendly poses further technical challenges.

■ DEVICES FOR BEHAVIORAL MONITORING

Response pads, keyboards, eye trackers, and accelerometer-based monitoring devices all have to be designed specifically for the MEG/EEG environment so that they do not produce electric, magnetic, or acoustic artifacts and thereby contaminate the recordings. Fiber-optic devices are ideal for both MEG and EEG environments.

To rule out the possibility of time-locked acoustic contamination from stimulus devices, one should run control recordings with the stimulus-presentation device (e.g., the passive-movement stimulator) working as in the real experiment but not actually connected to the subject. These control recordings are important to confirm that the brain responses are not elicited by concomitant acoustical noise or other inadvertent sources of artifacts.

■ PHANTOMS FOR MEG/EEG SOURCE ANALYSIS AND ARTIFACT REMOVAL

Physical phantoms were originally built as substitutes for living subjects' heads to learn about source localization accuracy of MEG/EEG recordings. In Chapter 1 we mentioned "dry" phantoms for MEG recordings, consisting of triangular current loops that are

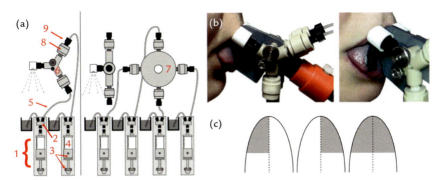

FIGURE 6.5. The main components of a gustometer. (a) Gustometer setup schematic: (1) pump module; (2) solenoid valve; (3) syringe holder and piston holder; (4) glass syringe; (5) tubing; (6) Y-connector; (7) multiway manifold; (8) inlet check valve; and (9) fitting. Left panel: Setup for up to two stimuli. Right panel: Setup for up to four stimuli. Manifold assembly is shown from a side view in the top left part of the panel. (b) Gustometer mouthpiece in situ (left image). Lateralized stimulation is possible via two separate spray heads placed on either side of a plastic separator. The right image shows lateralized stimulation locus using a colored liquid. Still images were extracted from a high-speed video recording (240 frames/s). (c) Possible types of tongue stimulation: left side, right side, and bilateral, respectively. Reproduced with permission from Andersen CA, Alfine L, Ohla K, Höchenberger R: A new gustometer: template for the construction of a portable and modular stimulator for taste and lingual touch. *Behav Res Methods* 2019, 51: 2733–2747.

equivalent to current dipoles in any spherical volume conductor that contains only concentric inhomogeneities (Ilmoniemi et al., 1985; for a history, see Oyama et al., 2015). However, for assessing EEG source localization accuracy, tissue conductivities also need to be considered.

An initial attempt to construct a naturally shaped phantom used a cadaver skull filled with conductive medium within which three current dipoles at known locations were energized. MEG signals were recorded with a single-channel third-order axial magnetometer, and EEG signals were picked up with 10–20 system electrodes cemented to the skull (Weinberg et al., 1986). A more recent head phantom comprised a 32-element current-dipole array immersed in saline–gelatin mixture within a cleaned human skull, covered by an artificial "scalp" consisting of layers of a partially conductive rubber latex (Leahy et al., 1998). The conductivities of these simulated "scalp," "skull," and "brain" tissues were titrated to resemble known human tissue conductivities that are notoriously difficult to measure (see Table 10.1). This time the MEG signals were collected with a "single-shot," whole-scalp, 122-channel neuromagnetometer and the EEG signals with 32 + 32 electrodes in two successive runs. The data were used to compare respective source localization results of MEG and EEG recordings for dipoles at different locations (and thereby necessarily of different signal-to-noise ratios). Noise in these phantom measurements, as in real MEG/EEG measurements, also includes errors in co-registration. On average, the source-localization errors were about double for EEG compared with MEG data. It has to be noted that since the conductivities of the cadaver-skull phantoms do not exactly match those of living brains and heads, the results cannot be considered as gold standards but rather indicate relative localization accuracies.

Over the years, MRI resolution has improved immensely, allowing fine parcellation of tissue layers and detailed forward models to be generated for individual subject heads. Therefore, physical head phantoms have no longer been used to assess the accuracy of MEG/EEG source localization.

However, more recently phantoms have been used for separating walking artifacts from brain signals recorded with portable EEG devices (see Chapter 9). For this purpose, a gelatin phantom head with embedded current sources was placed on a custom-built motion platform eliciting vertical sinusoidal motion on the phantom. ICA (Independent Component Analysis) decomposition separated out the various signals and identified increased spectral power across all canonical EEG frequency bands at head motion frequencies > 1.5 Hz and vertical displacements > 4 cm (Oliviera et al., 2016). Consequently, a new method—ICA decomposition with added Canonical Correlation Analysis (CCA)—was developed to remove walking artifacts (see Chapter 9) (Richer et al., 2020).

■ REFERENCES

Evans W, Kobal G, Lorig T, Prah JD: Suggestions for collection and reporting of chemosensory (olfactory) event-related potentials. *Chem Senses* 1993, 18: 751–756.

Feldman GM, Mogyorosi A, Heck GL, DeSimone JA, Santos CR, Clary RA, Lyall V: Salt-evoked lingual surface potential in humans. *J Neurophysiol* 2003, 90: 2060–2064.

Gardner EP, Costanzo RM: Spatial integration of multiple-point stimuli in primary somatosensory cortical receptive fields of alert monkeys. *J Neurophysiol* 1980, 43: 420–443.

Gopalakrishnan R, Machado AG, Burgess RC, Mosher JC: The use of contact heat evoked potential stimulator (CHEPS) in magnetoencephalography for pain research. *J Neurosci Methods* 2013, 220: 55–63.

Gotow N, Hoshi A, Kobayakawa T: Expanded olfactometer for measuring reaction time to a target odor during background odor presentation. *Heliyon* 2019, 5: e01254

Hesse MD, Nishitani N, Fink GR, Jousmäki V, Hari R: Attenuation of somatosensory responses to self-produced tactile stimulation. *Cereb Cortex* 2010, 20: 425–432.

Hummel T, Sekinger B, Wolf SR, Pauli E, Kobal G: "'Sniffin'-Sticks": olfactory performance assessed by the combined testing of odor identification, odor discrimination and olfactory threshold. *Chem Senses* 1997, 22: 39–52.

Hummel T, Kobal G: Chemosensory event related potentials to trigeminal stimuli change in relation to the interval between repetitive stimulation of the nasal mucosa. *Eur Arch Otolaryngol* 1999, 256: 16–21.

Hummel T, Kobal G, Gudziol H, Mackay-Sim A: Normative data for the "'Sniffin' Sticks" including tests of odor identification, odor discrimination, and olfactory thresholds: an upgrade based on a group of more than 3,000 subjects. *Eur Arch Otorhinolaryngol* 2007, 264: 237–243.

Ilmoniemi RJ, Hämäläinen MS, Knuutila J: The forward and inverse problems in the spherical model. In: Weinberg H, Stroink G, Katila T, eds. *Biomagnetism: Applications and Theory.* New York: Pergamon, 1985, 278–282.

Jousmäki V, Hari R: Somatosensory evoked fields to large-area vibrotactile stimuli. *Clin Neurophysiol* 1999, 110: 905–909.

Jousmäki V, Nishitani N, Hari R: A brush stimulator for functional brain imaging. *Clin Neurophysiol* 2007, 118: 2620–2624.

Jousmäki V: Gratifying gizmos for research and clinical MEG. *Front Neurol* 2021, 12: 814573.

Kettenmann B, Jousmäki V, Portin K, Salmelin R, Kobal G, Hari R: Odorants activate the human superior temporal sulcus. *Neurosci Lett* 1996, 203: 1–3.

Kobal G, Plattig KH: Metodische Anmerkungen zur Gewinnung olfaktorischer EEG-Antworten des wachen Menschen (objective Olfaktometrie). *Z EEG–EMG* 1978, 9: 135–145.

Kobal G: Pain-related electrical potentials of the human nasal mucosa elicited by chemical stimulation. *Pain* 1985, 22: 151e163.

Lambert GA, Mallos G, Zagami AS: Von Frey's hairs—a review of their technology and use—a novel automated von Frey device for improved testing for hyperalgesia. *J Neurosci Methods* 2009, 177: 420–426.

Lankinen K, Saari J, Hari R, Koskinen M: Intersubject consistency of cortical MEG signals during movie viewing. *NeuroImage* 2014, 92: 217–224.

Leahy RM, Mosher JC, Spencer ME, Huang MX, Lewine JD: A study of dipole localization accuracy for MEG and EEG using a human skull phantom. *Electroencephalogr Clin Neurophysiol* 1998, 107: 159–173.

Lötsch J, Hummel T: The clinical significance of electrophysiological measures of olfactory function. *Behav Brain Res* 2006, 170: 78–83.

Oliveira AS, Schlink BR, Hairston WD, König P, Ferris DP: Induction and separation of motion artifacts in EEG data using a mobile phantom head device. *J Neural Eng* 2016, 13: 036014.

Oyama D, Adachi Y, Yumoto M, Hashimoto I, Uehara G: Dry phantom for magnetoencephalography—configuration, calibration, and contribution. *J Neurosci Methods* 2015, 251: 24–36.

Pertovaara A, Reinikainen K, Hari R: The activation of unmyelinated or myelinated afferent fibers by brief infrared laser pulses varies with skin type. *Brain Res* 1984, 307: 341–343.

Piitulainen H, Bourguignon M, Hari R, Jousmäki V: MEG-compatible pneumatic stimulator to elicit passive finger and toe movements. *NeuroImage* 2015, 112: 310–317.

Richer N, Downey RJ, Hairston WD, Ferris DP, Nordin AD: Motion and muscle artifact removal validation using an electrical head phantom, robotic motion platform, and dual layer mobile EEG. *IEEE Trans Neural Syst Rehabil Eng* 2020, 28: 1825–1835.

Sun L, Okada Y: Vibrotactile piezoelectric stimulation system with precise and versatile timing control for somatosensory research. *J Neurosci Methods* 2019, 317: 29–36.

Tonoike M, Yamaguchi M, Kaetsu I, Kida H, Seo R, Koizuka I: Ipsilateral dominance of human olfactory activated centers estimated from event-related magnetic fields measured by 122-channel whole-head neuromagnetometer using odorant stimuli synchronized with respirations. *Ann N Y Acad Sci* 1998, 855: 579–590.

Weinberg H, Brickett P, Coolsma F, Baff M: Magnetic localisation of intracranial dipoles: simulation with a physical model. *Electroencephalogr Clin Neurophysiol* 1986, 64: 159–170.

CHAPTER 7

PRACTICALITIES OF DATA COLLECTION

Tell me and I forget. Teach me and I remember. Involve me and I learn.

BENJAMIN FRANKLIN

Creative experimentation propels our culture forward. That our stories of innovation tend to glorify the breakthroughs and edit out all the experimental mistakes doesn't mean that mistakes play a trivial role. As any artist or scientist knows, without some protected, even sacred space for mistakes, innovation would cease.

EVGENY MOROZOV

I n this chapter we provide a number of suggestions about optimization of MEG/EEG recording sessions to guarantee as good signal quality and as high a signal-to-noise ratio as possible.

■ GENERAL PRINCIPLES OF GOOD EXPERIMENTATION

It is always important (with the exception of sleep or intraoperative studies) to record MEG/EEG data from alert and cooperative subjects in as artifact- and noise-free conditions as possible. Cooperative subjects who are comfortable, yet alert, during the MEG/EEG recording session will yield optimal data that will contain fewer artifacts. An inviting, nonthreatening laboratory set-up with soft lighting and a comfortable chair can relax the subject in the laboratory environment, as can a calm, sympathetic, and professional experimenter.

Importantly, all subjects should be given the same instructions at the start of the study—as is already required by the approvals of institutional ethics committees—so that subjects' expectation of the experiment will be as similar as possible. To ensure uniform procedures for all subjects, it is recommended that all experimenters use a fixed protocol for running the experiments and explaining procedures to subjects, backed up by a written protocol that includes all necessary checklists and instructions. This consistency in protocol applies equally to experimenters within a lab and to those who are performing collaborative studies at partner sites.

It is better to divide the recording session to smaller "runs," consistent with COBIDAS (Committee on Best Practice in Data Analysis and Sharing) MEEG guidelines (Pernet et al., 2018, 2020), that can be repeated to examine the reliability of the phenomena of interest. Subjects who can relax and readjust their positions between runs are more likely to remain comfortable and vigilant for the entire recording session. In MEG sessions, the head position should, however, stay as similar as possible between the sessions, and especially between experimental conditions in the same session that will be directly compared in the planned data analysis. Instructions can be repeated at the start of each run to remind subjects about relaxing their muscles, minimizing blinking, and avoiding head and body movements. It is necessary to monitor the brain signals continually online for any artifacts or technical issues with the recording and to see whether additional instructions to the subject might be needed.

When the recording has commenced, special attention should be given to signal quality: some of the EEG electrodes might need to be adjusted (or regelled or rehydrated). MEG channels typically do not need adjustment during the recording provided that the SQUIDs have been properly tuned before the recording. Instead, OPMs need to be calibrated prior to each experiment by energizing them to produce a known field and then adjusting the sensor output to a preset value (Hill et al., 2020). Any deviations from the normal course of the experiment should be immediately recorded in a log so that anyone who subsequently analyzes the data is alerted for possible anomalies in the recording session, as well as for systematic problems across the entire experiment.

Some brain signals are strongly vigilance-dependent, and drowsiness will compromise signal quality. Thus it is extremely important to motivate the subject in advance, explaining that drowsiness or other deviations from the planned procedure may mar the data so that the subject's participation could be in vain. If drowsiness does set in during the recording session, talking to the subject between experimental runs may help in maintaining alertness. It is also important to keep the experimental runs as short as possible, meaning that the experimenter should know exactly what to do and when and then proceed quickly and efficiently with the experiment. Because stimulants, such as caffeine, can alter EEG activity, giving subjects caffeinated drinks to allow them to stay alert during the experiment might not be a good idea (see Chapter 11).

Given that many EEG and MEG studies require long periods of gaze fixation and voluntary suppression of eye blinking, some subjects may find that their eyes become dry during the experiment, especially if they wear contact lenses. Having the subject wear their prescription eyeglasses instead of contact lenses might be more comfortable, and MEG/EEG laboratories should have a set of nonmagnetic (for MEG and EEG–fMRI) eyeglass frames and an extensive set of lenses to be worn by subjects who need vision correction. Eye drops containing physiological (0.9%) sodium chloride can help to hydrate eyes during prolonged recording sessions.

The inability to fixate and see the environment sharply (e.g., due to myopia or because the visual field is featureless; see Lehtonen and Lehtinen, 1972) is one of the main reasons for increased posterior alpha activity (Chapter 11) that then may impair the quality of other signals of interest, especially visual-evoked responses. Naturally, the responses to visual stimulation will be significantly affected, mainly attenuated and delayed, if the subject cannot adequately see the stimuli.

■ REPLICABILITY CHECKS

The study design should always include some repetitions of stimuli and/or tasks to check data replicability. For example, evoked responses and the level of spontaneous activity might be different at the beginning and end of a session due to changes in vigilance. Moreover, additional resting-state blocks (of 1–2 min, with eyes open and eyes closed) are beneficial to give an idea about individual brain rhythms, their spectra, and reactivity to eye opening/closing.

One highly recommended and simple way to ensure that evoked responses are not contaminated by various artifacts and/or baseline shifts during data collection is to average the responses to odd and even stimuli separately and superimpose the two sets of responses on the screen to already see the replicability during data collection. It is also recommended that continuously recorded MEG/EEG data be stored even if evoked responses are averaged online.

Replicability of data was originally proposed as a criterion for publication of evoked-responses in both research and clinical data sets (Picton et al., 2000). Viewed from fMRI insights where signal replicability has been shown to differ between different brain areas and in fact to carry important information (Hasson et al., 2008), we may expect the variability of some less-well reproduced (longer latency) MEG/EEG responses to also carry information—for example about the subject's state—as long as the recordings are technically sound. Thus, one must ensure that the poor replicability is not due to noise in the recording but instead to real variability in brain function. Moreover, all early sensory responses—that tightly reflect the sensory input and are used to assess the integrity of afferent sensory pathways—should be clearly replicable before the recording can be considered reliable.

▪ EEG RECORDINGS: THE PRACTICE

Skin Preparation for Electrode-Impedance Measurement

General
It is a good idea to ask subjects to wash their hair (and skin) prior to arriving for an EEG study and to refrain from applying any cosmetic products on the skin or hair/scalp, such as makeup, moisturizer, hair conditioner, or hair spray/gel. In some cases, the hair may need to be (re)washed prior to the recording session, because the subject has used a shampoo that has a built-in conditioner. Hence, some investigators find it useful to have a (hairdresser's) sink in the EEG lab for this purpose.

Before beginning the study, the subject should remove jewelry and piercings, as items such as earrings can become caught in electrode caps and nets. Similarly, spectacles are removed while electrodes are being sited. Many EEG cap/net systems are manufactured in multiple sizes, so one of the first activities in the lab is to measure the circumference of the subject's head so that a suitable cap/net can be selected. At this same time, landmarks on the scalp, such as the vertex and inion, can also be identified and marked using a nonpermanent marker.

Skin Preparation for Electrode Application
Irrespective of which electrode system is used, putting tens or hundreds of electrodes quickly on a subject takes lots of practice and skill. New EEG personnel can be trained in electrode application by allowing them to initially put electrodes/caps/nets on a polystyrene hairdresser's dummy. The follow-up training might consist of "capping" other lab members. Subject comfort is very important during longer recording sessions, and it is important that all new experimenters have experienced being a subject as well, wearing the EEG electrodes and have actually completed an EEG recording session. They can then scrutinize, with good motivation, their own data and learn about signals and artifacts. During

long recording sessions, the electrode-fixation system, whether it be a rubber-band mesh, electrode cap, or alternate system, can begin to put pressure on parts of the scalp, and the subject's discomfort can be alleviated if the experimenter is well practiced in electrode application.

Before siting electrodes on the face or earlobes, the skin is mildly abraded (typically using exfoliating gel or cream) to remove the epidermal layer of the skin, then cleaned with an oil-removing substance (acetone or alcohol) to remove natural oils. Loose electrodes on the face and earlobes can be fixed with medical adhesive tape or glued on with a solid conducting paste.

Prior to today's high-density EEG caps, meshes, and nets, EEG electrodes were often glued to the scalp with collodion (an adhesive made from nitrocellulose, ethyl ether, and ethanol), which was dried using a hair dryer or source of compressed air, as electrodes were placed one by one. After the recording, the electrodes were removed by dissolving the collodion with acetone. Needless to say, the fumes from collodion and acetone were quite unpleasant for both subject and experimenter, which decreased the popularity of this method. Another electrode-fixation system, sometimes still used clinically, relies on fastening single electrodes to the scalp using gauze and relatively solid conductive paste. In the traditional and clinically widely used rubber-band nets, multiple electrodes can be quickly (with some experience) placed in the correct 10–20 locations as the rubber net stretches in equal proportions across the whole scalp.

Following skin preparation, impedances of less than 5 kΩ—or, in any case, less than 10 kΩ—can be easily obtained with the electrode systems described previously. Note that it is not a good idea to try to reduce electrode impedances below 2 kΩ (and it would be difficult, as well), as this will effectively create a "current bridge," or short-circuit, between the inputs of the EEG amplifier resulting in no measurable (or very tiny) EEG signals across the bridge. Bridging can also occur with overzealous skin abrasion or the rather liberal use of electrode gel.

Some modern EEG amplifier systems with extra high-input impedances are specifically designed to function with electrode impedances up to 50 to 70 kΩ or even 100 kΩ. Therefore, they can be used with scalp-electrode arrays that require little or no prior skin preparation, which is an advantage in EEG recordings of children and patients.

In many portable EEG systems, dry EEG electrodes are used with no additional skin preparation, resulting in high electrode impedances exceeding 100 kΩ. As already discussed in Chapter 5, the amplifiers in these portable systems have been specially designed to function with electrode impedances in this range.

Electrode-Impedance Measurement

Note that one measures *impedance*, which is the impediment of the electrode–skin interface to the flow of alternating current (AC), rather than the resistance to direct current (DC). Impedance measurement is more appropriate because EEG records signals produced by time-varying currents, such as brain rhythms. Moreover, applying steady voltages to the electrodes (e.g., via a regular resistance meter) would polarize them and potentially cause drifting and deteriorate the reliability of recorded slow brain potentials.

Commercial passive and active EEG systems typically have built-in impedance meters that pass a sinusoidal voltage across all electrodes, typically at around 20 Hz (which is in the middle of the EEG frequency range of interest) and measure the amplitude of the resulting voltages at each channel of the amplifier. The displayed impedances allow the experimenter to make adjustments, such as further skin abrasion or adding conductive medium. Some EEG systems allow the impedance values to be stored with the EEG data file. In other cases, the impedance values exceeding the manufacturer's recommendations need to be noted in a log or set of measurement notes, as artifacts and strange signals are typically more likely to occur at electrodes with much higher impedances relative to the reference.

In some commercial EEG systems, it is not possible to measure electrode impedances directly, but portable impedance meters are available for checking the impedances of all electrodes prior to plugging them in to the EEG amplifiers.

Electrode gel, paste, or solution tends to dry out as the experiment continues, particularly in a centrally heated or air-conditioned laboratory, progressively increasing the electrode impedances. Running portable air humidifiers in the laboratory to at least 30% humidity may reduce this problem. Thus it is advisable to check (and, if needed, adjust) all electrode impedances, including those of the reference and ground, at least once *during* the course of an experiment lasting longer than 30 min. In this way, any electrodes whose contacts are loose and impedances have increased to unacceptable levels can be adjusted. (If the impedance for a wet electrode has been very high, chances are that the EEG signals have been compromised. Electrodes such as this may need to be excluded from analyses, as we discuss in Chapter 10.) For EEG systems with nets and electrodes that make contact with the scalp via sponges soaked in KCl solution, experimenters might consider using a disposable operating-room cap whose inside has been sprayed with the solution; the resulting moist "microclimate" will prevent the conductive solution in the sponges from drying out. Even when using dry electrodes, at the very least, impedances should be checked at the start of the recording, and if the recording is longer than 30 minutes, at other times during the session.

■ MEG RECORDINGS: THE PRACTICE

The preparation of subjects for a MEG recording is quite straightforward. First the subjects must ensure that they have no magnetic material in/on the body or the clothing. Removing shoes, jewelry, hairpins, or combs and changing into laboratory scrubs will usually suffice, but one may also need to wash off liquid makeup and mascara as these may contain magnetic particles. Moreover, people wearing dental braces should not be studied unless the MEG is required for clinical purposes, since the braces introduce large artifacts into MEG recordings. When in doubt about the suitability of the subject for an MEG measurement, an easy preliminary screening procedure consists of making a short MEG measurement without attaching EEG electrodes or head position coils (described later) and examining the MEG signals online for any artifacts.

If a subject is participating in a study consisting of both MEG and fMRI recordings, the MEG recordings should be performed first, as it is possible that the subject might be magnetized in the MRI scanner (i.e., retain nonphysiological remanent magnetic fields for a prolonged period of time). If this order is not possible, the fMRI study and the subsequent MEG recording should be separated by at least 3 days (Gross et al., 2013). In some cases degaussing may help in removing magnetization induced by the MRI scanner as well as some other minor magnetic contaminants (see Mosher & Funke, 2020).

Even if no simultaneous EEG is recorded, it will be necessary to attach electrodes to the face to measure vertical and horizontal eye movements and blinks: one electrode above one eye, another below the same eye, one electrode lateral to the left eye, and another lateral to the right eye. Thus four electrodes (plus one ground electrode) are needed (Figure 7.1, right panel) to measure the electro-oculogram (EOG), the electrical signal generated by the eyes. Some experimenters try to reduce the number of electrodes and catch both vertical eye movements (and eye blinks) and horizontal eye movements with a single diagonal

EOG derivation, but it is better to have separate vertical and horizontal EOG channels (EOGv and EOGh), as it will greatly aid artifact identification and elimination (see Chapter 9). Similarly, we recommend simultaneous recording of the electrocardiogram— for example, simply between the two upper limbs—to identify heart-related contamination in the MEG/EEG signals.

Head position indicator (HPI) coils are attached to rigid parts of the scalp/face, such as the mastoids and forehead, according to the manufacturer's guidelines (Figure 7.1, right panel). If the subject is wearing an electrode cap, some of the HPI coils can be placed over the cap as the coils have to be accessible for digitization (Figure 7.1, left panel; and see description of digitization methods below). During the experiment, the HPI coils are activated by sending current to them so that they all will act as magnetic dipoles, producing very local magnetic flux just above them (see the magnetic dipole in Figure 1.3), allowing the coil locations (and the subject's head position) to be accurately determined by means of the MEG sensor array.

It is also possible to have continuous head-position monitoring by activating the coils at unique frequencies above the frequencies of interest in the MEG recording itself (e.g., at

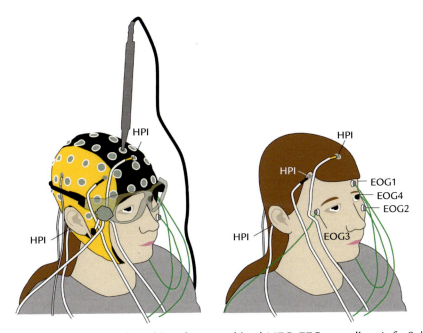

FIGURE 7.1. **Preparation of a subject for a combined MEG–EEG recording.** Left: Subject with an EEG-electrode cap and electrodes to measure eye movements and blinks (by means of EOG). For vertical EOG, electrodes are placed above and below one eye (see also right panel). Similarly, for horizontal EOG, two electrodes are placed on the temporal side of each eye. Here only the vertical EOG electrode on the lower aspect of the left eye is visible. A handheld probe for digitization of electrode locations and head-position indicator coils (HPIs) is displayed at the top; the probe is oriented perpendicular to the scalp as its tip touches an electrode (see main chapter text for operating principles of this digitization method). Right: The subject shown without the EEG cap to illustrate the EOG electrodes and HPI coils. Vertical EOG is recorded between electrodes EOG1 and EOG2 and horizontal EOG between electrodes EOG3 and EOG4.

around 330 Hz for sampling rates of 1 kHz) but still in the recording band. Such continuous monitoring may be necessary in infant and child recordings, as well as in studies of poorly cooperating patients. These additional non-brain signals can be removed from the raw data by either the MEG data acquisition system software itself or preprocessing software after the data files are exported for analysis.

Before the MEG measurement, the experimenter must follow the instrument-specific instructions to tune SQUIDs, or calibrate OPMs, so that they are ready for measurements. Moreover, when the subject is already placed in the measurement position, it is first necessary to carefully examine spontaneous MEG activity, as slow respiration-related or other movement-related slow fluctuations will indicate that the subject still has some magnetic material on or in the body.

■ MEASUREMENT OF MEG SENSOR AND EEG ELECTRODE POSITIONS

For neural source identification, we need to know exactly where the EEG electrodes and MEG sensors are located with respect to the subject's head (and therefore the brain). These position data can then be coregistered to the same individual's structural MRI to indicate where each electrode, or sensor, sits with regard to the underlying brain anatomy. Because of the time needed for siting the EEG electrodes and determining their relative positions, preparation time is typically clearly longer for an EEG than a MEG recording. The locations of the EEG electrodes are usually digitized *following* the completion of the EEG experiment, so that the subject does not get tired and the electrodes do not dry out and compromise signal quality.

In MEG recordings, one needs to know only the location of the whole sensor array, the MEG helmet, with respect to landmarks ("fiducial points") on the subject's head, because the individual sensors are at fixed locations. The locations of the HPI coils are digitized *prior* to commencing the MEG experiment because it is important to be sure that the localization procedure is functioning correctly.

In combined MEG/EEG recordings, the EEG-electrode locations should be digitized at the same time after the electrode impedances have been measured. Additional fiducial points and lines digitized on the scalp and face considerably improve the coregistration between MRI and MEG/EEG data sets (see, e.g., Mosher & Funke, 2020). These extra points on the top of the head are especially important if the soft tissues on the face and temporal areas have been compressed during MRI imaging, introducing inaccuracies to coregistration.

Several approaches are available for obtaining location information of EEG electrodes and MEG sensor arrays. For both MEG and EEG studies, additional fiducial points on the head are digitized, so that a 3D head-coordinate system can be constructed and the electrode/sensor locations can be coregistered with structural MRI data. Typical fiducial points, presented in the left panel of Figure 7.2, are the nasion (bridge of the nose, EEG electrode position Nz) and the left and right preauricular points that appear as a small indentation located just anterior to the tragus and can be easily felt with the fingers.

For SQUID MEG studies, the positions of the HPI coils are digitized together with fiducial points. A 3D head-coordinate system can then be constructed (see Figure 7.2 lower left), with the x-axis passing between the left and right preauricular points, the y-axis pointing toward the front along the inion–nasion line, and the z-axis pointing upward. Note that because the resulting coordinate system is orthogonal (by definition), *the z-axis does not necessarily pass through the vertex.* For EEG studies, however, the vertex (electrode Cz)

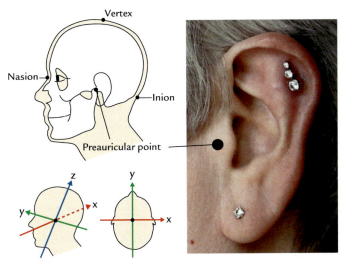

FIGURE 7.2. Fiducial points and coordinate axes. Left panels: Schematic left sagittal view of the head (top) shows fiducial points (black dots) at the nasion, inion, and the left preauricular point. The location of vertex is also indicated. Sagittal and axial views (bottom) of the head show the three orthogonal axes of the coordinate system: y-axis from inion to nasion, x-axis from left to right preauricular points, and z-axis from the crossing point of the x- and y-axes to the top of the head. Right image: A view of the ear showing the location of the preauricular point (black circle).

may be a useful additional fiducial point. Also note that the coordinate conventions may differ among different MEG and EEG manufacturers.

OPM sensors can be worn in either a flexible cap or in a rigid helmet. A 3D optical imaging system can be used to digitize both the subject's head surface and the OPM sensor positions in the cap or helmet. Infrared light can be projected onto the object of interest so that a camera at a known location detects the light (Zetter et al., 2019; Hill et al., 2020). These methods will likely improve in the future when the OPM devices become more popular.

In fMRI studies, two different 3D coordinate systems are commonly used: an older Talairach system, based on anchor points at the anterior and posterior commissures and an origin at the anterior commissure in the brain of a single subject postmortem, and a more recent MNI coordinate system, based on a large set of structural MRI images from healthy living individuals presented in a 3D standardized space. In both of these, the cardinal axes point in the same directions (x from left to right, y from back to front, and z from inferior to superior), but the systems differ in their sites of the origin and in the tilting of the cardinal axes with respect to the head, and thus transformations are needed to go between these coordinate systems. Moreover, the x, y, and z coordinates for the MEG/EEG recordings are *not* equal to the x, y, and z coordinates of the Talairach- or MNI-based 3D coordinate systems used in MRI, despite the same labels and similar directions for the axes. An additional feature to pay attention to is that in some (MRI) coordinate systems, axis directions may differ from those in the above coordinate systems, meaning that coordinate values will appear to have opposite signs.

The corresponding MEG/EEG fiducial points can be identified in MRI scans. In the past, some investigators placed radio-opaque markers (such as fish oil or vitamin E capsules) at these positions for a structural MRI scan performed with a field of view that accommodated the whole head. For this reason, when planning MEG/EEG studies, the investigators should know a priori whether they need to acquire a structural MRI scan that images *the whole head and not just the brain*. An alternative and more recent way is to use surface reconstruction of a high-resolution head MRI, with the ears included, and mark the fiducial points on the MRI volume itself.

Multiple methods—based on magnetic fields, ultrasound, or visible light—are at present available for digitization of EEG electrodes, fiducial points, and HPI coils. We already presented in Figure 7.1 an example of a *magnetic-field digitizing system* in which a stylus-shaped receiver picks up signals from a fixed magnetic source, which is typically located about 1 meter from the subject. As the operator needs to manually digitize each electrode location, this procedure can be time-consuming for larger EEG electrode arrays. A set of three or four HPI coils are usually attached to rigid parts of the face and head to also act as receivers that allow head movement to be tracked in space. In this way small head movements that occur during the digitization procedure can be corrected in the EEG electrode-location data. (Note that, in SQUID-based MEG, as detailed in the previous section, HPI coils are used in a different manner to help locate the sensor helmet with respect to the head and to track the subject's head position during the experiment.)

In an *ultrasonic electrode-digitizing system*, the principle of operation is the same as for the magnetic field–based systems: the strength of a signal from a set of ultrasonic sources at a fixed distance relative to the subject is measured at each electrode via a stylus-shaped device that has two receivers. Similar to the magnetic-field system, three additional receivers sited on the face allow for correction of head motion. Each EEG electrode is digitized individually. Ultrasonic systems are typically calibrated by the manufacturer.

For high-density-EEG electrode arrays, both of these electrode digitization methods are time-consuming and thus may become impractical. Instead, *photogrammetric* approaches allow electrode positions to be measured much more quickly. An older system, developed for the geodesic high-density EEG net, captured multiple visual images of the EEG electrode array via a set of 11 cameras in a single operation (Figure 7.3, left image) (Russell et al., 2005). For accurate localization, ideally each EEG electrode would be captured from at least three points of view. Post hoc semiautomated software estimated the positions of a subset of electrodes at selected strategic points on the net, so that the other electrode locations could then be estimated by interpolation. The operator could check the calculated electrode locations and make corrections and adjustments if needed. A newer way to perform photogrammetry is to move a handheld dual-camera array in continuous sequenced movements around the subject's head while the software automatically computes the electrode positions (Figure 7.3, right image). Operating the handheld photogrammetry tool requires some training and practice, not unlike that with using the magnetic-field-based digitization stylus in Figure 7.1.

An alternative method for electrode digitization is *optical 3D scanning* (Homölle & Oostenveld, 2019), which also automatically provides information about head shape. Moreover, MRI-compatible EEG electrodes can be visualized with structural MRI, and software algorithms can generate a 3D map of electrode positions within the structural MRI data set (Koessler et al., 2008), so that coregistration procedures are no longer needed to merge electrode locations with structural MRI data. However, this approach has only been used in very specialized multimodal imaging studies, as it would need MRI-compatible EEG and also have the EEG lab located very close to the MRI facility.

Head shapes and sizes vary widely between subjects. Head-shape information is needed to more accurately calculate electrode locations on the scalp and to facilitate matching of both EEG electrode locations and the MEG sensor array with the subject's own structural

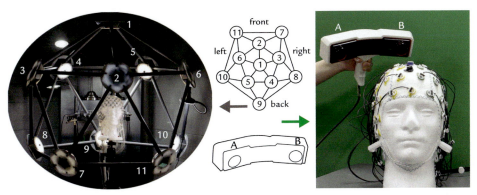

FIGURE 7.3. Digitization of EEG electrode positions. Left: Electrode digitization using a fixed-camera photogrammetry system is performed by placing the subject wearing an EEG cap in the center of an array consisting of 11 equidistant (or geodesic) cameras. Here a polystyrene head, viewed from front, "wears" an EEG net; the 11 cameras are numbered in the figure. Middle: The corresponding (gray arrow) 11-camera layout is shown schematically from a top view in the top schematic panel. The schematic at bottom depicts a portable 2-camera system shown in front view that corresponds to the system in the right image (green arrow). Right: Handheld 2-camera photogrammetry system that is moved in regular small movements around the subject's head in response to visual and acoustic prompts by the controlling software. (Social Neuroscience Laboratory, Indiana University, USA.)

MRI. With magnetic and ultrasonic approaches, the experimenter runs the receiver stylus over the subject's scalp in a series of repetitive movements in different directions. The obtained head-shape data sets can then be used in conjunction with the digitized electrode-location data to calculate the electrode locations more accurately, even when structural MRI images of the subject's head are not available.

All methods of electrode localization yield accurate data in the hands of experienced investigators but are prone to errors that may affect both the *accuracy* and the *precision* of the spatial location of the electrode or sensor. Accuracy of the electrode-location system based on magnetic fields can be compromised by the presence of large metallic objects in the measurement room (Russell et al., 2005) or on the floors directly above and below the laboratory. Moreover, if the distance between the magnetic, or ultrasonic, transmitter and receiver exceeds that recommended by the manufacturer, the signal-to-noise ratio of the location measurements will no longer be optimal as the signal measured at the stylus is decreased. The distance between the subject and the transmitter, as well as the distance between the stylus and electrode, should be kept constant and at manufacturer-recommended distances. With cup electrodes, the stylus is inserted into the hole of the electrode to touch the scalp, and with other electrode types the stylus tip should touch the top center of the electrode. Importantly, the axis of the stylus should be perpendicular to the head at each electrode location. In the fixed-camera photogrammetry system (Figure 7.3, left image), the subject's head must be positioned in the exact center of the array of cameras, as otherwise electrodes on one part of the head might not be sampled optimally relative to other locations. This problem does not arise with a hand-held dual-camera device (Figure 7.3, right image) where data are streamed to the localization software as the device is moved around the subject's head. To prevent errors in electrode localization, hair or electrode cables should not lie over the tops of the electrodes.

■ INFECTION CONTROL IN EEG AND MEG RECORDINGS

General

Light skin abrasion aims to break down the skin surface and may bring EEG electrodes into contact with blood, thus creating a potential risk for the transmission of serious infections, such as HIV, hepatitis, or Creutzfeldt–Jakob disease; these risks exist irrespective of whether or not the EEG laboratory is in a clinical environment (Putnam et al., 1992; Ferree et al., 2001). Some subjects may already have nonintact skin due to a noninfectious condition, such as psoriasis, or may come to the lab with scrapes or scratches. It should be noted that the risk of infection from drawing blood applies to experimenters as well. Sponges soaked in an appropriate ionic solution, dry electrodes, and MEMS-based sensors tend to minimize the likelihood of infection, as the skin does not need to be abraded.

Given the minor risk of infection following the completion of *any* EEG study, scalp EEG electrodes (and caps) and any other nondisposable items, such as hairbrushes the subject has used, should be cleaned with an appropriate hospital-grade disinfectant. Note that disinfectants can be corrosive and damage the EEG electrodes (and caps); thus it is wise to use specific solutions in concentrations recommended by electrode manufacturers. Disposable products, such as plastic syringes and blunted needles, should be discarded safely in biomedical waste containers that preclude reuse and prevent injury from sharp objects. Naturally other surfaces, or devices, such as response boxes or subject chairs, that have come into contact with the subject also need to be wiped down with disinfectant/detergent following the MEG/EEG study. Additionally, all experimenters must wash their hands immediately prior to, and also following, completion of the MEG/EEG recording. Many laboratories follow the practice of not allowing the consumption of food in the data-acquisition area.

In a clinical environment where patients are studied with *intracranial EEG*, scalp EEG electrodes may come into contact with blood on the patient's head, thereby increasing the potential risk of transmittable diseases. Note that conventional procedures of disinfection and sterilization are ineffective against the infectious particle, the prion, in Creutzfeldt-Jakob disease. At the time of writing (mid-2021), disinfecting the scalp EEG electrodes and other associated nondisposable items with sodium hypochlorite solution, an alkaline agent, was proposed to be effective against prions when used in appropriate concentrations (Putnam et al., 1992; Sakudo et al., 2011). In fact, bleach solutions (e.g., sodium hypochlorite) have traditionally been used to clean scalp EEG electrodes and laboratory surfaces before and after intracranial EEG recordings. For intracranial EEG studies, an additional good practice for the experimenter is to wear gloves.

COVID-19-Related Issues

At the time of writing (mid-2021), the COVID-19 pandemic had seriously affected EEG/MEG research worldwide; many research labs closed their doors, whereas diagnostic clinical EEG/MEG recordings continued to meet acute clinical needs.

According to current understanding, COVID-19 spreads via droplets in air containing SARS-CoV-2 virus particles from the breath of an infected person. The spread is also possible via contact with contaminated surfaces and materials. Thus the prevention of COVID-19 spread in an EEG/MEG research laboratory includes avoidance of contact with infected persons, mask wearing, maintaining social distance whenever possible, good hand hygiene, and the disinfection of caps, electrodes, and any other lab items that come into direct contact with the subject.

Recently, multiple articles and guidelines have proposed measures for safe EEG testing in clinical neurophysiology and neuropsychiatry laboratories (Bonner & Davidson, 2020a, 2020b; Desai et al., 2020; Grippo et al., 2020; Haines et al., 2020; San-Juan et al., 2020; Campanella et al., 2021; Canadian Society of Clinical Neurophysiologists [CSCN] et al., 2021). It is logical to also adopt similar practices in MEG and EEG research laboratories. COVID-19 safety guidelines will likely remain relevant until the pandemic has been controlled.

As new knowledge about COVID-19 accrues, these best practices may change. Researchers and subjects should monitor local pandemic statistics and follow up-to-date institutional and state/national safety guidelines. Most research-subject examinations are not urgent and can be postponed during disease peaks (although this may be problematic for longitudinal studies, where time intervals between successive visits are preplanned). In hospitals, decisions to perform clinical tests are made on the basis of risk–benefit assessments. For example, EEG recordings may be needed to aid diagnosis for acute admissions of suspected status epilepticus or for evaluation of post-traumatic or drug-related coma in either the emergency room or intensive care unit.

EEG and MEG laboratories can broadly follow recommendations for safe radiological examinations during the pandemic (Davenport et al., 2020). In brief, the laboratories should:

1. Acquire personal protective equipment to accommodate all laboratory members and research subjects so that face shields or goggles, masks, gloves, and other personal protective equipment can be used *according to institutional guidelines*.
2. Train all laboratory personnel to follow current COVID-19 safety guidelines.
3. Streamline subject flow to diminish unnecessary instances of nonsocial distancing.
4. Screen for COVID-19 symptoms when *scheduling* subjects for recordings, with *repeated screening in the laboratory prior to the study*, emphasizing that research subjects should only be examined if they are healthy, feel well, and have no respiratory symptoms.
5. Maintain regular routines for sanitization of EEG/MEG equipment and the lab facility (including all items coming into contact with the subject).
6. Develop a plan of what to do (consistent with institutional procedures) if a research subject or investigator should subsequently become COVID-19 positive.
7. Use common sense.

Close contact with the subject cannot be avoided during procedures involving EEG or ExG electrode placement, digitization of head position indicators and electrode locations, as well as digitization of the scalp surface. At all other times during the session, the experimenter can maintain social distance (> 2 m) from the subject. If individual EEG electrodes are used, viscous EEG paste and tape are suggested, as collodion use carries additional risks of aerosolization (Bonner & Davidson, 2020b; CSCN et al., 2021).

Given that exposure to viral load is also a consideration for COVID-19 infection, experimenters could consider reducing contact time with subjects. For example, for a given study, multiple experimenters could be rostered to run different subjects. Indeed, it is also important to remember to ventilate the test room(s) well between successive studies.

After the study is completed, all hard surfaces including, but not limited to, doorknobs, light switches, chairs, stools, beds, sinks/faucets, and counter spaces should be wiped down with disinfectants following product instructions for duration of surface contact. EEG/MEG equipment, electrodes and their cables, and all nondisposable items that have come into contact with the subject should be disinfected as per the specific manufacturer's COVID-19 safety recommendations and also general infection control protocols. All other test equipment and nondisposable supplies (response boxes, computer keyboards, computers, hairbrushes, or any other laboratory items) could be wiped/washed down with disinfecting wipes. Importantly, the procedures described here may be effective against other highly virulent diseases as well (Haines et al., 2020).

■ ELECTRICAL SAFETY

We have already seen how currents can flow very efficiently throughout the brain and the body. For this reason, international standards exist for the design of electromedical equipment such as MEG/EEG systems and their accessories. These standards ensure that, should the equipment become faulty, no harm will occur to the person connected to the device. The specific danger is not from the voltage but from the current passing through the body.

For brief (< 1 ms) DC pulses (such as those used in electrical somatosensory stimulation), the sensory threshold is about 1 mA and the pain threshold about 5 to 10 mA. AC is more dangerous than DC current because even tiny AC currents less than 10 mA can cause tetanic muscle contractions so that the person cannot open her or his hand and let go of a wire that is delivering the hazardous current. An AC current of 60 to 100 mA may be lethal as it may cause ventricular fibrillation; for DC currents, the threshold is 300 to 500 mA. These values apply to currents that pass through dry skin, say from a hand through the body to the (opposite) leg. If the hands are wet, skin impedance is much smaller, and the current delivered with the same voltage will be much higher.

Other consequences of unintended current flows include tissue heating and burning. For this reason, international safety standards (such as those of the International Electrotechnical Commission; https://www.iec.ch/homepage) for electromedical equipment dictate maximum leakage currents in microamperes (μA) through the person. The specified currents are small because the electromedical equipment may be used on patients during surgical procedures when the currents can find very low-resistance pathways through an open body cavity. In these cases, the current required to create ventricular fibrillation is lower than the milliampere-range currents we mentioned for skin-to-skin shock in an intact body.

It is thus important to understand what makes a current "like" to go through a person. The Ohm's and Kirchoff's laws indicate that the current always flows from higher to lower voltage (like water in a river) and divides proportionately according to the resistances of different possible paths. Thus, theoretically, we could hold (although we should never intentionally do so) a high-voltage wire, such as a power line, *provided that* the current that has a possible entry point to the body will not have an exit point at a lower voltage (Figure 7.4, bottom panel). Otherwise lethal current will flow through the body, as would happen if our hand is on the wire and we stand on wet ground without isolation (Figure 7.4, top panel). People often wonder why birds that sit on high-voltage power-line cables do not die from electric shocks. The reason is that both their feet are at the same voltage, and the body thus does not offer a low-resistance pathway to the current (Figure 7.4, both panels).

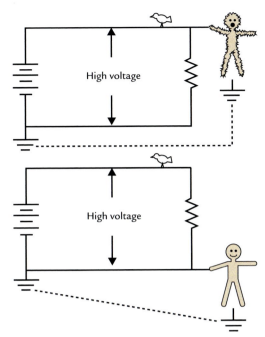

FIGURE 7.4. **Electrical safety and potential of electrical shock.** Top: A human touches a high-voltage power line with one hand while standing on the ground, thereby providing a low-resistance path (the human body) for the current. Thus a strong (even fatal) current can travel through the body. In contrast, the bird on the wire has both its feet at the same potential and thus does not experience a shock. Bottom: Here the human is touching the ground line of the high voltage circuit while standing on the ground. Because there is no voltage difference between the subject's hand and foot contact points, no current will flow through the body. Adapted and reproduced with permission from *Lessons in Electric Circuits*, Chapter 3 (http://www.allaboutcircuits.com/textbook/direct-current/chpt-3/importance-electrical-safety/).

The potential for electric hazards increases when a number of different devices are connected to the subject. For example, in intensive care units or operating rooms the patient may be connected to a cardiac monitor as well as to an EEG machine and may be undergoing electrocauterization at the same time. In a research EEG laboratory, as well, subjects may be connected to an EEG machine and have peripheral electrical stimulation cables connected to them. (In the case of transcranial magnetic stimulation [TMS]–EEG studies, specialized EEG amplifiers that have been designed to work with TMS stimulation are used. Similar design concerns apply to specialized EEG systems that are used in an MRI environment.) Similarly, MEG/EEG recordings in metal-wall chambers are especially vulnerable to electric hazards.

These considerations emphasize the necessity of using isolation between the subject and all electric recording, stimulation, and monitoring equipment. Moreover, *the subject should be grounded only at one point* to avoid the possibility of dangerous currents flowing through the body. The EEG amplifiers, stimulators, and other electronic devices should be connected to medical-grade isolation transformers according to the specifications set by the manufacturer.

■ REFERENCES

Bonner AM, Davidson P: Infection prevention: 2020 review and update for neurodiagnostic technologists. *Neurodiagn J* 2020a, 60: 11–35.

Bonner AM, Davidson P: Technical tips: keeping it clean during COVID-19. *Neurodiagn J* 2020b, 60: 195–207.

Campanella S, Arikan K, Babiloni C, Balconi M, Bertollo M, Betti V, Bianchi L, Brunovsky M, Buttinelli C, Comani S, Di Lorenzo G, Dumalin D, Escera C, Fallgatter A, Fisher D, Giordano GM, Guntekin B, Imperatori C, Ishii R, . . . Pogarell O: Special report on the impact of the COVID-19 pandemic on clinical EEG and research and consensus recommendations for the safe use of EEG. *Clin EEG Neurosci* 2021, 52: 3–28.

Canadian Society of Clinical Neurophysiologists (CSCN); Canadian Association of Electroneurophysiology Technologists (CAET); Association of Electromyography Technologists of Canada (AETC); Board of Registration of Electromyography Technologists of Canada (BRETC), Canadian Board of Registration of Electroencephalograph Technologists (CBRET); Appendino JP, Baker SK, Chapman KM, Dykstra T, Hussein T, Jones ML, Mezei MM, Mirsattari SM, Ng M, Nikkel J, Obradovic V, Phan C, Robinson L, Scott A, Tellez-Zenteno J, Van Niekerk M, Venance S, Moore F: Practice guidelines for Canadian neurophysiology laboratories during the COVID-19 pandemic. *Can J Neurol Sci* 2021, 48: 25–30.

Davenport MS, Bruno MA, Iyer RS, Johnson AM, Herrera R, Nicola GN, Ortiz D, Pedrosa I, Policeni B, Recht MP, Willis M, Zuley ML, Weinstein S: ACR statement on safe resumption of routine radiology care during the coronavirus disease 2019 (COVID-19) pandemic. *J Am Coll Radiol* 2020, 17: 839–844.

Desai U, Kassardjian CD, Del Toro D, Gleveckas-Marten N, Srinivasan J, Venesy D, Narayanaswami P, the AANEM Quality and Patient Safety Committee: Guidance for resumption of routine electrodiagnostic testing during the COVID-19 pandemic. *Muscle Nerve* 2020, 62: 176–181.

Ferree TC, Luu P, Russell GS, Tucker DM: Scalp electrode impedance, infection risk, and EEG data quality. *Clin Neurophysiol* 2001, 112: 536–544.

Grippo A, Assenza G, Scarpino M, Broglia L, Cilea R, Galimberti CA, Lanzo G, Michelucci R, Tassi L, Vergari M, Di Lazzaro V, Mecarelli O; SINC, LICE, and AITN: Electroencephalography during SARS-CoV-2 outbreak: practical recommendations from the Task Force of the Italian Society of Neurophysiology (SINC), the Italian League Against Epilepsy (LICE), and the Italian Association of Neurophysiology Technologists (AITN). *Neurol Sci* 2020, 41: 2345–2351.

Gross J, Baillet S, Barnes GR, Henson RN, Hillebrand A, Jensen O, Jerbi K, Litvak V, Maess B, Oostenveld R, Parkkonen L, Taylor JR, van Wassenhove V, Wibral M, Schoffelen JM: Good practice for conducting and reporting MEG research. *NeuroImage* 2013, 65: 349–363.

Haines S, Caccamo A, Chan F, Galaso G, Catinchi A, Gupta PK: Practical considerations when performing neurodiagnostic studies on patients with COVID-19 and other highly virulent diseases. *Neurodiagn J* 2020, 60: 78–95.

Hasson U, Yang E, Vallines I, Heeger D, Rubin N: A hierarchy of temporal receptive windows in human cortex. *J Neurosci* 2008, 28: 2539–2550.

Hill RM, Boto E, Rea M, Holmes N, Leggett J, Coles LA, Papastavrou M, Everton SK, Hunt BAE, Sims D, Osborne J, Shah V, Bowtell R, Brookes MJ: Multi-channel whole-head OPM-MEG: helmet design and a comparison with a conventional system. *NeuroImage* 2020, 219: 116995.

Homölle S, Oostenveld R: Using a structured-light 3D scanner to improve EEG source modeling with more accurate electrode positions. *J Neurosci Methods* 2019, 326: 108378.

Koessler L, Benhadid A, Maillard L, Vignal JP, Felblinger J, Vespignani H, Braun M: Automatic localization and labeling of EEG sensors (ALLES) in MRI volume. *NeuroImage* 2008, 41: 914–923.

Lehtonen JB, Lehtinen I: Alpha rhythm and uniform visual field in man. *Electroencephalogr Clin Neurophysiol* 1972, 32: 139–147.

Mosher JC, Funke ME: Towards best practices in clinical magnetoencephalography: patient preparation and data acquisition. *Clin Neurophysiol* 2020, 37: 498–507.

Pernet P, Garrido M, Gramfort A, Maurits N, Michel C, Pang E, Salmelin R, Schoffelen JM, Valdés-Sosa PA, Puce A: Best practices in data analysis and sharing in neuroimaging using MEEG. White paper 2018, https://osf.io/a8dhx/

Pernet P, Garrido M, Gramfort A, Maurits N, Michel C, Pang E, Salmelin R, Schoffelen JM, Valdés-Sosa PA, Puce A: Issues and recommendations from the OHBM COBIDAS MEEG committee for reproducible EEG and MEG research. *Nat Neurosci* 2020, 23: 1473–1483.

Picton TW, Bentin S, Berg P, Donchin E, Hillyard SA, Johnson R Jr, Miller GA, Ritter W, Ruchkin DS, Rugg MD, Taylor MJ: Guidelines for using human event-related potentials to study cognition: recording standards and publication criteria. *Psychophysiology* 2000, 37: 127–152.

Putnam LE, Johnson R Jr, Roth WT: Guidelines for reducing the risk of disease transmission in the psychophysiology laboratory. SPR Ad Hoc Committee on the Prevention of Disease Transmission. *Psychophysiology* 1992, 29: 127–141.

Russell GS, Jeffrey Eriksen K, Poolman P, Luu P, Tucker DM: Geodesic photogrammetry for localizing sensor positions in dense-array EEG. *Clin Neurophysiol* 2005, 116: 1130–1140.

Sakudo A, Ano Y, Onodera T, Nitta K, Shintani H, Ikuta K, Tanaka Y: Fundamentals of prions and their inactivation (review). *Int J Mol Med* 2011, 27: 483–489.

San-Juan D, Jiménez CR, Camilli CX, de la Cruz Reyes LA, Galindo EGA, Burbano GER, Penela MM, Perassolo MB, Valdéz AT, Godoy JG, Moreira AL, Kimaid PAT: Guidance for clinical neurophysiology examination throughout the COVID-19 pandemic. Latin American chapter of the IFCN Task Force–COVID-19. *Clin Neurophysiol* 2020, 131: 1589–1598.

Zetter R, Iivanainen J, Parkkonen L: Optical co-registration of MRI and on-scalp MEG. *Sci Rep* 2019, 9: 5490.

CHAPTER 8

DATA ACQUISITION, PREPROCESSING, AND SHARING

Every portrait that is painted with feeling is a portrait of the artist, not of the sitter.

OSCAR WILDE

Don't ever think that just because you do things differently, you're wrong.

GAIL TSUKIYAMA

FILTERING

MEG and EEG signals are recorded in analog form (as continuous-value signals), which, after proper amplification, need to be filtered to remove undesirable signal components with lower and higher frequencies relative to the signals of interest. The amplified analog signals then need to be transformed to digital form by data sampling (also called digitization or analog-to-digital conversion). To avoid the problem of aliasing, a very serious signal distortion that we describe later in this chapter, some filtering is *always* performed by analog circuitry in EEG/MEG equipment before the signal is digitized (see Chapter 5). Filtering can have dramatic effects on the data. Below we first discuss common types of filters and show their response characteristics before presenting examples of their effects on MEG/EEG signals.

Figure 8.1 displays the four main types of filters: low-pass, high-pass, band-pass, and band-stop (notch) filters. A low-pass filter will only pass, or allow, frequencies *below* a certain frequency. Conversely, a high-pass filter will only pass frequencies *above* a specified frequency. Low- and high-pass filters are typically used together to form band-pass filters that allow a desired range of frequencies, called a passband, to pass through the filter. A notch, or band-stop, filter will cut out activity in a particular narrow frequency range (e.g., around 50 Hz or 60 Hz) to eliminate power-line noise. Notch filters, however, produce discontinuities in the power spectrum of the MEG/EEG signal and hence should be used only if no other alternatives are available for reducing an unwanted signal and if signals of interest, such as gamma activity, do not occupy this frequency band. We discuss the respective low- and high-pass frequency limits for different filters later.

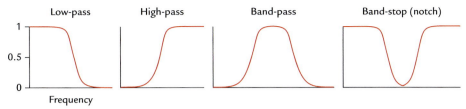

FIGURE 8.1. **Responses of different types of filters to signals of different frequencies.** The y-axis represents the signal in proportion to its maximum and the x-axis represents frequency. The low-pass filter passes only frequencies below a certain frequency (its "low-pass" frequency), whereas the high-pass filter passes frequencies above its "high-pass" frequency. A band-pass filter is a combination of low- and high-pass filters. A band-stop (or notch) filter attenuates activity over a narrow frequency range. Note that no filter is ideal in the sense that it would not attenuate any signals beyond its desired passband.

Analog high-pass and low-pass filters are essentially electric circuits consisting of resistors and capacitors. Hence they are called RC circuits. An RC circuit has a time constant, τ, which is the product of the resistance (in ohms) and capacitance (in farads). The time constant is expressed in seconds and indicates the time within which the signal returns to $1/e$ ($1/2.72$, i.e., 37%) of the original value following a transient input. The cut-off frequency, f, and τ are related so that $τ = 1/(2\pi f)$. For example, for $f = 0.1$ Hz signals to pass (relatively) unaffected through the filter, the time constant needs to be at least $1/(2\pi\ 0.1) = 1.6$ s.

Figure 8.2 illustrates the time constant principle in a square wave signal that has been passed through two types of filter. When a square-wave pulse (upper left panel) is fed to the high-pass circuit, the output shows a transient at the onset of the pulse and a similar transient but of opposite polarity at the offset of the pulse (middle left panel). After each transient the signal returns toward zero with time-constant-dependent decay τ. In contrast, a low-pass filter smooths and slows both the rising and decaying ends of the input square-wave pulse (lower left panel) with a time-constant-dependent rise and fall time.

In some cases, where very slow brain activity needs to be measured either to lengthy stimuli or in anticipation of stimuli or motor responses (see Chapter 17), direct current (DC) coupling may be used. In this context, DC refers to the absence of high-pass filtering (the time constant of the analog filtering circuit is effectively infinite so that the high-pass "cut-off" setting is 0 Hz), allowing ultraslow MEG/EEG signals to be recorded (see Chapter 5). As expected, with this type of recording set-up the amplifiers are more prone to drift, and slow artifacts may arise.

Each analog filter has a typical "roll-off characteristic" that describes how quickly activity is attenuated near the cut-off frequency as a function of frequency. Even though a filter is set to cut out activity beyond a particular frequency, say 40 Hz, the cut-off is never abrupt and some frequencies just below and just above the filter limit will still be present, but will drop, or roll off, at a particular rate.

Filter roll-off characteristics are usually expressed in units of dB/decade (a decade is the frequency range during which the frequency changes by a factor of 10), and they are calculated by taking the logarithm of the gain (ratio of output versus input voltage) as a function of signal frequency. Figure 8.3 schematically depicts a low-pass filter with a designated cut-off frequency of Fc (LP) and filter roll-off of 20 dB/decade. Note that frequencies just below Fc (LP), in the "passband," will also be attenuated (see –3 dB to 0 dB range

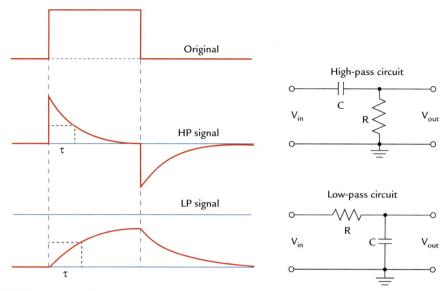

FIGURE 8.2. Modification of a square-wave pulse by analogue high-pass (HP) and low-pass (LP) filters consisting of resistor and capacitor circuits. Left: An original square-wave signal (top) fed through a HP filter (middle) loses its slow part and only the transients associated with the onset and offset of the square wave are maintained. The transients decay with a speed determined by the filter's time constant, τ, where τ = RC. Note that the transient at the offset goes negative (below the baseline) although the input signal had only positive values. In contrast, a LP filter (bottom) smooths the sharp onset and offset transients so that the signal both rises and decays slowly, again determined by the filter's time constant, τ. Right: Schematic diagrams showing the analog HP (top) and LP (bottom) filters, comprised of resistor and capacitor components (R and C, respectively); V_{in} and V_{out} refer to the input and output voltages of the circuit, respectively. The behaviors of these circuits may be more easily understood if one remembers that the capacitors pass high rather than low frequencies more easily. Thus, in the high-pass circuit, the high frequencies pass more easily than the low frequencies through the capacitor on the upper input line. In contrast, in the low-pass circuit, they more easily pass through the capacitor connected to ground.

of Figure 8.3). In the "stopband," frequencies higher than Fc (LP) have still been passed through the filter although clearly attenuated.

Typically, clinical EEG recordings are performed with band-pass filtering from 0.3 to 70 Hz, whereas in research settings where there may be interest in high-gamma activity as well, the band is often opened to, for example, 0.1 to 200 Hz, of course strictly depending on the signals of interest. Figure 8.4 illustrates the effects of applying different post hoc digital high- and low-pass filter settings to an EEG signal (trace 1). As the low-pass frequency is progressively decreased, the signal begins to lose its higher frequency components, or "fuzziness" (traces 2–4). Then as the low-pass frequency is progressively increased (traces 5–7), the lower frequencies in the signal are progressively flattened out.

Filter use has its pitfalls. Too narrow a filter may distort the MEG/EEG data because of *ringing*, which is artificial oscillations that occur around the filter's cut-off frequencies. Ringing can become very serious if the MEG/EEG passband is made too narrow (say, less than 4 Hz), which can be a problem for the narrow 50 or 60 Hz (notch) power-line-noise

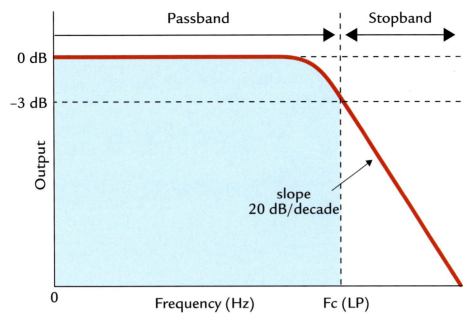

FIGURE 8.3. A low-pass filter and its roll-off slope. Output in decibels (dB) is plotted as a function of signal frequency, with the frequency passband shown with blue shading. The cutoff frequency of the low-pass (LP) filter Fc is shown at the –3-dB point. Note that above Fc there can still be a substantial amount of signal, and that in the immediate frequency range below Fc the signal amplitude already begins falling (from 0 dB). In this example, the filter roll-off is 20 dB/decade. A corresponding behavior will be seen for high-pass filters at their respective Fc.

filters. Such narrow filtering can also generate oscillatory activity from sharp transitions or discontinuities in the data. Similar problems can occur in both analog *and* digital (post hoc) filters.

Figure 8.5 demonstrates the consequences of using too narrow a filter on simulated MEG evoked-response data. The left panel depicts the activation time course of a current dipole in the auditory cortex 100 ms after sound onset. The original simulated response had a monophasic waveform (gray trace in the left panel) and a good dipolar spatial pattern (upper row of maps; compare with Figure 1.2). After heavy high-pass filtering (here at 6 Hz), the signal strength, as measured by the dipole moment, is decreased to almost half, and additional deflections of opposite polarity appear both before and after the main deflection (black trace in the left panel, Figure 8.5). Alarmingly, the field patterns now are dipolar also during these "ghosts" and look so "physiological" that one may think that the brain has really responded in this kind of triphasic manner (right lower maps). These real-looking ghosts may mislead the researcher into believing that the signal in a certain brain area has started much earlier than it has. In real ERP/ERF recordings, high-pass-filter cut-offs above 0.1 Hz distort the responses and are not recommended (Acunzo et al., 2012).

In the "40-Hz boom" of the 1990s, many MEG/EEG researchers applied very narrow filtering as they wished to visualize 40-Hz activity. It is quite likely, however, that not all these studies reported only 40-Hz brain activity but rather included filtering-generated oscillations due to sharp transitions in the data. Additionally, other physiological artifacts

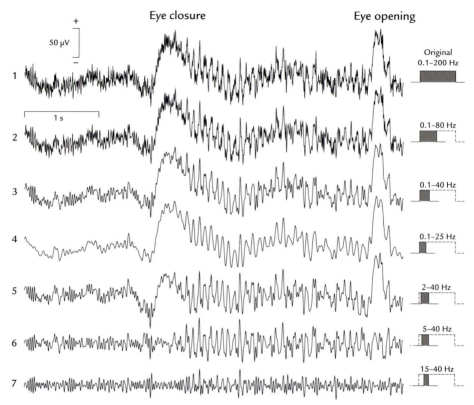

FIGURE 8.4. Effects of different filter settings on an EEG trace (Cz – average reference). A 5-s EEG recording (trace 1) was acquired with a passband of 0.1 to 200 Hz (sampling rate 500 Hz). In the traces below, the same EEG trace has been subjected to various post hoc digital filters. Traces 2 to 4 show the effects of decreasing low-pass frequency. Traces 5 to 7 depict the effects of increasing high-pass frequency. The filtering passband, relative to the original, is shown schematically at right. During the recorded epoch, the subject initially had the eyes open, and muscle artifact dominated the recording. Then she closed her eyes, which caused as a slow ocular artifact, followed by prominent alpha rhythm. At the end of the trace, the subject opened her eyes, with an associated ocular artifact. Data recorded in the Dual EEG Laboratory, Imaging Research Facility, Indiana University, USA.

can mar activity at these higher frequencies, and this is a real problem if they are only partially filtered out (see Chapter 9).

A filter can distort the signals also by delaying or advancing them, thereby causing latency and phase shifts. The amount of phase shift in the filtered data will vary as a function of frequency (similar to amplitude decreasing as a function of the filter's roll-off characteristic, see Figure 8.3). Importantly, in the time domain this will translate as latency shifts in event-related responses or in time–frequency plots, or as phase differences in frequency and coherence analyses, and it will also affect calculations of cross-frequency coupling of brain rhythms. Specifically, latency or phase lags can occur at low-pass filtering, and latency or phase leads can occur at high-pass filtering (Nilsson et al., 1993). This problem is not exclusive to analog circuitry and can also occur with digital filters used during data analysis. Most of these confounding effects can be avoided by post-hoc digital filters that do

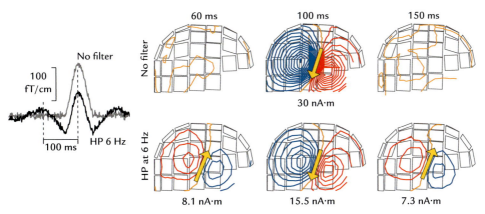

FIGURE 8.5. Effect of severe high-pass (HP) filtering on a simulated MEG response and associated field patterns. Left: The original simulated "auditory response" (gray trace); the signal starts flat and then has a monophasic deflection peaking at 100 ms. The black trace depicts the waveform (with some noise) after it has been heavily HP filtered at 6 Hz. Right: Magnetic field patterns shown at 60, 100, and 150 ms; the isocontour lines show the strength of the magnetic field in increments of 40 fT. The top row shows the patterns for the original signal, with a nice dipolar pattern at the peak of the signal at 100 ms; the arrow indicates the current dipole that best explains this pattern. At 60 and 150 ms the patterns show just noise. The bottom row shows the magnetic field patterns for the HP filtered signals. The strength of the source has decreased to almost half of the original amplitude (middle map), and this main response is both preceded and followed by dipolar field patterns of considerable strength, with current dipoles that adequately explain the patterns. Reproduced and modified with permission from Hari R: Magnetoencephalography: Methods and Clinical Aspects. In: Schomer DL and Lopes da Silva FH: *Niedermeyer's Electroencephalography: Basic Principles, Clinical Applications, and Related Fields.* 7th edition. New York: Oxford University Press, 2018.

not induce phase shifts, such as "acausal" filters that are run twice over the data—first in a forward and second in a reverse direction, thereby canceling any introduced time shifts (Acunzo et al., 2012). Still one has to be careful to apply the filters properly and check with test data, for example, that the filtered signals do not seem to move either forward or backward in time. For a discussion of pitfalls of filters in neurophysiological applications, see, for example, Widmann et al. (2015) and Yael et al. (2018).

Even with the best filters, phase shifts must be carefully examined whenever the response latency is essential for data interpretation. For example, in trying to find out the exact time when the earliest afferent input reaches the cortex, the properties of the applied filters should be controlled carefully (Ramkumar et al., 2013). One relatively easy way to do this is to apply square-wave inputs to the system to see how the selected filter modifies these well-defined signals (as already shown in Figure 8.2).

Given that the frequency range of the spontaneous MEG/EEG signal typically varies from 0 to 100 Hz, the scientific question or the data-analysis plan may dictate what filter settings are chosen for the recording. As digital filtering options are also available post hoc, it is useful to use a wider passband for the initial recording, say 0.01 to 200 Hz, so that phase shifts are not induced in the frequency ranges of interest in the raw data. This strategy would be useful for most visual, auditory, and somatosensory evoked responses as well (but see Chapters 13 and 15 for some exceptions where a wider passband is needed). At the analysis stage, a digital passband such as 0.1 to 40 Hz (to avoid line-frequency contamination) might be used as the final filtering cut. However, if one is interested in slow activity (such as sustained potentials/fields during long stimuli or slow baseline shifts during epileptic seizures) or in higher-frequency spontaneous or evoked activity in the gamma range, the recording passband needs to be adjusted accordingly.

The disadvantage of using too wide a passband at data acquisition is the large size of data files as a consequence of the necessary higher sampling frequencies (see next section). For example, to be recorded reliably, head-movement corrections in MEG data may require a recording passband of wider than 300 Hz and data digitization rates in the order of 1 kHz. However, the data can be down-sampled later.

With today's artifact-rejection software options, it is important to not only record the MEG/EEG signals of interest but to also capture unwanted (non-MEG/EEG) signal components more fully. In this way, software artifact rejection routines and/or additional digital filtering can identify and separate the wanted and unwanted signals more effectively. For example, too low a high-pass cut-off will cause artifacts due to electrical stimuli to spread in time so that they can mask short-latency brain responses. Thus other strategies must be used, such as not recording data for the duration of the artifact (e.g., for 5 ms) at all or recording signals at the acquisition phase with such a wide band that the stimulus artifacts remain brief and can be removed by setting the signal to equal zero for that time. In multimodal neuroimaging studies where EEG is recorded during fMRI scanning and/or TMS/tDCS stimulation, the filtering should not alter the appearance the large artifacts caused by stimulation and fMRI data acquisition, and it should not spread them in time. Otherwise even the best artifact-removal software will not abolish the artifacts, which if not dealt with will dwarf or completely hide the EEG signals. Filtering should not spread the large stimulation or fMRI data-acquisition artifacts to completely dwarf the EEG signal. These approaches are discussed, together with these artifacts, in Chapter 9.

Additional constraints that require an increase in filtering passband might occur from planned analyses, such as time–frequency analysis using wavelet-based decomposition. It is for this reason that it is always best to keep the measurement bandwidth wide at data acquisition and to limit the passband with post hoc filtering as needed. It is impossible to recover low- or high-frequency activity that has been filtered out during data acquisition. Disk space is inexpensive and worth the investment.

The choice of filtering passband has an intimate relationship with data sampling rate, which we discuss next.

■ DATA SAMPLING RATE

Amplification and analog-to-digital (AD) conversion in electronic circuits typically rescales signals to better match a dynamic range of 5 V (because the so-called transistor–transistor-logic circuits operate at voltage levels from 0 to 5 V). However, in some systems, alternative ranges might be used. Because of their small size, the MEG and EEG signals must be amplified by many orders of magnitude so that they can be adequately digitized without losing information for storage and subsequent processing. If the converted signals are too small, they use only a part of the dynamic range of the AD converter and thereby could have only a few possible discrete values. On the other hand, for some applications, such as ambulatory EEG and simultaneous EEG performed with fMRI or TMS, using only a part of the dynamic range for the brain signals could allow the entire signal (including prominent non-brain artifacts) to be recorded without "clipping" (i.e., the signal going beyond the dynamical range of the AD converter). Thus artifacts could be more easily identified and removed during data analysis. In these cases, the dynamic range of the amplifier naturally has to be large enough to provide adequate amplitude resolution for both brain and non-brain signals.

The resolution of an AD converter is expressed in bits, indicating how many different values the digitized signal can have, provided that the whole dynamic range is used. An 8-bit AD converter allows the distinction of $2^8 = 256$ different amplitude levels, a 12-bit converter 4,096 different levels, and a 16-bit converter 65,536 levels. If, for example, the signals were amplified so that the full dynamic range could cover 2 pT (= 2000 fT) for MEG and 2 mV (= 2000 μV) for EEG, a 12-bit AD converter would allow quantification in steps of ~0.5 fT and ~0.5 μV. When better resolution is needed, one should use an AD converter with more digitization steps or amplify the signal so that the full dynamic range is used.

Digitization (temporal sampling) rate determines the highest signal frequency that can be collected undistorted. According to the so-called Nyquist sampling criterion, the sampling frequency has to be *at least twice* the highest frequency in the data (at the absolute minimum), so that all frequencies of the signal can be accurately sampled. However, considerably higher sampling rates facilitate the accurate reproduction of signal shape.

That said, consideration should also be given to the particular MEG/EEG system analog filter roll-off characteristics before digitization, as these will determine the highest possible frequencies in the signal and allow a suitable data-acquisition rate to be chosen; if the slope is very shallow, the Nyquist frequency that allows the signals to be sampled without distortion may be considerably higher than the filter's low-pass cut-off frequency. We again emphasize that data should be sampled only after appropriate low-pass filtering of the original analog signal has occurred.

Aliasing (which literally means that different signals become indistinguishable from another) is effectively a distortion of the data, where a sampled signal may appear to have a completely different form compared with the actual measured signal, appearing to contain frequency components that are not really there. Aliasing can occur if the data (desired MEG or EEG signals, or artifacts) are sampled at a frequency that is too low, as is evident from Figure 8.6. The original signal (Figure 8.6, leftmost panel) can be rendered to be unrecognizable at sampling rates of less than twice the signal's frequency.

A clear everyday visual example of aliasing is the apparent backward movement of wagon wheels in old Western movies. The phenomenon arises when the time between successive film frames (changing at a 24-Hz rate) is longer than the time needed for the spoke of a wagon wheel to rotate to the position of the preceding spoke.

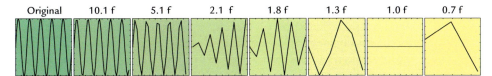

| Original | 10.1 f | 5.1 f | 2.1 f | 1.8 f | 1.3 f | 1.0 f | 0.7 f |

FIGURE 8.6. The phenomenon of aliasing. An original sinusoidal signal (leftmost panel) with frequency f was sampled at various digitization rates indicated relative to f. At frequencies above the Nyquist frequency (panels with sampling rates of 10.1 f, 5.1 f, and 2.1 f), the frequency content of the signal is preserved although the amplitude shows modulation compared with the original signal. At sampling rates below the Nyquist frequency, *aliased* signals with different frequencies emerge (all other panels). At a sampling rate equal to the original signal frequency, only a DC level will be seen (second panel from the right); the level would vary in value depending on when during the cycle the signal is being sampled.

In most MEG/EEG recordings, sampling at 500 Hz to 1 kHz (2 ms or 1 ms between data points) might be used with a low-pass filters set at 100 to 200 Hz. Higher low-pass filters might be appropriate, depending on the filter roll off. Other types of specialized recordings, such as brainstem evoked responses, require much wider recording bands (higher low-pass-filter settings) and accordingly higher sampling rates (see Chapters 13–15).

▪ SIMULATION OF EEG AND MEG DATA

Given the various issues noted with filtering and data sampling, it is useful to carefully scrutinize the entire pipeline from data acquisition to analysis using test data with known characteristics. Re-test is necessary if any part of the pipeline is changed. For data acquisition, signals with known characteristics can be inserted into the MEG/EEG sampling circuits. For this purpose, phantoms can be used (see Chapter 6). If this option is not available, a battery-operated signal generator can be connected to the EEG acquisition system to introduce sine and square-wave waveforms of known frequencies so that the effects of online filtering and of the AD input range can be visualized.

For data preprocessing or analysis phases, one may create artificial signals consisting of sinusoidal waveforms embedded in filtered colored noise (Puce et al., 1994). More recently, simulation packages, such as SEREEGA (Krol et al., 2018) and EEGSourceSim (Barzegaran et al., 2019), have become available for analyses that range from simple preprocessing steps to more complex source modeling procedures. For MEG, some groups have used simulated signals since the 1980s; for example, the evoked response MEG waveforms and field patterns of Figure 8.5 were generated by the manufacturer's simulation software.

▪ STANDARDIZATION OF DATA FORMATS AND ANALYSIS PIPELINES FOR DATA SHARING

Over the last decade, the culture of open science and multimodal data sharing has really strengthened in the neuroimaging community. At the same time, multiple big-data initiatives have emerged to advance both basic and clinical research. These large-scale efforts also include brain modeling and "in silico" simulation of some brain functions (e.g., the European Blue Brain and Human Brain Projects, and US Human Connectome and [privately-owned] Allen Institute initiatives). But the benefits of such large-scale "industrialized neuroscience" have also been questioned. Big data might not strictly be considered as knowledge per se, and they should be strategically developed in neuroscience within the context of appropriate progress in conceptual and theoretical understanding (see, e.g., Frégnac, 2017).

Big-data repositories coupled with high-capacity, cloud-based analysis platforms serve as sandboxes for the development and comparison of new analysis methods, and they also provide training material on experimental design and analysis. Large clinical data sets aid the search for biomarkers of various diseases, particularly in rare disorders where one research team or one country alone cannot collect a sufficient amount of data.

For the purposes of data and software sharing, data should follow agreed-on standardized file formats. Standardization is also highly beneficial in reading and writing publications and grant applications as many details can be omitted. In all instances, investigators should follow the current best-practice guidelines for data gathering and analysis (see, e.g., Picton et al., 2000; Duncan et al., 2009; Bagić et al., 2011; Jobert et al., 2012; Gross et al., 2013; Keil et al., 2014; Kane et al., 2017; Nichols et al., 2017; Hari et al., 2018; Pernet et al., 2020). These guidelines help generate best practices, design reproducible and replicable experiments, and more recently facilitate data sharing using an open-science approach (Niso et al., 2018).

The big data initiatives containing MEG data include (but are not limited to) the US-based Human Connectome Project (Larson-Prior et al., 2013), the UK-based Cam-CAN study (Cambridge Centre for Ageing Neuroscience) (Taylor et al., 2017), and the Canada-based Open MEG Archive (Omega) (Niso et al., 2016). Clinical scalp EEGs are available (e.g., Temple University Hospital; Obeid & Picone, 2016). Other sources of shared EEG data are available and will certainly increase in the future.

Brain Imaging Data Standard, BIDS

The Brain Imaging Data Standard (BIDS; see https://bids.neuroimaging.io/ and https://github.com/bids-standard/bids-specification) is a specification for how to organize neuroimaging data in a standardized manner in terms of data hierarchies, common directory and filenames, as well as documentation of experimental parameters (e.g., behavioral data logs, etc.) and metadata (including details of experimental tasks and data-recording systems). The first major effort in this direction was a grassroots working group for MRI file formats (Gorgolewski et al., 2016), where the comprehensive (parent) BIDS standard for structural and fMRI data was written based on the formats used in the open-science data repository OpenNeuro (https://openneuro.org/); MRI-BIDS also took into account the characteristics of many existing neuroimaging databases and the needs of various stakeholders, some of whom have now made open data a prerequisite of research funding or manuscript submission.

More recently, multiple BIDS daughter standards have emerged for electrophysiological data: MEG-BIDS (Niso et al., 2018), EEG-BIDS (Pernet et al., 2019), and invasive iEEG-BIDS (Holdgraf et al., 2019).

At the time of writing, the work continues to include eye tracking and other physiological recordings, as well as derivative standards for analyzed data.

A Bird's-Eye View of a Standardized Data Set Structure

Below we give an overview of the structure of a standardized BIDS data set, but researchers should always check current file-type specifications from recent BIDS-related publications and Github repositories with community-driven guides, tutorials, helper scripts, and Wiki resources available in MATLAB and Python. Users can also test new code on a set of empty data set files, and original data files may also be downloaded from multiple data sets.

File standards for MEG, EEG, and iEEG are fully compatible with the parent BIDS standard with which they share a number of common data descriptors, including Subject, Session, Technique, and Run. BIDS supports storage of stimulus files (including video) and annotations of events via a hierarchical event-descriptor extension. Specific metadata elements can be reported with the widely used JavaScript Object Notation (*.json*) and Tab Separated Value (*.tsv*) text file formats (shown in Figures 8.7 and 8.8).

Figure 8.7 displays the hierarchical directory structure for a typical MEG data set (which can also contain embedded EEG, EOG, and ECG data). The main "umbrella" structure that repeats itself is the subject directory, housing all related files of an individual across recording sessions. Each session directory will contain behavioral data, MRI data (anatomy), sensor digitization information and associated photos, event files, and the neurophysiological data themselves. Additional descriptor files (in *.csv* and *.json* formats) include lists of subject demographics, stimulus events, and experimental parameters. An identical hierarchy exists

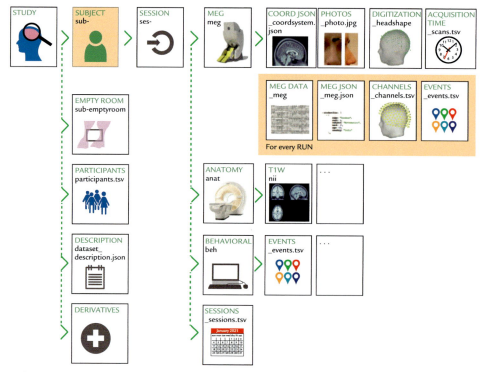

FIGURE 8.7. MEG data set: BIDS-compatible overall directory structure, generic filenames and file types. Schematic of directory tree (with directory attributes printed in uppercase green text and directory names in lowercase black text) showing the various data elements associated with an MEG study. The main study level contains a number of metadata elements (second column of icons) and a subject directory. This latter structure is repeated across all individuals in the study and contains a subdivision by "session." Further subdirectories include the MEG data itself and associated anatomical and behavioral data. MEG-BIDS associates all recordings with anatomical fiducial locations stored in a dedicated field of the MRI *.json* file, irrespective of whether source modeling will be performed in the data analysis pipeline. See main text for additional explanation. Reproduced with permission from Springer-Nature: Niso G, Gorgolewski KJ, Bock E, Brooks TL, Flandin G, Gramfort A, Henson RN, Jas M, Litvak V. Moreau JT, Oostenveld R, Schoffelen J-M, Tadel F, Wexler J, Baillet S: MEG-BIDS, the brain imaging data structure extended to magnetoencephalography. *Scientific Data* 2018, 5: 180110.

for EEG and iEEG data sets—with some differences. For example, MEG studies may contain empty room recordings, and iEEG studies may have intraoperative photos and CT (X-ray computerized tomography) and structural MRI volumes of implanted electrodes. Some studies may or may not have source localization information. Figure 8.8 displays some of the specific directory trees for a typical EEG data set, as well as the filenames (left column) and the contents of the various file types with associated variable names and exemplars in the "eeg" subdirectory (right column).

Multiple MEG/EEG software packages offer BIDS conversion tools/utilities, typically to be used at the time when data are being imported into the package for the first time.

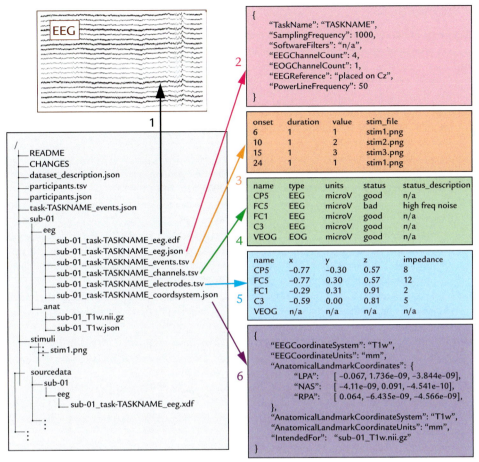

FIGURE 8.8. EEG data set: BIDS-compatible overall directory structure, generic filenames and file types, variable names, and exemplars. Bottom left: The light gray-shaded rectangle shows the BIDS directory tree and filenames for the various data types that are associated with an EEG data set that includes the EEG data itself (eeg directory), MRI-based anatomy (anat), and associated stimuli (for activation task studies). The contents of the six files of the "eeg" directory are revealed in the colored rectangles, numbered 1–6: 1 = raw EEG data; 2 = associated metadata; 3 = "events.tsv" file specifying all events occurring during recording session, referencing presented stimuli in the "stimuli" directory; 4 = "channels.tsv" file containing additional information about the raw EEG data, such as, filter settings and channel status (good/bad); 5 = "electrodes.tsv" file providing electrode locations; and 6 = "coordsystem.json" file providing the respective coordinate framework specification for interpreting electrode locations (e.g., with respect to a T1-weighted MRI scan). See main text for additional explanation. Reproduced with permission from Springer-Nature: Pernet C, Appelhoff S, Gorgolewski K, Flandin G, Phillips C, Delorme A, Oostenveld R: EEG-BIDS, an extension to the brain imaging data structure for electroencephalography. *Scientific Data* 2019, 6: 103.

▪ REFERENCES

Acunzo DJ, MacKenzie G, van Rossum MCW: Systematic biases in early ERP and ERF components as a result of high-pass filtering. *J Neurosci Methods* 2012, 209: 212–218.

Bagić AI, Knowlton RC, Rose DF, Ebersole JS: ACMEGS Clinical Practice Guideline (CPG) Committee: American Clinical Magnetoencephalography Society Clinical Practice Guideline 3: MEG-EEG reporting. *J Clin Neurophysiol* 2011, 8: 362–363.

Barzegaran E, Bosse S, Kohler PJ, Norcia AM: EEGSourceSim: a framework for realistic simulation of EEG scalp data using MRI-based forward models and biologically plausible signals and noise. *J Neurosci Methods* 2019, 328: 108377.

Duncan CC, Barry RJ, Connolly JF, Fischer C, Michie PT, Näätänen R, Polich J, Reinvang I, Van Petten C. Event-related potentials in clinical research: guidelines for eliciting, recording, and quantifying mismatch negativity, P300, and N400. *Clin Neurophysiol* 2009, 120: 1883–1908.

Frégnac Y: Big data and the industrialization of neuroscience: A safe roadmap for understanding the brain? *Science* 2017, 358: 470–477.

Gorgolewski KJ, Auer T, Calhoun VD, Craddock RC, Das S, Duff EP, Flandin G, Ghosh SS, Glatard T, Halchenko YO, Handwerker DA, Hanke M, Keator D, Li X, Michael Z, Maumet C, Nichols BN, Nichols TE, Pellman J, . . . Poldrack RA: The brain imaging data structure, a format for organizing and describing outputs of neuroimaging experiments. *Scientific Data* 2016, 3: 160044.

Gross J, Baillet S, Barnes GR, Henson RN, Hillebrand A, Jensen O, Jerbi K, Litvak V, Maess B, Oostenveld R, Parkkonen L, Taylor JR, van Wassenhove V, Wibral M, Schoffelen JM: Good practice for conducting and reporting MEG research. *NeuroImage* 2013, 65: 349–363.

Hari R, Baillet S, Barnes G, Burgess R, Forss N, Gross J, Hämäläinen M, Jensen O, Kakigi R, Mauguiere F, Nakasato N, Puce A, Romani GL, Schnitzler A, Taulu S: IFCN-endorsed practical guidelines for clinical magnetoencephalography (MEG). *Clin Neurophysiol* 2018, 129: 1720–1747.

Holdgraf C, Appelhoff S, Bickel S, Bouchard K, D'Ambrosio S, David O, Devinsky O, Dichter B, Flinker A, Foster BL, Gorgolewski KJ, Groen I, Groppe D, Gunduz A, Hamilton L, Honey CJ, Jas M, Knight K, Lachaux J-P, . . . Hermes D: iEEG-BIDS, extending the Brain Imaging Data Structure specification to human intracranial electrophysiology. *Scientific Data* 2019, 6: 102.

Jobert M, Wilson FJ, Ruigt GS, Brunovsky M, Prichep LS, Drinkenburg WH; IPEG Pharmaco-EEG Guidelines Committee. Guidelines for the recording and evaluation of pharmaco-EEG data in man: the International Pharmaco-EEG Society (IPEG). *Neuropsychobiology* 2012, 66: 201–220.

Kane N, Acharya J, Benickzy S, Caboclo L, Finnigan S, Kaplan PW, Shibasaki H, Pressler R, van Putten MJAM: A revised glossary of terms most commonly used by clinical electroencephalographers and updated proposal for the report format of the EEG findings. Revision 2017. *Clin Neurophysiol Pract* 2017, 2: 170–185.

Keil A, Debener S, Gratton G, Junghofer M, Kappenman ES, Luck SJ, Luu P, Miller GA, Yee CM: Committee report: publication guidelines and recommendations for studies using electroencephalography and magnetoencephalography. *Psychophysiology* 2014, 51: 1–21.

Krol LR, Pawlitzki J, Lotte F, Gramann K, Zander TO: SEREEGA: simulating event-related EEG activity. *J Neurosci Methods* 2018, 309: 13–24.

Larson-Prior LJ, Oostenveld R, Della Penna S, Michalareas G, Prior F, Babajani-Feremi A, Schoffelen JM, Marzetti L, de Pasquale F, Di Pompeo F, Stout J, Woolrich M, Luo Q, Bucholz R, Fries P, Pizzella V, Romani GL, Corbetta M, Snyder AZ, Consortium WU-MH: Adding dynamics to the Human Connectome Project with MEG. *NeuroImage* 2013, 80: 190–201.

Nichols TE, Das S, Eickhoff SB, Evans AC, Glatard T, Hanke M, Kriegeskorte N, Milham MP, Poldrack RA, Poline J-B, Proal E, Thirion B, Van Essen DC, White T, Yeo BTT: Best practices in data analysis and sharing in neuroimaging using MRI. *Nat Neurosci* 2017, 20: 299–303.

Nilsson J, Panizza M, Hallett M: Principles of digital sampling of a physiologic signal. *Electroencephalogr Clin Neurophysiol* 1993, 89: 349–358.

Niso G, Rogers C, Moreau JT, Chen LY, Madjar C, Das S, Bock E, Tadel F, Evans AC, Jolicoeur P, Baillet S: OMEGA: the Open MEG Archive. *NeuroImage* 2016, 124: 1182–1187.

Niso G, Gorgolewski KJ, Bock E, Brooks TL, Flandin G, Gramfort A, Henson RN, Jas M, Litvak V., Moreau JT, Oostenveld R, Schoffelen J-M, Tadel F, Wexler J, Baillet S: MEG-BIDS, the brain imaging data structure extended to magnetoencephalography. *Scientific Data* 2018, 5: 180110.

Obeid I, Picone J: The Temple University Hospital EEG Data Corpus. *Front Neurosci* 2016, 10: 196.

Pernet C, Appelhoff S, Gorgolewski K, Flandin G, Phillips C, Delorme A, Oostenveld R: EEG-BIDS, an extension to the brain imaging data structure for electroencephalography. *Scientific Data* 2019, 6: 103.

Pernet C, Garrido MI, Gramfort A, Maurits N, Michel CM, Pang E, Salmelin R, Schoffelen JM, Valdés-Sosa PA, Puce A: Issues and recommendations from the OHBM COBIDAS MEEG Committee for Reproducible EEG and MEG Research. *Nat Neurosci* 2020, 23: 1473–1483.

Picton TW, Bentin S, Berg P, Donchin E, Hillyard SA, Johnson R, Jr., Miller GA, Ritter W, Ruchkin DS, Rugg MD, Taylor MJ: Guidelines for using human event-related potentials to study cognition: recording standards and publication criteria. *Psychophysiology* 2000, 37: 127–152.

Puce A, Berkovic SF, Cadusch PJ, Bladin PF: P3 latency jitter assessed using 2 techniques: I. Simulated data and surface recordings in normal subjects. *Electroencephalogr Clin Neurophysiol* 1994, 92: 352–364.

Ramkumar P, Jas M, Pannasch S, Hari R, Parkkonen L: Feature-specific information processing precedes concerted activation in human visual cortex. *J Neurosci* 2013, 33: 7691–7699.

Taylor JR, Williams N, Cusack R, Auer T, Shafto MA, Dixon M, Tyler LK, Cam C, Henson RN: The Cambridge Centre for Ageing and Neuroscience (Cam-CAN) data repository: structural and functional MRI, MEG, and cognitive data from a cross-sectional adult lifespan sample. *NeuroImage* 2017, 144: 262–269.

Widmann A, Schröger E, Maess B: Digital filter design for electrophysiological data—a practical approach. *J Neurosci Methods* 2015, 250: 34–46.

Yael D, Vecht JJ, Bar-Gad I: Filter-based phase shifts distort neuronal timing information. *eNeuro* 2018, 5: e0261–17.2018.

CHAPTER 9

ARTIFACTS

All that glitters is not gold, all that glows is not silver.

ANONYMOUS

Garbage in, garbage out.

WILLIAM D. MELLIN, 1957

■ INTRODUCTION

MEG and EEG measurements are prone to unwanted signals in the form of both biological and nonbiological artifacts. To prevent and remove these enemies of clean signals, it is most important to sample them adequately, recognize their waveforms and spatial distributions, and understand their generation mechanisms. *Prevention of artifacts is always preferable to removing or compensating for them post hoc during data analysis.* Thus the main rules in obtaining clean data have been to (a) prevent artifacts from occurring in the first place, (b) reject MEG/EEG epochs contaminated by artifacts, and (c) correct or remove the remaining artifacts by postprocessing.

In some cases, artifacts may resemble the MEG/EEG signals of interest, which may not only confuse experimenters at data acquisition but also make the removal difficult, or sometimes even impossible during post-processing. Figure 9.1 depicts such an example of a faux "EEG signal." A semisolid mixture of jelly and condensed milk was connected to a set of EEG electrodes and amplifiers; this setup was stimulated by Tatum et al. (2011). The ions in the jelly/condensed milk medium can carry currents and therefore generate potential differences between electrodes. The proof is in the pudding! Three channels of "spontaneous EEG" are displayed, together with power spectral peaks in the EEG frequency range and quite realistic profiles of wavelet-filtered low and higher frequency activity.

Asking subjects to generate artifacts deliberately at the start of the recording session (while they also watch their own signals or receive verbal feedback on the artifacts) may help minimize physiological nonbrain artifacts during the actual recording. These initial artifactual exemplars might also form training materials for individualized artifact-reduction algorithms. BCI (brain–computer interface) forays with machine learning (ML) algorithms often do not consider artifacts (see Müller-Putz et al., 2008; Lotte et al., 2018), but they could benefit from this provision of learning exemplars for ML to use for data pre- and

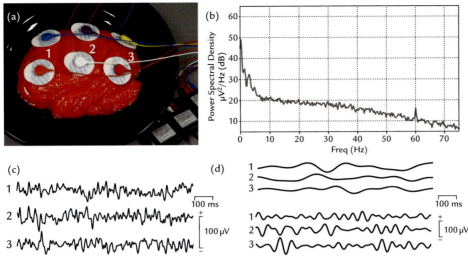

FIGURE 9.1. Non-physiological artifact. (a) A brain-shaped semi-solid mix of jelly/condensed milk has been connected to 3 differential amplifier inputs (channels 1, 2, 3) via wet Ag/AgCl electrodes (interelectrode impedances ~700 ohm, sampling frequency 500 Hz, passband 0.3–100 Hz, recording time of 2.5 min). The bowl was initially left untouched and then was briefly "jiggled" a couple of times to introduce some wobble in the sample and then was left to settle again before starting the recording. (b) Power-spectral density plot (from channel 1) displays a 1/f type distribution of "activity" with spectral peaks in the lower end of the EEG frequency range in the jelly/condensed milk mixture in its settled "resting state". A discrete peak of 60-Hz line noise is also visible. (c) A The recording displays "signal" of the mixture in its "resting state"; 1-s epoch of data (from all channels) presents a plausible "EEG signal". (d) Wavelet-filtered activity from the same epoch as in (c). Top 3 traces show activity in the 4–6 Hz range, whereas the bottom traces display activity in the 10–20 Hz range. Data recorded in the Social Neuroscience Laboratory, Indiana University, USA.

postprocessing (Chapter 10). Importantly, when the investigator continually monitors the subject and the recorded MEG/EEG signals during the experiment itself, some artifacts may be avoided by simply giving additional instructions to the subject between runs.

Physiological artifacts from the eyes, heart, and muscles arise because these organs also rely on electric signaling. These physiological currents can greatly interfere with MEG/EEG signals. In general, it is good to have—whenever possible—peripheral reference signals (e.g., electro-oculography [EOG], eye-gaze tracking, electrocardiogram, electromyogram, motion sensors) to better identify the suspected artifacts.

Table 9.1 lists some of these physiological artifacts and their typical amplitudes and frequencies relative to a typical EEG signal. Not only are these artifacts typically very much larger than the EEG signals, but also they may have overlapping frequency content. Portable EEG introduces additional challenges with abundant EMG contamination as the subjects move around, explore, and interact with their environment (discussed further in this chapter).

Nonphysiological MEG artifacts can arise from sources that are not in the subject's body but may be in the clothing, subject's chair, the stimulation and recording equipment, or even from outside the laboratory.

TABLE 9.1 Approximate amplitude and frequency contents of some common types of physiological signals

BODY PART	SIGNAL TYPE	FREQUENCY CONTENT	AMPLITUDE
Brain	Electroencephalogram (EEG)	0.5[a]–100 Hz	50–100 (500) µV
	Magnetoencephalogram (MEG)	0.5–100 Hz	2–500 fT
Heart	Electrocardiogram (ECG)	0.5–100 Hz	1 mV
	Magnetocardiogram (MCG)	0.5–100 Hz	2 pT
Muscle	Electromyogram (EMG)	10–5000[b] Hz	0.3–1 mV
	Magnetomyogram (MMG)	10–300 Hz	10 pT
Eyes	Electro-oculogram (EOG)	0–100 Hz	0.5–1 mV
	Magneto-oculogram (MOG)	0–100 Hz	2–5 pT

Note: Note the overlap in the main frequency content between EEG/MEG and other physiological signals and the large difference in amplitude between EEG/MEG and the other signals. The amplitudes are rough estimates. They can vary in different physiological and disease states and sensor locations, and they are especially dependent on the reference site (EEG) and the pickup coil configuration (MEG).

[a] This is the typical HP setting for clinical EEG, but if one is interested in, for example, sustained potentials, the high-pass filter may start from 0.03 Hz or one may even use direct coupling (DC). On the other hand, much higher EEG/MEG frequencies are often of interest.

[b] Note that these high EMG frequencies can only be picked up with needle electrodes directly inserted in the muscle. In surface EMG, the main frequency content is below 300 Hz.

One effective means to reduce artifacts is to use appropriate high-pass, low-pass, or bandpass filtering, *provided that the brain signals of interest are not in the same frequency band as the artifacts.* Otherwise, the EEG signals themselves would be diminished or abolished with the filtering.

A common procedure is to reject all artifact-containing epochs. This approach requires extra data to be collected at the outset to allow for a certain proportion of trials to be excluded from the subsequent analyses. Note, however, that if the artifacts are associated with certain brain states, this procedure may bias the results.

In this chapter, we describe the most commonly encountered artifacts and the ways to minimize them during data acquisition and to diminish their effect on the signals of interest during data analysis. We start with a brief overview of some frequently used artifact-removal and compensation methods (e.g., independent component analysis [ICA], canonical correlation analysis [CCA], signal-space separation [SSS], and signal-space projection [SSP]).

■ SOME COMMON ARTIFACT-REMOVAL METHODS

Blind Source Separation

"Blind" source separation refers to data-driven methods that attempt to separate a mixed signal into its separate components, or "sources," without considering any information about the sources themselves. Note that these sources do not refer to the neural current sources of MEG/EEG signals.

The most widely known blind source-separation method is ICA, which attempts to divide a set of mixed signals to components (sources) that are *independent* of each other in either time or space (Hyvärinen & Oja, 2000). Independence (ideally) means that knowing one of the components provides no information about the corresponding time courses (if the separation is performed in the time domain, "temporal ICA") or spatial distribution (if the separation is carried out in the spatial domain, "spatial ICA") of the other sources. The obtained independent components (ICs) will be either spatially or temporally uncorrelated, and their lack of correlation is implied by independence.

In ICA, the sources are separated without any information regarding the signals or the mixing process (Hipp & Siegel, 2013; Jonmohamadi et al., 2014). A classical and tangible example of the effective use of ICA is the separation of the voices of a number of speakers during a cocktail party (Figure 9.2) from the acoustic mix recorded using a number of microphones placed around the room (Bell & Sejnowski, 1995). Here the separation is based on the assumption that different voices are mixed linearly, which is also an appropriate assumption for MEG and EEG signals where N signal sources mix linearly to form an output that is recorded by a set of N sensors. The assumed number of sources is then equal to, or less than, the number of detectors (Brown et al., 2001). So, for example, for a 128-channel MEG/EEG recording, the maximum number of data projections, or ICs, would—in theory—be 128. However, the dimensionality of the analysis is reduced in advance, typically using principal component analysis (PCA) (Onton et al., 2006; Eichele

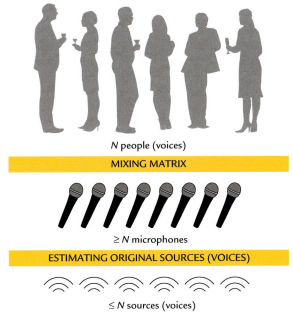

N people (voices)

MIXING MATRIX

$\geq N$ microphones

ESTIMATING ORIGINAL SOURCES (VOICES)

$\leq N$ sources (voices)

FIGURE 9.2. **The principle underlying ICA.** During a cocktail party, a set of N or fewer speakers will be talking at a given time. The collective speech signals are sampled by a set of at least N microphones that have been placed at different points around the room. The microphones constitute the mixing matrix. The individual sources corresponding to different speaker's voices can be extracted from the cocktail-party noise (summed output of all microphones) using an ICA algorithm. Note, however, that the transmission of signals is very different for sound and for MEG/EEG.

et al., 2011), as a large number of components can be unreliable in practice. On the other hand, a larger number of ICs may be more informative about the underlying physiology. For example, when ICA was applied with different numbers of components (dimensions) to an fMRI data set, hierarchically structured brain networks (e.g., somatosensory network, default network, and dorsal attention network) gradually fragmented into subnetworks when the dimensions were increased from 10 to 20 and 40 components (Pamilo et al., 2012).

As already noted, ICA assumes that source signals are statistically independent, which means that ICs have non-Gaussian distributions (Hyvärinen & Oja, 2000). Mathematical measures for non-Gaussianity are, for example, kurtosis (the fourth statistical moment) and negentropy (an information-theoretical quantity related to entropy). Other assumptions include linear mixing of source signals at the sensors, as well as stationarity of both the source signals and the mixing process (Vigario et al., 2000). Before ICA estimation, data need to be preprocessed by removing the mean signal and by whitening (i.e., removing correlations) (Chapter 10).

Although ICA does not preserve the scale or sign of the original (MEG/EEG) signals, the components can identify the spatiotemporal behavior of the putative signal sources. Some software packages generate the components in an order that reflects the decreasing order of the MEG/EEG variance accounted for by each component. Validation tests are available for investigating the reliability of ICs when the same analysis is rerun multiple times (Himberg et al., 2004).

ICA has proved useful in isolating and removing artifacts from MEG and EEG data (Vigario, 1997; Vigario et al., 2000; Brown et al., 2001), and it has also been used to differentiate between various brain signals and in searching for distinct evoked responses and different brain rhythms (Makeig et al., 1997; Huster & Raud, 2018). However, in these cases it is very difficult to know the "ground truth," that is, the real underlying neurophysiology, and thus the results must be interpreted in the context of all available neurophysiological knowledge.

Temporal rather than spatial ICA is usually applied in MEG/EEG analysis, although spatial ICA and ICA using spectral information have also been introduced (Hyvärinen et al., 2010; Ramkumar et al., 2012). For ICA to work optimally, both *the temporal and the spatial sampling* must adequately cover the signals of interest. ICA can produce individual components that may contain both the desired signal and unwanted artifacts, largely because they share the same topography or temporal structure. For example, both brain signals and artifacts can vary in a task-related manner, as happens when frontal EMG increases during a demanding cognitive task.

When common artifacts are searched for with ICA with the aim of removing them from MEG/EEG data, it is better to base the analysis on single-subject than group-level data as artifact morphology can differ across individuals and thus be difficult to identify and eliminate at a group level (see Chapter 10). In all cases, however, visual inspection of the ICA results is crucial, even when automated procedures are used (Chaumon et al., 2015). Within an individual subject, components can be identified by comparing their time courses with the MEG/EEG signals themselves, as well as by examining the components' scalp topographies and frequency contents. Having other signals in the recording, such as ECG, EOG, and EMG, might be helpful for identifying the exact temporal incidence for these artifacts in the MEG/EEG (see, e.g., Li et al., 2021).

Further in this chapter (see Figures 9.9 and 9.19), we present examples where artifacts have been successfully separated with ICA and removed from EEG signals. These types of analyses are best made on data that have *not* been digitally re-referenced and only after the removal of epochs with infrequent and large artifacts, such as subject movements. That said, these sorts of analyses have been applied well to conventional MEG/EEG studies performed in the laboratory when the subject is sitting and fixating eyes on a target. A number of semi-automated IC classifiers have been put forward to identify brain versus non brain signals, the latter consisting of artifacts related to the eyes, heart, muscles, line noise, and noise in individual recording channels (Nolan et al., 2010; Mognon et al., 2011; Winkler et al., 2014; Chaumon et al., 2015; Frølich et al., 2015; Pion-Tonachini et al., 2019). A large online repository of ICs trained on a large EEG database may be helpful for those who are learning to recognize artifactual ICAs (Pion-Tonachini et al., 2019).

Unlike regular ICA approaches that seek to minimize instantaneous correlations (i.e., with fixed zero delays), second-order blind identification (SOBI) calculates and compares cross-correlations at multiple user-specified time delays (Tang, Sutherland, & McKinney, 2005). Recommendations are available for the optimal use of SOBI, including a wide choice of time delays (Tang, Liu, & Sutherland, 2005).

Canonical correlation analysis is a multivariate version of the Pearson correlation (Hotelling, 1936), which was first used as a blind-source separation technique for fMRI data (Friman et al., 2002). CCA is also being used increasingly to extract relevant patterns of brain activity (e.g., Lankinen et al., 2014) and to remove artifacts such as eye blinks and muscle activity (Lin et al., 2018). CCA can also extract common features from multimodal data sets, such as MEG–fMRI and EEG–fMRI (Lankinen et al., 2018; Zhuang et al., 2020).

Signal-Space Projection and Separation Methods

Magnetic artifacts arising from outside the body were first efficiently removed from MEG signals with the SSP method (Uusitalo & Ilmoniemi, 1997). A more recent, highly effective method is (spatial) SSS and its temporally extended version, temporal SSS (tSSS) (Taulu et al., 2004; Taulu & Simola, 2006). These SSP and SSS methods are breakthroughs in MEG data analysis as they can remove, from multichannel MEG measurements, strong interference caused by both external noise sources and noise arising from the body itself.

SSP can be used for reducing both external magnetic artifacts entering the magnetically shielded room and artifacts arising from the body (Gramfort et al., 2014). SSP first empirically determines a distinct vector in signal space from multichannel MEG data collected during the recording session itself and an "empty-room" multichannel MEG measurement taken without the subject being present. The algorithm projects the MEG measurements onto a subspace orthogonal to the (empty-room) noise subspace. As the external interference typically remains quite stable inside the magnetically shielded room, the noise subspace can be removed from the data obtained during real MEG measurements. However, if the spatial interference patterns change, for example because new noise sources (e.g., equipment) are introduced inside the room, a new SSP operator must be computed.

When SSP is used to reduce in-body noise sources, such as EOG and ECG activity, the epochs from which the vector is computed are found from a multimodal data set that includes empty-room noise, as well as EOG and ECG artifacts.

The SSS method is based on the very basic physical properties of magnetic fields and the possibility of detecting MEG signals with the whole-scalp array from an almost spherical volume. SSS mathematically constructs the external and internal subspaces from spherical harmonics and reconstructs the sensor signals using only the internal subspace. The tSSS method works if the sources of brain signals and external interferences can be separated geometrically even if the brain signals are temporally correlated with any signal arising from nearby artifactual sources. One can divide the measured data into one set of elementary magnetic fields arising from sources inside the sensor helmet (Figure 9.3, yellow shading) and another set for fields arising from sources outside (Figure 9.3, red shading). Using the

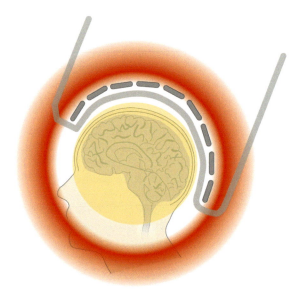

FIGURE 9.3. Volumes that can be separated with temporal signal-space separation analysis. Artifacts can be removed by the tSSS method between volumes inside and outside the head. The yellow (internal) volume contains the brain where the signals of interest are generated and the red (external) volume (extending outwards) contains artifactual sources. These internal and external volumes are uniquely defined although the sensor array does not constitute a full sphere. Adapted and reprinted from Taulu S, Hari R: Removal of magnetoencephalographic artifacts with temporal signal-space separation: demonstration with single-trial auditory-evoked responses. *Hum Brain Mapp* 2009, 30: 1524–1534. With permission from John Wiley & Sons.

basic physical properties of the magnetic fields (e.g., Maxwell's equations), the multichannel MEG signals can at any moment be uniquely decomposed into these two sets (Taulu et al., 2004), and the brain signals can be reconstructed by retaining only the elementary fields that correspond to sources inside the sensor helmet and thus likely arise from the brain.

Spatial SSS can separate brain signals from far-away (> 0.5 m) sources of external interference, and the tSSS removes nearby artifact sources (e.g., within the body). For a typical MEG measurement, spatial SSS can suppress external interference by a factor exceeding 100 (Taulu et al., 2005), so that the artifacts are suppressed even below the sensor noise while the brain signals are still retained in the reconstruction. However, some artifacts arising on the boundary of the inner and outer spheres (respective yellow and red areas in Figure 9.3), such as artifacts caused by eye movements, eye blinks, and facial muscle contractions, cannot—at least at present—be reliably removed by tSSS.

Using tSSS, single-trial auditory-evoked fields have been successfully recorded and their sources identified, although they were disturbed by purposefully introduced strong magnetic artifacts during the recording (Taulu & Hari, 2009). Additionally, tSSS has been shown to remove stimulus artifacts associated with a vagal nerve stimulation (Taulu & Simola, 2006; Cai et al., 2019) and deep brain stimulation (Kandemir et al., 2020). Figure 9.4 gives one such demonstrative example where the strong artifacts caused by a deep-brain stimulator were effectively removed by the tSSS treatment so that normal-appearing spontaneous activity became visible.

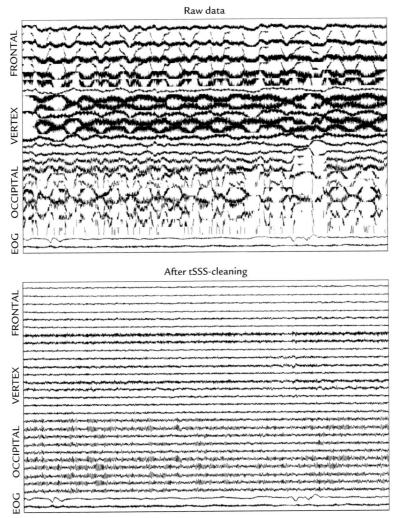

Raw data

After tSSS-cleaning

FIGURE 9.4. tSSS applied to real MEG data. The effect of tSSS artifact suppression on spontaneous MEG signals of a person who has an implanted deep-brain stimulator. Top: The original MEG signals recorded with multiple planar gradiometers from frontal, central (vertex) and occipital areas, with EOG on the two lowest traces. The MEG recording is contaminated by huge artifacts caused by periodic minute movements of the stimulator during respiration. Bottom: The same data after tSSS cleaning. The large artifacts have disappeared and even the normal posterior alpha rhythm can be seen. The duration of the traces is 30 s. Courtesy of Jyrki Mäkelä, Helsinki University Central Hospital, Finland. Reproduced and modified with permission from Hari R: Magnetoencephalography: Methods and Clinical Aspects. In: Schomer DL and Lopes da Silva FH: *Niedermeyer's Electroencephalography: Basic Principles, Clinical Applications, and Related Fields*. 7th edition. New York: Oxford University Press, 2018.

More recently, another method—oversampled temporal projection (OTP)—has been proposed for reducing uncorrelated MEG/EEG sensor random noise (Larson & Taulu, 2018). OTP makes no assumptions about the spatial or temporal composition of the artifacts, but it assumes that the noise and signals are not correlated and that they have been spatially oversampled. This method minimizes the spatial spread of artifacts. When OTP was evaluated side by side with tSSS, both OTP and tSSS effectively suppressed noise in MEG data. Further, there are benefits of using both methods jointly for low signal-to-noise ratio (SNR) data sets or for higher SNR data sets where single-trial responses will be analyzed (Clarke et al., 2020).

The combination of OTP and tSSS methods has also been found to be potentially useful for detecting high-frequency brain oscillations (Clarke et al., 2020)—an important consideration in clinical studies of epilepsy (Chapter 20).

Hence, (t)SSS and OTP methods have opened new possibilities for artifact reduction and signal identification in MEG investigations that were previously considered technically impossible, such as recordings from patients having implanted stimulators or metal objects.

Finally, artifacts in MEG/EEG traces can be "sparse"—that is, they can occur infrequently in time, but nevertheless mar the signals because they dominate the neurophysiological landscape. They can also occur very focally—in certain sensors (without being related to skin–electrode contact issues). The methods described above may not handle these optimally, and indeed trials with these sparse artifacts may often be rejected prior to using some automated artifact correction routine. The sparse time artifact removal (STAR) algorithm has been devised specifically to deal with these types of artifacts (de Cheveigné, 2016) and can be used in conjunction with the other methods. STAR works by first dividing the time-domain data into an artifact-free and an artifact-contaminated part. The artifact-free part is used to generate estimates of correlational relationships between all data elements (channels in sensor space or voxels in source space). Artifacts are corrected by exploiting and projecting information from one part of the data to the other.

■ EYE-RELATED ARTIFACTS

Eye Movements and Eye Blinks

Ocular artifacts arise because the eye is an electric dipole, with the cornea positively charged with respect to retina at the back of the eyeball (Figure 9.5a). This standing potential is due to polarization that develops because of anteriorly directed currents in the pigment epithelium of the retina (Arden & Kelsey, 1962a, 1962b), likely contributed to by currents in the photoreceptors.

During eye movements, the eyeball—that is, a charged electric dipole—moves within the volume conductor, and during eye blinks, the volume conductor surrounding the eye changes because of movements of the eyelids that, due to their moist inner surface, provide a well-conducting pathway for current flow. In both cases, the result is a clear eye-related artifact in MEG and EEG recordings. This generation mechanism is interesting as such, as it differs from the generation of MEG/EEG signals by local brain currents (current dipoles) that stay stable with respect to the volume conductor (head and body) but vary in strength due to neuronal activation. Figure 9.5 (panels b–d) illustrates the potential (EEG) and magnetic field (MEG) distributions related to both eye movements and eye blinks.

During *vertical eye movements*, the potentials (recorded with EOG) are of opposite polarities above and below the eyes, with rather symmetric spatial distribution (Figure 9.5b). Specifically, during upwardly directed eye movements, the skin above the eyes will be more positive and the skin on the cheeks more negative compared with the situation when the eyes gaze straight ahead. During downward eye movements, the polarities of the potentials are reversed (Figure 9.5b). These ocular artifacts in the vertical EOG (recorded between the upper and lower sides of the eye) are on the order of 0.5 mV.

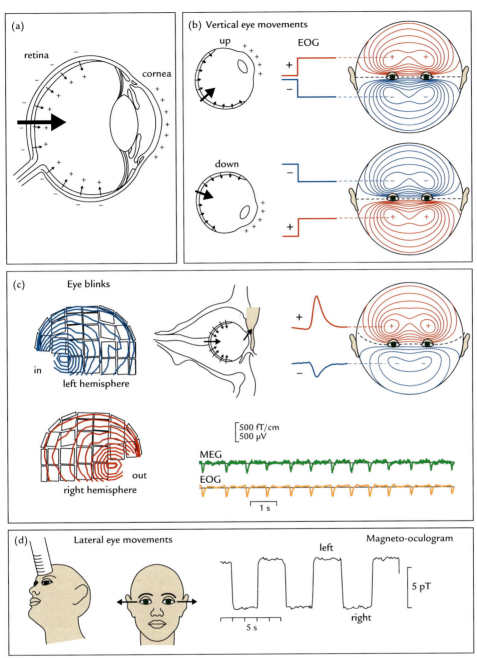

FIGURE 9.5. A schematic of the generation of ocular artifacts. (a) The eyeball can be viewed as a dipole, where the cornea is positively charged relative to the retina. (b) Upward and downward eye movements produce potential distributions that are rather symmetric with respect to eye level on the facial skin. The associated schematic EOG signals are shown for an electrode above and below the eyes. (c) During eyeblinks, the upper lid works as a sliding electrode, resulting in an asymmetric potential distribution on the face (at right) and very focal magnetic field patterns on the lateral sides of the orbits (at left). The two traces on the bottom right depict simultaneously recorded MEG (green) and EOG (yellow) signals,

From the MEG point of view, the vertical eye movements are equivalent to a vertically directed current dipole in the anterior part of the eye, resulting in signals where the magnetic field extremum can be seen on the lateral side of each orbit. For upward eye movements, the magnetic flux enters the head close to the left orbit and comes out close to the right orbit; for downward eye movements, the flux direction is the opposite.

For *eye blinks*, the situation is very similar to that of vertical eye movements. In EEG and EOG, the blinks are seen as deflections of about 0.5 mV in amplitude between electrodes above and below the eye (and thus about the same order as the signals related to eye movements, both considerably larger than the 10–100 μV EEG signals). The blink artifact has a rather stereotypical monophasic form that is similar in both EEG and MEG recordings (see Figure 9.5c and also Figures 9.9 and 9.10). The blinks last about 200 to 400 ms and tend to lengthen with drowsiness so that blink duration has been used as a marker of vigilance.

In EEG/EOG recordings, the potential distribution generated by eye blinks resembles that associated with upward-directed vertical eye movements, but in this case the distribution is asymmetric—stronger over the forehead than on the cheeks (Figure 9.5c). The corresponding magnetic field pattern has a very sharp entrance point on the lateral side of the left orbit and exit point on the lateral side of the right orbit (Figure 9.5c). The currents that best explain both the MEG and the EEG patterns during eye blinks are pointing toward the upper lid from the orbit, as shown in Figure 9.5c (Antervo et al., 1985; Hari et al., 1994).

The likely explanation for these findings is that, during eye blinks, the upper lid functions like a sliding electrode with good conductivity so that it will let the positive charges from the cornea move upward. This mechanism was originally suggested for EOG recordings by Barry and Jones (1965) and supported by the modeling of eye-blink MEG signals (Antervo et al., 1985); the neuromagnetic studies also supported the corneoretinal origin of the source currents, as both blink and eye-movement signals were larger during light than darkness (Katila et al., 1981; Antervo et al., 1985).

Concerning blink artifacts, we have to firmly reject the "Bell's phenomenon" explanation—still presented today in textbooks of clinical neurophysiology, based on the assumption that these artifacts are caused by upward rotations of the eyeballs. In EOG, a signal of about 20 μV corresponds to 1° of eyeball rotation (Schomer et al., 2018), meaning that a typical blink of about 500 μV would require an eyeball rotation on the order of 25°. Along similar lines, the magnetic MOG signals produced by 60° vertical eye movements were about double in amplitude when compared with eye-blink signals (Antervo et al., 1985), suggesting that if the blink signals were explained by eyeball movements, they should be about 30° in size. No such large eyeball movements have been reported in association with eye blinks. EEG recordings combined with magnetic search-coil monitoring of eyeball and eyelid positions have also clearly rejected the idea of Bell's phenomenon as the

---

FIGURE 9.5. **Continued**

during voluntary blinking. (d) Repetitive lateral left–right eye movements (at center) are associated with square-wave-shaped magnetic signals (at right) when recorded with an axial gradiometer above the frontal area (at left). Passband from DC to 3 Hz. Panels a and d adapted and reprinted from Katila T, Maniewski R, Poutanen T, Varpula T, Karp BJ: Magnetic fields produced by the human eye. *J Appl Phys* 1981, 52: 2565, with permission from AIP Publishing. Panel c adapted and reprinted from Antervo A, Hari R, Katila T, Ryhänen T, Seppänen M: Magnetic fields produced by eye blinking. *Electroencephalogr Clin Neurophysiol* 1985, 61: 247–253. With permission from Elsevier.

cause of eye-blink artifacts (Iwasaki et al., 2005). Additional support for the separate generation mechanisms of EEG artifacts caused by vertical eye movements and eye blinks arises from their different source models (Berg & Scherg, 1991).

Spontaneous eye blinks typically occur 15 to 20 times per minute. However, people are differentially sensitive to external stimuli, and they also have different blink rates that depend on not only an individual's need to remoisten the corneal surfaces (Ousler et al., 2008) but also the current cognitive load and social demand (Holland & Tarlow, 1975; Hirokawa et al., 2004). Importantly, people blink less while attending to a speaker or a video and more during pauses of the listened speech (Nakano & Kitazawa, 2010). Average blink rates may also vary in neurological and psychiatric patients relative to healthy subjects (Karson et al., 1984; Swarztrauber & Fujikawa, 1998; Tulen et al., 1999; Chan & Chen, 2004).

Abrupt, loud sounds and painful stimuli often elicit automatic blinks time-locked to the stimuli. Noxious stimuli applied to the face, such as carbon dioxide stimulation of the nasal mucosa (Huttunen et al., 1986), elicit reflexive blinks that even trained subjects cannot prevent. In such experiments, EOG monitoring is mandatory. Moreover, it is good experimental practice in any study to analyze the EOG signals within the same pipeline as MEG/EEG signals to be able to compare waveforms and amplitudes.

During *lateral eye movements*, the DC-coupled MEG recording (Figure 9.5d) shows nice, square wave–type signals that stay stable when the eyes are kept fixated to the left or right side. The MEG signal has opposite polarities between the upper and lower level of the eyes: for rightward movements, the flux enters the head above the eyes and exits the head beneath the eyes. For leftward eye movements, the MEG polarities are opposite. For rightward movements, EOG on the right side of the right eye is positive with respect to the left side of the left eye (Figure 9.6). During leftward horizontal eye movements, the polarities are reversed (compare also EEG signals related to lateral and vertical eye movements in Figure 9.6).

Note that the clinically often applied high-pass filtering at 0.5 Hz can considerably distort the waveforms of both eye-movement and blink-related signals so that the square wave–type signals related to eye movements (Figure 9.5d) start to decay according to the characteristics of the filter (cf. Figure 8.2), and the monophasic eye blinks can appear biphasic in the recording. Both eye-movement and eye-blink artifacts receive contributions from eyeball- and eye-lid movements in proportions that are difficult to estimate accurately.

Saccades and Microsaccades

Subtler ocular MEG/EEG artifacts can be produced by small fixational eye movements and eye drifts (particularly when the eyes are closed or when there is no preset location on which to fixate). Saccades are exploratory or willfully directed eye movements from one fixation point to another. Microsaccades—small, involuntary eye movements occurring when the subject attempts to fixate on a particular visual feature—typically occur at around 1 to 3 Hz; they may aid image stabilization and prevent image fading. Microsaccades tend to be on the order of fractions of a degree only, but can range up to 1°. That is the range where willful saccades can also occur (Engbert, 2006; Martinez-Conde et al., 2009), although these are typically larger, even tens of degrees in size. Given this size overlap between microsaccades and saccades, microsaccades have been operationally defined as "saccades that are produced while attempting to fixate" (Martinez-Conde et al., 2009).

The onset of a saccade and a microsaccade can be associated with a "saccadic spike" (Blinn, 1955), which in the EEG appears as an artifact of 10–30 ms duration and up to 100 μV in amplitude (Jäntti et al., 1983). Saccadic spikes are likely generated in facial, extraocular muscles (Beaussart & Guieu, 1977), and they can be detected as artifacts in both MEG

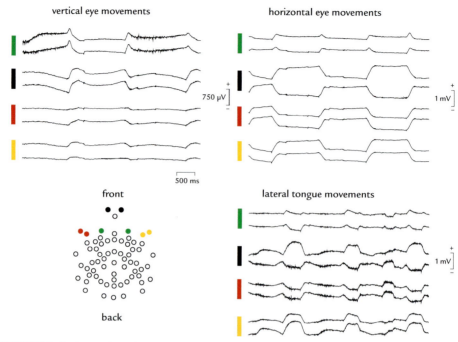

FIGURE 9.6. Examples of EEG artifacts associated with vertical and horizontal eye movements and tongue movements. EEG was recorded relative to the vertex while a subject made willful eye and tongue movements. The electrode map (bottom left) highlights eight parasagittal electrodes sited on the face above and below the eyes (green and black circles, respectively) and lateral to the eyes (red and yellow circles). Passband 0.1–200 Hz. Top left: During vertical eye movements the maximum deflections occurred in electrodes above and below the eyes (green and black electrodes). Some muscle activity is superimposed on these traces. Note the large (about 1 mV) size of these artifacts. In the green trace eyes up elicits a positive potential and eyes down a negative potential for electrodes above the eyes. The polarity is reversed in the black trace, as electrodes are sites below the eyes. Top right: Horizontal eye movements generate the biggest deflections in electrodes that are lateral to the eyes (red and yellow), with positive potentials occurring in the red trace to leftward movements and negative potentials to movements to the right. The opposite polarity is seen in the yellow traces from the other side of the head. The individual black traces show opposite polarities based on the relative positions of the low electrodes with respect to the eye movement. Bottom right: As the subject moves her tongue at regular intervals from side to side in the mouth, large artifacts and some superimposed EMG activity are seen on most channels. Note the similar polarity difference across the left and right sides, resembling the pattern seen for lateral eye movements. In this case however, as the tip of the tongue has the opposite polarity to the cornea, the polarities are reversed: leftward movements elicit negative potentials in the red traces, and movements to the right show positive potentials. Polarity is reversed in the yellow traces which come from electrodes on the other side of the head. The individual black traces show opposite polarities based on the relative positions of the low electrodes with respect to the tongue movement. Data recorded in the Dual EEG Laboratory, Imaging Research Facility, Indiana University, USA.

and EEG recordings (Carl et al., 2012). Microsaccades appear to contribute to the EEG signals of the posterior scalp by producing minute visual-evoked-response-type deflections 100 to 140 ms after the microsaccade (Dimigen et al., 2009). They thus resemble occipital lambda waves followed by about 80 ms exploratory saccades (Thickbroom et al., 1991; described for the first time in 1951 by Gastaut) and parieto-occipital responses following eye blinks by about 230 ms (Hari et al., 1994).

Infrared eye tracking combined with EEG recording has shown that electrical potentials related to saccades can occur in the 20- to 90-Hz range, thus overlapping with, and mimicking, beta and gamma EEG activity over the posterior scalp (Yuval-Greenberg et al., 2008) (Figure 9.7). The saccades that generated these EEG artifacts were only about 1° in size. Although the saccadic spike potentials were largest at frontal sites, near the eyes, they

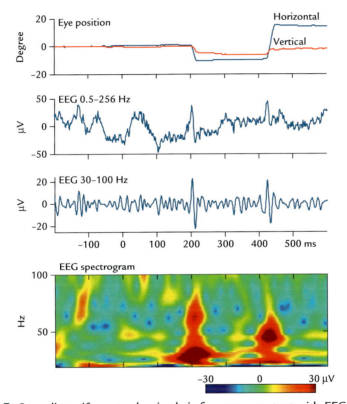

FIGURE 9.7. Saccadic artifacts overlap in their frequency content with EEG gamma activity. Top: Infra-red eye tracking shows a saccade with horizontal and vertical components (blue and red, respectively); extent of saccade in degrees is plotted as a function of time. Middle: Two EEG traces from channel CPz during the same time interval. The upper trace shows the original EEG (from 0.5 to 256 Hz), which is bandpass filtered from 30 to 100 Hz on the lower trace; the latter shows two clear spikes that coincide with the saccades shown in the top trace. Bottom: EEG spectrogram (frequency content of the original EEG signal as a function of time) with colors expressing signal amplitude. Prominent broadband activity (red hues) occurs at the same time as the saccades. Adapted and reprinted from Yuval-Greenberg S, Tomer O, Keren AS, Nelken I, Deouell LY: Transient induced gamma-band response in EEG as a manifestation of miniature saccades. *Neuron* 2008, 58: 429–441. With permission from Elsevier.

still produced clear EEG deflections even at the posterior scalp, starting about 22 ms after saccade onset (Keren et al., 2010). Similar high-frequency EEG artifacts were also associated with tiny saccadic eye movements, confirming the earlier observations that even very small eye movements can produce saccadic spike potentials. This artifact is clearly seen in simultaneous MEG magnetometer and EEG recordings, with spatial distributions consistent with extra-ocular source currents (Carl et al., 2012). Critically, while the gamma-band component of the saccadic spike is quite local regardless of saccade direction, the beta-band component's broader spatial extent can vary as a function of saccade direction (Gawne et al., 2017).

Microsaccades are the largest of three different types of spontaneous eye movement—the others being tremor and drift (Martinez-Conde, 2006). Tremor can occur at frequencies of ~90 Hz and show tiny excursions of ~8.5 s of arc, whereas drift is a random, slow, tiny eye movement that can occur between microsaccades and showing a tiny change of image over ~12 photoreceptors (given the very small size of tremor and drift, these will be unlikely to cause nuisance MEG/EEG signals).

Removal of Eye-Related Artifacts

Healthy subjects can be trained to minimize eye blinking during a recording session and to blink at particular times, such as during intertrial intervals in a task. Note, however, that asking subjects to inhibit eye movements and blinking and to just fixate on a target (typically a central cross) constitutes a secondary task that may interfere with the primary experimental task (Gratton et al., 1983; Croft et al., 2005), although having a secondary task may be a lesser evil in studies of low-level sensory processing. If blinking is related to some specific cognitive state, such as a pause in a video or listened speech (Nakano & Kitazawa, 2010), then removing blink artifacts and averaging all neural responses together—whether or not they were accompanied by blinks—means that we could potentially be averaging signals from different cognitive states. For visual studies, such pooling can also be problematic: if the blink occurs simultaneously with, or just before, stimulus onset, the subject may not have actually seen the stimulus at its onset. In these instances, evoked responses may be delayed with respect to the real stimulus onset or even be absent if the stimulus is brief.

The traditional way to avoid blink-related and gross eye-movement-related artifacts in MEG/EEG recordings has been to ask the subject to fixate on a designated point (usually a fixation cross at the center of the screen) and refrain from blinking as much as possible during stimulus presentation and task performance. (Most early MEG/EEG studies used averaging with low-pass filter cuts of around 40 Hz, so that the microsaccadic activity, discussed in the previous section, was not present in the analyzed data.) Epochs with coinciding eye artifacts were rejected from subsequent analyses. However, if MEG/EEG epochs coinciding with eye blinks and gross eye-movement artifacts are rejected, the experimental design must include enough trials to allow for the rejection of an a priori estimated trial number. This analysis procedure may also bias the results toward certain brain states when no eye movements or blinks take place.

Central gaze fixation may not always be feasible—particularly for infants and various patient populations. Nor is gaze fixation possible or even desirable in studies using naturalistic designs, such as viewing dynamic stimuli and movies, or in portable EEG studies.

Although it would be preferable not to have blink artifacts in the recording, eye-blink and eye-movement artifacts can be detected and corrected with multiple software routines (for an early review, see Croft & Barry, 2000). For any artifact removal to function properly, the artifacts must be correctly sampled and identified. Also, some sort of estimate,

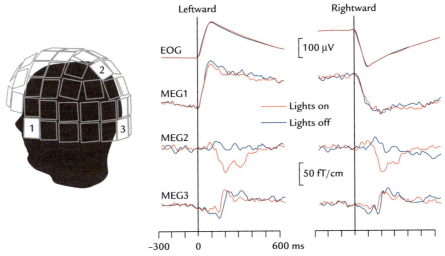

FIGURE 9.8. Saccade-related MEG signals. Left: The subject was performing ±10° horizontal saccades once every 3 s. The MEG helmet shows the locations of three planar MEG gradiometers from which signals are featured on right. Right: Horizontal EOG (top) shows clear signals during leftward and rightward saccades (with signal decays due to high-pass filtering). Sensor MEG1, located lateral to the left eye, shows very similar time courses. MEG2 located in the parietal midline does not see any eye-movement artifact (leftward and rightward saccades were balanced in the average) but a clear response (peak around 200 ms) that is abolished when the lights of the measurement room are shut off. MEG3, located on the low occipital midline, likely reflects activity from the cerebellum, independently of whether the lights are on or off. Passband 0.03–90 Hz, sampling rate 297 Hz. Adapted and reprinted from Jousmäki V, Hämäläinen M, Hari R: Magnetic source imaging during a visually guided [saccade] task. *Neuroreport* 1996, 7: 2961–2964. With permission from Wolters Kluwer Health, Inc.

or template, of the artifact must be generated, so that the artifact can be automatically removed from the MEG/EEG signal. Needless to say, the success of these approaches relies on the accurate detection of the artifact and will typically involve both automated processing and checking/intervention/adjustment by the experimenter. In MEG recordings, a third possibility might be to balance the artifacts caused by left- and right-directed saccades so that the subject will do an about equal amount of saccades to the left and right, thereby minimizing the influence of artifacts that are of opposite polarities but of the same size for both left- and right-sided saccades (Jousmäki et al., 1996); see Figure 9.8. This procedure would minimize artifacts related to horizontal saccades across the whole head and effectively over the posterior parts of the head where the saccade-related artifacts are small and the visual responses large. Note that in Figure 9.8 the clear signals in the posterior parietal midline (MEG2) and midoccipital area (MEG3) are not artifacts but are real brain signals.

Many algorithmic corrections of *eye blinks* and *eye movements* have assumed that the EEG contamination by ocular potentials is a linear function of EOG amplitudes (e.g., Plöchl et al., 2012), which is approximately valid for saccadic eye movements, whereas for larger movements, the EOG signal is a nonlinear sum of the positions of the eyeball and the eyelid covering the eyeball.

Another approach advocates correction of ocular EEG artifacts on the basis of pre-experiment eye-movement "calibration" runs (Croft & Barry, 2000). Here the EEG session commences with a calibration period that includes eye blinks as well as deliberate eye movements to a set of orthogonal points around a central fixation point. This procedure allows estimation of the sizes of eye-related signals in different EEG derivations as a function of the extent of eye movement.

In naturalistic task designs, depending on the extent of the possible eye movements, the collection of MEG/EEG data should include simultaneous infrared eye tracking, which, in fact, would be beneficial in most MEG/EEG studies, particularly when very slow signals or gamma activity will be analyzed. The eye-tracking signal could be used as a regressor in data analysis, although regression-based approaches for ocular artifact removal are more likely to over- or undercorrect individual artifact components (Plöchl et al., 2012). Alternatively, analyses performed in source space can facilitate the separation of ocular artifacts from saccades and microsaccades in MEG/EEG data (Hipp & Siegel, 2013).

Currently, blind source-separation techniques seem to provide the best automatic means to identify, and consequently remove, eye-movement and blink-related artifacts (Plöchl et al., 2012). Figure 9.9 depicts a sample of epoched EEG data from electrodes that

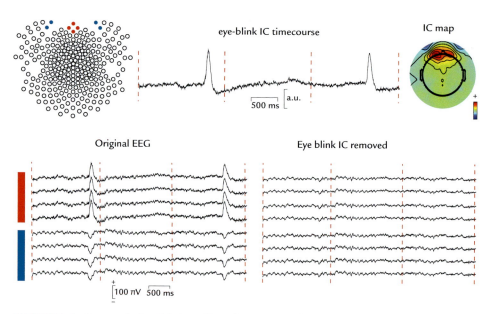

FIGURE 9.9. Removal of eyeblink artifacts from EEG with ICA. Epoched EEG data (Original EEG; bottom left; epochs separated by red vertical lines) recorded during visual stimulation in a healthy subject. Frontal electrodes are located above the eyes (red labels, in top left electrode map) and on the face below the eyes (blue labels) using 256-channel montage. (Note that the 2D representation has somewhat distorted the geodesic electrode positions, which appear to be lateral in this map.) Top middle trace shows the eyeblink IC time course, with the topographic IC map on the right. Bottom right panel shows the EEG traces after eye-blink removal. EEG was recorded with respect to the vertex. Passband 0.1–200 Hz, sampling rate 500 Hz; low-pass filtering at 45 Hz. Data recorded in the Social Neuroscience Laboratory, Indiana University, USA.

are above (red locations in the electrode array on top left) and below (blue locations) the eyes. The bottom left and right traces in the figure depict the same EEG data before and after removal of the eye-blink IC. The IC corresponding to eye blinks has a stereotypical anterior frontal and bilaterally symmetric scalp distribution (top right panel), with identical morphology and time course (top middle panel) to the eye blinks visible in the EEG. In principle, systematic lateral (and vertical) eye movements made during a visual activation task could also be removed from the EEG.

CCA has been used for removing eye-related artifacts in MEG/EEG data sets (Lin et al., 2018). SSP methods are also effective at characterizing and eliminating eye-blink artifacts. Figure 9.10 depicts the SSP projectors for eye blinks that have been generated for an MEG/EEG data set recorded with magnetometers, gradiometers, and EEG/EOG/ECG electrodes.

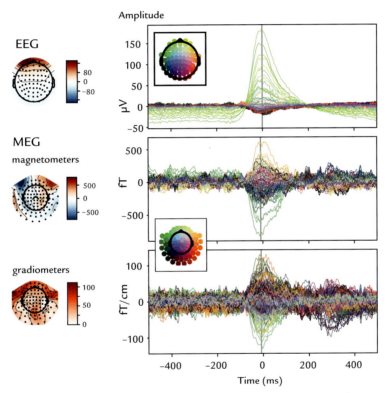

FIGURE 9.10. SSP projectors of eyeblink artifact for EEG and MEG. Scalp topographies (left) and time courses (right) with time zero centered at the blink's maximum amplitude (grey vertical line) for EEG electrodes (top), MEG magnetometers (middle) and gradiometers (bottom) are shown. The color-coded butterfly plots show the anterior topography of the blink artifact in EEG electrodes, magnetometers, and gradiometers, respectively. Respective units for color bars are microvolts, femtoteslas and femtoteslas/cm. Sensor arrays are depicted as black dots on scalp topographies and color dots (inset) on butterfly plots of time courses. Data in this single subject show blink durations of around 200 ms. SSPs were generated from 23 blinks. Data recorded in the Centre de Neuroimagerie de Recherche (CENIR and STIM platform), Institut du Cerveau et de la Moelle épinière (ICM), Sorbonne Université, Paris, France. Data analyzed in the Social Neuroscience Laboratory, Indiana University, USA.

Among the multiple other methods that have been applied, whether alone or in combination with each other, removing ocular artifacts from EEG signals has included the classical PCA. However, PCA easily clumps together activities that are not physiologically related. Consequently, PCA cannot always separate blink- or eye-related artifacts from, for example, oscillatory brain signals that are associated with the ocular activity.

To eliminate saccade-related EEG transients in studies of gamma-band activity, a correction algorithm named COSTRAP (for COrrection of Saccade-related TRAnsient Potentials) has been introduced (Hassler et al., 2011). Specifically, the average of horizontal and vertical EOG channels referenced to scalp electrode Pz, or "radial electro-oculogram (REOG)," is first calculated for the entire time series. Then using the first temporal derivative of the REOG signal, maxima and minima produced by the sharp edges of saccadic spikes are calculated and subjected to an amplitude threshold and a conservative temporal threshold of 3 spikes/s. Next, time courses from frontal EEG electrodes are generated to serve as templates for EOG removal from the EEG using an ICA-related approach whereby "virtual channels" with maximum saccadic potentials serve as templates for detecting and removing these signals from EEG derivations.

Irrespective of whether data are acquired using MEG or EEG, or whatever artifact-rejection methods are used, we advocate *always* recording vertical and horizontal EOG separately and subjecting these channels to the same analysis procedures, be it averaging or single-trial analyses. Often, only one variant of these artifact-removal methods is implemented in available analysis software, and the user may not necessarily have a choice as to which correction procedure to apply. In these cases, the user must have a clear understanding regarding how the implemented methods work.

■ MUSCLE ARTIFACTS

Generation and Recognition

Muscle contraction is regulated by electrical impulses that arrive via alpha motoneurons (from the anterior horn of the spinal cord) to the end plates on the muscle fibers, where they initiate muscle action potentials and muscle contraction. A *motor unit* consists of one alpha motoneuron and all the muscle fibers it innervates (Figure 9.11, left). The motor unit fires in an all-or-none fashion, with very little jitter between the contraction times of single muscle fibers (in fact, the jitter between contractions of muscle fibers belonging to the same motor unit exceeding about 50 μs speaks for a transmission defect, such as myasthenia gravis, in the nerve–muscle junction). The number of muscle fibers in a motor unit varies from four to six in eye muscles to hundreds in the large muscles of the back. The motor-unit potentials have different shapes, amplitudes, and durations depending on their size and the locations of the single muscle fibers with respect to the recording electrodes.

Weak muscle contraction results in EMG activity where the individual motor-unit potentials can be discerned (Figure 9.11, top right side trace). Only at intermediate and strong force levels (Figure 9.11, right middle and bottom traces) does an "interference" pattern emerge, with summation (and partial cancellation) of different motor-unit potentials.

Over 20 muscles in the face, head, and neck (some of them illustrated in Figure 9.12) are the most likely contaminants of EEG and MEG signals, and the artifacts they produce in MEG/EEG recordings can be quite variable in location, waveform, and frequency.

In scalp EEG recordings, facial and head muscle contractions are seen as myogenic artifacts in the 100-μV or 1-mV range, with a wide frequency spectrum from tens of hertz to a few hundreds of hertz depending on the muscle, its fiber types, and activation level and with

EMG

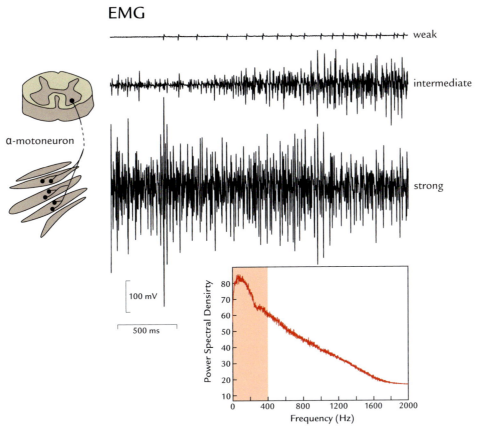

FIGURE 9.11. Schematic of a motor unit and a normal surface EMG from the right thenar during increasing contraction. Left: A motor unit comprises an α-motoneuron, with the soma located in the anterior horn of the spinal cord, and all muscle fibers it innervates (i.e., has contact with). Right: All muscle fibers of a single motor unit contract at the same time, thereby producing motor-unit potentials that during weak contraction are isolated in surface EMG (upper trace). During intermediate (middle trace) and strong (lower trace) contractions, the motor-unit potentials intermingle with the potentials of other motor units, thereby forming an interference pattern. The 3 EMG traces of 5-s duration reflect a progressively increasing muscle contraction; note that the vertical calibration bar here is 100 mV whereas it is typically 100 μV for EEG data. The power spectral density (μV^2/Hz) function (bottom) shows that the main activity occurs below 400 Hz (salmon shading). This activity peaks at around 50–100 Hz. Sampling rate 5 kHz, BP filter 5–2000 Hz. Data recorded in the Social Neuroscience Laboratory, Indiana University, USA.

a spatial pattern determined by the anatomical location of the muscle; the strongest EMG activity typically occurs at 20 to 80 Hz, thereby in the same frequency range as beta- and gamma-band signals that muscle activity thus may easily contaminate. Myogenic artifacts can widely distort the EEG recordings: the larger the muscles, the more strongly they are contracted. Figure 9.13 shows a 64-channel EEG recording during a deliberate attempt to generate a brief brow lift. In this case, all EEG derivations have been referenced relative to the vertex, and almost all of them show some artifact.

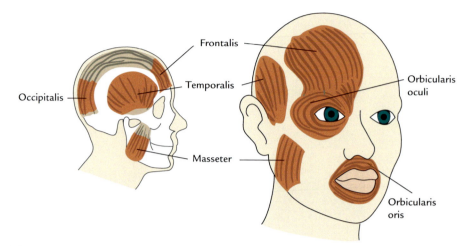

FIGURE 9.12. Some muscles of the head and face that can generate artifacts to MEG/ EEG recordings. Left: A sagittal schematic of the head and skull showing the locations of the frontalis, temporalis, occipitalis, and masseter (buccinator) muscles. The frontalis muscle is instrumental in brow raising, and temporalis and masseter muscles work antagonistically to open and close the jaw so that chewing and speaking are possible. Occipitalis is mainly responsible for moving the scalp back. Right: Schematic head showing the frontalis, temporalis, and masseter muscles, in addition to the orbicularis oris and orbicularis oculi muscles. Contraction of the ring-shaped orbicularis oculi muscle results in eye closure and blinking. Orbicularis oris controls movements of the mouth and lips. The depicted muscles are a small subset of all muscles that control the face, scalp, and neck, so that there are many potential muscular sources that can contaminate MEG/EEG signals.

Because motor-unit firing rates increase to about 10 to 20 Hz as the force increases, and because physiological tremor occurs at 8 to 12 Hz, firing of single motor units can obscure or even mimic alpha-range brain activity (Goncharova et al., 2003) and thus be visible in the ICA of the EEG data. An EEG study of two healthy subjects with complete neuromuscular blockade indicated that the scalp EEG was contaminated by myogenic activity in frequencies from 20 to 300 Hz; the authors even concluded: "Most of the scalp EEG recording above 20 Hz is of EMG origin" (Whitham et al., 2007, p. 1877). Mental effort increased 30–100 Hz EMG activity in scalp EEG, and scalp muscles are coactivated with simple hand actions, such as a button press (Whitham et al., 2008). These myogenic artifacts are least serious at the central electrode sites, and their ubiquity further stresses the importance of analyzing MEG/EEG signals in source rather than sensor space (see Chapter 10).

MEG recordings can also be contaminated by myogenic artifacts, but in source space muscular contamination of the MEG signals is not typically a problem, as the sources of the artifacts are much more superficial than those of any real brain signals. Still, a caveat to remember is that if the source is spatially extended, in source analysis it can appear to be deeper than it really is (see Chapter 10 and Figure 10.12).

As we have already noted, prior to starting the actual recording, showing subjects their EEG/MEG activity while they tense muscles and blink can help minimize these artifacts. Additionally, an attentive experimenter can potentially eliminate, or at least reduce, myogenic artifacts by asking the subject to relax the muscles in question. Despite these instructions, subjects may be unable to relax and release muscle tension. For example, they are

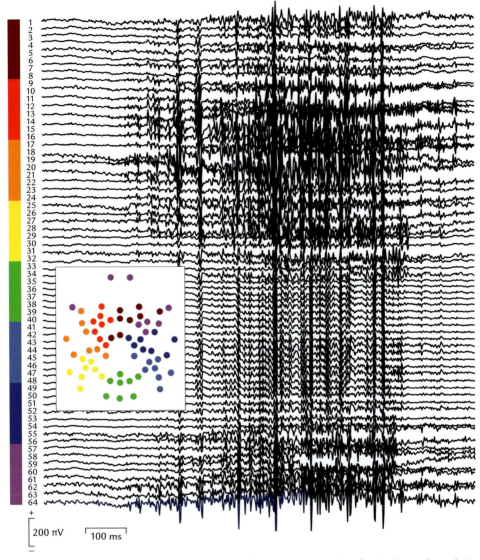

FIGURE 9.13. The effects of brow lift on EEG data. A 1.1-s epoch of a 64-channel geodesic EEG, recorded with respect to the vertex (passband 0.1–200 Hz), shows the effect of a quick brow lift. While artifacts appear throughout the entire 64-channel array, the maximum EMG contamination occurs on the face and frontal scalp (electrodes with red–orange and purple labels; see the left side of the traces). The inset shows a schematic geodesically arranged electrode map with color coding. Data recorded in the Dual EEG Laboratory, Imaging Research Facility, Indiana University, USA.

often unaware of muscle tension that arises when they make an active effort to provide the best possible performance on a task, or when they watch others' emotional or articulatory facial expressions and unconsciously mimic them (see Tamietto et al., 2009).

Some muscle artifacts might result from motor actions involving arms or legs, or when subjects cannot sit still and will continuously fidget and generate body movements, including periodic tremor, which can occur at different frequencies from about 10 Hz in physiological tremor, to about 4–6 Hz in Parkinson disease, and even slower (and often irregular) in hepatic encephalopathy.

EEG recorded with portable devices from subjects performing naturalistic upper-limb movements will likely contain prominent artifacts from neck and shoulder muscles. In addition, walking (or running) can produce movements of the portable EEG headset and electrodes (and/or sway if cables are present), as demonstrated in Figure 9.14. In the top set of traces, a regular artifact-free EEG is visible when the subject sits motionless, with eyes closed or open, whereas the lower traces are contaminated by the action of walking, with a predominant artifact produced by headset movement.

Walking or gait artifacts have been recorded from EEG electrodes without the presence of an EEG signal while the subject wore a swimming cap under a wig with conductive gel under the electrodes in addition to an accelerometer on the forehead (Kline et al., 2015). These artifacts increased in both amplitude and frequency when the subject walked faster. Artifact amplitude could vary on different locations of the head. The artifacts showed large intersubject variability and could not be abolished completely with different removal methods. Some subjects showed increased spectral power related to stepping frequency during "double support," that is, when both legs were in contact with the ground, and decreased spectral power during "single support," for instance, when only one leg contacts the ground at faster walking speeds. These spectral-power features of non-EEG walking artifact parallel those seen in some previous EEG studies of walking, suggesting that walking artifacts were not completely removed (Kline et al., 2015).

In some studies, motor activity is actually a variable of interest, for example, in investigations of corticokinematic coherence, where brain activity is studied relative to the execution of, for example, hand movements. In these cases, specific attention must be paid to potential muscular or movement artifacts. In MEG, head- and face-movement-related artifacts—accentuated on purpose by adding a magnetic wire to the scalp and tooth—can be dampened using tSSS to the extent that the artifacts do not affect amplitudes or waveforms of the computed corticokinematic coherence (Bourguignon et al., 2016) (see Chapter 17).

In addition to direct myogenic artifacts, tongue movements can create large glossokinetic artifacts in the frontotemporal EEG because the tip of the tongue carries a negative charge relative to the base. Hence, glossokinetic artifacts can be seen in the EEG both when the charged tongue moves (similar to the eyelid and eyeball situation described previously; see Figure 9.6, right bottom panel) and when the tongue comes into contact with the palate (Tatum et al., 2018). Similarly, if subjects speak or move their face during the recording, myogenic artifacts can arise from the tongue and from facial, occipital, and neck muscles. For MEG, artifacts from dental fillings can also occur during mouth movement. In geodesic EEG electrode arrays, the electrodes on the face and neck are especially vulnerable to myogenic artifacts.

Removal of Myogenic Artifacts

Again we stress that muscle artifacts are best avoided by ensuring that the experimental setup and performance requirements foster physical and behavioral comfort for subjects. Fortunately, typical muscle artifacts are easy to recognize in spontaneous MEG/EEG signals, although their frequency content can overlap with the brain signals of interest.

While muscle artifacts can be readily recognized, software-based corrections of EMG artifacts in EEG signals pose a particular challenge, as EMG activity varies greatly

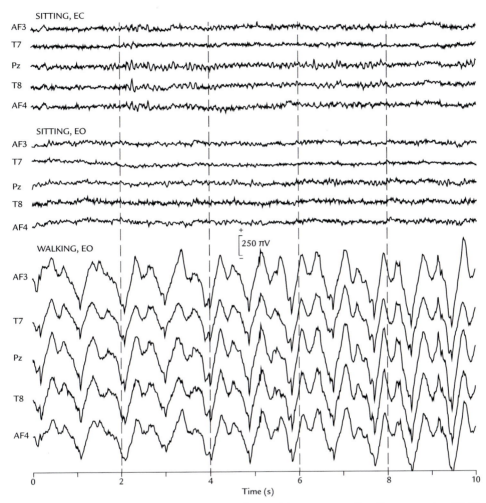

FIGURE 9.14. Walking artifact. A 5-channel portable EEG recording from putative 10-10 sites was artifact-free while the subject was sitting quietly in the laboratory, with eyes closed, EC (top 5 traces) and eyes open, EO (middle 5 traces). Prominent artifacts appeared when the subject was walking in the laboratory at a rate of about 1 step/s (bottom 5 traces). The regular artifact is likely caused by EEG headset movement (cable-free system with Bluetooth transmission), as was indicated by on-headset 3-axis accelerometer, gyroscope and magnetometer recordings (not shown). EEG was recorded from hydrophilic semi-dry polymer electrodes (moistened with glycerin solution) relative to the left mastoid (combined driven right leg/common mode sensing (DRL/CMS) reference; see Chapter 5). Sampling rate 128 Hz, passband 0.5–43 Hz (default notch filter at 60 Hz). Data recorded in the Social Neuroscience Laboratory, Indiana University, USA.

depending on recording location with respect to the underlying muscles and the strength of muscle contraction.

Figure 9.15 illustrates scalp topography, time courses, and spectral power of some EMG-related ICs during the course of an experiment. EMG activity can wax and wane at various stages of the recording session, evident in multiple ICs that each contain EMG

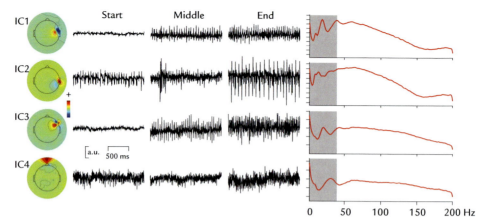

FIGURE 9.15. Independent components reflecting muscle artifacts with different scalp topographies and frequencies. Four ICs reflecting EMG activity during a 50-min recording session. The scalp distributions are quite focal and reflect EMG activity over parts of the frontal and temporal scalp (topographic maps at left). Three brief time courses of each IC are displayed at the start, middle, and end of the recording (middle panel). Muscle activity can progressively increase during the recording (IC1 and IC3), vary at different times (IC2), or remain relative constant (IC4). The power spectra (units of $\mu V^2/Hz$) for each IC (at right) show clear EMG activity that spreads up to 200 Hz in this 0.1 to 200 Hz recording (reference electrode at the vertex). The gray rectangles in the spectral plots highlight the typical EEG frequency range from 0 to 40 Hz. Data recorded in the Social Neuroscience Laboratory, Indiana University, USA.

activity. While ICA-based approaches can be a useful aid in removing certain artifacts, they cannot completely eliminate EMG activity from EEG data sets in sensor space (Delorme et al., 2007).

CCA has been used for reducing EMG-related MEG/EEG artifacts (Lin et al., 2018). In side-by-side tests using synthetic data sets, where the ground truth is known, CCA has been reported to outperform ICA (De Clercq et al., 2006; Gao et al., 2010) or to produce artifact correction that is comparable (nonperfect) to that obtained with SOBI (Urigüen & Garcia-Zapirain, 2015).

The method of "stride-time warping" has been proposed for removing gait artifact (Gwin et al., 2010). EEG data are recorded with other bodily signals, including lower limb EMG, video motion capture, and data on generated ground force. A channel-based template regression procedure is implemented; first the EEG data (time-locked to single gait cycles) are epoched to (left) heel-strike events and linearly time-warped so that the heel strike occurs at comparable latencies in each epoch. A gait-related artifact template is then created, for each channel and stride, by averaging 20 surrounding time-warped, stride-locked epochs (10 future and 10 past). The artifact template is linearly scaled for the best least-squares fit to the time-warped EEG signal and is then subtracted from the EEG data to reduce the ambulatory artifact. The "cleaned" EEG data are then reverse time warped to produce artifact-reduced, continuous time EEG channel signals.

The jury is still out as to what is the best method to suppress gait artifact. Clearly much more work needs to be performed, perhaps benchmarking a number of different approaches on the same data set.

■ CARDIAC ARTIFACTS

Generation and Recognition

The heart is a contracting smooth muscle that, like striated skeletal muscle, produces strong electric potentials on the body surface and magnetic fields outside the body. Electric and magnetic fields of the heart can be easily recorded and are known as the electrocardiogram (ECG) and magnetocardiogram (MCG), respectively. (In the literature they can also be referred to by the German-derived acronyms EKG and MKG, respectively.)

Figure 9.16 (left) shows a schematic cross section of heart, the associated cardiac vector (the net current direction during ventricular contraction), and a typical ECG trace (right) during a single heart cycle. The deflections of the ECG signal, labeled with letters from P to T, reflect the successive muscular events of the atria and ventricles (upper and lower chambers of the heart, respectively) as they pump blood through the body. The P wave reflects the depolarization (and therefore contraction) of the atria. The "QRS complex" reflects the depolarization (and contraction) of the ventricles, and the T wave reflects ventricular repolarization (and relaxation). Note that whereas in a nerve fiber (see Figure 2.2) the depolarization and repolarization phases are associated with current dipoles of opposite directions, in cardiac muscle the depolarization and repolarization currents have the same direction during both phases. The reason is that in the heart the repolarization progresses in a direction that is opposite to that of depolarization. Functionally, this repolarization order saves the heart from going into ventricular tachycardia—which could be fatal. Another feature that prevents tachycardia is that the cardiac muscle action potentials last for 100 to 200 ms (vs. about 1 ms in a nerve-cell axon) and therefore also prevent reactivation that is too frequent.

To best identify cardiac-cycle-related artifacts that can occur in both EEG and MEG, it is very useful to also monitor the ECG, with electrodes placed almost anywhere in the body, far away from each other, such as the two wrists or on each shoulder (lead I bipolar ECG configuration), or even one hand and one foot (leads II or III bipolar ECG configurations).

In MEG, the heartbeat-related artifact is left-hemisphere dominant and clearest in the lowest planar gradiometers of the helmet array (Jousmäki & Hari, 1996) (Figure 9.17). The artifact is a part of the MCG signal itself, just measured far away from the heart, because of its identical timing and width with the ECG signal (in Figure 9.17, compare lower ECG trace with MEG traces). Abnormally strong cardiac artifacts can be seen in the MEG/EEG

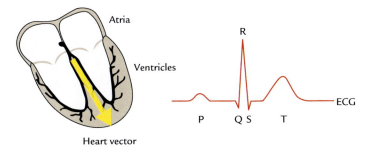

FIGURE 9.16. Electrical activity of the heart. Left: A schematic cross-section of the heart shows the upper and lower chambers (atria and ventricles). The position of the cardiac vector (yellow arrow) indicates the direction of the net current during the contraction of the ventricles. Right: A schematic of the ECG during a single heart cycle. Different deflections of the signal are labeled with letters from P to T. See text for description.

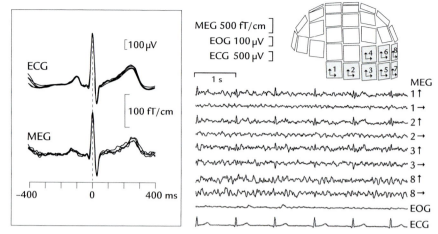

FIGURE 9.17. Cardiac artifacts in the MEG. Left: A comparison of the ECG signal and the associated artifact in planar-gradiometer MEG recordings. Several ECG cycles and simultaneous MEG artifacts are superimposed; both signals have the same timing and width. Right: A 5-s segment of MEG recorded from eight planar gradiometers over the left posterior scalp shows prominent cardiac artifacts at locations 1, 2, and 3 at the edge of the sensor array; the vertical and horizontal arrows on the right side of the traces indicate the directions of field gradients measured by the two orthogonal planar gradiometers at each sensor unit. EOG and ECG signals are displayed in the bottom traces. Adapted and reprinted from Jousmäki V, Hari R: Cardiac artifacts in magnetoencephalogram. *J Clin Neurophysiol* 1996, 13: 172–176. With permission from Wolters Kluwer Health, Inc.

of subjects suffering from ventricular hypertrophy of the heart, as their QRS complex and thus the main cardiac vector (reflecting contraction of the ventricles) is enlarged.

Another important cardiac-cycle-related artifact in MEG data results from the *ballistocardiogram* (Figure 9.18), which reflects small head and body movements along the body's longitudinal axis due to cardiac ejection of blood. The ballistocardiogram artifact peaks some 200 ms after the QRS peak of the ECG, and the waveform is much broader than that of the ECG/MCG. Ballistocardiographic artifacts can arise in MEG also if the subject's body or clothing contains magnetic material that then moves in synchrony with the cardiac cycle.

Ballistocardiographic artifacts become extremely large when the subject is within the strong magnetic field of an MRI scanner. Hence, ballistocardiographic artifacts are prominent in simultaneous EEG–fMRI recordings, and they manifest as comb-like streaks in time-frequency plots due to the harmonics produced by the heartbeat (Krishnaswamy et al., 2016).

In the EEG, the spatial distribution of the cardiac artifact is also asymmetric, so the artifacts are typically most visible on the left side of the neck and head (Dirlich et al., 1997) (see also Figure 9.19, ICA topographic map). In babies, the cardiac artifact in EEG recordings may be diminished or even eliminated by changing the child's head orientation with respect to the body.

Previously, EEG was sometimes recorded with respect to a two-electrode noncephalic reference where each individual's prominent ECG artifacts would be abolished by unique adjustments of a variable resistor (described in Chapter 5). However, elimination of ECG

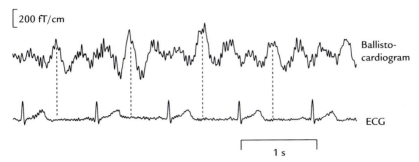

FIGURE 9.18. Ballistocardiogram. An MEG trace showing a prominent ballistocardiogram artifact (top) with a fixed relationship to the ECG (bottom); the ballistocardiographic artifact peaks about 200 ms (vertical line) after the peak of the QRS complex in the ECG. Reproduced and modified with permission from Hari R: Magnetoencephalography: Methods and Clinical Aspects. In: Schomer DL and Lopes da Silva FH: *Niedermeyer's Electroencephalography: Basic Principles, Clinical Applications, and Related Fields.* 7th edition. New York: Oxford University Press, 2018.

by adjusting the two resistors may not always be successful, as the heart's position in the chest (and orientation of the net cardiac vector) varies across individuals and also according to respiratory phase, sometimes requiring even repositioning of the reference electrodes. As we have already stated, it is always preferable to use a single reference point, so from this perspective a noncephalic reference would not be recommended.

That said, portable EEG systems must operate in extreme conditions, where a mobile subject can experience many sources of electrical interference that are not present in the laboratory. Therefore, some investigators have proposed using active amplification with driven right leg/common-mode sensing (DRL/CMS) configurations (see Chapter 5) to help mitigate nonbrain signals in portable EEG studies (Nordin et al., 2018).

A pulsatile artifact can also occur in the EEG if the electrode overlies a blood vessel in the scalp. This artifact is usually clearly visible during online monitoring, and it can be eliminated by moving the EEG electrode a small distance. In intracranial EEG recordings performed during surgery, a pulsatile artifact can warn the neurosurgeon of the proximity of a blood vessel and allow electrode position to be adjusted. In chronically implanted patients, however, such artifacts can mar the recording and cannot be remedied as the electrodes are secured in place by suturing.

Removal of Cardiac Artifacts

As the cardiac artifact is stereotypic in waveform and spatial distribution, it can be effectively identified and removed using ICA, as it typically appears as a well-defined individual IC (Figure 9.19).

Figure 9.20 depicts SSP projectors of the ECG artifact in EEG electrodes, MEG magnetometers and planar gradiometers, with a total duration of ~400 ms. SSP is another effective means of removing this artifact from MEG and EEG signals.

Ballistocardiographic (BCG) artifacts can be suppressed using software or hardware, either during the recording itself or post hoc. Typically, a template or model of the artifact is generated from the EEG corrupted by MRI and BCG artifacts and sampled at high rates, say > 5 kHz (Koskinen & Vartiainen, 2009). More recent removal methods do not require

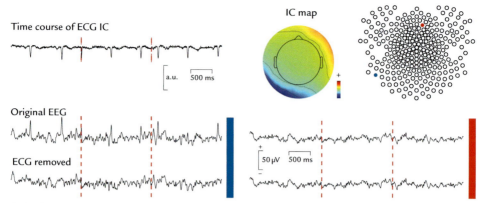

FIGURE 9.19. Removal of ECG artifact from the EEG by ICA. Epoched EEG data from a healthy subject (passband 0.1–200 Hz, vertex reference) (bottom of figure). The IC time course (top left) shows a clear ECG-like signal, where the P wave, QRS complex, and T wave can be identified. A topographic IC map in the middle top portion of the figure shows the largest artifact over the left neck and lower posterior scalp. As noted in the text, the polarities of ICs are irrelevant. The lower left part of the figure displays EEG data from an electrode on the left side of the neck (blue) with ECG artifact and an electrode anterior to the vertex on the right scalp (red) without the artifact; see the electrode map at the top right. The upper and lower traces display EEG before and after removal of the ECG IC, respectively. Data recorded in the Social Neuroscience Laboratory, Indiana University, USA.

such high sampling rates (Krishnaswamy et al., 2016). Precise synchronization between the MRI scanner and EEG system is required so that the timing of gradient pulses corresponding to each acquired slice can be accurately modeled.

▪ RESPIRATION-RELATED ARTIFACTS

Generation and Recognition

Slow fluctuations at the frequency of respiration can occur in the MEG signal in the presence of even tiny metallic fragments in a subject's body or clothing. One very frequent source of this kind of artifact is the upper button of the trousers as it moves during normal respiration; thus unbuttoning often helps, although it is better to use totally nonmagnetic clothing. This kind of artifact is easy to notice in online monitoring during the experiment.

Slow MEG artifacts assumed to be directly related to respiration have been described but so far with unknown origin (Rodin et al., 2005). It is possible that magnetized nanoparticles in the lungs, airborne in urban environments from traffic and combustion (Maher et al., 2016), might cause detectable respiration-related MEG artifacts, although magnetopneumographic identification of lung contamination is based on recording of the remanent magnetic field after magnetization of the chest area.

Respiration does not usually cause artifacts to EEG recordings, although respiration-related sway of poorly anchored electrode cables can elicit slow drifts in one or multiple derivations. Sometimes, a reference electrode placed on the nose may sample respiration-related artifacts, presumably related to nostril flaring.

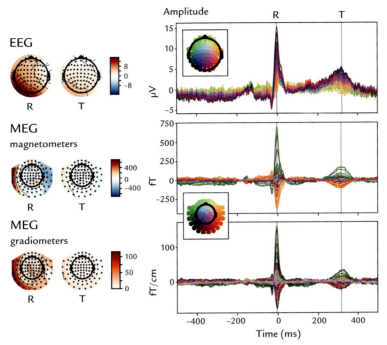

FIGURE 9.20. Identification of ECG artifact in EEG and MEG data by the SSP method. Left: Scalp topographies of the SSP projectors at R and T wave maxima in the ECG are shown for EEG, magnetometer MEG, and planar-gradiometer MEG data, color-coded in units of µV, fT, and fT/cm, respectively. Note the clearly different spatial distributions for magnetometer and planar-gradiometer MEG (for an explanation, see Figure 5.15). Sensors are depicted as black dots on scalp topographies. Right: SSP projector waveforms. Sensor positions appear as colored dots (insets) on butterfly plots of time courses. Waveforms demonstrate a clear hemispheric asymmetry in morphology. Single-subject data generated from over 500 heartbeats. Data recorded in the Centre de Neuroimagerie de Recherche (CENIR and STIM platform), Institut du Cerveau et de la Moelle épinière (ICM), Sorbonne Université, Paris, France. Data analyzed in the Social Neuroscience Laboratory, Indiana University, USA.

Removal of Respiration Artifacts

The best way to prevent respiration artifacts occurring during MEG recordings is to ensure that the subject does not have any magnetic material in the body or in the clothing. If the slow respiration-related shifts are present in MEG/EEG recordings, one may try to dampen them by high-pass filtering in postprocessing. ICA may also capture some aspects of prominent respiration artifacts. However, similar to high-pass filtering, these "blind" approaches risk also eliminating slow brain activity, which itself may be a variable of interest.

If ECG signals are recorded concurrently with MEG/EEG data, the respiratory cycle can be modeled by the ECG-derived respiration (EDR) technique (Moody et al., 1986; Varone et al., 2021). EDR is based on variations of ECG signals during the respiratory cycle, caused by chest movements and the associated changes of the heart vector. It is also possible to use a respiratory belt in addition to the EEG and ECG recordings, so that the respiratory signal can be monitored directly. Respiratory artifacts could be removed using correlational or regression-based approaches.

■ SWEATING

Generation and Recognition

Sweating can be a problem in EEG recordings as it is accompanied by electrodermal changes, high-amplitude slow (< 0.5 Hz) potentials that can contaminate measurements of slow event-related potentials (e.g., Picton & Hillyard, 1972; Corby et al., 1974). These artifacts disappear on cessation of sweating—sometimes requiring that the subject be cooled with a fan during the recording session. Figure 9.21 displays a portable EEG recording where a sweaty brow produced large signal fluctuations in two frontal traces, whereas EEG from bilateral central and occipital sites was unaffected by the artifact. Should the subject sweat more profusely, the artifact would be present in other EEG electrodes as well. In perimenopausal women, the occurrence of "hot flushes" may cause similar slow fluctuations in the EEG.

Whether sweating can cause artifacts in MEG has not—according to our knowledge—been specifically studied. Until now we have only heard anecdotal reports that such artifacts might occur in MEG if the subject feels hot during the recording (which will be unlikely as most air-conditioned magnetically shielded rooms tend to be quite cool).

Removal of Sweating Artifacts

Ideally, a comfortable temperature in the laboratory or shielded room will minimize the likelihood of dealing with a sweating subject, as will mild abrasion of the skin. Moreover, post hoc high-pass filtering can diminish this artifact provided that one is not interested in slow responses, such as sustained potentials associated with sensory stimuli or preparation for movements (see Chapters 17 and 18).

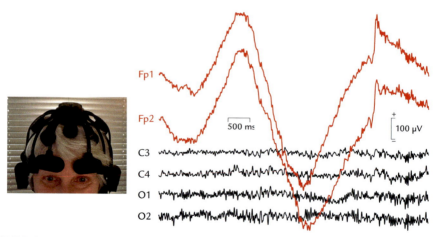

FIGURE 9.21. Sweating artifact. Portable EEG traces from six 10–20 sites in a subject with a sweaty brow. Traces from the bilateral frontal, central and occipital scalp are shown over a 5-s interval. Both frontal traces show very large and slow baseline sway. EEG recorded from dry Ag/AgCl "spider" or "finger" electrodes with respect to A1. Sampling frequency 500 Hz, passband 0.5–100 Hz, post-hoc filtering from 0.5 to 40 Hz. Data courtesy of Dr. Ben Ramsden in the Lab in Electrical Brain Activity, Indiana University, USA.

■ NONPHYSIOLOGICAL ARTIFACTS

The most common nonphysiological artifacts in MEG/EEG include power-line noise and various artifacts that emanate from surrounding equipment. Artifacts can also be generated by high-voltage power tools. Large MEG fluctuations can arise from the motion of far-away large metallic objects, such as elevators, cars, trams, and trains, or even chairs in the room just outside the magnetically shielded room.

Sometimes, problems with electrode connections, cable malfunctions or simply unacceptably high impedances for EEG electrodes can produce broadband "colored" noise (e.g., white noise). This noise, when filtered, can potentially masquerade as a realistic EEG signal (see Figure 9.1 and also Tatum et al., 2011).

Power-Line Noise and Its Removal

A noticeable, and very common, nonphysiological artifact is "line" (power-line) noise that arises from the alternating current supplied to electrical wall outlets and is visible in both EEG and MEG recordings. Depending on the country, the line noise occurs at either 50 or 60 Hz and at their harmonics. In the time domain, the signal is typically sinusoidal (see Figure 9.22, upper panel) and often also contains harmonics that can be easily seen in power spectra. The line noise is particularly accentuated in EEG electrode pairs that have an impedance mismatch (and impaired common-mode rejection), in electrodes that make poor contact with the scalp (and have a high impedance), and if the EEG equipment has grounding problems. The lower panel of Figure 9.22 displays concurrent 50-Hz line noise in MEG magnetometers and planar gradiometers and in EEG electrodes.

As line noise can sometimes be difficult to eliminate, much care must be paid to all cables that connect the measurement device with stimulators, response pads, and monitoring devices. Turning off fluorescent lighting and moving other equipment and cabling away from EEG leads and amplifiers can diminish the line artifact. Similarly, making sure that the electrode impedances remain optimal throughout the EEG recording session, as described in Chapter 7, will also help reduce this problem.

If line noise cannot be eliminated during the recording, its removal must be tackled during data processing, preferably prior to the main analysis.

On occasion, line noise may arise from sources outside the laboratory. Equipment using high power or voltages in other parts of the building may create intermittent, but large, artifacts in EEG traces. These sources include arc welders and other high-voltage, construction-related equipment. Additional problems can occur when EEG recordings are performed in the intensive-care unit or operating room, where drips, pumps, and ventilators can create various artifacts (Klass, 1995). Keeping the EEG cables and amplifiers as far away as possible from these devices is helpful in minimizing the artifacts, as is also anchoring the cables to the subject's shoulder with a clip or tape to prevent cable sway.

It is particularly important to minimize line-noise artifacts if high-frequency brain signals, such as gamma activity, are of interest. The scalp topography of line noise can change during the course of an EEG recording, as electrode impedances gradually change relative to one another and the reference electrode. Therefore, the spatial topography of line noise usually differs from that of most brain rhythms. Line-noise issues could also cause issues in naturalistic environments where portable EEG systems with dry electrodes are being used.

60-Hz line noise

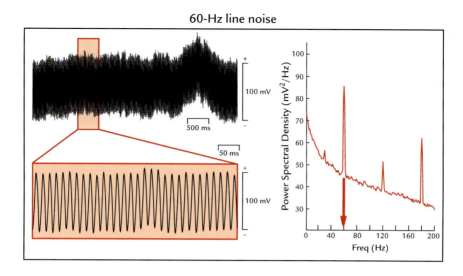

50-Hz line noise

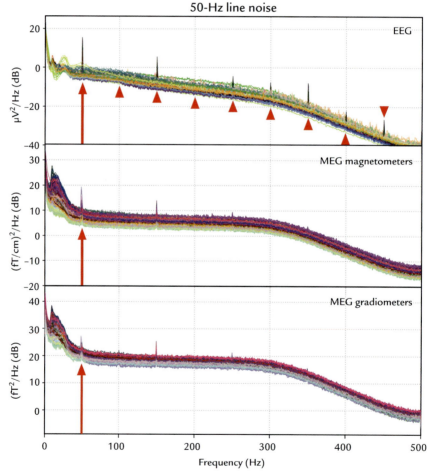

FIGURE 9.22. **Power-line noise.** Top: 60-Hz line noise in EEG data. A 5-s epoch from an electrode making poor contact with the scalp shows a prominent 60-Hz artifact (top left

A number of *power-line noise removal* options are available, some of them instantiated in existing MEG/EEG analysis software packages.

If line noise cannot be prevented, a post hoc digital notch filter that does not introduce phase shifts, set to the appropriate line frequency (and its harmonics, if necessary), can work, although it will introduce discontinuities in the power spectrum and distortions in the data.

If CCA- and ICA-based approaches are applied to remove line noise, the variable nature of this type of noise can lead the artifact to appear in multiple components. If all these artifact-containing components were discarded, real brain signals could be lost as well as they are often mixed with the noise. This problem is most serious in low-density/portable EEG recordings, which already suffer from low dimensionality.

The *discrete Fourier transform (DFT) filter* of the Fieldtrip Toolbox has been suggested for the removal of power-line noise and its harmonics (Oostenveld et al., 2011). By calculating sine/cosine components on short data epochs (e.g., 1 s), changes in line-noise characteristics at a particular measurement sensor can be better handled. Estimated sine and cosine components at the desired frequencies are subtracted from the amplitude spectrum. As one of the assumptions of the filter is that the noise has constant amplitude, this artifact may not be completely eliminated if line-noise amplitude changes within the epoch, and its amplitude fluctuations may affect neighboring frequencies in the power spectrum (Leske & Dalal, 2019).

A regression-based approach for line-noise removal has been developed as part of the EEGLAB suite. Its main steps include passing a sliding window across the data and transforming the signals into the frequency domain using a set of multitapers with predetermined spectral resolution. A frequency-domain regression model then estimates the amplitude and phase of a set of selected deterministic sinusoids (which includes line-noise harmonics), tests them statistically, and after some additional checks subtracts these line-noise estimates from the data. The noise can be removed from either the raw EEG itself or ICs (Bigdely-Shamlo et al., 2015). This approach may also have similar issues as the DFT filter: if the amplitude of the noise is variable, the power-line noise might not be completely removed.

Line noise and its harmonics can be removed without distortion of neighboring frequencies. For example, MEG/EEG data can be sent through two parallel streams, where the artifact is removed by spectral and spatial approaches, and then these two outputs are combined. This algorithm requires only one parameter that specifies the number of spatial components to reject from the artifact contaminated stream (de Cheveigné, 2020).

FIGURE 9.22. **Continued**

trace), with its characteristically "fuzzy" appearance. The lower left trace displays a magnified section of the artifact (red box from top trace), demonstrating a regular sinusoidal waveform whose spectral peak is at 60 Hz (right panel). Sampling frequency 1 kHz, passband 0.1–200 Hz. Data from the Social Neuroscience Laboratory, Indiana University, USA. Bottom: 50-Hz line noise in MEG/EEG power spectra. Prominent peaks at 50 Hz and its harmonics in all MEG and EEG channels are visible. The red full arrow, shown in the EEG and MEG signal boxes, indicates 50-Hz activity. Harmonics of 50 Hz have been annotated by arrowheads in the EEG box. Sampling frequency 1 kHz, passband 0.1–300 Hz. Recorded in the Centre de Neuroimagerie de Recherche (CENIR and STIM platform), Institut du Cerveau et de la Moelle épinière (ICM), Sorbonne Université, Paris, France.

Response-Box Artifacts

Only nonmagnetic response pads should be used with MEG recordings, and in neither MEG nor EEG recordings should the response pads themselves cause any sound.

Some response boxes, such as numerical keypads, can introduce artifacts in the EEG signal because of capacitance changes associated with key presses. While the artifact as such can be stereotypical, it may occur in the recording epoch with variable timing (onset and also duration) depending on the subject's behavioral responses (Figure 9.23, left panel). It is thus recommended that only specific MEG- and EEG-compatible response boxes be used to avoid these types of artifacts.

Artifacts Related to EEG Electrodes and MEG Sensors

A number of different artifacts can arise from improperly applied EEG electrodes. One type of artifact appears as a very slow baseline drift (Figure 9.23, middle panel). These "bad electrode" artifacts can be eliminated by reapplying the electrode or by improving the contact between the electrode and the scalp. Persistence of this artifact usually indicates a (partly) broken electrode wire, requiring replacement or repair. Pop will occur in improperly applied electrodes and is thought to occur when a buildup of charge between the electrode surface and conducting medium is suddenly released. Drift and pop can appear more frequently as the electrode gel or conductive solution dries out as the experiment progresses.

In both EEG and MEG recordings, artifacts can be created by the experimenter's movements around the subject. In EEG, this problem can be exaggerated in colder climates,

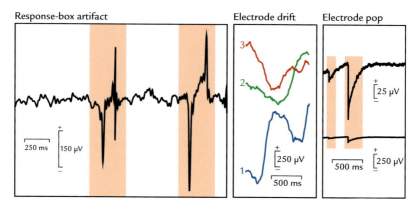

FIGURE 9.23. **Response-box and EEG electrode artifacts.** Left panel: EEG from a single channel in a task where the subject has made 2 button presses on a non-MEG/EEG compatible response box. Two prominent artifacts appear (red shading) as the subject responds in the activation task. The artifact is caused by a changed capacitance at the time of button press and release. Passband 0.1–100 Hz. Data recorded in the Social Neuroscience Laboratory, Indiana University, USA. Middle and right panels: EEG electrode drift and pop. Left: Drift in an EEG electrode manifests as large excursions in amplitude (see calibration bars). Three epochs (1, 2, and 3) separated by less than 1 s are shown. Right: Electrode pop typically consists of a large-voltage transient whose return back to baseline will depend on the filters being used. Here an EEG electrode pops (red shading) releasing accumulated electric charge. The same trace is displayed at two different gains to display the artifact and the EEG signal. Passband 0.1–200 Hz. Data recorded in the Dual EEG Laboratory, Imaging Research Facility, Indiana University, USA.

where heating in winter leads to drier air in the laboratory, thereby creating a problem with static electricity. As noted, additional humidification in the laboratory can diminish this problem, and, of course, unnecessary movements in the recording environment have to be avoided. Ideally, the experimenter should not be located near the subject during the recording.

In MEG experiments, the measurement gantry is very sensitive to vibrations, many of which may arise from the subject's own movements, which can be transferred to the sensor helmet via the floor; direct touch to the arm holders and gantry; or outside sources. If an experimenter or a caregiver must be with the subject inside the shielded room (e.g., during a pain experiment as depicted in Figure 6.2), they need to sit as still as possible in nonmagnetic clothing, without touching any part of the MEG device unless absolutely necessary.

In earlier MEG systems based on a SQUID (superconducting quantum interference device), *flux-trap* artifacts, limited to some channels, could appear as abrupt up-and-down shifts of the MEG channel. The problem could be eliminated by retuning the channel using procedures specific to the MEG device. Fortunately, the SQUID sensors of today are so stable that the flux-trap problem is almost nonexistent unless magnetic material is brought close to the sensors. If one of the SQUIDs is "broken," it cannot be replaced until the next service break (which may take place only once per year). Meanwhile, care must be taken that one does not spread the poorly behaving channel's artifacts to other channels by means of data-analysis methods. Specifically, this channel would need to be eliminated from further analyses (see Chapter 10).

If continuous head-position information is requested, sinusoidal currents at different frequencies are fed to the head-position-indicator (HPI) coils continuously. During preprocessing, these HPI coil signals are analyzed to compute head position information, typically at time intervals of 100–500 ms. The HPI coil frequencies (which are visible in the raw unfiltered MEG data; see, e.g., Figure 2 in Jas et al., 2018) are selected to fall outside the brain signal frequency range of interest and can thus be removed by bandpass (or low-pass) filtering before subsequent analysis.

EEG Artifacts Caused by fMRI Scanning and Noninvasive Brain Stimulation

Many EEG studies performed simultaneously with MRI scanning or noninvasive brain stimulation come with substantial technical challenges. To aid artifact removal and data analysis, the exact timing of MRI pulse sequences and brain stimulation events must be timestamped in the EEG file.

We have already discussed the special EEG electrodes that can be used within the MR environment (see Chapter 5). MRI pulse sequences cause substantial artifacts in EEG recordings. Thus early EEG–fMRI studies alternated acquisition of EEG and fMRI data, or they triggered the fMRI data acquisition with an EEG event, such as an epileptic spike (Ives et al., 1993; Warach et al., 1996). These strategies avoided MRI gradient artifacts, exploiting the known time lags of the hemodynamic responses. Today, the high dynamic range of EEG amplifiers allows the recording of both the EEG and the large MRI gradient artifacts (up to over 400 times the size of EEG signals) without clipping. Because the MRI pulse sequences are predictable and repetitive, the current artifact removal algorithms commonly learn to recognize the artifact before using some template-based removal strategy to extract a clean EEG signal. Template methods can include a moving average filter, cubic spline interpolation, or hierarchical clustering (for a recent comprehensive review, see Bullock et al., 2021). Alternatively, blind source-separation methods (ICA, CCA, etc.) can be applied. Once the MRI gradient artifact has been removed, other artifacts can be better handled.

For example, the magnet's helium pump causes artifacts that spread widely across the frequency spectrum. One solution is to switch off the helium pump during a simultaneous EEG–fMRI recording, which causes heating in the magnet, results in greater helium use, and also risks damaging the MRI scanner. Fortunately, the helium pump artifact (as well as the ballistocardiogram artifact, see Figure 9.18) can be removed, if the tiny movements of the scanner and body are monitored with extra sensors, such as carbon wire loops (van der Meer et al., 2016).

Transcranial magnetic stimulation (TMS) applies brief, but strong, magnetic pulses (~1 tesla or more) that create very large transient artifacts in the simultaneously recorded EEG. TMS can also polarize the EEG electrodes, and the large capacitors of the TMS equipment can cause (exponential) recharging artifacts in the EEG. Other artifacts (e.g., focal muscle contraction at TMS stimulation site) are also an issue. Over the years, hardware and software solutions have reduced some of these artifacts (reviewed by Rogasch et al., 2017; Varone et al., 2021).

In transcranial direct current stimulation (tDCS) and transcranial alternating current stimulation (tACS), small currents (up to 2 mA) are delivered to the scalp via two electrodes positioned bifrontally on opposite hemispheres or in an anterior-posterior cross-hemispheric configuration. tDCS is often applied with a steady current for minutes, but in tACS the stimulation varies rapidly and can, for example, be adjusted in real time to ongoing EEG activity (5–40 Hz). These stimuli can contaminate the simultaneous EEG recordings in different ways, and several artifact removal methods are currently under development (Gebodh et al., 2019; Kohli & Casson, 2019).

How to Ensure the Signals Come From the Brain

Many decades ago, the cerebral versus noncerebral origins of different MEG/EEG signals were frequently discussed. For example, there was skepticism in the early 1980s that the 100-ms auditory response—despite the dipolar field pattern of the MEG signals over the supratemporal auditory cortex (Hari et al., 1980)—could arise from the auditory cortex. Specifically, the responses were proposed to be long-latency muscle artifacts. Two observations finally convinced the skeptics: (a) biting on a nonmagnetic eraser increased facial muscle tension but did not enhance the response, in contrast to what would have occurred if the response was of muscular origin, and (b) the response was unilaterally abolished in a stroke patient with temporal lobe injury (Mäkelä & Hari, 1992).

The view that sustained EEG potentials to long tones (Hari et al., 1980) and vibratory stimuli (Hari, 1980) were of cerebral origin was challenged by a dissertation reviewer. The reviewer's assumption that the sustained responses reflect electrodermal responses arising at the electrode–skin interface was rebutted by showing that the sustained potentials remained unchanged although the skin under the scalp electrode was scratched by a needle to the bleeding point.

As another example, the first MEG responses to observed painful electric stimulation of the tooth were argued not to be due to pain afferents, but rather to concomitant stimulation of tactile afferents from the gum. As no MEG responses were elicited when the same stimuli were applied to a devitalized (dead) tooth (Hari et al., 1983), it became obvious that the response was really produced by pain afferents.

As we have already noted, recording physiological signals, such as EOG, ECG, EMG, respiration, and limb movements in conjunction with MEG/EEG can help identify many physiological artifacts. However, such extra recordings are not always possible, particularly with some commercial EEG systems. In those cases, monitoring the EEG data during the recording session can help identify sudden signal changes, such as the onset of putative physiological and nonphysiological artifacts. Video monitoring of the subject during the EEG recording can be useful to identify artifacts, especially in infants or patients.

■ REFERENCES

Antervo A, Hari R, Katila T, Ryhänen T, Seppänen M: Magnetic fields produced by eye blinking. *Electroencephalogr Clin Neurophysiol* 1985, 61: 247–254.

Arden GB, Kelsey JH: Changes produced by light in the standing potential of the human eye. *J Physiol* 1962a, 161: 189–204.

Arden GB, Kelsey JH: Some observations on the relationship between the standing potential of the human eye and the bleaching and regeneration of visual purple. *J Physiol* 1962b, 161: 205–226.

Barry W, Jones GM: Influence of eye lid movement upon electro-oculographic recordings of vertical eye movements. *Aerospace Med* 1965, 36: 855–858.

Beaussart M, Guieu JD: Artefacts. In: Rémond A, ed. *Handbook of Electroencephalography and Clinical Neurophysiology*. Amsterdam: Elsevier 1977, 11A: 80–96.

Bell AJ, Sejnowski TJ: An information-maximization approach to blind separation and blind deconvolution. *Neural Comput* 1995, 7: 1129–1259.

Berg P, Scherg M: Dipole models of eye movements and blinks. *Electroencephalogr Clin Neurophysiol* 1991, 79: 36–44.

Bigdely-Shamlo N, Mullen T, Kothe C, Su K-M, Robbins KA: The PREP pipeline: standardized preprocessing for large-scale EEG analysisfc. *Front Neuroinform* 2015, 9: 1–20.

Blinn KA: Focal anterior temporal spikes from external rectus muscle. *Electroencephalogr Clin Neurophysiol* 1955, 7: 299–302.

Bourguignon M, Whitmarsh S, Piitulainen H, Hari R, Jousmäki V, Lundqvist D: Reliable recording and analysis of MEG-based corticokinematic coherence in the presence of strong magnetic artifacts. *Clin Neurophysiol* 2016, 127: 1460–1469.

Brown GD, Yamada S, Sejnowski TJ: Independent component analysis at the neural cocktail party. *Trends Neurosci* 2001, 24: 54–63.

Bullock M, Jackson GD, Abbott DF: Artifact reduction in simultaneous EEG-fMRI: a systematic review of methods and contemporary usage. *Front Neurol* 2021, 12: 622719.

Cai C, Kang H, Kirsch HE, Mizuiri D, Chen J, Bhutada A, Sekihara K, Nagarajan SS: Comparison of DSSP and tSSS algorithms for removing artifacts from vagus nerve stimulators in magnetoencephalography data. *J Neural Eng* 2019, 16: 066045.

Carl C, Açık A, König P, Engel AK, Hipp JF: The saccadic spike artifact in MEG. *NeuroImage* 2012, 59: 1657–1667.

Chan RCK, Chen EYC: Blink rate does matter: a study of blink rate, sustained attention, and neurological signs in schizophrenia. *J Nervous Ment Dis* 2004, 192: 781–783.

Chaumon M, Bishop DV, Busch NA: A practical guide to the selection of independent components of the electroencephalogram for artifact correction. *J Neurosci Methods* 2015, 250: 47–63.

Clarke M, Larson E, Tavabi K, Taulu S: Effectively combining temporal projection noise suppression methods in magnetoencephalography. *J Neurosci Methods* 2020, 341: 108700.

Corby JC, Roth WT, Kopell BS: Prevalence and methods of control of the cephalic skin potential EEG artifact. *Psychophysiology* 1974, 11: 350–360.

Croft RJ, Barry RJ: Removal of ocular artifact from the EEG: a review. *Neurophysiol Clin* 2000, 30: 5–19.

Croft RJ, Chandler JS, Barry RJ, Cooper NR, Clarke AR: EOG correction: a comparison of four methods. *Psychophysiology* 2005, 42: 16–24.

de Cheveigné A: Sparse time artifact removal. *J Neurosci Methods* 2016, 262: 14–20.

de Cheveigné A: ZapLine: A simple and effective method to remove power line artifacts. *NeuroImage* 2020, 207: 116356.

De Clercq W, Vergult A, Vanrumste B, Van Paesschen W, Van Huffel S: Canonical correlation analysis applied to remove muscle artifacts from the electroencephalogram. *IEEE Trans Biomed Eng* 2006, 53: 2583–2587.

Delorme A, Sejnowski T, Makeig S: Enhanced detection of artifacts in EEG data using higher-order statistics and independent component analysis. *NeuroImage* 2007, 34: 1443–1449.

Dimigen O, Valsecchi M, Sommer W, Kliegl R: Human microsaccade-related visual brain responses. *J Neurosci* 2009, 29: 12321–12331.

Dirlich G, Vogl L, Plaschke M, Strian F: Cardiac field effects on the EEG. *Electroencephalogr Clin Neurophysiol* 1997, 102: 307–315.

Eichele T, Rachakonda S, Brakedal B, Eikeland R, Calhoun VD: EEGIFT: group independent component analysis for event-related EEG data. *Comput Intell Neurosci* 2011: 129365.

Engbert R: Microsaccades: a microcosm for research on oculomotor control, attention, and visual perception. *Prog Brain Res* 2006, 154: 177–192.

Friman O, Borga M, Lundberg P, Knutsson H: Exploratory fMRI analysis by autocorrelation maximization. *NeuroImage* 2002, 16: 454–464.

Frølich L, Andersen TS, Mørup M: Classification of independent components of EEG into multiple artifact classes. *Psychophysiology* 2015, 52: 32–45.

Gao J, Zheng C, Wang P: Online removal of muscle artifact from electroencephalogram signals based on canonical correlation analysis. *Clin EEG Neurosci* 2010, 41: 53–59.

Gastaut Y: [A little-known electroencephalographic sign: occipital points occurring during opening of the eyes]. *Rev Neurol (Paris)* 1951, 84: 635–640.

Gawne TJ, Killen JF, Tracy JM, Lahti AC: The effect of saccadic eye movements on the sensor-level magnetoencephalogram. *Clin Neurophysiol* 2017, 128: 397–407.

Gebodh N, Esmaeilpour Z, Adair D, Chelette K, Dmochowski J, Woods AJ, Kappenman ES, Parra LC, Bikson M: Inherent physiological artifacts in EEG during tDCS. *NeuroImage* 2019, 185: 408–424.

Goncharova, McFarland DJ II, Vaughan TM, Wolpaw JR: EMG contamination of EEG: spectral and topographical characteristics. *Clin Neurophysiol* 2003, 114: 1580–1593.

Gramfort A, Luessi M, Larson E, Engemann DA, Strohmeier D, Brodbeck C, Parkkonen L, Hämäläinen MS: MNE software for processing MEG and EEG data. *NeuroImage* 2014, 86: 446–460.

Gratton G, Coles MG, Donchin E: A new method for off-line removal of ocular artifact. *Electroencephalogr Clin Neurophysiol* 1983, 55: 468–484.

Gwin JT, Gramann K, Makeig S, Ferris DP: Removal of movement artifact from high-density EEG recorded during walking and running. *J Neurophysiol* 2010, 103: 3526–3534.

Hari R: Evoked potentials elicited by long vibrotactile stimuli in the human EEG. *Pflügers Arch* 1980, 384: 167–170.

Hari R, Aittoniemi K, Järvinen ML, Katila T, Varpula T: Auditory evoked transient and sustained magnetic fields of the human brain: localization of neural generators. *Exp Brain Res* 1980, 40: 237–240.

Hari R, Kaukoranta E, Reinikainen K, Huopaniemi T, Mauno J: Neuromagnetic localization of cortical activity evoked by painful dental stimulation in man. *Neurosci Lett* 1983, 42: 77–82.

Hari R, Salmelin R, Tissari S, Kajola M, Virsu V: Visual stability during eyeblinks. *Nature* 1994, 367: 121–122.

Hassler U, Barreto NT, Gruber T. Induced gamma band responses in human EEG after the control of miniature saccadic artifacts. *NeuroImage* 2011, 57: 1411–1421.

Himberg J, Hyvärinen A, Esposito F: Validating the independent components of neuroimaging time-series via clustering and visualization. *NeuroImage* 2004, 22: 1214–1222.

Hipp JF, Siegel M: Dissociating neuronal gamma-band activity from cranial and ocular muscle activity in EEG. *Front Hum Neurosci* 2013, 7: 338.

Hirokawa K, Yagi A, Miyata Y: Comparison of blinking behavior during listening to and speaking in Japanese and English. *Perc Motor Skills* 2004, 98: 463–472.

Holland MK, Tarlow G: Blinking and thinking. *Perc Motor Skills* 1975, 41: 403–406.

Hotelling H: Relations between two sets of variates. *Biometrika* 1936, 28: 321–377.

Huster RJ, Raud L: A tutorial review on multi-subject decomposition of EEG. *Brain Topogr* 2018, 31: 3–16.

Huttunen J, Kobal G, Kaukoranta E, Hari R: Cortical responses to painful CO_2 stimulation of the nasal mucosa. *Electroencephalogr Clin Neurophysiol* 1986, 64: 347–349.

Hyvärinen A, Oja E: Independent component analysis: algorithms and applications. *Neural Netw* 2000, 13: 411–430.

Hyvärinen A, Ramkumar P, Parkkonen L, Hari R: Independent component analysis of short-time Fourier transforms for spontaneous EEG/MEG analysis. *NeuroImage* 2010, 49: 257–271.

Ives JR, Warach S, Schmitt F, Edelman RR, Schomer DL: Monitoring the patient's EEG during echo planar MRI. *Electroenceph Clin Neurophysiol* 1993, 87: 417–420.

Iwasaki M, Kellinghaus C, Alexopoulos AV, Burgess RC, Kumar AK, Han YH, Lüders HO, Leigh RJ: Effects of eyelid closure, blinks, and eye movements on the electroencephalogram. *Clin Neurophysiol* 2005, 116: 878–885.

Jäntti V, Aantaa E, Lang H, Schalén L, Pyykkö I: The saccade spike. *Adv Otorhinolaryngol* 1983, 30: 71–75.

Jas M, Larson E, Engemann DA, Leppäkangas J, Taulu S, Hämäläinen M, Gramfort A: A reproducible MEG/EEG group study with the MNE software: recommendations, quality assessments, and good practices. *Front Neurosci* 2018, 12: 530.

Jonmohamadi Y, Poudel G, Innes C, Jones R: Source-space ICA for EEG source separation, localization, and time-course reconstruction. *NeuroImage* 2014, 101: 720–737.

Jousmäki V, Hämäläinen M, Hari R: Magnetic source imaging during a visually guided [saccade] task. *Neuroreport* 1996, 7: 2961–2964.

Jousmäki V, Hari R: Cardiac artifacts in magnetoencephalogram. *J Clin Neurophysiol* 1996, 13: 172–176.

Kandemir AL, Litvak V, Florin E: The comparative performance of DBS artefact rejection methods for MEG recordings. *NeuroImage* 2020, 219: 117057.

Karson CN, Burns RS, LeWitt PA, Foster NK, Newman RP: Blink rates and disorders of movement. *Neurology* 1984, 34: 677–678.

Katila T, Maniewski R, Poutanen T, Varpula T, Karp PJ: Magnetic fields produced by the human eye. *J Appl Physics* 1981, 52: 2565–2571.

Keren AS, Yuval-Greenberg S, Deouell LY: Saccadic spike potentials in gamma-band EEG: characterization, detection and suppression. *NeuroImage* 2010, 49: 2248–2263.

Klass DW: The continuing challenge of artifacts in the EEG. *Am J EEG Technol* 1995, 35: 239–269.

Kline JE, Huang HJ, Snyder KL, Ferris DP: Isolating gait-related movement artifacts in electroencephalography during human walking. *J Neural Eng* 2015, 12: 046022.

Kohli S, Casson AJ: Removal of gross artifacts of transcranial alternating current stimulation in simultaneous EEG monitoring. *Sensors (Basel)* 2019, 19: 190.

Koskinen M, Vartiainen N: Removal of imaging artifacts in EEG during simultaneous EEG/fMRI recording: reconstruction of a high-precision artifact template. *NeuroImage* 2009, 46: 160–167.

Krishnaswamy P, Bonmassar G, Poulsen C, Pierce ET, Purdon PL, Brown EN. Reference-free removal of EEG-fMRI ballistocardiogram artifacts with harmonic regression. *NeuroImage* 2016, 128: 398–412.

Lankinen K, Saari J, Hari R, Koskinen M: Intersubject consistency of cortical MEG signals during movie viewing. *NeuroImage* 2014, 92: 217–224.

Lankinen K, Saari J, Hlushchuk Y, Tikka P, Parkkonen L, Hari R, Koskinen M: Consistency and similarity of MEG- and fMRI-signal timecourses during movie viewing. *NeuroImage* 2018, 173: 361–369.

Larson E, Taulu S: Reducing sensor noise in MEG and EEG recordings using oversampled temporal projection. *IEEE Trans Biomed Eng* 2018; 65: 1002–1013.

Leske S, Dalal SS: Reducing power line noise in EEG and MEG data via spectrum interpolation. *NeuroImage* 2019, 89: 763–776.

Li Y, Wang PT, Vaidya MP, Flint RD, Liu CY, Slutzky MW, Do AH: Electromyogram (EMG) removal by adding sources of EMG (ERASE)—a novel ICA-based algorithm for removing myoelectric artifacts from EEG. *Front Neurosci* 2021, 14: 597941.

Lin C-T, Huang C-S, Yang W-Y, Singh AK, Chuang C-S, Wang Y-K: Real-time EEG signal enhancement using canonical correlation analysis and Gaussian mixture clustering. *J Healthc Eng* 2018, 2018: 5081258.

Lotte F, Bougrain L, Cichocki A, Clerc M, Congedo M, Rakotomamonjy A, Yger F: A review of classification algorithms for EEG-based brain–computer interfaces: a 10 year update. *J Neural Eng* 2018, 15: 031005

Maher BA, Ahmed IA, Karloukovski V, MacLaren DA, Foulds PG, Allsop D, Mann DM, Torres-Jardón R, Calderon-Garciduenas L: Magnetite pollution nanoparticles in the human brain. *Proc Natl Acad Sci U S A* 2016, 113: 10797–10801.

Makeig S, Jung T-P, Bell AJ, Ghahremani D, Sejnowski TJ: Blind separation of auditory event-related brain responses into independent components. *Proc Natl Acad Sci U S A* 1997, 94: 10979–10984.

Mäkelä JP, Hari R: Neuromagnetic auditory evoked responses after a stroke in the right temporal lobe. *Neuroreport* 1992, 3: 94–96.

Martinez-Conde S: Fixational eye movements in normal and pathological vision. *Prog Brain Res* 2006, 154: 151–176.

Martinez-Conde S, Macknik SL, Troncoso XG, Hubel DH. Microsaccades: a neurophysiological analysis. *Trends Neurosci* 2009, 32: 463–475.

Mognon A, Jovicich J, Bruzzone L, Buiatti M: ADJUST: an automatic EEG artifact detector based on the joint use of spatial and temporal features. *Psychophysiology* 2011, 48: 229–240.

Moody GB, Mark RG, Bump MA, Weinstein JS, Berman AD, Mietus JE, Goldberger Al: Clinical validation of the ECG-derived respiration (EDR) technique. *Comput Cardiol* 1986, 13: 507–510.

Müller-Putz G, Scherer R, Brunner C, Leeb R, Pfurtscheller G: Better than random: a closer look on BCI results. *Int J Bioelectromagn* 2008, 10: 52–55.

Nakano T, Kitazawa S: Eyeblink entrainment at breakpoints of speech. *Exp Brain Res* 2010, 205: 577–581.

Nolan H, Whelan R, Reilly RB: FASTER: fully automated statistical thresholding for EEG artifact rejection. *J Neurosci Methods* 2010, 192: 152–162.

Nordin AD, Hairston WD, Ferris DP: Dual-electrode motion artifact cancellation for mobile electro-encephalography. *J Neural Eng* 2018, 15: 056024.

Onton J, Westerfield M, Townsend J, Makeig S: Imaging human EEG dynamics using independent component analysis. *Neurosci Biobehav Rev* 2006, 30: 808–822.

Oostenveld R, Fries P, Maris E, Schoffelen JM: FieldTrip: open source software for advanced analysis of MEG, EEG, and invasive electrophysiological data. *Comput Intell Neurosci* 2011: 156869.

Ousler GW 3rd, Hagberg KW, Schindelar M, Welch D, Abelson MB: The Ocular Protection Index. *Cornea* 2008, 27: 509–513.

Pamilo S, Malinen S, Hlushchuk Y, Seppä M, Tikka P, Hari R: Functional subdivision of group-ICA results of fMRI data collected during cinema viewing. *PLoS One* 2012, 7: e42000.

Picton TW, Hillyard SA: Cephalic skin potentials in electroencephalography. *Electroencephalogr Clin Neurophysiol* 1972, 33: 419–424.

Pion-Tonachini L, Kreutz-Delgado K, Makeig S: ICLabel: an automated electroencephalographic independent component classifier, dataset, and website. *NeuroImage* 2019, 198: 181–197.

Plöchl M, Ossandón JP, Konig P: Combining EEG and eye tracking: identification, characterization, and correction of eye movement artifacts in electroencephalographic data. *Front Hum Neurosci* 2012, 6: 278.

Ramkumar P, Parkkonen L, Hari R, Hyvärinen A: Characterization of neuromagnetic brain rhythms over time scales of minutes using spatial independent component analysis. *Hum Brain Mapp* 2012, 33: 1648–1662.

Rodin E, Funke M, Haueisen J: Cardio-respiratory contributions to the magnetoencephalogram. *Brain Topogr* 2005, 18: 37–46.

Rogasch NC, Sullivan C, Thomson RH, Rose NS, Bailey NW, Fitzgerald PB, Farzan F, Hernandez-Pavon JC: Analysing concurrent transcranial magnetic stimulation and electroencephalographic data: a review and introduction to the open-source TESA software. *NeuroImage* 2017, 147: 934–951.

Schomer DL, Epstein CM, Herman ST, Maus D, Fisch BJ: Recording principles: Analog and digital principles; polarity and field determinations; multimodal monitoring; polygraphy (EOG, EMG, ECG, SAO2). In: Schomer DL, Lopes da Silva F, eds. *Niedermeyer's Electroencephalography*, 7th ed. New York: Oxford University Press, 2018: 104–153.

Swarztrauber K, Fujikawa DG: An electroencephalographic study comparing maximum blink rates in schizophrenic and nonschizophrenic psychiatric patients and nonpsychiatric control subjects. *Biol Psychiatry* 1998, 43: 282–287.

Tamietto M, Castelli L, Vighetti S, Perozzo P, Geminiani G, Weiskrantz L, de Gelder B: Unseen facial and bodily expressions trigger fast emotional reactions. *Proc Natl Acad Sci U S A* 2009, 106: 17661–17666.

Tang AC, Liu J-Y, Sutherland MT: Recovery of correlated neuronal sources from EEG: the good and bad ways of using SOBI. *NeuroImage* 2005, 28: 507–519.

Tang AC, Sutherland MT, McKinney CJ: Validation of SOBI components from high-density EEG. *NeuroImage* 2005, 25: 539–553.

Tatum WO, Dworetzky BA, Schomer DL: Artifact and recording concepts in EEG. *J Clin Neurophysiol* 2011, 28: 252–263.

Tatum WO, Reinsberger C, Dworetzky B: Artifacts of recording and common errors in interpretation. In: Schomer DL, Lopes da Silva FH, eds. *Niedermeyer's Electroencephalography: Basic Principles, Clinical Applications, and Related Fields*, 7th ed. New York: Oxford University Press, 2018: 266–316.

Taulu S, Hari R: Removal of magnetoencephalographic artifacts with temporal signal-space separation: demonstration with single-trial auditory-evoked responses. *Hum Brain Mapp* 2009, 30: 1524–1534.

Taulu S, Kajola M, Simola J: Suppression of interference and artifacts by the signal space separation method. *Brain Topogr* 2004, 16: 269–275.

Taulu S, Simola J: Spatiotemporal signal space separation method for rejecting nearby interference in MEG measurements. *Phys Med Biol* 2006, 51: 1759–1768.

Taulu S, Simola J, Kajola M: Applications of the signal space separation method. *IEEE Trans Signal Process* 2005, 53: 3359–3372.

Thickbroom GW, Knezevic W, Caroll WM, Mastaglia FL: Saccade onset and offset lambda waves: relation to pattern movement visually evoked potentials. *Brain Res* 1991, 551: 150–156.

Tulen JHM, Azzolini M, de Vries JA, Groeneveld WH, Passchier J, van de BJM: Quantitative study of spontaneous eye blinks and eye tics in Gilles de la Tourette's syndrome. *J Neurol Neurosurg Psychiatry* 1999, 67: 800–802.

Urigüen JA, Garcia-Zapirain B: EEG artifact removal—state-of-the-art and guidelines. *J Neural Eng* 2015, 12: 031001.

Uusitalo MA, Ilmoniemi RJ: Signal-space projection method for separating MEG or EEG into components. *Med Biol Eng Comput* 1997, 35: 135–140.

van der Meer JN, Pampel A, Van Someren EJW, Ramautar JR, van der Werf YD, Gomez-Herrero G, Lepsien J, Hellrung L, Hinrichs H, Moller HE, Walter M: Carbon-wire loop based artifact correction outperforms post-processing EEG/fMRI corrections—a validation of a real-time simultaneous EEG/fMRI correction method. *NeuroImage* 2016, 125: 880–894.

Varone G, Hussain Z, Sheikh Z, Howard A, Boulila W, Mahmud M, Howard N, Morabito FC, Hussain A: Real-time artifacts reduction during TMS–EEG co-registration: a comprehensive review on technologies and procedures. *Sensors (Basel)* 2021, 21: 637.

Vigario RN: Extraction of ocular artefacts from EEG using independent component analysis. *Electroencephalogr Clin Neurophysiol* 1997, 103: 395–404.

Vigario R, Särelä J, Jousmäki V, Hämäläinen M, Oja E: Independent component approach to the analysis of EEG and MEG recordings. *IEEE Trans Biomed Eng* 2000, 47: 589–593.

Warach S, Ives JR, Schlaug G, Patel MR, Darby DG, Thangaraj V, Edelman RR, Schomer DL: EEG-triggered echo-planar functional MRI in epilepsy. *Neurology* 1996, 47: 89–93.

Whitham EM, Lewis T, Pope KJ, Fitzgibbon SP, Clark CR, Loveless S, DeLosAngeles D, Wallace AK, Broberg M, Willoughby JO: Thinking activates EMG in scalp electrical recordings. *Clin Neurophysiol* 2008, 119: 1166–1175.

Whitham EM, Pope KJ, Fitzgibbon SP, Lewis T, Clark CR, Loveless S, Broberg M, Wallace A, DeLosAngeles D, Lillie P, Hardy A, Fronsko R, Pulbrook A, Willoughby JO: Scalp electrical recording during paralysis: quantitative evidence that EEG frequencies above 20 Hz are contaminated by EMG. *Clin Neurophysiol* 2007, 18: 1877–1888.

Winkler I, Brandl S, Horn F, Waldburger E, Allefeld C, Tangermann M: Robust artifactual independent component classification for BCI practitioners. *J Neural Eng* 2014, 11: 035013.

Yuval-Greenberg S, Tomer O, Keren AS, Nelken I, Deouell LY: Transient induced gamma-band response in EEG as a manifestation of miniature saccades. *Neuron* 2008, 58: 429–441.

Zhuang X, Yang Z, Cordes D: A technical review of canonical correlation analysis for neuroscience applications. *Hum Brain Mapp* 2020, 41: 3807–3833.

CHAPTER 10

ANALYZING THE DATA

One man's rubbish may be another's treasure.

ATTRIBUTED TO HECTOR URQUHART, 1860S

Kāda dzija, tāda drēbe. [The type of yarn determines the cloth.]

LATVIAN PROVERB

■ INTRODUCTION

Science aims to find new features, regularities, and relationships in the world. It moves forward by basing the next steps on solid new pieces of evidence provided by the members of the scientific community. Scientists doing experimental work thus first have to obtain reliable new results and then convince the rest of the scientific community.

In our opinion, the first three rules of data analysis are to (a) look at the data, (b) look at the data, and (c) look at the data! This important scrutiny should have already started during data collection, so that the signals of interest could be successfully separated from artifacts and noise.

It is highly recommended to display the original MEG/EEG data from single subjects in publications, in addition to group data, so that the reader will immediately obtain an idea about the quality of the data on which the new findings rely. It is also necessary to demonstrate the replicability of the results both within and across subjects.

Here we discuss principles of more commonly used MEG/EEG data analysis approaches. As MEG and EEG excel at temporal accuracy, whereas fMRI (functional magnetic resonance imaging) and PET (positron emission tomography) are poor in temporal information, we should seize the opportunity to focus on temporal dynamics in MEG/EEG research rather than worrying too much about whether the absolute source locations are accurate to a few millimeters. We discuss these ideas in more detail further in this chapter.

The MEG/EEG data analysis landscape is complex and depends as much on experimental design as on the types of attributes that experimenters want to extract from their data. One major distinction can be made between evoked-response and resting-state studies, as we discussed in Chapter 4. Induced activity occurring in relation to the stimulus need not be rigidly time-locked to the external event but may well be systematically influenced by mental operations, in addition to the simultaneously present evoked responses that have been so ubiquitous in past literature. Both these types of stimulus-related activity can be examined in terms of their frequency content, not unlike analyses of resting-state (spontaneous) MEG/EEG. In both evoked-response and resting-state MEG/EEG studies, the main purpose is to characterize the underlying brain rhythms and oscillatory content and scrutinize their scalp topography and source currents. (For recent guidelines on resting-state studies, see Babiloni et al., 2020). The data from various analysis approaches form grist for the mill for functional connectivity (FC) and brain network analyses—a dramatic contrast from the studies of the twentieth century where the main focus was on the activity of local brain regions.

From the analysis point of view, the main difference between evoked-response and resting-state studies is that evoked responses are typically (but not necessarily) averaged to improve the signal-to-noise ratio, which facilitates, for example, reliable source analysis, whereas the resting-state data are not averaged. That said, both types of data set typically must be broken down (i.e., segmented) so that data analysis may remain computationally tractable. Investigators can study the desired experimental variable in either sensor- or source-space; we discuss the related potential pitfalls in this chapter. Second, they can analyze the spontaneous and stimulus-driven, single-trial data in the time or frequency domain, or often preferably in both, largely depending on the research question.

Many data visualization schemes share common elements across resting-state and evoked-response studies, but certain types of analyses may have highly specific needs for displaying the results. Many of these possibilities can be learned by reading existing literature.

Irrespective of the experimental design and analysis plan, the data quality requirements are largely identical for resting-state or task-related (evoked) MEG/EEG recordings.

■ DATA INSPECTION AND PREPROCESSING

Prior to performing any analyses, the measured data must always be visually inspected for artifacts. For example, in direct current recordings or in recordings using very long time constants, the amplifiers tend to drift to either the positive or negative input limit and the (automatic) resets will cause large signal jumps that, after normal filtering, may be difficult to discern (Chapters 8 and 9).

Given that currently more and more laboratories are conducting high-density recordings of MEG/EEG data, it is inevitable that some subjects' data may include "bad channels" due to malfunctioning sensors, noisy amplifiers, or broken connections (see Chapter 9). Such bad channels must be removed from the data as a first step in *any* analysis. Following artifact rejection and other preprocessing steps, these channels can be replaced by interpolated data from neighboring channels, but with caution. Interpolation routines only work well if the bad channels have a complete set of well-functioning neighbors; that is, they are away from the edge of the cap/net, and they are not all concentrated in one cluster. Some software developers indicate that in high-density EEG recordings the number of bad channels should constitute less than 10% of the total number. A word of caution is warranted for recordings carried out with portable EEG systems, which typically use a low number of electrodes, because signal interpolation may not be an option.

Sometimes questions arise on initial inspection of the data: Is one channel "bad," or does it contain artifacts in large numbers of trials? If so, what type of artifact is it? A high-amplitude signal in just one MEG sensor in a sensor helmet indicates that its source cannot be inside the brain because it otherwise should be visible in multiple sensors, and we thus are likely dealing with a bad channel or an external artifact. Similarly, EEG signals that show exceptionally large-amplitude excursions typically indicate poor skin–electrode contact, and these electrodes would usually be earmarked as bad channels. High-density recordings can aid in the recognition of focal or abnormal signal topographies that are produced, or influenced, by physiological artifacts, such as contraction of head muscles, subtle eye movements, or signals related to heart electrical activity or blood-vessel pulsation.

■ ANALYSIS OF AVERAGED DATA

Evoked Versus Induced Activity

Stimuli that the subject can perceive *evoke* activity in the brain and may or may not be seen in the MEG/EEG record. If the evoked activity is phase- (or time-) locked to the stimulus, it can be uncovered by stimulus-locked averaging (see Figure 10.1, left-side traces). It is also possible that each stimulus will *induce* EEG/MEG activity, which, despite being the same frequency each time, is not exactly phase-locked to the stimulus (see Figure 10.1, right-side traces). Due to this time jitter, conventional time-locked averaging would not uncover the induced activity (Figure 10.1, right bottom line). Practically, both evoked and induced activity can co-occur, resulting in *total* activity, which is their sum. Induced activity can therefore be estimated by subtracting evoked activity from the estimate of total activity (see, e.g., Tallon-Baudry et al., 1996). Induced activity can be seen by first either rectifying (to examine amplitude) or squaring (to examine power) the signals in the frequency band of interest and thereafter averaging them with respect to the event.

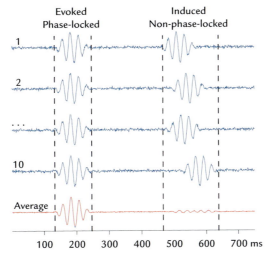

FIGURE 10.1. **Evoked versus induced activity.** Simulated waveforms have been averaged across 10 trials. On the left, the oscillatory activity is phase-locked in all trials to a stimulus delivered at time zero (blue traces from 1 to 10). On the right, similar induced oscillatory activity is elicited by the stimulus but without phase-locking relative to stimulus onset. The phase-locked activity results in a strong averaged response, whereas the non-phase-locked signals cancel out in the average waveform that remains close to noise level (red trace). Adapted and reprinted with permission from Hermann CS, Grigutsch M, Busch BA: EEG oscillations and wavelet analysis. In: Handy TC, ed. *Event-Related Potentials: A Methods Handbook.* Cambridge, MA: MIT Press, 2005: 229–259.

Spontaneous or *ongoing brain activity* is always present irrespective of whether or not a subject performs a task, and it can influence how evoked and induced responses evolve and how they are related to perception and cognition (see, e.g., Busch et al., 2009). Further in this chapter (and in Chapter 11), we examine how spontaneous, induced, and evoked activity vary and interact.

Signal-to-Noise Considerations

The MEG/EEG signals of interest may be quite small; thus, the accuracy of any further analysis can be improved by increasing the signal-to-noise ratio. For evoked responses, this is best achieved by collecting a large number of responses per condition and averaging them using an appropriate filtering bandwidth. For resting-state analyses, the total duration of the recording period will largely depend on the types of analyses to be performed (see below).

Signal averaging is based on the assumption that the recorded time-varying signal $x(t)$ comprises a distinct signal embedded in noise, that is, $x(t) = s(t) + n(t)$, where $s(t)$ is the signal of interest, repeating identically from one trial to another; and $n(t)$ represents the total noise. Thus averaging N responses would improve the signal-to-noise ratio by $\sqrt{N}$ provided that the noise remains stationary and the state of the subject (and thereby the signal of interest) stays about the same. Therefore, averaging two responses would improve the signal-to-noise ratio by a factor of 1.41 (41%) compared with a single response, averaging 10 responses by a factor of 3.16 (216%), averaging 50 responses by a factor of 7.07 (607%), and averaging 100 responses by a factor of 10 (900%).

Noise arising from multiple internal and external sources actually sums as squares, so the total noise is the square root of the sum of squared individual noise values. Thus the largest noise source by far dominates the total noise. In MEG, noise is expressed as a function of the frequency, using units of fT per square root of the frequency band measured in hertz (i.e., $fT/\sqrt{Hz}$). So, for example, a $5\,fT/\sqrt{Hz}$ noise level of an MEG device is practically negligible when the "brain noise" (brain's spontaneous activity that in many cases is itself the signal of interest) is $60\,fT/\sqrt{Hz}$, as can be easily seen by computing the total noise, which is $\sqrt{(60^2 + 5^2)} = \sqrt{3{,}625} = 60.2\,fT/\sqrt{Hz}$. Here the instrument has added noise by only 0.3%. If the signal to be measured is only $10\,fT/\sqrt{Hz}$, then the corresponding total noise would be $\sqrt{(10^2 + 5^2)} = \sqrt{125} = 11.2\,fT/\sqrt{Hz}$, an 11.8% increase to the total noise by the instrument. Note that when the signal frequency band is increased, the total noise increases in proportion to the square root of the bandwidth (provided that the noise is about the same at all frequencies).

Spontaneous MEG/EEG activity (here being discussed as "noise") is strongest at frequencies below 30 Hz but much lower at frequencies above 100 to 200 Hz. Thus at these higher frequencies any hardware improvements could have an important effect on signal quality. Importantly, in multichannel MEG devices, noise that is coherent across several channels can be removed computationally, as the sensor array provides information about its spatial distribution.

Sometimes the term *noise floor* is used to refer to the sum of all noise sources in the measurement system. For a SQUID–neuromagnetometer, the noise floor would be affected by the SQUID (superconducting quantum interference device) noise itself, thermal noise arising from the wires and other components in the cooled part of the system, and importantly also the properties of the flux transformer. An excellent example of the dramatic lowering of the noise floor of a single-channel axial gradiometer is presented in Chapter 15 (see Figure 15.8 for recording of single-trial, 600-Hz oscillatory responses).

Segmentation

Typically, continuous MEG/EEG data are acquired during a recording session, irrespective of whether it is a resting-state or task-related design. To make the data analysis problem computationally tractable, the continuous record is "cut up" into segments. For task-related designs, the segments (or) epochs consist of a prestimulus or a pre-event period, followed by a period long enough to contain the particular activity of interest. Typical prestimulus baselines are longer than 100 ms, and in studies where very slow evoked responses are examined, they are even longer, for example, 500 ms. Longer baselines may be appropriate for certain types of analyses, as described further in this chapter. This consideration will impact experiment duration. Typically, the signal level should have returned to the baseline level at the end of the analysis epoch. If this is not the case, one should consider increasing the baseline duration or at least ensure that the activity at the end of the epoch is reliable brain activity and not some random or artificial fluctuation.

It is important to consider the potential trade-off between epoch length and artifact-rejection criteria. For example, longer epochs are more likely to be contaminated by artifacts, such as eye blinks, and thus a considerable amount of data may be wasted if all artifactual trials are rejected from further analysis. A good baseline period is relatively flat and shows good replicability between multiple single trials or evoked responses.

Amplitude and Latency Measures

Evoked responses are characterized by peak amplitudes (with respect to prestimulus baseline; see Figure 10.2) and latencies (with respect to stimulus onset, or relative to a motor event) are commonly measured. The amplitudes and latencies (for peaks and troughs) may be measured from the averaged responses with semiautomated algorithms within predesignated latency ranges, for example, from 80 to 140 ms for visual-evoked responses that peak around 100 ms, or the first 10 ms of the response for auditory brainstem responses. In clinical settings, the measured peak amplitude and latency values are compared with normative values, and in research laboratories, they typically form the inputs for a statistical analysis of group-level data.

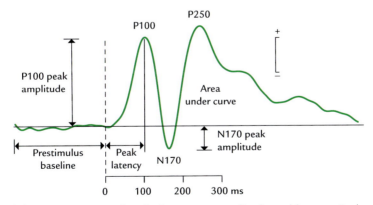

FIGURE 10.2. Measurement of evoked response amplitude and latency. Peak amplitudes of an evoked response are measured relative to a prestimulus baseline, and peak latencies are measured relative to stimulus onset (dashed vertical line). Response size can also be gauged by the area under the curve. In this example, three evoked response peaks are labeled according to the naming convention described in Chapter 14 for visual evoked responses.

We again remind that signal averaging is based on the assumption that the single responses differ from each other only by noise. If this is not the case, for example because of latency jitter or amplitude changes associated with something like varying vigilance, the averaged response is more like a weighted envelope of the single responses. A good internal quality control of the results is to superimpose all single-trial responses and then avoid response averaging if the response variability would violate the principles of averaging.

If an analyzed evoked response is judged to be absent or abnormal, the first step is to check that the measurement is replicable (easiest by superimposing two traces from identical experimental runs and ensuring that the prestimulus baseline is featureless). In MEG recordings, even a small difference in head position with respect to the sensor array between trials may have a big effect on evoked-response amplitudes. For example, if a certain sensor first sits over the zero line of a field pattern, it may after head rotation or other movement pick up larger signals in which the latencies can differ as well. Consequently, response averaging or comparison may not be feasible even *across the same subject's successive measurements* (as long as the analyses are made in sensor space).

Some investigators also measure peak-to-peak amplitudes and latencies, for example, from the peak of P100 to the (trough of) N170 in Figure 10.2. However, problems may arise as the neural generators of successive deflections of the evoked response typically differ. One may also measure the area under the curve (AUC) to assess the integrated magnitude of a response; this measure is particularly useful for the later parts of the response, which may be so broad that no clear peak can be identified or if the waveforms vary a lot across individuals.

If the response amplitudes are very different between subjects—as often happens in ECoG (electrocorticography) or SEEG (stereoencephalography EEG), where signal amplitudes are influenced greatly by local proximity to neuronal generators—it is possible to normalize the response amplitudes and express them as z-scores (Babo-Rebelo et al., 2022). This procedure "levels the playing field" and allows statistical analyses to be performed without violating test assumptions so that the results of a small number of individual subjects do not end up dominating the data set.

Topographic Maps

In a 2D display of the resting state of task-related EEG data, topographic scalp voltage maps can depict interpolated voltages between the electrode locations at any time point (see Figure 5.10). Most typically, such maps are displayed at times of response peaks and troughs. Animations of these maps can give useful insights to the organization of the activity. The scalp maps can be superimposed on 3D plots of the head surface (see Figure 18.4) and then examined from different sides of the head during animated rotation While not as esthetic, the 2D topographic map remains the most useful, as all EEG signals can be seen in one view.

Taking the second spatial derivative of the topographic scalp voltage map produces a Laplacian, or current source density (CSD), map, which putatively displays exit and entry points for scalp currents (Giard & Peronnet, 1999), although the CSD is not based on measures of actual current flow in the brain. These CSD maps are thus very different from intracortical CSD recordings, obtained with microelectrodes from different cortical depths to identify current sources and sinks within the cortex (Schroeder et al., 1990). However, the scalp CSD plots are interesting because they are "reference free," meaning that the CSD profile does not change as a function of the selected reference electrode. CSD presentation of EEG scalp topography is also advantageous for calculating measures of coherence (see further discussion). For a detailed examination of the scalp CSD and related issues, see Tenke and Kayser (2012).

For MEG data, 2D or 3D topographic maps of the flux exiting and entering the head are routinely generated, and maps may also be displayed for response power (see further sections in this chapter). In all cases (for both MEG and EEG data), however, this kind of interpolated map is just for visualization, and the data analysis (e.g., source identification) relies on the real measured data and the sensor locations. If one is using an MEG array where each sensor unit houses two orthogonal planar gradiometers, and if the analysis will be at the signal (and not the source) level, then it may be useful to compute "vector sums" for single sensors; for two orthogonal signals s_1 and s_2, the vector sum is $\sqrt{(s_1^2 + s_2^2)}$. This measure has lost the directional information of the local source currents and thus is insensitive to minor differences in head position. Importantly, the vector sums of averaged responses from the two orthogonal sensors do not equal the averages of vector sums of single responses, and only the former are feasible for MEG signal analysis.

■ ANALYSIS OF UNAVERAGED DATA

Interest in quantifying the spontaneous features of the EEG is not new. Prior to the availability of computers, clinical neurophysiologists literally counted the number of cycles or used calibrated "frequency rulers" on a particular part of the EEG trace to determine the dominant frequency of the background activity and of abnormal slowing or epileptic discharges, as well as their possible hemispheric lateralization. Their primary goal was to characterize EEG activity and thereby produce differential diagnoses for various brain disorders (see Chapter 20). Since those times, many different computerized analysis methods have mushroomed. We can only briefly feature some of these methods in this next section.

Brain Microstates

Since the early 1970s, global field power (GFP) and global dissimilarity (GD) of scalp EEG were advocated as measures that were less susceptible to problems relating to reference electrodes (Chapter 5) (Lehmann, 1971; Lehmann & Skrandies, 1980; Murray et al., 2008; Pourtois et al., 2008). GFP is the root mean square of the EEG signals across all electrode sites, and GD is the standard deviation of the voltage topographic map across the entire electrode array; both measures are calculated for each time point in the poststimulus epoch. High GFP values associated with low GD values with a similar spatial topography indicate the presence of a reliable brain signal and have been used as robust measures of response latencies and amplitudes.

Scrutiny of the GFP and GD scalp distributions led to proposals that the brain has quasi-stable "microstates" that last for tens to hundreds of milliseconds as potential "basic building blocks" of certain neural computations (Lehmann et al., 1987). Specifically, four or five "prototypic microstates" and their expression and sequence have been extracted during mentation and certain clinical disorders (Khanna et al., 2015; Michel & Koenig, 2018). Low GFP values occurring in the presence of high GD with the same topography signal the transition from one microstate to another. Although EEG brain microstates have been associated with resting-state networks as identified using fMRI (Michel & Koenig, 2018), their functional significance has to date remained elusive. Perhaps the brain microstates should be more closely tied to discussions of the very rich temporospatial signatures of the EEG/MEG data that have been examined in cortical fingerprinting (for MEG, see, e.g., da Silva Castanheira et al., 2021; for EEG/fMRI, see, e.g., Meir-Hasson et al., 2014), which may provide a framework to better understand some of these larger, recurring global patterns.

MEG/EEG Signal Level and Power

Measurements of electrical signals played a central role in electrical engineering well beyond neurophysiology and included careful characterization of the signal's frequency content. Already in the nineteenth century, Albert Michelson—recipient of the 1907 Nobel Prize in Physics—devised a mechanical "harmonic analyzer" that was composed of gears, springs, and levers capable of performing Fourier analysis (Hammack et al., 2014). Whereas the earliest EEG machines were merely recording and display devices, in 1938 Grass and Gibbs described an ingenious hardware system that generated reliable power spectra of EEG signals. EEG was recorded onto 35-mm film run in a loop through an optoelectric analyzer that they had built. Power spectra obtained from three subjects who were reading or just resting with eyes open and closed showed clear differences in the alpha peak as a function of condition (Grass & Gibbs, 1938)—similar to what we are used to seeing today (see also Chapter 11).

The immense technical challenges incurred for hardware-generated power spectra probably dampened enthusiasm for examining EEG signals in this way. Thus, it was only in the 1960s, when computers were developed with enough memory and power for complex mathematical computations, that spectral analysis of EEG data became more popular. It then became easy to compute Fourier transforms by treating the EEG signal as a linear sum of single-frequency sinusoids.

In any setting, the calculation of amplitude or power spectra requires data epochs of sufficient length to ensure that all frequencies of interest are adequately represented; the longer the epoch, the better the frequency resolution and the less will a certain frequency "leak" (i.e., spread) to neighboring frequencies. Today, aggregate measures such as the median frequency and spectral-edge frequency are often tracked in the operating room or intensive-care unit (Chapter 20). Median frequency is the frequency at which the power in the spectrum has been divided in half, and spectral-edge frequency is defined as the frequency below which 95% of the spectral power occurs (Purdon et al., 2015). Many researchers today use the efficient computer algorithm known as the fast Fourier transform (FFT) to obtain amplitude and power spectra or associated signal-phase information. These basic analyses form the starting point for a number of frequency-domain analyses that we discuss subsequently.

Event-Related Desynchronization/Synchronization and Temporal Spectral Evolution

Event-related desynchronization (ERD) and synchronization (ERS) were popularized by Pfurtscheller and coworkers (for a review, see Pfurtscheller & Lopes da Silva, 1999) to quantify changes in the *power* of task-related EEG rhythms at one time relative to a "baseline" period at another time. In this analysis, the MEG/EEG signals are first bandpass filtered to the frequency band of interest, their amplitudes are squared across all epochs, and then a moving window is used to calculate the average power as a function of time. ERD and ERS are expressed as percentage power changes relative to a baseline period preceding the event, with the event a sensory stimulus or a motor action.

To evaluate ERD or ERS changes reliably, the MEG/EEG signal should be examined for at least several seconds before and after the event of interest. ERD and ERS can co-occur in a given MEG/EEG channel location but across different frequency bands. In choosing the suitable frequency band, one may first need to examine the exact power-spectral peaks of individual subjects as subjects typically have different peak frequencies in their brain rhythms (Haegens et al., 2014). Most typical ERDs occur for the posterior alpha rhythms during visual tasks and for the lower frequency component of mu rhythm during sensori-motor tasks (Pfurtscheller & Lopes da Silva, 1999), although ERD (and ERS) can occur also in other frequencies.

Although ERD and ERS are widely applied, two comments are appropriate. First, we do not currently have any direct evidence about real neuronal synchronization versus desynchronization underlying these phenomena. Therefore, it might be better to describe these changes in brain rhythms as *enhancements* and *suppressions*. Second, computing the power of brain signals might not be the most feasible approach because all evoked responses are expressed as signal amplitudes. Therefore, it will be difficult to directly compare changes in ERD/ERS and evoked responses. To remediate this problem, Salmelin and Hari (1994) introduced temporal spectral evolution (TSE), which is otherwise similar to ERS/ERD but the signals are rectified (to compute amplitude) and not squared (to compute power). The advantage of TSE is that evoked-response amplitudes and the changes of background activity can be readily compared using the same units.

Time–Frequency Analyses

Time–frequency analyses go one step further by computing and visualizing the spectral and amplitude (or power) content of the signal as a function of time simultaneously for all frequencies of interest. Fourier transforms, Hilbert transforms, and wavelet-based approaches (Wacker & Witte, 2013; Gross, 2014) are commonly used to calculate MEG/EEG signal power (or amplitude) and phase as a function of time; these methods are mathematically equivalent (Bruns, 2004). Wavelet-based approaches probably have been most widely used in time–frequency analysis.

Wavelets are functions of discrete duration, generated by multiplying (typically a sinusoidal) "carrier" function by an "envelope" function, which is typically a Gaussian of known width and zero mean (Figure 10.3). These so-called Morlet or Gabor wavelets are the most commonly used in time–frequency analysis of MEG/EEG signals. Wavelets can improve spectral estimation in real-life situations where data are not of infinite length and Fourier analysis would (in theory) not provide sharp spectral peaks from single frequencies. Data windowing with wavelets can sharpen the spectral peaks of data of finite length. However, the time–frequency representations still suffer from uncertainty: if the time is represented precisely, then the frequencies cannot be represented so precisely, and vice versa. For more details on wavelets and analysis of neurophysiological data, see Samar (1999) and Morales and Bowers (2022).

For a typical time–frequency analysis, a set of wavelets (each at a different frequency) is constructed to cover the whole frequency range of interest. The wavelet functions act as selective bandpass filters: a wavelet of a particular frequency and number of cycles is slid over the MEG/EEG signal at each time point, yielding a set of wavelet coefficients for each frequency. As the wavelet function has a discrete length, the wavelet coefficients depict activity around that particular time point in the data epoch. Hence, features in MEG/EEG data can be visualized in both time and frequency. This type of approach can be used for task-related or resting-state epoched data. For the latter data type, what constitutes a "baseline" for analysis, however, may be challenging to specify.

A common way of displaying a time–frequency analysis output is to plot the frequency of activity (on the *y*-axis) as a function of time (on the *x*-axis) (Tallon-Baudry

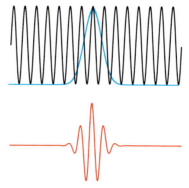

FIGURE 10.3. An example of a wavelet. A sinusoid (black trace) weighted by a Gaussian function (blue trace) yields a wavelet (red curve). Here the wavelet has five cycles.

et al., 1996), relative to a pre-event baseline (Figure 10.4). This approach allows "narrowband" or "broadband" oscillations to be clearly seen; narrowband oscillations are confined to only a narrow fraction of the frequency range defining a particular MEG/EEG band, whereas broadband oscillations denote activity that occurs over a substantial part of one (or more) frequency band(s) of interest (Lopes da Silva, 2013; see also Figure 11.8, right panels).

A number of normalization strategies are used for time–frequency analyses, and the choice partly depends on the analysis goal. The traditional procedure is to first compute the mean and standard deviation of power at each frequency at the prestimulus

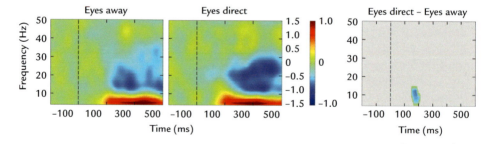

FIGURE 10.4. Time–frequency plots. Left two panels: Frequency of EEG signals during a visual task with two conditions: a face gazing away (Eyes away) and at the subject (Eyes direct) as a function of time. Vertical color scale indicates power in dB. The two conditions show very similar profiles of activity: a prolonged increase below 10 Hz (in theta and alpha bands) and a prolonged decrease in the beta band up to 30 Hz after the stimulus onset (vertical broken line). Passband of the original recordings was 0.1–200 Hz. Data are from a nine-electrode cluster centered on the left sensorimotor scalp. Right panel: Statistically significant difference between the two conditions, as assessed by a bootstrap method, in the theta and alpha ranges for a brief period at around 200 ms. Adapted and reprinted from Rossi A, Parada FJ, Kolchinsky A, Puce A: Neural correlates of apparent motion perception of impoverished facial stimuli: a comparison of ERP and ERSP activity. *NeuroImage* 2014, 98: 442–459. With permission from Elsevier.

baseline. This mean is then subtracted from all time points and at each frequency in the epoch. Finally, these baseline-centered values are divided by the standard deviation. This approach assumes an "additive model," where stimulus-induced power adds onto existing power at the same frequencies. Another common analysis strategy is to calculate percentage changes of poststimulus MEG/EEG power with respect to prestimulus baseline, based on an "EEG gain model," where a stimulus is assumed to *proportionally* increase or decrease the amplitude of existing oscillatory EEG activity (Grandchamp & Delorme, 2011). This approach, however, does not distinguish between effects that occur in the pre- or the poststimulus period. Additionally, this measure overestimates magnitudes of ERS and underestimates ERD. This issue can be minimized in part by normalizing the poststimulus power (or amplitude) by prestimulus baseline in single trials (Hu et al., 2014). In practice, examination of evoked and induced activity will need both average and single-trial calculations to separate these two types of brain activity.

If the aim is to keep similar precision across frequencies, the number of cycles of the wavelet function can be altered across the frequency range, given the reciprocal relationship between time and frequency. Hence, as frequency increases, the number of cycles of the wavelet function can be increased to try to preserve frequency precision.

Figure 10.5 (left panels) shows two wavelet functions of different lengths and their associated frequency spectra (middle panels). The time–frequency plots (right panels) show that the longer wavelet allows the two frequency bands of activity to be separated in the bottom plot (horizontal white dashed line), whereas the shorter wavelet in the upper plot does not. However, increasing the number of wavelet cycles can generate unstable measures at those higher frequencies and runs the risk of spreading oscillatory activity into the prestimulus period. Thus, a trade-off strategy needs to be adopted for optimal frequency–time precision (see Cohen, 2014). For example, a linear increase from three wavelet cycles at 3 Hz to eight cycles at 100 Hz has been used (Busch et al., 2009).

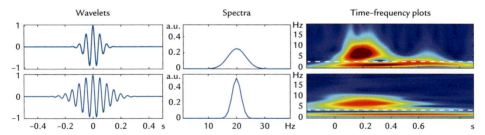

FIGURE 10.5. Resolution differences in time–frequency analyses as a function of wavelet length. Left: Two wavelet functions of different lengths. Middle: The associated power spectra, with a narrower power spectrum for the longer than the shorter wavelet. Right: The time–frequency plots show that the longer wavelet allows the two frequency bands of activity to be separated at the lower frequency (white dashed line), whereas the shorter wavelet does not (white dashed line). Note that the apparent durations of the activity at the two frequency bands are affected as well. Adapted and reprinted from Hermann CS, Rach S, Vosskuhl J, Strüber D: Time–frequency analysis of event-related potentials: a brief tutorial. *Brain Topogr* 2014, 27: 438–450. With permission from Springer.

An alternative way to improve spectral estimation in time–frequency analysis is to use the multitaper method, which refers to multiplying the data with tapering (windowing) functions that are zero at each end of an epoch of interest (see Cohen, 2014, for an excellent explanation of this approach). Windowing is the standard procedure when computing Fourier spectra on MEG/EEG data to avoid introducing discontinuities and therefore additional components in the spectra. Figure 10.3 already illustrated tapering of a wavelet by a Gaussian function. The multitaper time–frequency analysis uses a set of orthogonal functions of different frequencies called (Slepian) tapers (see Slepian, 1978), with which the MEG/EEG data are first multiplied and then averaged across all tapered signals to improve spectral estimation.

Cohen (2014) noted three situations where the multitaper time–frequency analysis is advantageous over other types of approaches: (1) for noisy data or small numbers of trials; (2) for single-trial analysis, especially for frequencies > 30 Hz; and (3) for scrutinizing high-frequency activity > 60 Hz. On the flip side, multitaper analysis might not be optimal at frequencies < 30 Hz or if the exact timing needs to be determined for the high-frequency MEG/EEG signals (due to the relatively low temporal precision of the multitaper method).

Nonparametric statistical analyses, such as permutation and bootstrapping tests, can be used to examine whether an observed change in the time–frequency analysis is statistically significant relative to the pre-event baseline in a particular condition or relative to other experimental conditions (Maris & Oostenveld, 2007; Groppe et al., 2011). Given that MEG/EEG data sets typically include signals from many channels and experimental conditions, as well as many time points in each experimental trial, problems may arise with multiple comparisons and the generation of false-positive observations (Groppe et al., 2011; Siegel et al., 2012). To avoid this problem, different types of false discovery statistics can be implemented, based on family-wise error (FWE) and false discovery rate (FDR), and each method is suited to pulling out different types of effects from the MEG/EEG data (Groppe et al., 2011).

Phase Resetting and Models of Evoked Activity

There is still an ongoing discussion regarding the relationship between evoked, induced, and total activity. Sayers and colleagues (1974) originally noted that no EEG power increases take place in the poststimulus period, despite the presence of a clear evoked response. They reasoned that some type of rearrangement of neural activity had taken place to produce the synchronized evoked activity following the stimulus. The idea of "phase resetting," that is, the phase of ongoing neural oscillations is realigned or "reset" by the onset of the stimulus, was proposed to explain these findings (Sayers et al., 1974). In agreement with the phase-resetting hypothesis, phase variance of certain frequency components was reported to decrease in the poststimulus period (Lopes da Silva, 2006).

The idea of phase resetting has not been without its critics, with a vigorous debate occurring over the years and an alternative "evoked model" being proposed. To appreciate the theoretical differences between the two models, their basic features need to be compared (see Shah et al., 2004; Sauseng et al., 2007, for reviews on this topic). The phase-resetting model proposes that (a) the ongoing MEG/EEG oscillations, at the dominant frequency seen in the evoked response, must be present in the prestimulus period; (b) a stimulus-induced phase shift ("phase concentration") results in phase synchrony at the dominant evoked-response frequency across experimental trials; and (c) the power is not increased during the poststimulus period.

In contrast, the evoked model proposes that (a) stimulus induces power increase in the poststimulus period, (b) a (likely) stimulus-elicited phase change produces synchronization of activity, and (c) ongoing MEG/EEG oscillations at the dominant evoked-response frequency need not be present at the time of stimulus presentation. In other words, the evoked response to the incoming stimulus is a neural population response.

At the time of writing (2022), the jury was still out, and both mechanisms could likely play a role in the generation of event-related brain activity (see Shah et al., 2004; Sauseng et al., 2007). It is plausible that invasive recordings of ongoing field potential and multiunit activity, combined with simultaneous recordings of noninvasive (both single-trial and averaged) EEG signals, will be needed to tease out the generation mechanisms of evoked and induced activity. These complex processes potentially involve relationships between oscillatory activity across different frequency bands, which we briefly explore in the section on cross-frequency coupling (CFC).

Still, the distinction between phase resetting and phase locking needs to be made when discussing oscillatory MEG/EEG activity (Canavier, 2014). An incoming discrete, brief sensory stimulus can transiently reset the phase of ongoing oscillatory MEG/EEG activity. Strictly speaking, phase-locked activity is periodic activity that is elicited to a quasiperiodic input. These two signals thus have a measurable relationship between their respective phases. We use the term *phase locking* in the rest of this book to refer to relationships between different types of periodic activity in MEG/EEG signals.

Cross-Frequency Coupling

In both resting-state and task-related experiments, synchronized activity occurring between neural populations can occur within the same MEG/EEG frequency band or link activity across different frequency bands. Frequencies in a lower MEG/EEG band can modulate the amplitude, frequency, or phase of a higher frequency MEG/EEG signal, a phenomenon known as cross-frequency coupling (CFC). CFC has been demonstrated in neurophysiological recordings ranging from invasive studies of single units and field potentials to scalp EEG and MEG. Four forms of CFC have been described in neurophysiological data: phase–amplitude, phase–phase, phase–frequency, and amplitude–amplitude coupling. These forms of coupling are denoted using power instead of amplitude in Figure 10.6.

We briefly discuss phase–amplitude CFC subsequently and highlight some ways of visualizing and quantifying CFC. A number of reviews are available on this topic (Jensen & Colgin, 2007; Cohen, 2008; Canolty & Knight, 2010; Aru et al., 2015; Hyafil et al., 2015). While most investigators use "amplitude" when describing forms of CFC, "power" (squared amplitude) has also been used in, for example, phase–power coupling (Jensen & Colgin, 2007).

Irrespective of which CFC phenomenon is being assessed or which method is used to calculate the CFC measure, estimates of the signal at each frequency to be related must first be extracted from the MEG/EEG data between pairs of sensors (or brain regions). This analysis can be initiated by generating a bandpass-filtered MEG/EEG data set at each desired frequency range. Then, phase or amplitude measures are extracted from each filtered data set, and specific calculations are performed for the CFC type of interest. If there is no a priori hypothesis for a relationship between two particular frequencies of interest (a very bad idea for many reasons!), the analysis will require an extremely large set of comparisons between measures at different frequencies, involving significant computation time and resources, as well as creating statistical problems with multiple comparisons.

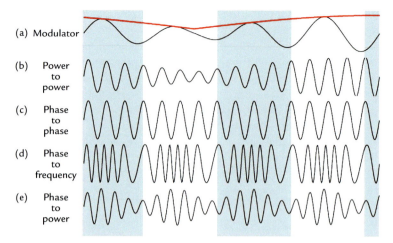

FIGURE 10.6. Types of CFC. Four different types of CFC. Here the term *power* is used to depict the type of cross-frequency coupling, but corresponding coupling can also be described with respect to amplitude. In power-to-power CFC (trace b), the power (or amplitude) of the higher frequency signal is modulated by the power (or amplitude) envelope of the lower frequency signal (trace a, red line). Other types of CFC can occur between phases and signal levels, such as phase-to-phase CFC (c), phase-to-frequency CFC (d), and phase-to-power (e). See text for further explanation. Adapted and reprinted from Jensen O, Colgin LL: Cross-frequency coupling between neuronal oscillations. *Trends Cogn Sci* 2007, 11: 267–269. With permission from Elsevier.

Consider, for example, a toy EEG data set in sensor space with 16 electrodes (or in source space with 16 voxels) where frequencies from 4 to 50 Hz would be investigated, for example, in 1-Hz steps using a set of wavelet functions. For a given sensor pair (or pair of voxels), an analysis of theta–alpha coupling alone would require 24 pairings given by four frequencies in the theta range (4, 5, 6, and 7 Hz) and six frequencies in the alpha range (8, 9, 10, 11, 12, and 13 Hz), so that the theta–alpha couplings would be between frequencies (in Hz) of 4–8, 4–9, 4–10, 4–11, 4–12, 4–13, 5–8, 5–9, 5–10, 5–11, 5–12, 5–13, 6–8, 6–9, 6–10, 6–11, 6–12, 6–13, 7–8, 7–9, 7–10, 7–11, 7–12, 7–13. In other words, $m \times n$ calculations would be needed, where m and n refer to frequency bands in the theta and alpha range, respectively.

If the recording array has p channels, or voxels, this would potentially set up $p!/(2!(p-2)!)$ combinations (pairs) of the channels, and at each measurement sensor or voxel pair both the lower (m) and higher (n) frequency couplings with respect to the other measurement sensor/voxel would need to be assessed. Hence, to assess theta–alpha coupling between 16 measurement sensors would require 5,760 data comparisons across the frequency couplings, that is, $2 \times m \times n \times 16!/(2!\ 14!)$. Generating this many comparisons carries the risk of an increased number of false-positive observations. This is a just a toy example, whereas high-density recordings of MEG/EEG data in 64, 128, or 256 channels are used in cognitive neuroscience, and the coupling of theta activity is often examined with the (relatively wide) gamma range (and not in 1-Hz bands). Thus, it is strongly recommended that CFC methods only be used in hypothesis-driven analyses as the number of calculations can quickly become prohibitive.

In *phase–amplitude coupling* (PAC), the amplitude of a high-frequency oscillation in one site (sensor/brain region) is modulated by the phase of a lower frequency rhythm in

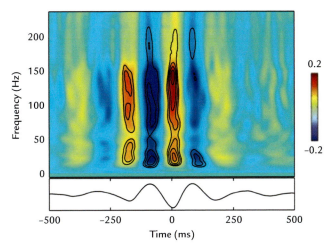

FIGURE 10.7. Phase–amplitude coupling. Theta-range electrocorticographic signal (bottom trace) is coupled to gamma activity displayed in the time–frequency plot (top), where the gamma activity peaks correspond to the troughs of theta activity. The color scale depicts amplitude in arbitrary units. Adapted and reprinted from Canolty RT, Knight RT: The functional role of cross-frequency coupling. *Trends Cogn Sci* 2010, 14: 506–515. With permission from Elsevier.

another site. For example, for theta–gamma PAC—which appears to be the most common form of PAC reported in the literature (Hyafil et al., 2015)—the phase of theta activity would modulate the amplitude of gamma activity. Theta–gamma coupling can occur not only between brain regions but also within a single brain region (Lisman & Jensen, 2013). Figure 10.7 depicts theta–gamma coupling where the presence of gamma activity (upper plot) is contingent on troughs in theta activity (lower plot).

In PAC, the higher frequency rhythm is said to be "nested" in the lower frequency signal, also referred to as "nested oscillations" (Lisman & Idiart, 1995; Chrobak & Buzsaki, 1998).

Different methods have been used to quantify PAC, many of them originally applied to invasively recorded field-potential animal and human data. Tort and colleagues (2010) demonstrated similar CFC phenomena across eight methods, although some approaches were more resistant to noise than others. The initial step is to bandpass filter the MEG/EEG signals to the respective two frequency ranges of interest for the two signal sources that are being compared. For the lower frequency signal (e.g., theta rhythm), the instantaneous phase information is extracted. For the higher frequency signal of interest that occurs at a different measurement sensor/brain region, the amplitude envelope and phase of the variations at the lower frequency are quantified relative to the phase of the lower frequency at the other sensor/brain region (Tort et al., 2010).

Phase-locking value (PLV) has been used to quantify PAC where the low-frequency phase extracted from the signal at the first site is compared with the phase of the low-frequency amplitude envelope at the second site. A PLV of 1 indicates that the phase series are exactly locked, whereas a value of zero indicates that they are completely desynchronized. PLV has been said to be less prone to noise relative to other PAC methods (Tort et al., 2010).

PAC can be visualized in phase–amplitude plots where the amplitude envelope of the higher frequency signal is expressed as a function of the lower frequency signal's phase. Several other indices are available to quantify cross-frequency interactions in PAC, for example, the modulation index and the phase-lag index (PLI) (Canolty & Knight, 2010; Tort et al., 2010).

Much of the reported CFC phenomena, particularly related to PAC, have been recorded invasively in humans and animals. We would argue that CFC calculations on MEG/EEG data should be made in source rather than sensor space based on similar arguments made regarding the measurement of certain measures of FC and its artificial inflation in sensor space (see below; for more detail on this issue, see illustrative examples from Schaworonkow & Nikulin, 2022).

■ MEASURES OF ASSOCIATION AND CONNECTIVITY

To understand brain function it is essential to learn, beyond the activated brain regions and their activation sequence, about their anatomical and/or functional connectivity. A decade ago, studies of *functional connectivity* (FC) became popular after a large body of data was amassed on the *functional segregation* of brain areas (Friston, 2011). FC indicates *the presence of a statistical relationship* between two signals that covary, either simultaneously or with a fixed time lag. Even a strong FC does not assume or demonstrate any physical connection between the brain areas generating the two signals. Thus, in principle, both signals could be driven by a third party *that has not been included in the analysis*. Thus, FC does not imply a causal relationship between the signals. Note that FC differs from *effective connectivity*, which refers to the causal influence of one neural signal to another. Both measures are dynamic, which creates many challenges for the thorough and valid analysis of these ever-changing phenomena.

It is also worth mentioning that while the demonstration of anatomical connectivity between the functionally coupled areas is desirable, even if such data are available from, for example, individual diffusion tensor imaging data, caution must be exercised as *long-distance connectivity is very sparse* in human and macaque brains (Markov et al., 2013; Rosen & Halgren, 2021).

Functional Connectivity

Functional connectivity in neuronal networks—revealing correlations and interactions of activation, but without causal links—can be studied by various measures, such as dynamic imaging of coherent sources (Gross et al., 2001). Dynamic FC can be applied to fMRI data, but a major drawback is the temporal sparseness of the data even when sampling fMRI data simultaneously with other higher temporal resolution physiological signals (see Hutchison et al., 2013; Martin et al., 2021). Among the many variables affecting fMRI FC measures are task demands and also various brain–body interactions associated with the subject's vigilance and cognitive and affective states (Martin et al., 2021). Here the temporal richness of MEG/EEG data provides significant advantages, as does the technical ease of obtaining nonbrain physiological signals simultaneously. Indeed, in the 1950s, prior to the invention of computers and digital sampling and analysis techniques, *analog* FC measures (i.e., cross-correlation methods) were applied to study the covariation of two EEG traces. These results emerged from the collaboration of EEG pioneers such as Mary Brazier and others (at the Massachusetts General Hospital in Boston, MA) with information theory pioneer Norbert Wiener, who was working on his already influential theory of prediction (Wiener, 1956). These computations were generated by analog devices based on complex electric circuit-based solutions (for a historical review, see Barlow, 1977).

Today, the calculation of FC measures of neurophysiological signals provides continual grist for the network-science mill. Below, we cover some of the more commonly used measures of FC in MEG/EEG analysis. The interested reader can also benefit from the comprehensive reviews of Bastos and Schoffelen (2016) and O'Neill et al. (2018).

It is prudent to remember that oscillatory rhythms can be quite different in character in noninvasive MEG/EEG and invasive intracranial EEG (iEEG) recordings and thus may produce different results in FC computations (Lopes da Silva, 2013). It is the consistency of the relative timing (i.e., phase difference) between brain signals that can identify the existence of coupled activity across recording locations.

MEG/EEG FC measures can be broadly grouped into *nondirected* and *directed* measures (left and right sides, respectively, of Figure 10.8) (Bastos & Schoffelen, 2016). Nondirected FC, such as correlation, identifies a relationship but does not indicate who drives whom. In contrast, directed FC identifies the direction of the relationship (i.e., think of a horse pulling a cart). Therefore, one neural source will be seen as driving another's behavior, where this potentially causal relationship is determined statistically. A second broad-brush division within directed and nondirected FC measures is that of model-based versus model-free approaches. For example, in a model-based approach the FC measure might assume linearity of the data or some other attribute. A final broad division differentiates time-domain from frequency-domain methods (upper vs. lower part, respectively, of Figure 10.8). Below we briefly discuss the different computational methods highlighted in the figure, starting from correlation (a time-domain measure) and coherence (a frequency-domain measure) to examine relationships between different MEG/EEG signals or between MEG/EEG and physiological signals from the body (see Chapter 16).

Correlation and Coherence

We start our brief tour of nondirected model-based FC methods with two coupling measures, *correlation* and *coherence*. Correlation is a (time-domain) measure that determines the degree to which two variables covary (with values between –1 and 1), whereas coherence is computed in the frequency domain. Correlation and coherence behave somewhat comparably both in principle and in simulated and real EEG/MEG data sets.

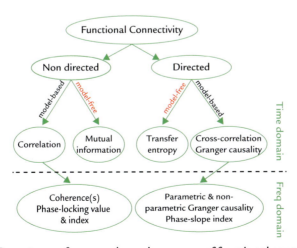

FIGURE 10.8. Some types of commonly used measures of functional connectivity. See main text for explanation. Modified with permission from Bastos AM, Schoffelen JM: A tutorial review of functional connectivity analysis methods and their interpretational pitfalls. *Front Syst Neurosci* 2016. 9: 175.

Measures of MEG/EEG *correlation* are sensitive to both phase and polarity of the signals but are independent of changes in signal amplitude (see Guevara & Corsi-Cabrera, 1996). Correlation calculations were much favored in the neurophysiological literature the mid-twentieth century when computational resources were limited for studying brain functional relationships. Correlation is a model-based method with the assumptions that the two sets of signals are continuous variables, are normally distributed, have equal variances, have observations that can be paired, and have no outliers.

Coherence is a frequency-domain measure that assesses the stability in relative timing between two MEG/EEG signals (Goldstein, 1970). It indicates linear dependence between two signals as a function of frequency and has a magnitude ranging from 0 to 1.

A coherence value of 1 indicates complete synchrony or a perfect linear relationship between two signals at a certain frequency during a certain period of time. Synchrony refers to two signals changing at the same frequency and with the same phase lag (Singer, 1999). In contrast, a coherence value of zero indicates an absence of temporal relationship between the two signals. Note that MEG/EEG signals may show high coherence values at some frequencies and low values at others. Coherence serves as a nondirected, model-based measure of FC (see Figure 10.8, left side) with similar assumptions to correlation.

Whereas coherence is the preferred method in scrutinizing the stability of the relationship between two signals, correlation is useful when the focus is on the waveforms themselves and on the nature of the temporal coupling between the two signals (Guevara & Corsi-Cabrera, 1996). Importantly, coherence measures are sensitive to the relative phases of the two signals but do not depend on power level. As coherence is calculated with squared signals, information about signal polarity is lost—which does not happen in calculations of correlation.

Note the difference between "coherence" and "coherency." Coherency refers to the normalized cross-spectrum at a specific frequency of interest. It is a complex number whose magnitude ranges from 0 to an angle indicating phase lag between the two signals. In the literature, these terms can often be unintentionally intermixed.

A known issue with MEG/EEG coherence calculations is that artificially inflated results can occur if the sensors, even far apart, see the same source. For example, the extrema of magnetic field patterns and electric potential distributions can be easily 8–12 cm apart for a *tangential* current source, especially if the source is *deep*, and thus EEG measurements, or MEG recordings with magnetometers or axial gradiometers, may pick up activity of the same source even when the signal polarities are opposite. Alternatively, if the sensors are close to each other, for example, in high-density scalp EEG recordings, coherence can increase simply because both sensors see activity from the same *superficial* source. Even invasive EEG recordings are not completely immune to this problem, although intracranial coherence measures across large distances, for example, between frontal and occipital sites, typically show lower coherence values than those for scalp EEG (Nunez et al., 1997; Thatcher, 2012). Therefore, it has been suggested that one should distinguish between different spatial scales when discussing synchronized activity: short range (millimeter scale; intracranial microelectrodes), intermediate range (~1- to 3-cm scale), and long range (10- to 25-cm scale; scalp EEG) (Nunez et al., 2001).

Retaining the imaginary part of the complex number of coherence, that is, *imaginary coherence*, allows relationships between signals to be assessed by removing these confounding effects of synchronization at 0° and 180° lags caused by volume conduction in EEG and/or active reference electrodes. However, even with these methods, spurious correlations may arise between brain areas (Palva et al., 2018), which calls for extreme care in connectivity analyses. An additional nuisance contribution to coherence measures comes from ongoing rhythmic interactions between hemispheres; this effect can be eliminated by subtracting the imaginary coherence measures between homologous hemispheric channels or regions (Nolte et al., 2004; Sanchez Bornot et al., 2018). For a side-by-side comparison of imaginary coherence relative to a number of other FC methods (which are discussed further in this section), see Sanchez Bornot et al. (2018).

Measures of *partial coherence* assess the stability between two signals of interest after the contributions of a third known signal have been removed. It was first used for analysis of seizure propagation by Gersch and Goddard (1970) and could disentangle the contribution of various thalamic nuclei to cortical brain rhythms (Lopes da Silva et al., 1980). An alternative is the measure of partial directed coherence that allows assessment of short-lived interactions between neuronal populations while indicating the direction of current flow (Sameshima & Baccala, 1999). This method can identify the directionality of the coupling between brain and the moving body part (see Chapter 17), implying that corticokinematic coherence mainly reflects proprioceptive feedback from the body to the brain.

Phase-Locking Factor, Phase-Locking Value, and Phase-Lag Index

Phase-locking factor (PLF; see Tallon-Baudry et al., 1996) expresses the average degree of signal synchrony within a given sensor at a particular epoch in time across a series of experimental trials. Hence, the PLF is the average of the phase-coherence values across trials, with 1 denoting a perfect correspondence of activity at a given frequency across trials and zero indicating effectively no synchrony at that particular frequency and time point. PLF can be calculated using Fourier- or wavelet-based approaches, and statistical significance can be assessed using bootstrap or permutation analyses. PLF can identify evoked activity and potentially separate it from induced activity, as only the former will have a consistent phase relationship to the stimulus.

While it is of interest to quantify (e.g., by means of PLF) how synchronized activity recorded from one sensor varies during an experiment, in most instances it is more informative to measure to what degree activity is synchronized across different sensors or different brain regions. Synchrony between two signal sources is commonly quantified with PLV (Lachaux et al., 2002; Le Van Quyen & Bragin, 2007) by measuring the phase at each frequency and time point. Unfortunately, the PLV computed from EEG data can be readily contaminated by volume conduction. This problem is particularly serious for deep sources, as the signals originating from the same source occur at multiple locations at the same time. Here the *imaginary part* of the PLV can be useful because it reveals signals that have a phase lag, which cannot arise from the same source (Sadaghiani et al., 2012).

Finally, an example of a nondirected, model-based FC measure that deals with the effects of common sources is the PLI. It is based on an examination of the distribution of instantaneous nonzero (or non-180°) phase lags (at a particular frequency) between two signals that are asymmetric in their phase distributions, meaning that they have a preference for certain phase lags (Stam et al., 2007). PLI is known to suffer from small-magnitude synchronization effects: small perturbations can turn phase lags into phase leads and vice versa. One improvement may be the weighted PLI (wPLI), which weighs the phase lags based on the imaginary component of the cross-spectrum of the two signals (Vinck et al., 2011).

Mutual Information

Unlike the methods discussed above, mutual information (MI) is a model-free, nondirected FC method based on ideas from information theory (see Shannon, 1948). It can pull out such linear and nonlinear dependencies between two signals that may not be evident in covariance (or linear calculations of correlation). MI measures the average number of bits (or shannons) that can be predicted from two time series. MI is zero if the two considered random variables are independent. It ignores the temporal structure in the data, therefore shuffling data point order should not make a difference to the result. Practically, the time series is analyzed using a moving time window over which the MI measure is calculated for each point in time (Paluš, 1997). MI measures are symmetric, meaning that the mutual information is equal for XY and YX, where X and Y are two EEG or MEG signals, and it cannot be known which time series is the cart and which the horse. This can be remediated with time-delayed MI by first lagging one time series relative to the other, calculating the MI measures, and then repeating the same procedure after introducing the time lag to the second time series (e.g., Wilmer et al., 2012).

One limitation with most of these FC methods is that they can only be used to examine relationships between two random variables, for example, MEG/EEG signals between two active brain sources or two types of neurophysiological coupling or rhythm. Recently, a new method has been proposed to examine the MI of *multiple rhythms*—allowing a more complete CFC analysis to be constructed between multiple sources of rhythmic activity (Ibáñez-Molina et al., 2020). These approaches will be important for future work in network science dealing with multilayered brain networks (e.g., Mandke et al., 2018).

We now turn to our directed FC measures (the right side of Figure 10.8).

Transfer Entropy

Transfer entropy (TE) is a method based on information theory, proposed as an asymmetric cousin of MI to show—at least in principle—the directionality of the functional connection (Schreiber, 2000). Similar to MI, TE is model free and is computed in the time domain. Several approaches have been generated to make the demanding calculations computationally tractable. For example, one approach—known as binning or embedding—constrains the data to a certain number of delays in the selected time window. Since the optimal values for the embedding parameter for a given situation are unknown, the calculated TE values may be erroneous (for reviews on TE, see Montalto et al., 2014; Cekic et al., 2018). A MATLAB-based software package is available for calculating TE (Montalto et al., 2014) and mutual information (Lindner et al., 2011).

Transfer entropy has been computed for both EEG and MEG data (some early examples were given by Vicente et al., 2011; Wibral et al., 2011), as well as in examining coupling between neural and vascular data (Lüdtke et al., 2010). A more recent TE approach, called phase TE, was developed for examining connectivity between different neural sources with potential CFC relationships in (bandpass-filtered) MEG/EEG signals (Lobier et al., 2014).

Cross-Correlation

Cross-correlation between two time series can be computed by shifting one of two MEG/EEG signals in time, then computing the correlation measure, and repeating this process over multiple time lags. If both signals are similar enough in temporal structure (e.g., both contain oscillatory patterns), cross-correlation may infer directionality of information flow. However, in the presence of complex bidirectional interactions, cross-correlograms are difficult to interpret as they may lack a clear dominant peak and contain both positive and negative lags (Bastos & Schoffelen, 2016). Other methods, such as Granger causality (see below) may be able to provide a solution to the problem.

Granger Causality

Granger causality—originally developed for assessing statistical links between economic variables (Granger, 1969)—estimates statistically directed interactions between two signals, X and Y, with the ability to separate unidirectional interactions from signal X to Y versus from signal Y to X.

Granger causality can be calculated in both time and frequency domains. Time-domain calculations use an autoregressive (AR) framework, where future values of a time series are modeled as a weighted combination of the past values. In a *univariate* AR model, the values of time series X are predicted as a weighted combination of past values of Y, whereas in the *bivariate* AR model the values of time series X are predicted on past values of Y and also by past values of time series X. If the ratios of the variances for the residuals in transitioning from univariate to bivariate models are > 1 (leading to Granger causality values > 0), Y is said to Granger cause X. In time-domain analysis of EEG/MEG data, estimates of instantaneous power and phase, obtained from, for example, continuous wavelet transforms, allow the interactions of brain networks to be studied on very short timescales (O'Neill et al., 2018).

Frequency-domain Granger causality (Geweke, 1982), although computationally intensive, can be more easily related to other frequency-domain measures, such as coherence and partial directed coherence (see Baccalá & Sameshima, 2006). For its calculation, both a frequency-dependent spectral transfer matrix and the covariance of the AR model's residuals are estimated. (For analysis pipelines for calculating variants of parametric or nonparametric Granger causality, see Bastos & Shoffelen, 2016.)

It has to be noted that even if Granger causality measures would strongly imply causal connections between two signal sources, the results cannot rule out the possibility that a third party could drive both of these sources. One also has to remember that Granger causality, as with other methods in this section, addresses FC, which is the statistical dependence of signals, without indicating whether the information flows in a certain direction between the studied sources.

A new measure, the phase-slope index (PSI), was developed because Granger causality is known to inadequately deal with mixtures of independent sources that also differ in frequency content (Nolte et al., 2008). A multivariate version of PSI was reported to perform better than the regular PSI for simulated and real data. For example, in the MEG data of 61 subjects, directed alpha-band FC was identified between the visual network and other resting-state networks, specifically the dorsal attention and frontoparietal networks (Basti et al., 2018).

Functional Connectivity: Quo Vadis?

Many of our FC (and CFC) analysis methods for characterizing rhythmic activity are based on the assumptions that the MEG/EEG signals are sinusoidal. Yet, as we have already noted in Chapter 4, in a number of cases rhythmic brain activity is *not* sinusoidal (e.g., mu rhythm that comprises at least two distinct frequency components that themselves can look sinusoidal). This issue has encouraged the development of algorithms that take into account the shape of the rhythmic activity (reviewed by Cole & Voytek, 2017). Importantly, the overall shape (and additional frequency content) of the modulating rhythm can affect computations of CFC. A procedure and software have been proposed for a cycle-by-cycle analysis of nonsinusoidal neural oscillations to first test for the presence of oscillatory activity and then characterize the waveform's symmetry, which can have implications for biophysical and statistical modeling (Cole & Voytek, 2019). Increasing the density of spatial sampling might in some cases allow the components of the periodic (nonsinusoidal) signal to be identified and separated.

A somewhat related discussion in the literature centers on contrasting "transient bursty" versus "rhythmically sustained oscillatory" activity, which may well be different and idiosyncratic for each canonical frequency band (for a discussion, see Jones, 2016; van Ede et al., 2018; Zich et al., 2020). At any rate, distinction between these phenomena has implications for understanding the *underlying physiology* and not just for improving data analysis.

It is also now very evident that whole-brain FC changes can occur across different timescales (for a review, see Sadaghiani & Wirsich, 2020). Here brain rhythms of different frequencies, similar to those we describe in the context of multisensory processing (see Figure 16.6), as well as CFC (see above) might support complex FC between brain regions. Practically, this could be instantiated by cortical rhythms operating at different frequencies and with varied spatial scales of coupling between brain areas and different cortical layers. Within this "oscillatory multiplexing," the same information might be transferred on multiple frequency bands to different destinations. Additionally, high-level brain regions, such as the prefrontal cortex, send feedback signals to "lower-level" early sensory brain regions, which is also the basic principle of predictive coding (see Chapter 18). These findings have also led to the idea of "oscillopathies"—disruptions or absence of certain essential cortical rhythms as a function of brain lesions (Helfrich & Knight, 2019). As we have already noted, FC is dynamic and may therefore give a very different view of human brain function than the vistas obtained from temporally sparse fMRI data. The dynamic nature of FC is a multidimensional jigsaw puzzle, but for MEG and EEG analysis offers exciting avenues for interpreting the complex, often nonlinear, interactions between different brain rhythms and brain areas (see Chapter 22).

Effective Connectivity

Effective connectivity, as stated above, identifies causal links between specific brain regions (or sources) by using both structural (anatomical) and functional data in analyses. Causal links are directional; in other words, one region is said to causally change the activity of the other. A real challenge is to identify the reciprocal connections between brain areas and their layer-specific connection patterns in the cortex.

Technically speaking, the directed FC methods we described above, such as transfer entropy and Granger causality, would fall under the effective connectivity umbrella—because they calculate the influence of one brain structure on another. We have briefly discussed these methods in the previous section, together with the potential pitfalls of using them in sensor space and making inferences about causality.

Dynamic Causal Modeling
Dynamic causal modeling (DCM) is a popular method for assessing effective connectivity (Kiebel et al., 2008). It was initially used with fMRI data (David & Friston, 2003) but was further developed to handle MEG/EEG data (David et al., 2003; Kiebel et al., 2008). DCM aims to generate spatiotemporal dynamic model(s) of effective connectivity between brain regions, taking into account various biophysical parameters at a number of spatial scales with appropriate statistical evaluation. A set of potential models of hypothesized interconnections between brain areas of interest are first specified. These different models are typically formulated on previous literature and then fitted to the data to generate parameters and estimate evidence. Finally, the models are contrasted using a Bayesian statistical comparison to determine which of the proposed models best account for the experimental data. In DCM, computations proceed in source space (see Source Modeling section).

Graph-Theoretical Analysis
Graph-theoretical analysis (Bullmore & Sporns, 2009) has been applied to the study of brain structure and function only relatively recently, although it as a mathematical approach first appeared in the nineteenth century (Sporns, 2010). The critical elements of the graph

are "nodes," and they are linked together (or not) by connections that are called "edges." Various mathematical measures can be generated to express the density and clustering of nodes and their relative configuration and relationship with neighboring nodes (Rubinov & Sporns, 2010). In both structural and functional brain-related graph analyses, gray matter regions and their (existing white matter) connections most typically have been expressed as nodes and edges, respectively. Recently, however, a novel approach has reversed these assignments, where now gray and white matter are edges and nodes, respectively. Novel measures of "edge FC" and "edge time series" have been shown to be reliable across multiple sessions in the same individuals—an approach that may be fruitful in looking for biomarkers of brain disease (Faskowitz et al., 2020).

From a FC perspective, graph-theoretical analysis allows networks of brain regions sharing common activity profiles to be identified. This approach generates a connectivity matrix for individual subject or group data. The type of connectivity matrix generated depends entirely on the inputted measure—connectivity matrices can be "unweighted" or "weighted," that is, indicate the presence of or the strength of an existing connection, respectively. Additionally, connectivity matrices can also be "nondirected" or "directed." The directed option indicates which region likely sends input to another—a requirement for an analysis of effective connectivity.

Previously, we also mentioned potential effects of one brain region on another, which can be either direct (e.g., A influences C) or indirect via another brain structure (where A influences B, which influences C). These interactions can be investigated with graph-theoretical analysis using directed FC measures to identify direct connections from A to C and also *two-step connections* from A to B to C. This latter triangular connection pattern, where three nodes (or brain regions) are linked is a very specific example of a "motif"—a particular type of subset of connection pattern (Rubinov & Sporns, 2010).

The published graph-theoretical analyses of MEG/EEG have to date mainly expressed data in *sensor space*, using FC measures described in this chapter to generate connectivity matrices. It is not clear how certain graph-theoretical measures are affected by potentially artificially inflated FC measures calculated from sensor space data (see previous discussions). Studies explicitly comparing the same data side by side in both source and sensor space are needed to better understand this problem.

On the Practicalities of Connectivity Analyses

For performing effective-connectivity or network analyses on MEG/EEG data in source space, the problem is made more tractable by subdividing the structural brain data set into tissue parcels or regions, using automated algorithms from freely available open-source academic software. A number of common automating "parcellation" schemes exist and have been evaluated side by side for MRI-based resting-state network data (see for example de Reus & van den Heuvel, 2013; Arslan et al., 2018; Eickhoff et al., 2018; Bryce et al., 2021). We discuss challenges for data analyses with respect to parcellation schemes in more detail in Chapter 21.

■ SOURCE MODELING

Forward and Inverse Problems in MEG and EEG

Much of today's cognitive and systems-neuroscience research is focused on FC analyses. We have already discussed in detail the shortcomings of working in sensor space. Therefore, we recommend examining MEG/EEG data in source space for computing FC measures and performing physiologically based analyses related to generators of brain signals.

The *forward problem* refers to the calculation of the electric or magnetic fields, $E(r)$ or $B(r)$, respectively, given a known primary current distribution $J_p(r)$ within the brain (here r is the location vector). In practice, one places a known source into a known location in the brain and solves the "forward" problem by generating the associated EEG and MEG signals.

To go in the opposite direction—from measured MEG/EEG signals to the actual source currents in the brain—we need to solve the *inverse problem*. As discussed previously (Chapter 3), in the unconstrained form, the inverse problem has no unique solution as the distribution of the magnetic field or electric potential at the surface of the head could arise from any number of current configurations within the head.

Traditionally, the MEG literature was the main body of work dealing with the inverse problem (for a review, see Hämäläinen et al., 1993), so in this section we first discuss the neural source analysis of MEG data.

The inverse problem can be constrained by information related to the individual subject's anatomy, for example, based on high-resolution structural MRI from which the cortical mantle can be computed and used as the site of possible source–current locations. Altogether, MRI and computerized tomographic images can provide the raw data for the generation of realistic head models for both MEG and EEG analyses. EEG can supplement MEG in pinpointing radial and deep currents (see Chapter 3).

Head Models

A homogeneous spherical model of the head was originally proposed by Mary Brazier (1949) for interpreting sources of EEG signals, but this was a poor approximation of the head given that tissue conductivities—which vary widely in the head (Table 10.1)—dampen and smear the EEG signal distribution on the scalp. Hence, two-layer models, consisting of an outer shell and a central core (Geisler & Gerstein, 1961), and three-layer models representing brain, skull, and scalp (Rush & Driscoll, 1968) were introduced. Today, models based on six tissue types (skin, skull compacta, skull spongiosa, cerebrospinal fluid, gray matter, and white matter) are not uncommon (Schrader et al, 2021).

For MEG, as we discussed in Chapter 3, the uniform conducting single-shell sphere model still remains an extremely useful approximation, and even head models with realistic shapes can consist of one homogeneous volume because magnetic fields are *not* distorted by differences in tissue conductivities. However, for EEG the more complex head models need to take into account different tissue conductivities and thicknesses, relying on the values that are available in the literature (see Table 10.1). However, ideally, more accurate measurements of tissue conductivities in *individual subjects* are needed. Electrical impedance tomography (Holder, 1992) performed during scalp EEG recordings could ultimately achieve this purpose (Dabek et al., 2016); however, this measurement method still has many challenges.

Two main choices are available for realistic head models: a boundary-element model (BEM) or a finite-element model (FEM). The input for both methods is a high-resolution structural MRI scan of the *head* (not brain) and sometimes additional scans to aid in better defining the cortical surface (see Chapter 22 for a commentary on issues relating to brain parcellation schemes). BEM and FEM both first segregate the various tissues of the head/brain from one another, but they express the results in a different way. BEM will generate a set of surfaces (built up from meshes with triangular elements of variable size to accommodate the representation of curvatures) that correspond to boundaries at the scalp surface,

TABLE 10.1 Values of Absolute Conductivity of Different Tissues in the Human Head (In Units of Siemens/m)

TISSUE TYPE	GEDDES AND BAKER (1967)	OOSTENDORP ET AL. (2000)	GONCALVES ET AL. (2003)	GUTIERREZ ET AL. (2004)	LAI ET AL. (2005)	MCCANN ET AL. (2019)
Scalp	0.43	0.22	0.33	0.749	0.33	0.41
Skull (overall)	0.006–0.015	0.015	0.0081	0.012	0.0132	0.02
Skull: outer compact						0.005
Skull: spongiform						0.048
Skull: inner compact						0.007
CSF	–	–	–	1.79	–	1.71
Brain	0.12–0.48	0.22	0.33	0.313	0.33	–
Gray matter						0.47
White matter						0.22

CSF = cerebrospinal fluid.

Adapted and reprinted from Hallez H, Vanrumste B, Grech R, et al. Review on solving the forward problem in EEG source analysis. *J Neuro Eng Rehab* 2007, 4: 46, and McCann H, Pisano G, Beltrachini L. Variation in reported human head tissue electrical conductivity values. *Brain Topogr* 2019, 32: 825–858.

outer skull, brain gray matter, and the like; however, generating a surface for the cerebrospinal fluid (CSF) layer covering the cortex may be a challenge and may require MRI scans with other pulse sequences. FEM is a volume, rather than a surface, and its basic building block is thus the voxel. FEMs can be advantageous when fMRI data will be directly related to source-space MEG or EEG data. BEM might be preferred when computation needs to be made more tractable because the computed meshes are a way to reduce dimensionality of the data set. For a review comparing BEMs and FEMs, see Hallez et al. (2007).

Single-Dipole Model

The standard model for currents giving rise to MEG and EEG signals is a local current dipole. In EEG analysis, the dipole (see Chapter 3) must be specified with six parameters: three location coordinates (x, y, and z) and three components of dipole strength, one along each coordinate axis. In MEG analysis, only five free parameters are needed—three for location and two for strength—as radial currents do not produce an external magnetic field (in an ideal sphere) and thus can be neglected (see Figure 1.4).

On the basis of the measured MEG/EEG data, the dipole parameters can be found, or "the dipole is fitted," by a nonlinear least-squares search that was first applied to MEG signals by Tuomisto and colleagues (1983). In a least-squares search, one compares the measured field pattern with a field pattern produced by an ideal current dipole and then computes differences between the field values point by point; the differences are squared, and the dipole location that produces the *smallest sum* of the squared difference values is assumed to be the site of an equivalent current dipole (ECD) that best explains the measured signal pattern. For a point-like current dipole, the field strength decreases inversely as the function of the square of the distance.

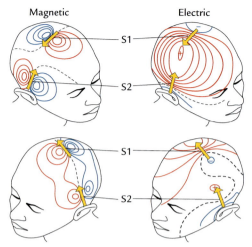

FIGURE 10.9. Relative sensitivities of MEG and EEG. Source areas and MEG (magnetic) and EEG (electric) signal distributions associated with stimulation of the left peroneal nerve. MEG patterns indicate clearly separate sources in the contralateral (right) foot SI cortex (source S1) and in bilateral SII cortices (sources S2), whereas the strongest EEG response (seen in the right top panel) is far from the activated cortices. See text for explanation.

The current dipole model can be used to identify multiple, simultaneously active sources that are separated by a few centimeters from each other if they are parallel to one another, or even close to dipoles if they differ in timing and orientation. For example, Figure 10.9 shows somatosensory-evoked magnetic fields from the first and second somatosensory cortices SI and SII, with a distinct field pattern for each source (a unilateral SI and bilateral SII sources). In this case the orientations of the sources are particularly favorable for MEG, whereas the electric potential distributions are smeared and largely overlapping, which makes it difficult to find the underlying sources. Instead, the first guess on the basis of the EEG scalp distribution would be a radial dipole in the parietal cortex clearly outside the SI and SII cortices.

Goodness of Fit and Confidence Limits of the Model

A goodness-of-fit value g can be used to describe how well the field pattern of an ECD, determined by means of a least-squares search, agrees with the measured data. In other terms, g indicates how much variance of the measured signals the model can explain; thus it is a measure similar to the R^2 used in linear regression analysis as the measure of explained variance. If $g = 1$, the model agrees completely with the measurement. If $g = 0$, the model is irrelevant and does not describe the measurements any better than a zero field would. The goodness-of-fit value can deviate from 1 if the data are very noisy or if the source does not behave like a local current dipole. Here it is important to remember that *one can locate an incorrect model source with extremely good precision* (Figure 3.7), so that the source seems to be reliable, for example, in repeated measurements.

The estimated dipole location always has some inaccuracy that can be quantified by calculating confidence limits for the location in 3D space, for example, along the longitudinal direction (in the direction of the ECD), in the transverse direction (perpendicular to the dipole), and along its depth (along the location vector). Figure 10.10 shows activations

MEG   EEG

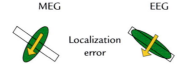

Localization error

FIGURE 10.10. **Localization errors of MEG and EEG.** A schematic presentation of local-ization errors of a current dipole (yellow arrow) situated perpendicular to a cortical sheet (white rectangle). The green ovals depict two-dimensional confidence areas for MEG and EEG source localization, indicating that MEG localizes the source more accurately in the di-rection transversal to the current direction (i.e., along the cortical sheet), and EEG identifies the source best in the direction along the current.

(current dipoles) schematically for a short piece of cortex, with the 2D confidence limits depicted around the yellow arrow that indicates source strength and direction. For MEG, the confidence limits are smallest in the direction transverse to the dipole orientation and about double along the dipole and in the direction of depth, whereas for EEG the con-fidence limits are smallest along the direction of the dipole. Thus, MEG is at its best in discriminating source changes along a cortical strip (in a wall of a fissure), for example, in discriminating finger representations along the central sulcus, whereas EEG is better in dis-criminating activity between two adjacent walls of a cortical fissure (Figure 10.10).

We must remember that the distance of the measurement site to the source determines the details we are able to see in the underlying field patterns. Figure 10.11 illustrates that when the magnetic signal produced by two parallel current dipoles in a sphere is measured on the surface, the pattern clearly deviates from that produced by a single dipole (Figure 10.11, dashed blue line). However, when the measurement is performed 2 cm outside the surface, the minor details of the summation pattern of the two dipoles are no longer visible, and the distribution resembles that produced by a single dipole (red solid line). Consequently, when a single dipole is used to explain the field produced by two dipoles, such as those in Figure 10.11, the ECD is deeper and stronger than the actual sources be-cause it needs to explain the field pattern and strength produced by two dipoles. This mod-eling error is only weakly reflected in the goodness-of-fit measure g, and thus it is typically not possible to differentiate between one dipole versus two parallel dipoles that are less than 2 cm away. However, using the anatomy of the cortical mantle as a constraint for pos-sible dipole locations would help.

If the brain activation is very extended (i.e., a set of multiple small dipoles in a region of cortex), as is shown in Figure 10.12, a single-dipole model can give misleading results. In the middle panel, the ECD is considerably deeper than the horizontally extended layer, whereas in the right panel, the ECD is more superficial than the center of gravity of the layer because the active areas close to the measurement sensor contribute more to the signal than do the deeper parts that are further away from the sensor.

Spatial Resolution

Given the nonuniqueness of the inverse problem that affects both MEG and EEG, skeptics often doubt the possibilities of accurately localizing any sources of MEG/EEG signals. In Figure 3.7, we made a distinction between accuracy and precision of source localization. *Spatial resolution* of MEG/EEG is often confused with these measures, although it should refer to the ability to distinguish between two (or more) sources. One example is the dif-ferentiation between sources of electrical stimulation of different fingers. If the fingers are

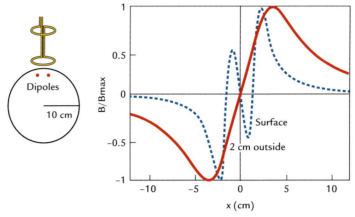

FIGURE 10.11. The effect of recording distance on the details of the measured magnetic field pattern. Left: Two parallel tangential current dipoles are located 2 cm apart from each other in a sphere with a radius of 10 cm. Right: If the MEG signals could be recorded immediately at the surface of the sphere, the summation of the patterns of the two dipoles would result in quite a complex pattern (blue dashed line). These details have been lost in a recording made 2 cm above the surface (red solid line), indicating that at that distance it is very difficult to discern the fine details of the underlying source currents. Reproduced and modified with permission from Hari R: Magnetoencephalography: Methods and Clinical Aspects. In: Schomer DL and Lopes da Silva FH: *Niedermeyer's Electroencephalography: Basic Principles, Clinical Applications, and Related Fields.* 7th edition. New York: Oxford University Press, 2018.

stimulated at different times, their separate sources in the somatosensory cortex can be differentiated with MEG at submillimeter resolution. The reason is that the distinction now goes in the direction perpendicular to the source currents where the confidence limits for source location based on MEG recordings are the smallest (as shown in Figure 10.10). Moreover, the signal-to-noise ratio of the early evoked responses can be increased easily just by increasing the number of averaged responses.

The spatial resolution of MEG depends on several factors, such as the strength and depth of the source, the noise level, and how well the measurement locations cover the most informative parts of the field pattern (Hari et al., 1988). The configuration of the flux transformer also affects the ultimate spatial resolution of the recordings. The best signal sensitivity is obtained by a magnetometer that has no compensation coils. However, the magnetometer is also very sensitive to various sources of noise, and it thus behaves well only in well-shielded environments, but even there it can easily pick up biological noise arising, for example, from the heart or the eyes.

Differences in the spatial resolution between different instruments accentuate when the depth of the source increases because the measured signals drop with flux-transformer-dependent rate (Figure 5.15, bottom panel); deep local sources typically cannot be localized with an accuracy better than ±1 cm on the basis of the MEG signals only (Figure 10.13) but see the discussion on detection of deep sources in Chapter 22. Therefore, it is preferable to make the measurements within a shielded room with a first-order gradiometer rather than to use second- or third-order gradiometers in a noisy environment. The interpretation of the results is more straightforward and less vulnerable to errors if the noise is prevented rather than mathematically compensated for.

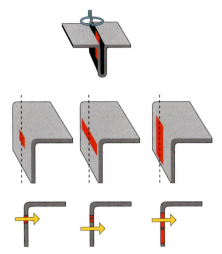

FIGURE 10.12. Modeling an extended activation patch in the wall of a cortical fissure with a single current dipole. The schematic (top) shows an activated patch within fissural cortex and a planar gradiometer placed directly over it. The middle row shows different configurations of the activated patch, and the bottom row shows the location of the equivalent current dipole in a side view. When the activated area is less than 2 cm in diameter (left), the equivalent dipole pinpoints accurately its center. When the activated area is extended in horizontal direction (middle), the equivalent current dipole will overestimate the depth. When the activation extends to the direction of depth (right) the equivalent current dipole is more superficial than the center of gravity of the activated patch because the areas close to the sensors contribute more to the signals picked up outside the head. Adapted and reprinted from Hari R: On brain's magnetic responses to sensory stimuli. *J Clin Neurophysiol* 1991, 8: 157–169. With permission from Wolters Kluwer Health, Inc.

On-scalp devices, such as optically pumped magnetometers (OPMs), offer promise for increased spatial resolution because the sensors are closer to the brain than are the traditional low-temperature SQUID arrays; however, this advantage depends on the sensor noise and is true mainly for superficial currents. One issue hampering both signal-to-noise and spatial resolution is the potential sensor movement in semiflexible OPM helmets (Zetter et al., 2019; Hill et al., 2020). In traditional SQUID-based MEG measurements, the subject's head movements can be either continuously tracked and corrected (Uutela et al., 2001) or—more effectively—the head position can be fixed with a custom-made head cast that fits snugly into the rigid MEG (Meyer et al., 2017). The flexible head cast has even enabled layer-specific inferences to be made about brain activity (Bonaiuto et al., 2018).

Source Extent

Source extent will always be rather illusory, for not only MEG/EEG signals but also fMRI activations. In fMRI, brain activations are identified by statistical thresholding (usually between-condition differences), which means that improving the signal-to-noise ratio of the measured signals will inevitably lead to more extensive activation blobs (which has been also demonstrated experimentally).

When MEG/EEG signals are modeled with single-current dipoles, the assumption is that the current is very local, and thus no estimates are directly obtained for the extent of

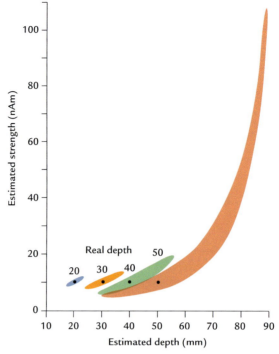

FIGURE 10.13. Dependence of the estimated current-dipole strength on the real source depth. A 10-nAm current dipole was placed into different depths (from 20 to 50 mm) of a sphere with radius of 10 cm, and the strength and depth of an equivalent current dipole were estimated. The colored areas show the 95% confidence limits for these estimates, indicating that the deeper the real source, the more uncertainty exists in its estimated strength and depth. Adapted and reprinted from Hari R, Joutsiniemi S-L, Sarvas J: Spatial resolution of neuromagnetic records: theoretical calculations in a spherical model. *Electroencephalogr Clin Neurophysiol* 1988, 71: 64–72. With permission from Elsevier.

activation. However, some hints can be obtained from the source strengths. For example, a dipole moment of 20 nAm (nanoampere meter) can be compared with dipole moments associated with single postsynaptic potentials that are approximately 20 fAm in size (although dependent on the axon diameter; cf. Vvedensky et al., 1985). Thus, about a million synapses should be simultaneously active to produce a response on the order of 20 nAm. Of course, this is very clearly a lower limit approximate because opposite currents cancel out to a large extent in the activated brain area.

Another estimate can be obtained by comparing the dipole moment with current density measurements obtained from animal cortex, which are of the order of 100 to 250 nA/mm^2. Assuming this estimate over an effective thickness of 1 mm, Hari (1990) estimated that a dipole moment of 10 nAm would correspond to 40 mm^2 of active cortex, in other words 0.25 nAm/mm^2. This value is about the same magnitude as the estimate of about 0.7 nAm/mm^2 of cortical tissue suggested and in part also measured in turtle, pig, and monkey (Murakami & Okada, 2015).

The MEG signal size per tissue area may increase in some special cases. For example, the spreading depression is associated with increased current flow due to opening of large Ca2$^+$ channels (Tottene et al., 2011), likely contributed by the glia. On the other hand, highly synchronous discharges during epileptic seizures would also be associated with considerably higher current densities.

Effect of Synchrony

Synchrony is an important variable for the determination of the net current. For example, epileptogenic tissue with very synchronous activity produces much stronger net currents than normally functioning tissue does.

It follows from basic statistics that if we have in a certain area N_s identical elements (neurons) that are synchronous and N_{as} neurons that are asynchronous, the signal sizes produced by these elements are related by $N_s / \sqrt{N_{as}}$, and therefore the percentage contribution of the synchronous elements to the total signal would be $100 * N_s / (N_s + \sqrt{N_{as}})$ (Hari et al., 1997). Figure 10.14 shows results of this kind of calculation assuming that

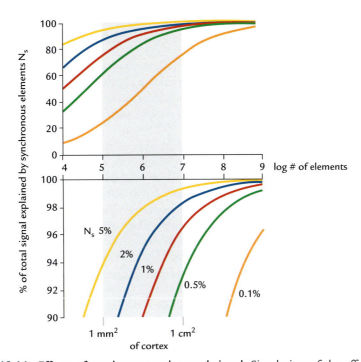

FIGURE 10.14. **Effects of synchrony on the total signal.** Simulation of the effects of synchrony. The bottom panel shows enlarged the upper part of the top panel. The horizontal axes on both plots show the log number of elements in the studied neuronal populations, ranging from 10^4 to 10^9. From these, 10^5 would correspond to the number of pyramidal cells in 1 mm^2 of cortex and 10^7 would correspond to 1 cm^2 of cortex. All elements are assumed to have similar time courses. The traces of different colors refer to different proportions of synchronous elements (from 0.1% to 5%) when the other elements are asynchronous. The vertical scale shows how much of the total signal (sum of signals produced by both synchronous and asynchronous elements) is explained by the synchronous elements. See text for further explanation. Adapted and reprinted from Hari R, Salmelin R, Mäkelä JP, Salenius S, Helle M: Magnetoencephalographic cortical rhythms. *Int J Psychophysiol* 1997, 26: 51–62. With permission from Elsevier.

pyramidal neurons (10^5 per 1 mm^2 of cortex) act as the synchronous or asynchronous oscillatory elements. It turns out that 5% synchronous neurons in 1 mm^2 of cortex would explain 94% of the total signal. Similarly, just 0.5% synchronous neurons in 1 cm^2 of cortex would explain 93% of the total signal. The results suggest that surprisingly small synchronous populations could be responsible for the main signals that we record with MEG and EEG. In real life, this proportion and the contributing synchronous elements vary as a function of them.

Multidipole Models, Distributed Models, and Beamformers

When a single current-dipole model is not adequate to explain the data, one may use multidipole models or distributed models, the latter of which consists of a large number of minute current dipoles.

The multidipole model assumes several current dipoles that maintain their positions and, optionally, also their orientations throughout the time interval of interest. However, the dipoles are allowed to change their amplitudes smoothly as a function of time. The user can define the number of dipoles or use some algorithms to suggest the suitable number on the basis of unexplained variance.

When several sources overlap both temporally and spatially, a multidipole model may be problematic because of interactions between nearby, but opposite, dipoles. It is then important to take into account the spatiotemporal course of the signals as a whole, instead of considering each time sample separately; such an approach was first taken in EEG analysis (for a review, see Scherg, 1990).

One can also search for more general solutions of the neurophysiological inverse problem. For example, distributed models consider grids of dipoles across a volume of tissue. The minimum-norm estimate (MNE) (Hämäläinen & Ilmoniemi, 1994) assumes that out of the various possible source currents, the most likely solution has the smallest norm. Classical MNE prefers very superficial current estimates since those closest to the sensor array will be the smallest ones. Thus, improved variations are depth-weighted MNE (Ioannides et al., 1990) and dynamic statistical parametric mapping (Dale et al., 2000), which employs source spaces that are constrained to the individual's cerebral cortex, as well as standardized low-resolution electromagnetic tomography (Pascual-Marqui, 2002). The available MNE software handles mixed MEG and EEG data sets (Gramfort et al., 2014), but one caveat—true for all estimates of distributed sources—is the blurring of the source estimates so that even a local source can have an extent of up to a few centimeters, depending on the method employed (see, e.g., Hämäläinen & Hari, 2002).

Another approach that has been used in both MEG and EEG source modeling is beamforming in its various variants (Hillebrand & Barnes, 2005; Grech et al., 2008; Kim & Davis, 2021). Beamforming was originally developed for sonar, radar, and microwave communications applications (Widrow & Stearns, 1985; Van Veen & Buckley, 1988) to allow separation and estimation of signals from a desired location, despite the presence of overlapping signals and noise arising from other nearby locations. In MEG/EEG data analysis, a beamformer constructs a set of spatial filters, with different weights for each element (voxel) in the brain, with the assumption that no two distant cortical areas generate coherent local field potentials or magnetic fields over long timescales. Beamformer methods have been used for modeling of oscillatory behavior, as well as for examining phenomena such as ERS and ERD (Hillebrand & Barnes, 2005). One benefit of beamforming is that the number of sources do not need to be specified a priori, and the result is typically quite an extensive source volume. On the other hand, beamformers easily produce ghost sources or collapse closely located sources together. Three commonly used variants of beamformer methods are linearly constrained minimum-variance (LCMV), multiple-signal classification (MUSIC), and synthetic-aperture magnetometry (SAM) (for a recent tutorial on differences between these, see Kim & Davis, 2021).

Distributed versus single- or multidipole models represent two extreme ends of the source-modeling scale currently used with MEG and EEG data. The MNE, with its variants, is an optimal estimate when minimal prior information is assumed or used. The dipole model is preferable when one can assume that a relatively small patch of the cortex produced the measured signal. However, for many investigations such prior knowledge (or guesses) may not be available.

Figure 10.15 shows that the chosen analysis model largely determines the result of the analysis, whether the source appears very local or is very distributed. The main message here is that local current dipoles are no less "physiological" than distributed models, whose appearance may be more attractive. For both a distributed current (top, left) and local current (top, right), the field patterns (second row) and dipole models (third row) are identical, as is also the MNE-based solution (two bottom rows). These results imply that the analysis method largely determines the appearance of the output of the source-modeling procedure. Each analysis method is based on some assumptions that also affect the physiological conclusions that can be made.

As we noted, source modeling using the methods described here can also be performed on EEG data, but given that EEG is greatly affected by tissue conductivities, more accurate models of the head/brain are needed.

Hypothesis Testing With Predetermined Source Locations

Yet another approach applied in MEG analysis is to test hypotheses about source locations by computationally placing local current sources in certain locations, defined on the basis of the subject's anatomical MRI, and then asking how well these sources would explain the measured MEG patterns. This approach, which is based on forward calculations, has been used to explore activation of human hippocampus and thalamus during various tasks by placing the source in several volume elements and then comparing the computed and measured results (Tesche, 1996, 1997). The problem is that MEG's spatial resolution is poor for deep sources, and thus it is difficult—on the basis of these analyses only—to be confident about accurate source location.

■ STATISTICAL CONSIDERATIONS

Group Effects

Every individual brain has a characteristic neurophysiological signature. How should the interindividual variability in evoked responses be represented? If only the time courses are of interest, one can either superimpose all subjects' responses with, or without, the grand-average waveform. If grand averages are presented, then confidence intervals or other measures of variation (e.g., the standard error of mean) around the grand-average waveforms are a must. For MEG, grand averages from particular sensor locations are not a good idea because the individual subjects' responses depend strongly on the relative positions of the sensors and the brain. However, MEG source waveforms may be grand averaged, provided that they appear rather similar in visual inspection across subjects.

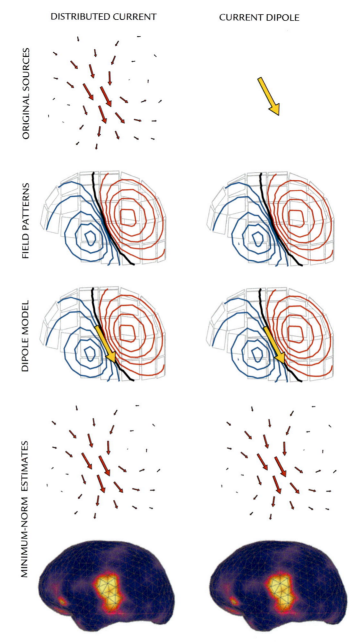

DISTRIBUTED CURRENT

CURRENT DIPOLE

ORIGINAL SOURCES

FIELD PATTERNS

DIPOLE MODEL

MINIMUM-NORM ESTIMATES

FIGURE 10.15. **How analysis method can affect the results of source estimation.** When simulated local distributed current (top left) and a current dipole (top right) were placed into the auditory cortex, both produced similar dipolar magnetic field patterns (second row). The dipole model resulted in ECDs (yellow arrows) at the same place and of same size (third row), and the minimum-norm analysis resulted in similar estimates of distributed currents (two bottom rows). See text for further explanation. Adapted and reprinted from Hämäläinen M, Hari R: Magnetoencephalographic characterization of dynamic brain activation: basic principles, and methods of data collection and source analysis. In: Toga A, Mazziotta J, eds. *Brain Mapping: The Methods*, 2nd ed. Boston: Elsevier, 2002: 227–253. With permission from Elsevier ©2002.

Importantly, if the peak latencies of averaged evoked responses vary greatly between individuals, the whole effect or response may disappear, or be altered, in the across-group average. This effect is similar to what can happen in a single subject's cross-trial average of non-phase-locked responses (shown schematically in Figure 10.1). For example, during infant development, the response latencies and morphology change substantially, and the latencies of somatosensory responses, especially, vary with the subject's height (and limb length). Thus, the subject group should be as homogeneous as possible regarding these variables. In other cases, age and limb length can be used as covariates in the data analysis.

One problem in group-level analysis is that the very strong responses of a single person can dominate the group average, as often occurs when intracranial ECoG or iEEG data are combined across subjects. Whether this is the case can often be quickly checked by superimposing the signals of interest from all subjects (which should be done in any case). If there is no reason to exclude these outliers from the data set (e.g., nothing irregular occurred during data acquisition), one could consider transforming the data to reduce variance before final analyses; for example, outliers can be much less serious in amplitude than power (squared signal) measures. When effects of experimental conditions are studied, intraindividual normalization may sometimes be applied to allow all subjects to contribute (almost) equally to the group-level results. For example, one could use response strength at a certain interstimulus interval as the reference and then examine only percentage changes in response size at other interstimulus intervals (without comparing the original signal sizes).

An alternative approach for dealing with group data that contain large interindividual variability is to perform analyses of variance (ANOVA), making sure that variances across subjects and experimental condition are similar. Here, the "sphericity test" can be useful in addressing the similarity of variances. Sphericity ranges from zero to 1 and is violated if the value deviates from 1. Depending on this value, different correction factors can be applied to effectively reduce the false-positive error rate and make the statistical test more conservative.

The amplitude and peak measures and parametric statistical approaches discussed here were used in the past when data from only a small number of (EEG) sensors were available due to the technological limits of the time. Some of these methods may be applicable to data recorded with today's portable EEG devices, which also use small numbers of sensors. Today, with high-density recordings, these analyses are useful if data of the current study need to be compared with the previous literature. For example, if one were to study activity of the auditory cortex, the hypotheses could be focused on sensors that have been previously described to show the most prominent activity. However, when using high-density recordings, one first must have a hypothesis—as in any research—and know what to search for because otherwise an additional problem of "cherry-picking" may arise if the researcher, for example, focuses on only the largest signals in the data set.

Whole-Head Analysis of Evoked Responses

Analysis approaches considering the entire set of channels (or source space) resemble those routinely used in fMRI data analyses. They are attractive as they can avoid issues related to cherry-picking (see above). Full whole-head analyses also allow results of previous studies focusing on single scalp/brain areas to be reconciled. A number of available freeware packages are available for this type of analysis, in both parametric and nonparametric form (see Baillet et al., 2011, for a survey of more commonly used software packages).

Some whole-head EEG/MEG analysis approaches use a general linear model (GLM) in a two-stage analysis—with individual-subject effects identified at the first level and group effects examined at the second level (Litvak et al., 2011; Pernet et al., 2011). Figure 10.16

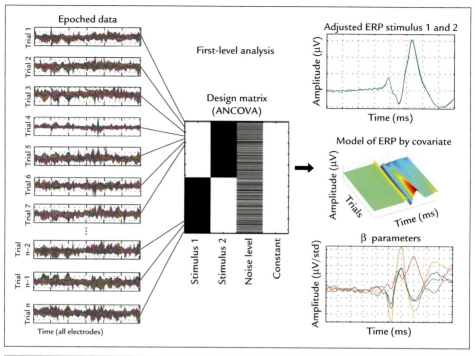

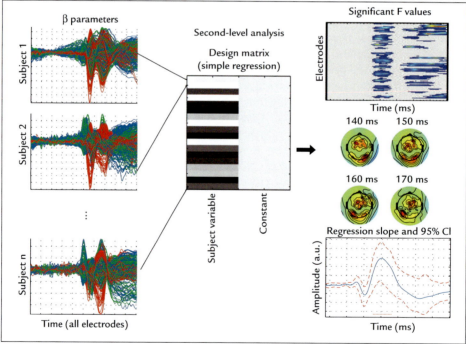

FIGURE 10.16. Stages in analysis of whole-head evoked response EEG data. Top: In the first-level analysis, the epoched EEG data of each subject, comprising all trials, are analyzed to obtain estimates of beta parameters that reflect the effects of experimental conditions coded in the design matrix. The design matrix includes a specification of codes for the effect of stimulus 1 and stimulus 2 (stimulus conditions), and the noise level across all stimuli.

presents the approach behind this analysis. At the first level (top panel of figure), single trials from all subjects and conditions are specified in a design matrix, and parameters of a GLM are estimated for each subject at each time point and each channel independently. At the second level of analysis (lower panel of figure), estimated beta parameters from the first-level analyses across all subjects are used to estimate the effects of various experimental variables. Significant spatiotemporal main and interaction effects between conditions can be identified using bootstrapping methods or permutation testing, which are attractive as they make no assumptions regarding the normality of the data.

The researcher should always design experiments to answer a research question, be it about the function of a circumscribed brain region (e.g., hand somatosensory cortex) or related to the overall brain response to a certain stimulus. The whole-scalp analysis will always reveal a far richer structure in the data than would be observed with the conventional analyses described previously in this chapter (see Chapter 19; Figure 19.4). Whole-head analysis is needed, for example, for studying hemispheric differences, for sequencing of temporal processing, or for clinical applications where the sources and effects of brain abnormality are not known in advance. In the MEG community, whole-head analysis has been used since the emergence of whole-scalp-covering magnetometers in 1990s.

MEG Signal Detectability and Statistical Power in Group Studies

Effect of Source Current Orientation and Location
Although MEG in principle sees only tangential currents, many currents in the real brain are "tilted" with respect to the scalp and thus should be visible in MEG recordings. The simulations in Figure 10.17 (Hillebrand & Barnes, 2002) show that most parts of the cortex, except for the mesial cortex, in fact do likely produce MEG signals, although the required source strength depends on the brain area. It is very difficult to correctly sample the deep medial regions.

Sensor Sensitivity, Number of Trials, Group Size, Effect Size, and Statistical Power
The smaller is the signal of interest the more data one has to collect to demonstrate statistically significant effects. On the other hand, even negligible differences between two groups can be made statistically significant by increasing the N and thereby the statistical power of the analysis. Thus one has to decide—preferably *prior to the analysis*—what effect size (the strength of the phenomenon under study) is meaningful for further interpretations. For example, if one is interested in the effects of latitude on the height of fourth graders, it is possible to collect so many subjects for height measurements that even a 0.1-mm group

---

FIGURE 10.16. Continued

Bottom: In the second-level analysis, the beta parameter(s) of experimental condition(s) for each subject, generated from the first-level analysis, are tested for significance across subjects. Statistically significant results can be displayed in various ways, including a display of significant *F* values as a function of channel and time (top right), or as topographic maps at various points in time, or as amplitude time courses with confidence intervals. Regression slopes and their 95% CIs are plotted on the bottom right. Reprinted with permission from Pernet CR, Chauveau N, Gaspar C, Rousselet GA: LIMO EEG: a toolbox for hierarchical LInear MOdeling of ElectroEncephaloGraphic data. *Comput Intell Neurosci* 2011: 831409. doi: 10.1155/2011/831409.

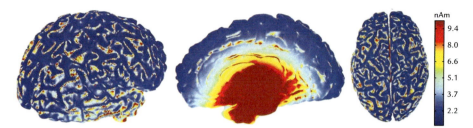

FIGURE 10.17. Source strength needed for MEG detection of current dipoles in different parts of the cortex. See text for explanation. Adapted and reprinted from Hillebrand A, Barnes GR: A quantitative assessment of the sensitivity of whole-head MEG to activity in the adult human cortex. *NeuroImage* 2002, 16: 638–650. With permission from Elsevier.

difference may become statistically significant, but this will certainly not help to reveal the mechanisms of growth.

Effect sizes are reported together with values of statistical significance (e.g., *F* values and *p* values) that themselves do not adequately indicate the real significance of a phenomenon. One should avoid "*p*-hacking," which is testing so many relationships that at least one of them becomes statistically significant, then report it and forget the nonsignificant ones. Naturally, post hoc tests conducted on statistically significant main and interaction effects will also have to be corrected for multiple comparisons. If the data are not normally distributed, nonparametric analyses or Bayesian statistics can be used. We recommend the "Ten Simple Rules for Effective Statistical Practice" (Kass et al., 2016), and the COBIDAS MEEG (magnetoencephalography and electroencephalography) guidelines (Pernet et al., 2020) for further reading.

If sensor-wise MEG/EEG evoked responses are compared statistically between conditions, one has to remember that the "noise" (arising mainly from the underlying spontaneous activity) varies according to the brain region. Additionally, the sensors—due to their position and due to the geometry of the volume conductor—are differentially sensitive to neural currents at different locations in the brain (see Chapter 3). In source space, the analyses are often more straightforward, but then it is important to consider signal detectability, which—together with the amount of data collected from each individual and with the size of the studied group of subjects—is closely related to the measurements' statistical power.

Unfortunately, the specific questions of "*How many subjects and how many trials do I need in a certain experiment?*" have only the answer: "It depends" (Boudewyn et al., 2018; Chaumon et al., 2021). It depends on the many factors mentioned above—signal detectability with respect to source orientation, noise levels, group size, and effect size. But it is also dependent on the replicability of the signals in single individuals (e.g., that the subject stays similarly engaged in the task throughout the recording and does not get drowsy), as well as on the result variability from subject to subject when group data are of interest.

One recent study systematically examined the effect of the number of trials and subjects on statistical power in MEG sensor-level signals in a resting-state MEG dataset of 89 subjects (Chaumon et al., 2021). "Evoked activity" was injected into half of the data set by inserting a 10-nAm current dipole at a particular time point in the data epoch. Monte Carlo–like simulations were performed on a range of trials and subjects. A statistical comparison between epochs "with" and "without" evoked activity detected significant differences at the sensor level with classical paired *t* tests across subjects, using amplitude, squared amplitude, and GFP measures. Group-level differences varied substantially, by not only anatomical location but also chosen power measure (Figure 10.18).

The anatomical location of the source can substantially affect its detectability and therefore the statistical power of group-level studies. Sources can be expressed in terms of their position variability, that is, how much the spatial location of the dipole varies across the group of subjects. A distribution of position variability was constructed by first placing the dipole in one location in the standardized 3D (MNI) space and then examining its position in each subject's native space. A source in the fusiform gyrus had a relatively low cross-subject position variability, and it produced reliable power across all three measures despite its large distance from MEG sensors (Figure 10.19). In contrast, the sources in the superior occipital gyrus had relatively high cross-subject variability, and they resulted in variable statistical power across measures, even though they were close to the sensors (Figure 10.19). The source positions and orientations can covary, as happens, for example, for sources in sulci versus convexial cortex, which makes it difficult to assess the independent impact of these variables. Additional simulations where the source position and orientation were controlled *independently* of the individual anatomy confirmed the strong effects of source orientation and source distance from the sensors, as expected. The major effect on source detectability came from orientation variability (when source position was kept constant) and less so from position variability (when source orientation was kept constant).

According to this study no overall recommendations for the ideal number of trials and subjects can be made without considering each study case by case (Chaumon et al., 2021). For example, in network-based FC investigations, experiments should be designed to reliably detect the *weakest of all sources of interest* based on previous knowledge of the involved brain structures. For studies investigating new scientific questions, it may not be possible to predict what and where the weakest sources of interest would be, and their signal-to-noise ratios are not known in advance.

▪ COMMON PITFALLS IN DATA ANALYSIS AND INTERPRETATION

Here we briefly reiterate some of the most important points with respect to data analysis and interpretation:

- *Data analysis*: The main lines of analysis should be planned during the *design* of the MEG/EEG study, considering detectability of sources and effect sizes. Some analysis methods may impose additional constraints on the properties or type of MEG/EEG data to be acquired.
- *Reference electrode and the scalp EEG distribution*: Reference electrodes should never be physically linked during data acquisition; instead, use single-electrode references and digitally re-reference after data acquisition.
- *Appropriate bandpass filtering and data sampling*: During data acquisition, use filtering that will adequately sample the signals of interest and not remove or distort real effects or introduce phase or latency shifts in the data. If artifact-removal methods are used, unwanted signals may need to be sampled in their entirety, and thus a wider filter passband at acquisition may be needed.
- *Computing FC measures*: Do not compute FC measures (e.g., coherence) between signals that actually reflect activity of the same source. Thus, work in source rather than sensor space whenever possible and be aware of the potential and field

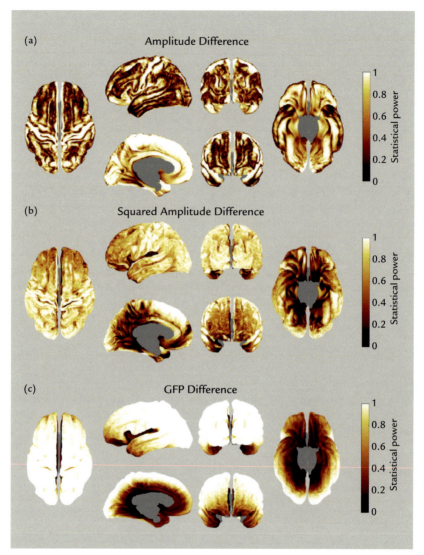

FIGURE 10.18. Estimates of statistical power across the cortical surface for detecting sensor-level MEG signal generated by a single 10-nAm current dipole. In a simulated experiment with 25 subjects, with 50 trials each, the dipole was placed at every possible cortical location and the resulting MEG signal was compared with a no-stimulus condition. Simulations used pre-processed MEG resting-state data from the Human Connectome Project. Three power measures are displayed on brains depicting superior, left lateral, left medial, anterior, posterior, and inferior views. (a) Amplitude difference. Relatively high statistical power values are seen within major sulci and on the medial wall. (b) Squared amplitude difference. The statistical power is relatively lower in medial and inferior regions. (c) GFP difference. Relatively higher statistical power is seen for superficial neocortical sources, and low statistical power occurs for deep sources. Adapted and reprinted from Chaumon M, Puce A, George N: Statistical power: Implications for planning MEG studies. *NeuroImage* 2021, 233: 117894. With permission from Elsevier.

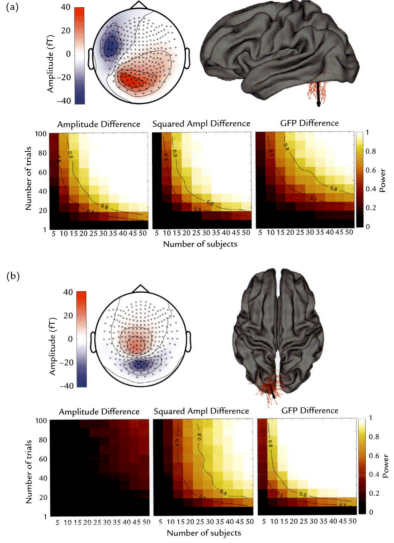

FIGURE 10.19. Detecting group-level differences in MEG sensor-level signals for two sources at different anatomical positions. (a) A source with low cross-subject position variability in the fusiform gyrus. Top left: Isocontour map of the magnetic field averaged across 89 subjects for current dipoles located in the fusiform gyrus. Black circles denote MEG sensor positions on the 2D schematic head viewed from top. The color bar indicates the strength of magnetic field exiting (red) and entering (blue) the head in femtoteslas (fT). Top right: Lateral view of the brain, with red arrows representing positions of simulated individual dipoles. The bold black arrow displays the average dipole across subjects. Lower panel: Statistical power as a function of the number of subjects and trials for tests on simple amplitude differences (left), squared-amplitude differences (middle; Ampl refers to amplitude) and global field power (GFP) differences at this location. The statistical power (color-coded, see scale on the right) was estimated by Monte Carlo simulations. The isocontour lines highlight power estimates of 0.5 and 0.8. (b) Corresponding visualization for a source with relatively high cross-subject position variability in the superior occipital gyrus. See panel a for notations and the main text for further explanation. Adapted and reprinted from Chaumon M, Puce A, George N: Statistical power: Implications for planning MEG studies. *NeuroImage* 2021, 233: 117894. With permission from Elsevier.

patterns associated with the sources. (Measures of effective connectivity require computation in source space.)

- *Source models*: Use physiologically plausible and appropriate models to test your hypotheses. Beware of taking source analyses to their limits; for example, with Bayesian methods that rely on prior information, one can easily model noise.

■ REFERENCES

Arslan S, Ktena SI, Makropoulos A, Robinson EC, Rueckert D, Parisot S: Human brain mapping: a systematic comparison of parcellation methods for the human cerebral cortex. *NeuroImage* 2018, 170: 5–30.

Aru J, Aru J, Priesemann V, Wibral M, Lana L, Pipa G, Singer W, Vicente R: Untangling cross-frequency coupling in neuroscience. *Curr Opin Neurobiol* 2015, 31: 51–61.

Babiloni C, Barry RJ, Basar E, Blinowska KJ, Cichocki A, Drinkenburg W, Klimesch W, Knight RT, Lopes da Silva F, Nunez P, Oostenveld R, Jeong J, Pascual-Marqui R, Valdés-Sosa P, Hallett M: International Federation of Clinical Neurophysiology–(IFCN)—EEG Research Workgroup: recommendations on frequency and topographic analysis of resting state EEG rhythms. Part 1: Applications in clinical research studies. *Clin Neurophysiol* 2020, 131: 285–307.

Babo-Rebelo M, Puce A, Bullock D, Hugueville L, Pestilli F, Adam C, Lehongre K, Lambrecq V, Dinkelacker V, George N: Visual information routes in the posterior dorsal and ventral face network studied with intracranial neurophysiology and white matter tract endpoints. *Cereb Cortex* 2022, 32: 342–366.

Baccalá LA, Sameshima K: Comments on "Is partial coherence a viable technique for identifying generators of neural oscillations?" Why the term "Gersch Causality" is inappropriate: common neural structure inference pitfalls. *Biol Cybern* 2006, 95: 135–141.

Baillet S, Friston K, Oostenveld R: Academic software applications for electromagnetic brain mapping using MEG and EEG. *Comput Intell Neurosci* 2011, 2011: 972050.

Barlow JS: The early history of EEG data-processing at the Massachusetts Institute of Technology and the Massachusetts General Hospital. *Int J Psychophysiol* 1977, 26: 443–454.

Basti A, Pizzella V, Chella F, Romani GL, Nolte G, Marzetti L: Disclosing large-scale directed functional connections in MEG with the multivariate phase slope index. *NeuroImage* 2018, 175: 61–175.

Bastos AM, Schoffelen JM: A tutorial review of functional connectivity analysis methods and their interpretational pitfalls. *Front Syst Neurosci* 2016, 9: 175.

Bonaiuto JJ, Meyer SS, Little S, Rossiter H, Callaghan MF, Dick F, Barnes GR, Bestmann S: Lamina-specific cortical dynamics in human visual and sensorimotor cortices. *eLife* 2018, 7: e33977.

Boudewyn MA, Luck SJ, Farrens JL, Kappenman ES: How many trials does it take to get a significant ERP effect? It depends. *Psychophysiology* 2018, 55: e13049.

Brazier M: The electrical fields at the surface of the head during sleep. *Electroencephalogr Clin Neurophysiol* 1949, 1: 195–204.

Bruns A: Fourier-, Hilbert- and wavelet-based signal analysis: are they really different approaches? *J Neurosci Methods* 2004, 137: 321–332.

Bryce NV, Flournoy JC, Guassi Moreira JF, Rosen ML, Sambook KA, Mair P, McLaughlin KA: Brain parcellation selection: an overlooked decision point with meaningful effects on individual differences in resting-state functional connectivity. *NeuroImage* 2021, 243: 118487.

Bullmore E, Sporns O: Complex brain networks: graph theoretical analysis of structural and functional systems. *Nat Rev Neurosci* 2009, 10: 186–198.

Busch NA, Dubois J, VanRullen R: The phase of ongoing EEG oscillations predicts visual perception. *J Neurosci* 2009, 29: 7869–7876.

Canavier CC: Phase-resetting as a tool of information transmission. *Curr Opin Neurobiol* 2014, 31: 206–213.

Canolty RT, Knight RT: The functional role of cross-frequency coupling. *Trends Cogn Sci* 2010, 14: 506–515.

Cekic S, Grandjean D, Renaud O: Time, frequency, and time-varying Granger-causality measures in neuroscience. *Stat Med* 2018, 37: 1910–1931.

Chaumon M, Puce A, George N: Statistical power: implications for planning MEG studies. *NeuroImage* 2021, 233: 117894.

Chrobak JJ, Buzsaki G: Gamma oscillations in the entorhinal cortex of the freely behaving rat. *J Neurosci* 1998, 18: 388–398.

Cohen MX: Assessing transient cross-frequency coupling in EEG data. *J Neurosci Methods* 2008, 168: 494–499.

Cohen MX: *Analyzing Neural Time Series: Theory and Practice.* Cambridge, MA: MIT Press, 2014.

Cole SR, Voytek B: Brain oscillations and the importance of waveform shape. *Trends Cogn Sci* 2017, 21: 137–149.

Cole S, Voytek B: Cycle-by-cycle analysis of neural oscillations. *J Neurophysiol* 2019, 122: 849–861.

Dabek J, Kalogianni K, Rotgans E, van der Helm FC, Kwakkel G, van Wegen EE, Daffertshofer A, de Munck JC: Determination of head conductivity frequency response in vivo with optimized EIT–EEG. *NeuroImage* 2016, 127: 484–495.

Dale AM, Liu AK, Fischl BR, Buckner RL, Belliveau JW, Lewine JD, Halgren E: Dynamic statistical parametric mapping: combining fMRI and MEG for high-resolution imaging of cortical activity. *Neuron* 2000, 26: 55–67.

da Silva Castanheira J, Orozco Perez HD, Misic B, Baillet S: Brief segments of neurophysiological activity enable individual differentiation. *Nat Commun* 2021, 12: 5713.

David O, Cosmelli D, Hasboun D, Garnero L: A multitrial analysis for revealing significant corticocortical networks in magnetoencephalography and electroencephalography. *NeuroImage* 2003, 20: 186–201.

David O, Friston KJ: A neural mass model for MEG/EEG: coupling and neuronal dynamics. *NeuroImage* 2003, 20: 1743–1755.

de Reus MA, van den Heuvel MP: The parcellation-based connectome: limitations and extensions. *NeuroImage* 2013, 80: 397–404.

Eickhoff SB, Yeo BTT, Genon S: Imaging-based parcellations of the human brain. *Nat Rev Neurosci* 2018, 19: 672–686.

Faskowitz J, Esfahlani FZ, Jo Y, Sporns O, Betzel RF: Edge-centric functional network representations of human cerebral cortex reveal overlapping system-level architecture. *Nat Neurosci* 2020, 23: 1644–1654.

Friston KJ: Functional and effective connectivity: a review. *Brain Connect* 2011, 1: 13–36.

Geddes LA, Baker LE: The specific resistance of biological material—a compendium of data for the biomedical engineer and physiologist. *Med Biol Eng* 1967, 5: 271–293.

Geisler CD, Gerstein GL: The surface EEG in relation to its sources. *Electroencephalogr Clin Neurophysiol* 1961, 13: 927–934.

Gersch W, Goddard GV: Epileptic focus location: spectral analysis method. *Science* 1970, 169: 701–702.

Geweke J: Measurement of linear dependence and feedback between multiple time series. *J Am Stat Assoc* 1982, 77: 304–313.

Giard MH, Peronnet F: Auditory-visual integration during multimodal object recognition in humans: a behavioral and electrophysiological study. *J Cogn Neurosci* 1999, 11: 473–490.

Goldstein S: Phase coherence of the alpha rhythm during photic blocking. *Electroencephalogr Clin Neurophysiol* 1970, 29: 127–136.

Goncalves SI, de Munck JC, Verbunt JP, Bijma F, Heethaar RM, Lopes da Silva F: In vivo measurement of the brain and skull resistivities using an EIT-based method and realistic models for the head. *IEEE Trans Biomed Eng* 2003, 50: 754–767.

Gramfort A, Luessi M, Larson E, Engemann DA, Strohmeier D, Brodbeck C, Parkkonen L, Hämäläinen MS: MNE software for processing MEG and EEG data. *NeuroImage* 2014, 86: 446–460.

Grandchamp R, Delorme A: Single-trial normalization for event-related spectral decomposition reduces sensitivity to noisy trials. *Front Psychol* 2011, 2: 236.

Granger CWJ: Investigating causal relations by econometric models and cross-spectral methods. *Econometrica* 1969, 37: 424–438.

Grass AM, Gibbs FA: A Fourier transform of the electroencephalogram. *J Neurophysiol* 1938, 1: 521–526.

Grech R, Cassar T, Muscat J, Camilleri KP, Fabri SG, Zervakis M, Xanthopoulos P, Sakkalis V, Vanrumste B: Review on solving the inverse problem in EEG source analysis. *J Neuroeng Rehabil* 2008, 5: 25.

Groppe DM, Urbach TP, Kutas M: Mass univariate analysis of event-related brain potentials/fields: I. A critical tutorial review. *Psychophysiology* 2011, 48: 1711–1725.

Gross J: Analytical methods and experimental approaches for electrophysiological studies of brain oscillations. *J Neurosci Methods* 2014, 228: 57–66.

Gross J, Kujala J, Hämäläinen M, Timmermann L, Schnitzler A, Salmelin R: Dynamic imaging of coherent sources: studying neural interactions in the human brain. *Proc Natl Acad Sci U S A* 2001, 98: 694–699.

Guevara MA, Corsi-Cabrera M: EEG coherence or EEG correlation? *Int J Psychophysiol* 1996, 23: 145–153.

Gutierrez D, Nehorai A, Muravchik CH: Estimating brain conductivities and dipole source signals with EEG arrays. *IEEE Trans Biomed Eng* 2004, 51: 2113–2122.

Haegens S, Cousijn H, Wallis G, Harrison PJ, Nobre AC: Inter- and intra-individual variability in alpha peak frequency. *NeuroImage* 2014, 92: 46–55.

Hallez H, Vanrumste B, Grech R, Muscat J, De Clercq W, Vergult A, D'Asseler Y, Camilleri KP, Fabri SG, Van Huffel S, Lemahieu I: Review on solving the forward problem in EEG source analysis. *J Neuroeng Rehabil* 2007, 4: 46.

Hämäläinen M, Hari R: Magnetoencephalographic characterization of dynamic brain activation: basic principles, and methods of data collection and source analysis. In: Toga A, Mazziotta J, eds. *Brain Mapping: The Methods*, 2nd ed. Amsterdam: Academic Press, 2002: 227–253.

Hämäläinen M, Hari R, Ilmoniemi RJ, Knuutila JET, Lounasmaa OV: Magnetoencephalography—theory, instrumentation, and applications to noninvasive studies of the working human brain. *Rev Mod Phys* 1993, 65: 413–497.

Hämäläinen M, Ilmoniemi R: Interpreting magnetic fields of the brain: minimum norm estimates. *Med Biol Eng Comput* 1994, 32: 35–42.

Hammack B, Kranz S, Carpenter B: *Albert Michelson's Harmonic Analyzer: A Visual Tour of a Nineteenth Century Machine That Performs Fourier Analysis*. Articulate Noise Books, 2014. (See also the video by Bill Hammack showing the Harmonic Analyzer at work: https://www.youtube.com/watch?v=GyYflzRVu6M)

Hari R: The neuromagnetic method in the study of the human auditory cortex. In: Grandori F, Hoke M, Romani G, eds. *Auditory Evoked Magnetic Fields and Potentials*. Advances in Audiology, Vol 6. Basel, Switzerland: Karger, 1990: 222–282.

Hari R, Joutsiniemi SL, Sarvas J: Spatial resolution of neuromagnetic records: theoretical calculations in a spherical model. *Electroencephalogr Clin Neurophysiol* 1988, 71: 64–72.

Hari R, Salmelin R, Mäkelä JP, Salenius S, Helle M: Magnetoencephalographic cortical rhythms. *Int J Psychophysiol* 1997, 26: 51–62.

Helfrich RF, Knight RT: Cognitive neurophysiology of the prefrontal cortex. *Handb Clin Neurol* 2019, 163: 35–59.

Herrmann CS, Rach S, Vosskuhl J, Struber D: Time-frequency analysis of event-related potentials: a brief tutorial. *Brain Topogr* 2014, 27: 438–450.

Hill RM, Boto E, Rea M, Holmes N, Leggett J, Coles LA, Papastavrou M, Everton SK, Hunt BAE, Sims D, Osborne J, Shah V, Bowtell R, Brookes MJ: Multi-channel whole-head OPM-MEG: helmet design and a comparison with a conventional system. *NeuroImage* 2020, 219: 116995.

Hillebrand A, Barnes GR: A quantitative assessment of the sensitivity of whole-head MEG to activity in the adult human cortex. *NeuroImage* 2002, 16: 638–650.

Hillebrand A, Barnes GR: Beamformer analysis of MEG data. *Int Rev Neurobiol* 2005, 68: 149–171.

Holder DS: Electrical impedance tomography (EIT) of brain function. *Brain Topogr* 1992, 5: 87–93.

Hu L, Xiao P, Zhang ZG, Mouraux A, Iannetti GD: Single-trial time-frequency analysis of electrocortical signals: baseline correction and beyond. *NeuroImage* 2014, 84: 876–887.

Hutchison RM, Womelsdorf T, Allen EA, Bandettini PA, Calhoun VD, Corbetta M, Della Penna S, Duyn JH, Glover GH, Gonzalez-Castillo J, Handwerker DA, Keilholz S, Kiviniemi V, Leopold DA, de Pasquale F,

Sporns O, Walter M, Chang C: Dynamic functional connectivity: promise, issues, and interpretations. *NeuroImage* 2013, 80: 360–378.

Hyafil A, Giraud AL, Fontolan L, Gutkin B: Neural cross-frequency coupling: connecting architectures, mechanisms, and functions. *Trends Neurosci* 2015, 38: 725–740.

Ibáñez-Molina AJ, Soriano MF, Iglesias-Parro S: Mutual information of multiple rhythms for EEG signals. *Front Neurosci* 2020, 14: 574796.

Ioannides AA, Bolton JPR, Clarke CJS: Continuous probabilistic solutions to the biomagnetic inverse problem. *Inverse Probl* 1990, 6: 523–542.

Jensen O, Colgin L: Cross-frequency coupling between neuronal oscillations. *Trends Cogn Sci* 2007, 11: 267–269.

Jones SR: When brain rhythms aren't "rhythmic": implication for their mechanisms and meaning. *Current Opin Neurobiol* 2016, 40: 72–80.

Kass RE, Caffo BS, Davidian M, Meng XL, Yu B, Reid N: Ten simple rules for effective statistical practice. *PLoS Comput Biol* 2016, 12: e1004961.

Khanna A, Pascual-Leone A, Michel CM, Farzan F: Microstates in resting-state EEG: current status and future directions. *Neurosci Biobehav Rev* 2015, 49: 105–113.

Kiebel SJ, Garrido MI, Moran RJ, Friston KJ: Dynamic causal modelling for EEG and MEG. *Cogn Neurodyn* 2008, 2: 121–136.

Kim JA, Davis KD: Magnetoencephalography: physics, techniques, and applications in the basic and clinical neurosciences. *J Neurophysiol* 2021, 125: 938–956.

Lachaux JP, Lutz A, Rudrauf D, Cosmelli D, Le Van Quyen M, Martinerie J, Varela F: Estimating the time-course of coherence between single-trial brain signals: an introduction to wavelet coherence. *Neurophysiol Clin* 2002, 32: 157–174.

Lai Y, van Drongelen W, Ding L, Hecox KE, Towle VL, Frim DM, He B: Estimation of in vivo human brain-to-skull conductivity ratio from simultaneous extra- and intra-cranial electrical potential recordings. *Clin Neurophysiol* 2005, 116: 456–465.

Lehmann D: Multichannel topography of human alpha EEG fields. *Electroencephalogr Clin Neurophysiol* 1971, 31: 439–449.

Lehmann D, Ozaki H, Pal I: EEG alpha map series: brain micro-states by space-oriented adaptive segmentation. *Electroencephalogr Clin Neurophysiol* 1987, 67: 271–288.

Lehmann D, Skrandies W: Reference-free identification of components of checkerboard-evoked multi-channel potential fields. *Electroencephalogr Clin Neurophysiol* 1980, 48: 609–621.

Le Van Quyen M, Bragin A: Analysis of dynamic brain oscillations: methodological advances. *Trends Neurosci* 2007, 30: 365–373.

Lindner M, Vicente R, Priesemann V, Wibral M: TRENTOOL: a Matlab open source toolbox to analyse information flow in time series data with transfer entropy. *BMC Neurosci* 2011, 12: 119.

Lisman JE, Idiart MA: Storage of 7 ± 2 short-term memories in oscillatory subcycles. *Science* 1995, 267: 1512–1515.

Lisman JE, Jensen O: The theta-gamma neural code. *Neuron* 2013, 77: 1002–1016.

Litvak V, Mattout J, Kiebel S, Phillips C, Henson R, Kilner J, Barnes G, Oostenveld R, Daunizeau J, Flandin G, Penny W, Friston K: EEG and MEG data analysis in SPM8. *Comput Intell Neurosci* 2011, 2011: 852961.

Lobier M, Siebenhühner F, Palva S, Palva JM: Phase transfer entropy: a novel phase-based measure for directed connectivity in networks coupled by oscillatory interactions. *NeuroImage* 2014, 85: 853–872.

Lopes da Silva FH: Event-related neural activities: what about phase? *Prog Brain Res* 2006, 159: 3–17.

Lopes da Silva F: EEG and MEG: relevance to neuroscience. *Neuron* 2013, 80: 1112–1128.

Lopes da Silva FH, Vos JE, Mooibroek J, Van Rotterdam A: Relative contributions of intracortical and thalamo-cortical processes in the generation of alpha rhythms, revealed by partial coherence analysis. *Electroencephalogr Clin Neurophysiol* 1980, 50: 449–456.

Lüdtke N, Logothetis NK, Panzeri P: Testing methodologies for the nonlinear analysis of causal relationships in neurovascular coupling. *Magn Reson Imaging* 2010, 28: 1113–1119.

Mandke K, Meier J, Brookes MJ, O'Dea RD, Van Mieghem P, Stam CJ, Hillebrand A, Tewarie P: Comparing multilayer brain networks between groups: introducing graph metrics and recommendations. *NeuroImage* 2018, 166: 371–384.

Maris E, Oostenveld R: Nonparametric statistical testing of EEG- and MEG-data. *J Neurosci Methods* 2007, 164: 177–190.

Markov NT, Ercsey-Ravasz M, Lamy C, Ribeiro Gomes AR, Magrou L, Misery P, Giroud P, Barone P, Dehay C, Toroczkai Z, Knoblauch K, Van Essen DC, Kennedy H: The role of long-range connections on the specificity of the macaque interareal cortical network. *Proc Natl Acad Sci U S A* 2013, 110: 5187–5192.

Martin CG, He BJ, Chang C: State-related neural influences on fMRI connectivity estimation. *NeuroImage* 2021, 244: 118590.

McCann H, Pisano G, Beltrachini L. Variation in reported human head tissue electrical conductivity values. *Brain Topogr* 2019, 32: 825–858.

Meir-Hasson Y, Kinreich S, Podlipsky I, Hendler T, Intrator N: An EEG finger-print of fMRI deep regional activation. *NeuroImage* 2014, 102(Pt 1):128–141.

Meyer SS, Bonaiuto J, Lim M, Rossiter H, Waters S, Bradbury D, Bestmann S, Brookes M, Callaghan MF, Weiskopf N, Barnes GR: Flexible head-casts for high spatial precision MEG. *J Neurosci Methods* 2017, 276: 38–45.

Michel CM, Koenig T: EEG microstates as a tool for studying the temporal dynamics of whole-brain neuronal networks: a review. *NeuroImage* 2018, 180: 577–593.

Montalto A, Faes L, Marinazzo D: MuTE: a MATLAB toolbox to compare established and novel estimators of the multivariate transfer entropy. *PLoS One* 2014, 9: e109462.

Morales S, Bowers ME: Time-frequency analysis methods and their application in developmental EEG data. *Dev Cogn Neurosci* 2022, 54: 101067.

Murakami S, Okada Y: Invariance in current dipole moment density across brain structures and species: physiological constraint for neuroimaging. *NeuroImage* 2015, 111: 49–58.

Murray MM, Brunet D, Michel CM: Topographic ERP analyses: a step-by-step tutorial review. *Brain Topogr* 2008, 20: 249–264.

Nolte G, Bai O, Wheaton L, Mari Z, Vorbach S, Hallett M: Identifying true brain interaction from EEG data using the imaginary part of coherency. *Clin Neurophysiol* 2004, 115: 2292–2307.

Nolte G, Ziehe A, Nikulin VV, Schlögl A, Krämer N, Brismar T, Müller K-R: Robustly estimating the flow direction of information in complex physical systems. *Phys Rev Lett* 2008, 100: 234101.

Nunez PL, Srinivasan R, Westdorp AF, Wijesinghe RS, Tucker DM, Silberstein RB, Cadusch PJ: EEG coherency: I. Statistics, reference electrode, volume conduction, Laplacians, cortical imaging, and interpretation at multiple scales. *Electroencephalogr Clin Neurophysiol* 1997, 103: 499–515.

Nunez PL, Wingeier BM, Silberstein RB: Spatial-temporal structures of human alpha rhythms: theory, microcurrent sources, multiscale measurements, and global binding of local networks. *Hum Brain Mapp* 2001, 13: 125–164.

O'Neill GC, Tewarie P, Vidaurre D, Liuzzi L, Woolrich MW, Brookes MJ: Dynamics of large-scale electrophysiological networks: A technical review. *NeuroImage* 2018, 180: 559–576.

Oostendorp TF, Delbeke J, Stegeman DF: The conductivity of the human skull: results of in vivo and in vitro measurements. *IEEE Trans Biomed Eng* 2000, 47: 1487–1492.

Paluš M: Detecting phase synchronization in noisy systems. *Phys Lett A* 1997, 235: 341–351.

Palva JM, Wang SH, Palva S, Zhigalov A, Monto S, Brookes MJ, Schoffelen JM, Jerbi K: Ghost interactions in MEG/EEG source space: a note of caution on inter-areal coupling measures. *NeuroImage* 2018, 173: 632–643.

Pascual-Marqui RD: Standardized low-resolution brain electromagnetic tomography (sLORETA): technical details. *Methods Find Exp Clin Pharmacol* 2002, 24(Suppl D): 5–12.

Pernet C, Garrido MI, Gramfort A, Maurits N, Michel CM, Pang E, Salmelin R, Schoffelen JM, Valdés-Sosa PA, Puce A: Issues and recommendations from the OHBM COBIDAS MEEG Committee for Reproducible EEG and MEG Research. *Nat Neurosci* 2020, 23: 1473–1483.

Pernet CR, Chauveau N, Gaspar C, Rousselet GA: LIMO EEG: a toolbox for hierarchical LInear MOdeling of ElectroEncephaloGraphic data. *Comput Intell Neurosci* 2011, 2011: 831409.

Pfurtscheller G, Lopes da Silva FH: Event-related EEG/MEG synchronization and desynchronization: basic principles. *Clin Neurophysiol* 1999, 110: 1842–1857.

Pourtois G, Delplanque S, Michel C, Vuilleumier P: Beyond conventional event-related brain potential (ERP): exploring the time-course of visual emotion processing using topographic and principal component analyses. *Brain Topogr* 2008, 20: 265–277.

Purdon PL, Sampson A, Pavone KJ, Brown EN: Clinical electroencephalography for anesthesiologists: Part I: Background and basic signatures. *Anesthesiology* 2015, 123: 937–960.

Rosen BQ, Halgren E: A whole-cortex probabilistic diffusion tractography connectome. *eNeuro* 2021, 8: ENEURO.0416-20.2020.

Rubinov M, Sporns O: Complex network measures of brain connectivity: uses and interpretations. *NeuroImage* 2010, 52: 1059–1069.

Rush S, Driscoll DA: Current distribution in the brain from surface electrodes. *Anesth Analg* 1968, 47: 717–723.

Sadaghiani S, Scheeringa R, Lehongre K, Morillon B, Giraud AL, D'Esposito M, Kleinschmidt A: Alpha-band phase synchrony is related to activity in the fronto-parietal adaptive control network. *J Neurosci* 2012, 32: 14305–14310.

Sadaghiani S, Wirsich J: Intrinsic connectome organization across temporal scales: new insights from cross-modal approaches. *Netw Neurosci* 2020, 4: 1–29.

Salmelin R, Hari R: Spatiotemporal characteristics of sensorimotor neuromagnetic rhythms related to thumb movement. *Neuroscience* 1994, 60: 537–550.

Samar VJ: Wavelet analysis of neuroelectric waveforms. *Brain Lang* 1999, 66: 1–6.

Sameshima K, Baccalá LA: Using partial directed coherence to describe neuronal ensemble interactions. *J Neurosci Methods* 1999, 94: 93–103.

Sanchez Bornot JM, Wong-Lin KF, Ahmad AL, Prasad G: Robust EEG/MEG based functional connectivity with the envelope of the imaginary coherence: sensor space analysis. *Brain Topogr* 2018, 31: 895–916.

Sauseng P, Klimesch W, Gruber WR, Hanslmayr S, Freunberger R, Doppelmayr M: Are event-related potential components generated by phase resetting of brain oscillations? A critical discussion. *Neuroscience* 2007, 146: 1435–1444.

Sayers BM, Beagley HA, Henshall WR: The mechanism of auditory evoked EEG responses. *Nature* 1974, 247: 481–483.

Schaworonkow N, Nikulin VV: Is sensor space analysis good enough? Spatial patterns as a tool for assessing spatial mixing of EEG/MEG rhythms. *NeuroImage* 2022, 253: 119093.

Scherg M: Fundamentals of dipole source analysis. In: Grandori F, Hoke M, Romani GL, eds. *Auditory Evoked Magnetic Fields and Electric Potentials*. Advances in Audiology Series, Vol. 6. Basel, Switzerland: Karger, 1990: 40–69.

Schrader S, Westhoff A, Piastra MC, Miinalainen T, Pursiainen S, Vorwerk J, Brinck H, Wolters CH, Engwer C: DUNEuro—a software toolbox for forward modeling in bioelectromagnetism. *PLoS One* 2021, 16: e0252431.

Schreiber T: Measuring information transfer. *Phys Rev Lett* 2000, 85: 461–464.

Schroeder CE, Tenke CE, Givre SJ, Arezzo JC, Vaughan HG Jr: Laminar analysis of bicuculline-induced epileptiform activity in area 17 of the awake macaque. *Brain Res* 1990, 515: 326–330.

Shah AS, Bressler SL, Knuth KH, Ding M, Mehta AD, Ulbert I, Schroeder CE: Neural dynamics and the fundamental mechanisms of event-related brain potentials. *Cereb Cortex* 2004, 14: 476–483.

Shannon CE: A mathematical theory of communication. *Bell Syst Tech J* 1948, 27: 379–423.

Siegel M, Donner TH, Engel AK: Spectral fingerprints of large-scale neuronal interactions. *Nat Rev Neurosci* 2012, 13: 121–134.

Singer W: Neuronal synchrony: a versatile code for the definition of relations? *Neuron* 1999, 24: 49–65.

Slepian, D: Prolate spheroidal wave functions, Fourier analysis, and uncertainty–V: the discrete case. *Bell Syst Tech J* 1978, S7: 1371–1430.

Sporns O: *Networks of the Brain*. Cambridge, MA: MIT Press, 2010.

Stam CJ, Nolte G, Daffertshofer A: Phase lag index: assessment of functional connectivity from multi channel EEG and MEG with diminished bias from common sources. *Hum Brain Mapp* 2007, 28: 1178–1193.

Tallon-Baudry C, Bertrand O, Delpuech C, Pernier J: Stimulus specificity of phase-locked and non-phase-locked 40 Hz visual responses in human. *J Neurosci* 1996, 16: 4240–4249.

Tenke CE, Kayser J: Generator localization by current source density (CSD): implications of volume conduction and field closure at intracranial and scalp resolutions. *Clin Neurophysiol* 2012, 123: 2328–2345.

Tesche CD: Non-invasive imaging of neuronal population dynamics in human thalamus. *Brain Res* 1996, 729: 253–258.

Tesche CD: Non-invasive detection of ongoing neuronal population activity in normal human hippocampus. *Brain Res* 1997, 749: 53–60.

Thatcher RW: Coherence, phase differences, phase shift, and phase lock in EEG/ERP analyses. *Dev Neuropsychol* 2012, 37: 476–496.

Tort AB, Komorowski R, Eichenbaum H, Kopell N: Measuring phase-amplitude coupling between neuronal oscillations of different frequencies. *J Neurophysiol* 2010, 104: 1195–1210.

Tottene A, Urbani A, Pietrobon D: Role of different voltage-gated Ca^{2+} channels in cortical spreading depression: specific requirement of P/Q-type Ca^{2+} channels. *Channels (Austin)* 2011, 5: 110–114.

Tuomisto T, Hari R, Katila T, Poutanen T, Varpula T: Studies of auditory evoked magnetic and electric responses: modality specificity and modelling. *Il Nuovo Cimento* 1983, 2D: 471–494.

Uutela K, Taulu S, Hämäläinen M: Detecting and correcting for head movements in neuromagnetic measurements. *NeuroImage* 2001, 14: 1424–1431.

van Ede F, Quinn AJ, Woolrich MW, Nobre AC: Neural oscillations: sustained rhythms or transient burst-events? *Trends Neurosci* 2018, 41: 415–417.

Van Veen BD, Buckley KM: Beamforming: a versatile approach to spatial filtering. *IEEE ASSP Magazine* 1988, 5: 4–24.

Vicente R, Wibral M, Lindner M, Pipa G: Transfer entropy-a model-free measure of effective connectivity for the neurosciences. *J Comput Neurosci* 2011, 30: 45–67.

Vinck M, Oostenveld R, van Wingerden M, Battaglia F, Pennartz CM: An improved index of phase-synchronization for electrophysiological data in the presence of volume-conduction, noise and sample-size bias. *NeuroImage* 2011, 55: 1548–1565.

Vvedensky V, Hari R, Ilmoniemi R, Reinikainen K: Physical basis of neuromagnetic fields. *Biophysics* 1985, 30: 154–158.

Wacker M, Witte H: Time-frequency techniques in biomedical signal analysis: a tutorial review of similarities and differences. *Methods Inf Med* 2013, 52: 279–296.

Wibral M, Rahm B, Rieder M, Lindner M, Vicente R, Kaiser J: Transfer entropy in magnetoencephalographic data: quantifying information flow in cortical and cerebellar networks. *Prog Biophys Mol Biol* 2011, 105: 80–97.

Widrow B, Stearns SD: *Beamformers With Superresolution: Adaptive Signal Processing*. Upper Saddle River, NJ: Prentice Hall, 1985.

Wiener N: The theory of prediction. In: Beckenbach EF, ed. *Modern Mathematics for the Engineer: First Series*. Originally published by New York: McGraw-Hill, 1956. Reprinted in its entirety by Dover Publications Inc., Mineola, NY, 2013 [pp 165–190].

Wilmer A, de Lussanet M, Lappe M: Time-delayed mutual information of the phase as a measure of functional connectivity. *PLoS One* 2012, 7: e44633.

Zetter R, Iivanainen J, Parkkonen L: Optical co-registration of MRI and on-scalp MEG. *Sci Rep* 2019, 9: 5490.

Zich C, Quinn AJ, Mardell LC, Ward NS, Bestmann S: Dissecting transient burst events. *Trends Cogn Sci* 2020, 24: 784–788.

SECTION 3

CHAPTER 11

BRAIN RHYTHMS

Rhythm is something you either have or don't have, but when you have it, you have it all over.

—ELVIS PRESLEY

There is music wherever there is rhythm, as there is life wherever there beats a pulse.

—IGOR STRAVINSKY

■ INTRODUCTION

In this section of the book, we provide examples of MEG and EEG studies to illustrate the wide spectrum of possibilities for investigating the neurodynamics of human brain function. Instead of providing a comprehensive coverage of the existing literature, we present examples of various spontaneous, evoked (including event-related) and induced MEG/ EEG signals that importantly have increased our understanding of the human brain's sensory, motor, cognitive, and affective functions. We have leaned considerably toward our own studies and experiences, given that we are more aware of their pitfalls and challenges and hopefully can provide the reader with better educational insights with these examples.

We want to repeatedly emphasize that the major contribution of MEG and EEG recordings is in the accurate timing information they provide. Although it is also important to know from which brain region the signals arise, at some stages the focus on source locations has gone too far. For example, MEG has been referred to as "magnetic source imaging," although the main contribution definitely is the accurate timing information, given that such information cannot be obtained by fMRI or PET. Consequently, a lot of effort has been put into minor improvements of the source models for both MEG and EEG, although it is difficult to know how accurate the results are because the correct source locations are in most cases unknown.

Converging evidence related to source locations needs to be obtained from different avenues, including patient studies of the effects of well-defined lesions of the supposed source areas, electric and magnetic stimulation of these same regions in healthy volunteers, and by comparing the results with intracranial recordings obtained from both humans and nonhuman primates.

The human brain is a rich repository of multiple neurophysiological rhythms that occur spontaneously in the ongoing MEG/EEG, are elicited or dampened by sensory stimuli, or are associated with motor events or with cognitive or affective processing. Somewhat surprisingly, the frequencies of brain rhythms are preserved across a large variety of mammals in whom the brain volumes vary by a factor of 17,000, ranging from the mouse to the elephant (Buzsáki et al., 2013) (see Figure 11.1). One likely reason for this similarity of frequencies, independent of the animal's size, may be related to intrinsic biophysical properties of neurons and microcircuits that generate the rhythms and impose the temporal limits for synchrony depending, for example, on the timing between pre- and postsynaptic firing. Another intriguing constraint comes from the mechanics of the skeletal muscles where the properties of myosin and actin filaments—that define muscle contraction speed—have remained largely similar across mammals (Buzsáki et al., 2013). It therefore seems that the body with its direct interactions with the world primarily dictates some fundamental aspects of timing in our brains (Hari & Parkkonen, 2015).

Here we briefly overview rhythmic MEG and EEG activity in the frequency bands that were introduced in Chapter 4. The dominant frequencies have been traditionally calculated from interpeak intervals of successive deflections in the filtered data (in the past, special rulers existed for this purpose) and today more conveniently from frequency spectra or wavelet analyses. The width of the spectral peak provides information about the consistency of the frequency, because the peaks broaden if the main frequency fluctuates, for example if the subject becomes drowsy.

The reactivity of different brain rhythms is of interest in many studies and can be quantified by monitoring changes in the amplitude or power of the specific rhythm (see Chapter 10 for analysis methods common to both MEG and EEG). It is also possible to average either the original rhythms or their envelopes (i.e., time-varying peak or root-mean-square values) of signal amplitude or power, with respect to external stimuli or internal cues. Naturally, if the brain rhythm is not exactly phase-locked to the stimulus, it disappears during averaging of the original signals, similarly as happened to the induced brain rhythms in Figure 10.1. Notably, averaging the envelopes always results in positive nonzero values that do not depend on the phase of the rhythm.

If the averaged activity triggered by the stimulus can be subtracted from the overall MEG/EEG signal, it leaves behind the *induced* activity that is modified by the stimulus or task but is not exactly time-locked to these events (see Chapter 10 and Figure 10.1). Unaveraged (single-trial) MEG/EEG data, which include both evoked responses and rhythmic activity, can be nowadays effectively analyzed, as we demonstrate in this and later chapters.

Whereas stimulus-locked evoked responses typically concentrate within a time window of less than a second, cortical rhythms can be modulated over periods of several seconds or even minutes (Ramkumar et al., 2012), showing stimulus- and task-related suppressions ("desynchronizations") and enhancements ("synchronizations") as we discussed in Chapter 10.

■ ALPHA RHYTHM OF THE POSTERIOR CORTEX

The classical EEG alpha rhythm as defined by Hans Berger and by Lord Adrian (see Chapter 4 and Figure 4.1) typically refers to sinusoidal oscillations at around 10 Hz (range 8–13 Hz, 50–100 μV) in the human posterior cortex. As we noted earlier, the terms *alpha rhythm* and *alpha activity* have often been used more generically, causing some confusion in the literature. The classical posterior alpha rhythm has a strong relationship to visual input so that eye opening in healthy, sighted subjects suppresses the rhythm (Figure 11.2). However, prominent alpha activity can appear even when the eyes are open if the visual

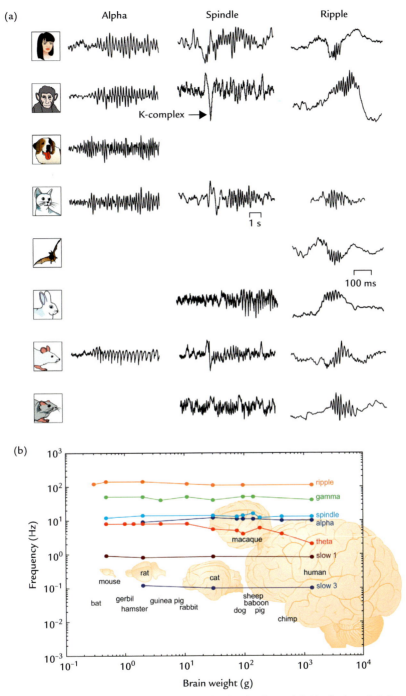

FIGURE 11.1. **Across-species preservation of brain rhythms.** (a) Similarity of alpha oscillations, sleep spindles, and hippocampal ripples in different mammals ranging from humans to rodents. (b) Brain-rhythm frequency stays relatively constant as a function of brain weight (in grams) across several orders of magnitude for different mammals. Note the log–log scale. Reprinted from Buzsáki G, Logothetis N, Singer W: Scaling brain size, keeping timing: evolutionary preservation of brain rhythms. *Neuron* 2013, 80: 751–764. With permission from Elsevier.

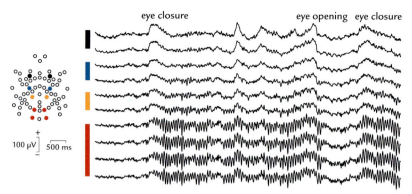

FIGURE 11.2. **Alpha reactivity.** A 5-s EEG epoch from a subject who initially had his eyes open; signals are shown from ten selected derivations from a 64-channel EEG data set. Eye closure is indicated by the prominent slow artifact in the frontal channels (black and blue circles on electrode map and black and blue bars next to EEG traces), after which rhythmic alpha appears on the posterior scalp (red circles on electrode map and red bar next to EEG traces). The alpha terminates on eye opening and restarts once the eyes are closed again. Eye movements also occur during eye closure (as shown by the frontal channels). Data recorded in the Dual EEG Laboratory, Imaging Research Facility, Indiana University, USA.

input is monotonous or the subject is in darkness or is myopic and is not using normal visual correction. These features are consistent with the original idea of the posterior alpha rhythm reflecting a type of "resting state" in the visual system.

Poor reactivity of the posterior alpha to eye opening versus closing may be a sign of a diffuse brain disorder. In adult subjects, the peak of the alpha frequency can vary by 1 to 2 Hz during various tasks with different cognitive load and also during serial recordings (Oken & Chiappa, 1988; Haegens et al., 2014).

Alpha rhythm typically responds strongly to visual stimulation. Figure 11.3 (left panel) demonstrates EEG from a subject with very persistent posterior alpha rhythm seen even when her eyes are open. The rhythm is briefly suppressed following the onset of a visual stimulus (a face presented for 500 ms) but has already started to return prior to the delivery of the next stimulus. Activity of selected single trials (left panel) and all trials in the experiment (right panel) show that the alpha suppression is consistent during a long recording session comprising more than 900 stimulus presentations.

The traces in Figure 11.4 depict amplitude envelopes (levels of instantaneous amplitude) of 9 to 13-Hz MEG activity of a single subject passively viewing black-and-white drawings of everyday objects (left panel) and naming them covertly (middle panel) or overtly (right panel). The recordings are from planar gradiometers that react most strongly to neural events just under the sensor (see Figure 5.15). During passive viewing, the stimuli elicited clear suppression in the occipital cortex (as seen by the steep decrease in the signal from sensor 1). This effect was strengthened during covert and especially overt naming in the same location: the occipital suppression lasted much longer and was also associated with enhancement–suppression sequences in frontal and central (sensorimotor) areas (sites 2–5) (Salmelin et al., 1994). These findings are consistent with the view that alpha-band suppressions in task-related active brain regions can be associated with alpha-band enhancements in nontask-related brain regions (Pfurtscheller & Lopes da Silva, 1999; Knyazev et al., 2011).

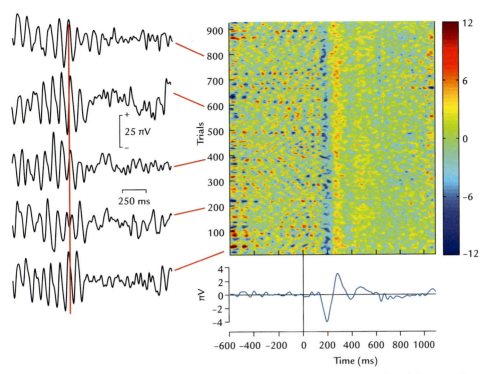

FIGURE 11.3. Alpha suppression. Several 1700-ms EEG epochs are displayed from an electrode on the posterior occipitotemporal scalp during visual stimulation. Left: The selected epochs show rhythmic alpha. During the 600-ms pre-stimulus period (stimulus delivery indicated by the red vertical line), alpha is prominent but is suppressed about 100 ms after stimulus delivery and returns at the end of the epoch. Right: The top plot shows activity from all trials of the recording session time-locked to stimulus presentation at time zero; the color bar at right indicates amplitude in microvolts. Alpha and its suppression time-locked to the stimulus are seen throughout the entire recording session. The plot at bottom right shows averaged activity, with a clear visual evoked response, with the first prominent deflection peaking around 200 ms. This response can also be clearly seen in the single trials in the plot at top right. Because stimulus presentation was deliberately randomized so as not to lock with alpha phase, the prominent prestimulus alpha has cancelled out in the averaged signal. Data recorded in the Social Neuroscience Laboratory, Indiana University, USA.

The characteristics of the posterior alpha rhythm change across the lifespan. In infants as young as three or four months, a reactive posterior rhythm occurs at around 4 Hz, and its mean frequency increases to about 6 Hz at 12 months of age and to about 8 Hz at 36 months; by 6 to 12 years it can reach adult alpha frequencies of 10 Hz, with considerable interindividual differences (for a review, see Riviello et al., 2011). Given these large developmental changes in the posterior rhythm, labels such as "theta" or "alpha" may be a source of confusion in this literature. It is thus necessary to document, in addition to the main frequencies and their topographies, the age of the subjects to make clear what exactly is being studied. In healthy senescence, the frequency of the posterior alpha rhythm tends to slightly decrease.

Already over half a century ago, intracranial EEG recordings from implanted depth electrodes showed that multiple distinct sites produce alpha-like oscillations in the posterior

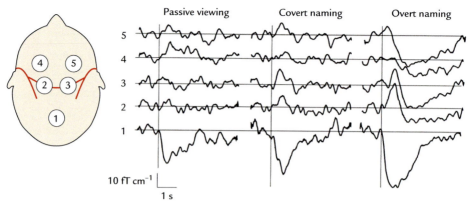

FIGURE 11.4. Changes of MEG alpha level of a single subject during picture viewing. The traces show amplitude envelopes (levels) of 9 to 13 Hz MEG signals as a function of time, recorded by planar gradiometers at the indicated five locations. Amplitude is given in units of fT/cm. The subject was either passively viewing (left panel) black-and-white line drawings of everyday objects presented for 100 ms once every 5 s or naming them covertly (middle panel) or overtly (right panel). About 100 single traces were first filtered digitally from 9 to 13 Hz and their amplitude envelopes were averaged. Reprinted by permission from Salmelin R, Hari R, Lounasmaa OV, Sams M: Dynamics of brain activation during picture naming. *Nature* 1994, 368: 463–465. Copyright Macmillan Publishers Ltd.

cortex (Perez-Borja et al., 1962). According to MEG recordings, the sources of posterior ~10 Hz alpha oscillations are concentrated predominantly in the parieto-occipital and calcarine sulci. These two posterior alpha subclusters differ in their current orientations, with stronger activity in the parieto-occipital than the calcarine cluster (Hari et al., 1997). Even within these subclusters, several sources with independent temporal behaviors are active simultaneously (Lü et al., 1992; Salmelin & Hari, 1994a), supporting the idea of a multitude of neuronal sources of the posterior alpha rhythm.

We still know remarkably little about the role and generator mechanisms of different EEG/MEG rhythms (Cohen, 2017). Several views have been presented about the functional significance of alpha-band activity (for reviews, see Palva & Palva, 2007; Klimesch, 2012; Bazanova & Vernon, 2014). Adrian and Matthews (1934) originally proposed that alpha activity is a cortical idling rhythm, but this idea has been repeatedly challenged in favor of functional roles related to information coding, the support and modulation of attentional states, and facilitation of communication between different neuronal populations (for a didactic review, see Lopes da Silva, 2013). Specifically, inhibition at specific phases of alpha oscillations has been suggested as a timing mechanism for pulsed information transfer (Jensen & Mazaheri, 2010; Klimesch, 2012).

A very interesting role for alpha (and beta) frequencies was recently suggested on the basis of lamina-specific recordings of spikes and field potentials in monkey cortex while the monkeys were evaluating the predictability of visual stimuli. In the framework of predictive coding (see Chapter 18), a "predictive routing" model was proposed to account for the findings (Bastos et al., 2020): low-frequency alpha and beta could prepare cortical areas for processing predicted inputs by inhibiting stimulus-elicited gamma rhythms and spiking. Consequently, unpredicted stimuli might be associated with less alpha and beta rhythmicity and more gamma rhythms and spikes. Clearly, much further work needs to be performed to clarify the range of potential functional roles between these slower modulatory rhythms and gamma activity.

■ MU RHYTHM OF THE SENSORIMOTOR CORTEX

We have already mentioned the Rolandic arc-shaped mu rhythm and shown its frequency spectra (see Chapter 4 and Figures 4.2 and 4.3). MEG and EEG recordings agree with the pioneering intracranial recordings of Jasper and Penfield (1949), showing that the mu rhythm has at least two frequency components, one around 10 Hz and the other around 20 Hz; however, these two components are not exact harmonics and often show different time courses (Tiihonen et al., 1989). Henry Gastaut originally named the rhythm *mu* to refer to the motor system as he observed it in scalp EEG over the motor cortex (Gastaut, 1952). In MEG recordings, mu seems to predominantly originate from areas close to the hand primary sensorimotor cortex (Tiihonen et al., 1989), which may be related to the large representation of the hand in the sensorimotor homunculus. Interestingly, the sources of the 20-Hz mu component tend to be *anterior* (with respect to the course of the central sulcus) to those of the 10 Hz component (Figure 11.5), suggesting that they receive contributions from the precentral motor cortex (Salmelin & Hari, 1994b); see also source clusters in Figure 17.3 (lower panel).

During voluntary movements, the Rolandic mu rhythm is first suppressed (depending on the movements, this suppression can start even 0.5–2 s prior to the movement). Following movement completion, mu rhythm phasically increases, forming "rebounds" that typically peak about 0.5 s after a transient movement. For the 20-Hz component, the rebounds follow the somatotopic organization of body parts along the precentral gyrus, shifting from the most medial position for foot movements via the hand area to the most lateral location for mouth movements, in good agreement with sites of somatosensory responses to stimulation of the same body parts (Salmelin et al., 1995). In contrast, the sources of the 10-Hz component remained clustered close to the hand region, regardless of the body part moved. The 10- and 20-Hz components of the mu rhythm thus apparently reflect, at least in part, activity of separate functional networks: the 10-Hz rhythm is predominantly somatosensory, and the 20-Hz rhythm mainly reflects motor function.

Mu can often be seen as waxing and waning local activity over the sensorimotor scalp in resting subjects (see Figure 4.2). In traditional clinical EEG recordings, mu rhythm was visible only in a minority (from 5 to 15%) of all recordings, and it was often considered to be pathological (Fisch, 1999; Riviello et al., 2011). The likelihood of EEG mu detection has been increased with the use of spectral analysis with motor tasks that enhance mu reactivity and the use of high-density EEG arrays.

As we discuss in Chapter 17, the 20-Hz component of the mu rhythm during isometric contractions is synchronous with surface EMG from the contracted muscle.

■ TAU RHYTHM OF THE AUDITORY CORTEX

An alpha-like rhythm, 8 to 10 Hz *tau* has been observed in MEG recordings (see Figure 11.6), with neural sources located in the supratemporal auditory cortex (Tiihonen et al., 1991; Lehtelä et al., 1997; Weisz et al., 2011). Thus tau is best visualized in planar-gradiometer MEG recordings just over the auditory cortices (Tiihonen et al., 1991; Lehtelä et al., 1997). Tau is suppressed by sounds but unaffected by eye opening/closing, which clearly differentiates it from the parieto-occipital alpha (see the frequency spectrum in Figure 11.6). These findings would agree with the idea that tau rhythm is a resting rhythm specific to the auditory cortex.

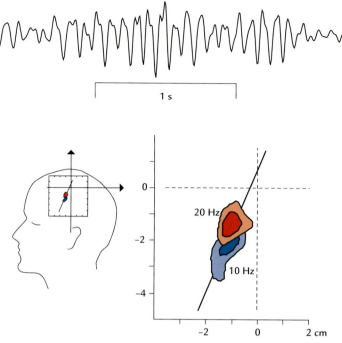

FIGURE 11.5. Sources of the Rolandic mu rhythm. Top: An MEG trace recorded with a planar gradiometer over the sensorimotor cortex shows clear arch-shaped mu rhythm over a 2.5 s interval (the same trace is also depicted on the cover of this book). Bottom: Isodensity maps of the locations of equivalent current dipoles used to model the ~10-Hz (blue) and ~20-Hz (red) components of the mu rhythm; the maps are superimposed on the left sensorimotor cortex of the schematic head on the left. Both contour maps are based on about 5,000 single dipoles that were found during the rebounds that followed self-paced movements of the right thumb, performed once every 5 s. The expansion of the same figure at right shows that the two components of mu do not share a common location. The sources of the 10-Hz component are located slightly more lateral and posterior with respect to the sources of the 20-Hz component; the line approximates the course of the central sulcus. Adapted and reprinted from Salmelin R, Hari R: Spatiotemporal characteristics of sensorimotor neuromagnetic rhythms related to thumb movement. *Neuroscience* 1994, 60: 537–550. With permission from Elsevier.

Tau is best seen when the subject is drowsy and when the parieto-occipital alpha has already slightly decreased or disorganized (as described later in this chapter, tau would likely be seen during sleep stage 1a). Figure 11.7 shows this phenomenon schematically. During the awake state (Figure 11.7, top panel), the sources giving rise to occipital alpha are much stronger than the sources for tau, whereas during drowsiness the situation is reversed (Figure 11.7, bottom). Thus the strongest 10-Hz-range activity is seen in the frontocentral midline as could be expected from the respective orientations of these two sources (Hari, 2011). It is interesting to note that an "alpha shift" from posterior to anterior EEG scalp has been suggested as an EEG indicator of decreased vigilance (Bente, 1964). These findings agree with the phenomenon as such but also provide information about the generator mechanisms. We need not necessarily propose any "spread" or "traveling" of alpha activity,

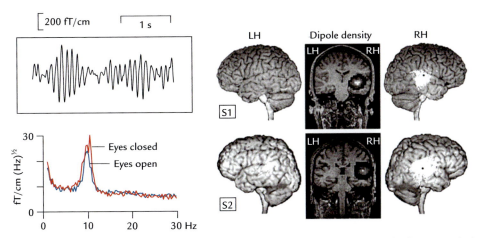

FIGURE 11.6. Tau rhythm and its sources. Left top: An example of tau rhythm recorded with planar MEG sensors over the right Sylvian fissure. Left bottom: Frequency spectrum of the tau rhythm in a single person, showing a clear peak at about 10 Hz and no effect of eye opening/closing. Adapted and reprinted from Tiihonen J, Hari R, Kajola M, Karhu J, Ahlfors S, Tissari S: Magnetoencephalographic 10-Hz rhythm from the human auditory cortex. *Neurosci Lett* 1991, 129: 303–305. With permission from Elsevier. Right: Source locations of 6.5 to 9.5 Hz spontaneous oscillations for two subjects (one in each row), projected onto surfaces and coronal sections of individual brains. The black dots visible on the right hemisphere (RH) in the middle of the clusters of white dots (each indicating the site of one current dipole) are source locations for N100m to sound onsets. The dipole densities (coronal sections in the middle) are presented as contour plots, where the highest dipole densities are displayed in white and the lowest in black. LH refers to the left hemisphere and RH to the right. Adapted and reprinted from Lehtelä L, Salmelin R, Hari R: Evidence for reactive magnetic 10-Hz rhythm in the human auditory cortex. *Neurosci Lett* 1997, 222: 111–114. With permission from Elsevier.

because the changed anteroposterior topography of the EEG oscillations can be explained by the changed relative strengths of the parieto-occipital "alpha" and temporal-lobe "tau" sources.

The existence of *several rhythms with partially overlapping frequencies in the alpha range* (see also Weisz et al., 2011) emphasizes the importance of testing the reactivity of these multiple brain rhythms so that (each) observed rhythm can be characterized correctly in terms of its frequency, topography, generation site, and reactivity. This thorough scrutiny should also be performed for investigations and claims relating to traveling waves of alpha activity.

■ BETA RHYTHMS

We first make a distinction between beta rhythms that are regular oscillations often around 20 Hz and beta activity that can be less rhythmic and incorporates a broader range of frequencies between 14 and 30 Hz and is present during attentive wakeful behavior. Notably, there is considerable evidence for the existence of multiple beta rhythms (for a review, see Cannon et al., 2014) that vary by both frequency and generation site. Some investigators use 40 Hz as the upper limit of the beta range (see Chapter 4), which can create some

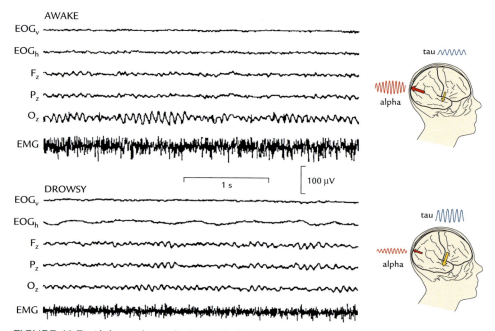

FIGURE 11.7. Alpha and tau during wakefulness and drowsiness. Left panels: Expanded EEG segments from three midline locations and submental EMG recorded from a subject who was awake (top) and drowsy (bottom); the traces are extracted from Figure 11.11 ("drowsy" refers to sleep stage 1a). Right: Schematic presentation of EEG changes in midline sites when the subject is awake (top) and parieto-occipital alpha is the dominant source, and when the subject is drowsy (bottom) when alpha sources have diminished and tau sources are dominant. See the text for further explanation. Adapted and reprinted from Hari R: Magnetoencephalography: methods and applications. In: Schomer DL, Lopes da Silva FH, eds. *Niedermeyer's Electroencephalography: Basic Principles, Clinical Applications, and Related Fields*, 6ᵗʰ ed. Philadelphia, PA: Lippincott Williams & Wilkins, 2011: 865–900.

confusion as to what is considered beta versus gamma activity. Consistent with existing best-practice guidelines, we advocate the use of 30 Hz as the demarcation point between beta and gamma so that 40-Hz rhythms, which may show individual variations in peak frequency, can all be included in the gamma range (see Babiloni et al., 2020; Pernet et al., 2020). Of course, it is again better to indicate the exact frequency of the activity of interest, rather than label it only as beta or gamma.

In the clinical EEG sphere, rhythmic beta is best known as *drug beta* or *benzo buzz*, which arises from the administration of benzodiazepines and is clearly identifiable in the anterior scalp (see frontal channels in Figure 20.1). The likely reason for this distribution is that the main sources are located in the fissural portion of the primary motor cortex (Jensen et al., 2005). Rhythmic beta-range activity also exists in the Rolandic cortex as a part of the mu rhythm (as we have already discussed) as well as in other parts of the sensorimotor system, for example in the basal ganglia and thalamus, supplementary motor cortex, and cerebellum.

Invasive recordings in humans have shown functional coupling (increased coherence) between the primary sensorimotor cortex (S1 and M1, and the mu rhythm therein) and the supplementary motor area (SMA) during voluntary movements: almost 1 s prior to the movement, coherence in beta activity started to increase between SMA and S1–M1 (across a frequency range of 0–33 Hz) and peaked 0.3 s after the movement (Ohara et al., 2001).

Invasive recordings in monkeys have shown that maintained motor contractions require directed beta activity *from* primary somatosensory cortex *to* both motor cortex and inferior posterior parietal cortex, suggesting that synchronized beta oscillations can bind activity within multiple parts of the sensorimotor system (Brovelli et al., 2004). The synchronized beta activity extends beyond the cerebral cortex. For example, beta (and alpha) range activity in human thalamus (in nucleus ventralis intermedius) was coherent with pathological hand tremor at 3 to 6 Hz and/or with EMG frequencies of 8 to 27 Hz (Marsden et al., 2000). Additionally, as we discuss in Chapter 17, beta-range activity in the motor cortex is coherent with that in the spinal motoneuron pool and with activity in distal and proximal muscles (for reviews, see Salenius & Hari, 2003; Baker, 2007).

The collective work has led to the idea that beta oscillations function to maintain the status quo in certain brain areas, especially in the sensorimotor system, to support motor control and cognition (Engel & Fries, 2010). In the motor cortex, this interpretation would be in line with the original association of the Rolandic mu rhythm to immobility (Gastaut, 1952). It should be noted that inhibition is extremely important in the motor system for the selection of the most suitable movement given the presence of many possibilities ("motor equivalence").

■ THETA RHYTHMS

Theta rhythms are 4 to 7.5 Hz oscillations (although some investigators draw the line at 8 Hz) that can be related to drowsiness and sleep, brain pathology, cognitive operations, and hedonic functions (in infants). Predominant activity in the theta range is normal in certain stages of development (Riviello et al., 2011). Much animal work has been related to theta rhythms in hippocampus and the relationship of theta to higher frequencies. The proposed cognitive functions of theta include encoding and retrieval of spatial information from episodic memory (Hasselmo & Stern, 2014) and the maintenance of working memory (Hsieh & Ranganath, 2014). Given that gamma activity is often strongest at the peak of the local theta cycle, theta has been proposed to enable the effective "packaging" of information (Colgin, 2013) by gating of signal transfer (Raghavachari et al., 2001; Lisman & Jensen, 2013), thereby facilitating communication and functional coupling across cortical regions segregated by distance (Colgin, 2013; Cavanagh & Frank, 2014).

Theta-band oscillations around 4–8 Hz, matching syllabic rate, also occur during processing of heard speech (Peelle & Davis, 2012, 2013; Bourguignon et al., 2013); these frequencies are also visible in the acoustic envelope of natural speech (Chandrasekaran et al., 2009; Elliott & Theunissen, 2009).

■ GAMMA RHYTHMS

Considerable variability exists in how the higher frequency EEG/MEG bands are defined. Some authors consider the gamma band to be expanded up to 600 Hz and to include functionally different sub-bands, such as a low-gamma band from 30 to 60 Hz, a high-gamma band from 60 to 200 Hz (including "ripples" at 100–200 Hz), and an ultrafast band from 200 to 600 Hz (Uhlhaas et al., 2011). The leftmost panel of Figure 11.8 depicts these different subtypes of gamma, and the rightmost panels display examples of "narrowband" and "broadband" gamma activity.

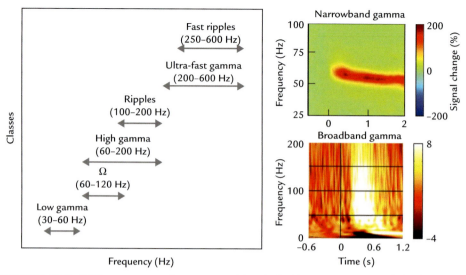

FIGURE 11.8. Different types of gamma activity. Left: Frequency spans of six classes of gamma activity. Note that scalp EEG will typically detect only the lower frequency classes of gamma, whereas MEG and electrocorticography recordings can detect the faster activity. Adapted and reprinted from Uhlhaas PJ, Pipa G, Neuenschwander S, Wibral M, Singer W: A new look at gamma? High- (> 60 Hz) gamma-band activity in cortical networks: function, mechanisms and impairment. *Prog Biophys Mol Biol* 2011, 105: 14–28. With permission from Elsevier. Right top: An example of narrowband MEG gamma activity (red stripe) in response to an inwardly moving circular sinusoidal grating presented at time zero. Vertical color scale shows percentage signal change of gamma activity. Modified and reprinted from van Pelt S, Boomsma DI, Fries P: Magnetoencephalography in twins reveals a strong genetic determination of the peak frequency of visually induced gamma-band synchronization. *J Neurosci* 2012, 32: 3388–3392. Right bottom: Broadband gamma activity recorded between two intracranial EEG electrodes in parietal cortex to the presentation of a Mooney face stimulus at time zero. The color scale depicts normalized amplitude (relative to pre-stimulus baseline). Adapted and reprinted from Lachaux JP, George N, Tallon-Baudry C, Martinerie J, Hugueville L, Minotti L, Kahane P, Renault B: The many faces of the gamma band response to complex visual stimuli. *NeuroImage* 2005, 25: 491–501. With permission from Elsevier.

Compared with invasive intracranial EEG recordings that show both local and global gamma-range activity (for a review, see Buzsaki & Wang, 2012), fast and ultrafast gamma rhythms—which can receive contributions from action potential spikes as well (Arnulfo et al., 2020)—are greatly attenuated in human scalp EEG recordings. The reasons for this attenuation include potential distortions by the skull and scalp (Srinivasan et al., 1996) but also the possibility of very local and nondipolar source configurations (Tallon-Baudry et al., 1999). According to intracranial animal work, multiple types of gamma rhythms can co-exist or occur in isolation (for a review, see Buzsaki & Wang, 2012).

The quite well-known 40-Hz rhythm (Gray et al., 1989) appears to be a special case of activity in the gamma range. It is the omnipresence of this frequency band that has likely resulted in misinterpretations that steady-state MEG/EEG evoked responses in both auditory and visual modalities (see Chapters 13 and 14) would show "resonances" at stimulation rates of about 40 Hz. In physics, a resonance means a tendency of the system to react with larger amplitude to a specific (stimulation) frequency. In the brain, however, the clear enhancement of the steady-state responses at stimulation frequencies of about 40 Hz results from the overlap of successive evoked response deflections at these specific stimulation rates, whereas the single responses are actually *not* enhanced at 40 Hz, although the steady-state response is (see Figure 13.7 and Figure 14.11 and the related discussions in Chapters 13 and 14). However, the enhancement of the steady-state response at about 40 Hz indicates that responses to individual stimuli contain 40-Hz frequencies that then superimpose just at this stimulation rate.

Increases and modulations of 30- to 100-Hz gamma activity have been reported during various motor, perceptual, and cognitive tasks, including attention-dependent signal selection, feature binding, multisensory integration, sensorimotor coordination, manipulation of contents of working memory, and the formation of long-term memories (for reviews, see Fries et al., 2007; Herrmann et al., 2010; Whittington et al., 2011; Sedley & Cunningham, 2013). Based on the behavioral and neurophysiological findings, gamma oscillations have therefore been suggested to have either facilitatory or inhibitory roles in perception and cognition. Given these complex findings, a set of models consistent with the different possible roles for gamma have been proposed to provide a basis for future experiments. Sedley and Cunningham (2013) proposed that gamma activity (supported by brain circuitry displayed in Figure 11.9, panel a), can be locally generated without input from other cortical regions and is fed forward to other brain regions (panel b). Alternatively, (either top-down or bottom-up) cortical inputs—both increased and decreased—can generate local gamma activity, which can be excitatory (panel c), or inhibitory (panel d).

■ DELTA-BAND ACTIVITY AND ULTRA-SLOW OSCILLATIONS

When recorded with "normal" clinical filter settings (0.3–70 Hz), delta-band activity (< 3.5 Hz) occurs in healthy adults only during deep sleep. Instead, an awake person's delta-range activity is considered a sign of brain pathology, related, for example, to stroke, brain trauma, or serious brain infection, such as encephalitis. In these disorders, delta is often asymmetric across the hemispheres.

Ultra-slow (or infraslow) fluctuations (i.e., activity < 1 Hz or as low as 0.1 Hz) were originally described in rabbit motor and visual cortices in the form of rhythmic activity around 0.1 Hz and below 0.03 Hz (Aladjalova, 1957). Ultra-slow EEG rhythms have been described in humans during sleep (Achermann & Borbely, 1997) but also in awake subjects performing a somatosensory detection task, leading the authors to suggest that these slow fluctuations reflect changes in the excitability of cortical networks and thereby affect an awake subject's ability to detect stimuli (Monto et al., 2008). Invasive recordings in humans have also shown ultra-slow activity in the thalamus (Hughes et al., 2011). This type of slow activity is currently of much interest because its time course is in the same range as that of fMRI-signal fluctuations (Damoiseaux et al., 2006).

Ultra-slow fluctuations can be recorded only when the amplifiers have long time constants or are DC-coupled. Note, however, that such recordings are extremely prone to various artifacts arising from movements, electrode polarization, and more (see also Figure 5.4 and related text on full-band EEG recordings in Chapter 5). Therefore, delta-band activity must be first definitively dissociated from artifacts related to eye movements, respiration, and voluntary actions. Ideally these bodily signals should be monitored while performing an MEG/EEG study.

Note that epileptic discharges can be associated with changes in DC level that are filtered out in a typical clinical recording.

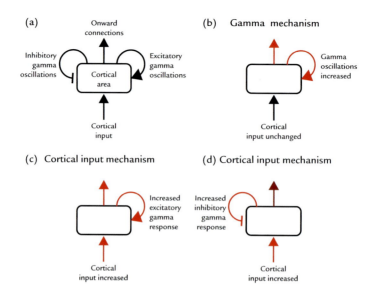

FIGURE 11.9. Different models for generation of gamma activity. (a) A schematic depicts a cortical area with inhibitory (left) or excitatory (right) feedback connections within itself as well as possible input from, and output to, other brain regions. (b) The cortical area can *increase* (indicated by red lines) gamma-band activity locally and send the output to other brain regions without requiring external input from other brain regions. (c) Increased cortical input can increase local excitatory gamma activity in the cortical area that sends output onto other brain regions. (d) Increased cortical input can increase local inhibitory gamma in the cortical area as it sends output to other brain regions. In all cases (b) through (d), the gamma activity has increased equally, but it will produce different effects locally as well as at the output region. Reproduced with permission from Sedley W, Cunningham MO: Do cortical gamma oscillations promote or suppress perception? An under-asked question with an over-assumed answer. *Front Hum Neurosci* 2013, 7: 595.

■ COUPLING BETWEEN DIFFERENT BRAIN RHYTHMS

During tasks and rest, different brain rhythms can interact by exhibiting cross-frequency coupling where modulations of the faster rhythms are typically coupled to the slower rhythm, and theta–gamma and alpha–gamma interactions are commonly observed (see Chapter 10). A number of reviews describe, discuss, and debate the various types of interactions between brain rhythms (Canolty & Knight, 2010; Aru et al., 2015; Hyafil et al., 2015).

It has been proposed that narrowband gamma activity (see Figure 11.8) elicited by visual stimuli would provide feedforward signals (originating from superficial cortical layers and targeting layer 4), whereas alpha- and beta-band rhythms would function as feedback signals (Michalareas et al., 2016). Information transfer and timing of activity would be accomplished by the coupling of alpha activity to gamma and theta activity to gamma (Lisman & Jensen, 2013). Overall, gamma activity displays complex interactions with other brain rhythms, which likely produces coupled activity across brain networks. These types of interactions are likely to be at the root of multilayered resting-state network behavior both in hemodynamic and neurophysiological studies (Mantini et al., 2007; Engel et al., 2013; Singer, 2013).

▪ CHANGES IN BRAIN RHYTHMS DURING SLEEP

As an individual becomes drowsy and eventually falls asleep, her or his MEG/EEG undergoes a series of predictable changes (Loomis et al., 1935a, 1935b) that correlate with known sleep stages (Dement & Kleitman, 1957a). These well-described stages are used in sleep laboratories around the world to study individuals with sleep disorders (Chang et al., 2011).

During a normal night's sleep, an individual will transition through four to five sleep cycles, each including nonrapid-eye-movement (NREM) sleep (stages 1–4) followed by a period of rapid-eye-movement (REM) sleep. Each cycle typically lasts around 90 min, although REM periods become relatively longer and periods of slow wave NREM sleep become shorter through the night. An average adult spends about 75% of total sleep time in NREM sleep and 25% in REM (Fisch, 1999). In contrast, infants can spend up to 50% of their time in REM sleep, and this proportion gradually decreases with development until it, at around two years of age, stabilizes at the same level as that of an adult (Riviello et al., 2011).

MEG and EEG records show typical features during different stages of vigilance and sleep (Lu et al., 1992), illustrated for one subject in Figure 11.10. MEG was recorded with planar gradiometers over the right temporal lobe and EEG from a few midline channels; EOG and submental EMG signals are shown as well. As the subject drowses (Stage 1a), the 10-Hz posterior alpha activity is first more prominent than during the awake stage, and as the subject moves toward falling asleep, the occipital alpha starts to become disorganized. At the same time, the MEG sensors over the temporal lobe show accentuated tau rhythm. "Sharp waves" in EEG (also called vertex waves or vertex sharp transients) appear prominently at the vertex—indicating Stage 1b light sleep.

K-complexes are the hallmarks of Stage 2 sleep. In EEG recordings, K-complexes have a diffuse scalp distribution, with a clear vertex maximum, thereby resembling both vertex sharp waves (mentioned above) and evoked vertex potentials to abrupt sounds (see Chapter 13). In contrast, early MEG recordings indicated multiple local sources for the K-complexes (Numminen et al., 1996). However, source analysis of MEG or scalp EEG has not succeeded in identifying the exact brain sources *that seem to be* generating the K-complexes (Wennberg & Cheyne, 2013). *Consistent with these observations, in intracranial recordings* the sources of K-complexes appear to be widely distributed. Likely sources include bilateral mesial and deep brain areas, which therefore likely result in considerable cancellation of MEG signals. (For a similar cancellation for sources in the mesial foot area preceding simultaneous movements of both feet, see Chapter 17.) A recent MEG study has proposed the generators of K-complexes involve the anterior cingulate cortex as a part of the brain's saliency network (Ioannides et al., 2019).

Stage 2 sleep also exhibits sleep spindles that in the EEG are typically seen over the (fronto)central scalp. Spindles can occur either in isolation or in association with K-complexes, typically occurring immediately after them. These spindle-shaped waxing-and-waning 0.5- to 3-s bursts of rhythmic 11–16 Hz activity are triggered by the bursting of thalamocortical neurons (Schönauer & Pölchen, 2018). The inhibitory nature of sleep spindles is implied from observations that they dampen processing of sounds (Dang-Vu et al., 2011). Accordingly, GABA-ergic drugs can enhance the occurrence of spindles.

Classically, a distinction has been made between anterior slower and posterior faster spindles, which could reflect two different generators. However, recent intracranial recordings indicated that the frequency variation can be large in both anterior and posterior spindles (Gonzalez et al., 2022).

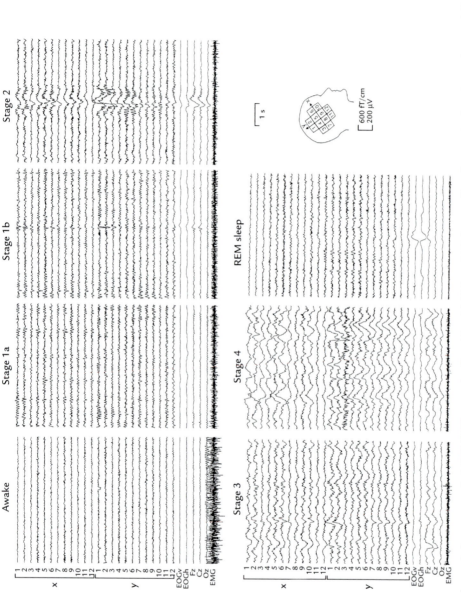

FIGURE 11.10. Awake and sleep stages in MEG/EEG records. Combined MEG and EEG recording from a single subject during different stages of sleep. The MEG was recorded with a 24-channel planar gradiometer placed over the lateral side of the right hemisphere (schematic head). The two signals obtained from the two orthogonal gradiometer channels at each sensor location are plotted separately (12 uppermost traces along the x direction and 12 subsequent traces in the y direction; for coordinate axes, see the schematic head). The next two traces show vertical (EOGv) and horizontal (EOGh) electro-oculograms, and the next three traces are scalp EEG signals recorded from occipital (Oz), central (Cz), and frontal (Fz) midline. The lowest trace depicts surface EMG from submental muscles located under the chin. Vertical calibration bars reflect MEG and EEG signal strengths in fT/cm and µV, respectively. For further details, see text. Adapted and reprinted from Lu S-T, Kajola M, Joutsiniemi S-L, Knuutila J, Hari R: Generator sites of spontaneous MEG activity during sleep. *Electroencephalogr Clin Neurophysiol* 1992, 82: 182–196. With permission from Elsevier.

Interestingly, the spindle density (number of spindles per unit time during NREM sleep) correlates with the consolidation of both declarative and procedural (motor) memories (Marshall et al., 2020; Lutz et al., 2021). Sleep spindles can be related to the strengthening of synaptic connections (Schönauer & Pölchen, 2018), and they could reflect brain activity underlying reorganization of short-term hippocampus-related memories to long-term distributed cortical memories that are not hippocampus dependent (Marshall et al., 2020). The MEG/EEG community could pay more attention to sleep spindles and potentially contribute to research related to general learning abilities as well as memory consolidation in memory disorders, including early Alzheimer's disease (Weng et al., 2020).

As sleep deepens, MEG/EEG signals show strong slowing, with delta activity becoming more prominent. In Stage 3 sleep, 20% to 50% of the activity is in the delta range, and the proportion of delta increases to greater than 50% in Stage 4 sleep. For this reason, deep sleep is often called *slow-wave sleep*, which is in stark contrast to the so-called *paradoxical sleep* or REM sleep that displays general flattening with faster activity as well as characteristic eye movements (Aserinsky & Kleitman, 1953; Dement & Kleitman, 1957b). Dreaming occurs predominantly during REM sleep.

Various sleep disorders, resulting in excessive daytime sleepiness, affect 0.05% to 5% of the U.S. population at any given time (Sleepiness, 1997). Sleep deprivation disrupts normal sleep cycles or "sleep architecture" and it is often used as an "activation procedure" for clinical EEG studies to provoke epileptic discharges that can identify the type of seizure disorder or even signal a possible epileptic focus (see Chapter 20 for seizure disorders).

Sleep apnea, where frequent arousal occurs during the night because of periods of obstructed breathing, affects an estimated 4% and 2%, respectively, of middle-aged men and women in the United States (National Heart, Lung, and Blood Institute, 1995). Polygraphic recordings typically include EEG, EOG, a respiration belt, and oxygen saturation monitoring (see Figure 11.11) and are used to identify the disrupted sleep architecture and the type of sleep disorder. Additional EMG electrodes are placed most commonly on submental muscles (under the chin), so that the loss of muscular tonus during REM sleep can be easily detected. Analysis of EEG and accompanying EOG and EMG data allows the sleep cycles in that individual to be documented and hopefully the sleep disorder to be diagnosed. Routine polygraphic sleep studies are classical examples of recording "embodied" brain activity. They continue to provide a rich information source related to an individual's state of consciousness and awareness.

Figure 11.11 presents a demonstrative example of a polygraphic recording of a 58-year-old man who was studied due to persistent insomnia, snoring, and difficulties in staying asleep (see the figure legend for the description of each trace in the record). The EEG changes reflect transitions from deeper sleep stages to a more shallow one—as also indicated by the arousal marker (green line above the sixth trace). The polygraphic recording documented a serious obstructive sleep apnea, with the turquoise-shaded boxes showing periods of abnormally shallow breathing (hypopnea). A second bout of hypopnea is followed by awakening, as shown by muscle artifacts in EEG traces and increased activity in the EMG trace. (This individual had 52 hypopneic or apneic—cessation of breathing—events per hour, where the upper limit of normal is 4.)

Polygraphy can also be diagnostic for other sleep disorders, such as narcolepsy or cataplexy. In narcolepsy, an individual can suddenly enter REM sleep while awake, and in cataplexy, muscle tone is paroxysmally lost during strong emotions, such as anger, or happiness involving laughter, so that the individual may drop to the ground. Narcoleptic subjects

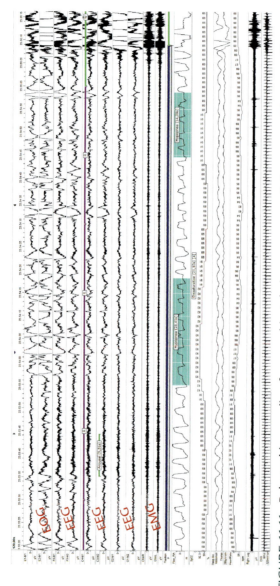

FIGURE 11.11. Polygraphic recording from a subject during assessment of sleep apnea. The traces (from top to bottom) depict two EOG channels, six EEG channels, two submental EMG channels, patient position, nasal respiratory flow, oxygen saturation (with a pulse oximeter on a fingertip), two channels of activity from respiration belts, surface EMG from the right leg (m. tibialis), and ECG. Sleep stages have been scored in 30-s epochs (starting from left). One spontaneous arousal interval is marked (see the purple marker line above fifth trace, and the arousal marker with green line above the sixth trace), and it is followed by decreased respiratory flow (hypopnea), which results in 4%-unit oxygen desaturation. Hypopnea is indicated by the turquoise shading on the respiration trace. The latter period of hypopnea does not decrease the oxygen saturation, but in the right end of the traces the patient wakes up—as is indicated by the "fuzziness" in the EEG and MEG traces resulting from the increased muscle activity—likely because of the hypopnea. Courtesy of Anniina Alakuijala, Department of Clinical Neurophysiology, Helsinki University Hospital, Finland.

easily fall asleep as the EEG electrodes are being placed for the clinical EEG recording, but after these naps they can stay awake for the actual study, which thus may be turn out to be nondiagnostic.

■ EFFECTS OF ANESTHETICS AND OTHER DRUGS ON EEG/MEG

In 1847 John Snow described changes in consciousness and bodily function during ether anesthesia (Snow, 1847). Ninety years later, Guedel (1937) published a now-classic volume that systematically described respiratory, muscular, and autonomic signs of progressively deeper anesthesia to inhaling ether, from induction and maintenance of general anesthesia to anesthetic overdose. EEG has been looked to for monitoring anesthetic depth since the early days (Gibbs et al., 1937), and noninvasive human EEG recordings were first performed in the operating room over 75 years ago (Brazier & Finesigner, 1945).

The major problem in interpreting EEG changes during increasingly deeper anesthesia is that different anesthetic agents produce markedly different electrophysiological signatures (Sloan, 1998; Purdon et al., 2015). Additional variability occurs because the anesthetized person is typically administered a combination of drugs: analgesics to prevent pain, relaxants to prevent muscle contraction, and anesthetic(s) to abolish sensation and induce unconsciousness. The routine clinical use of mixtures of agents, as well as the nonspecificity of EEG changes for any agent, have made it difficult to provide a generalized measure of anesthetic depth, although multiple depth-of-anesthesia monitors and algorithms are available (Roche & Mahon, 2021). Nonspecificity of electrophysiological changes regarding the inducing pharmacological agent are problematic also for various psychedelics, despite the rapidly growing literature and interest in this area. In addition to other effects in brain and body, for example in the cardiovascular and sensorimotor systems, psychedelics can modify brain connectivity (Barnett et al., 2020). In the future, improved analysis methods might open interesting new windows to these altered states of consciousness and their neurobiological basis.

In general, EEG activity slows down, and evoked responses diminish and become delayed as the anesthetic depth increases to surgical levels. However, during the induction of anesthesia, the EEG can indicate arousal—known as *paradoxical excitation*—with low-voltage beta activity being the dominant signal. In contrast, the phenomenon of burst suppression can be seen during profound surgical anesthesia and consists of periods of effectively no discernable activity interspersed with high-amplitude mixed-frequency activity. An MEG example of burst suppression is shown in Figure 11.12 in an enflurane-anesthetized dog (Jäntti et al., 1995); the study was primarily carried out to demonstrate that nonphysiological artifact-free MEG activity can be recorded during artificial ventilation.

Still to this day we are missing a reliable *generalizable* neurophysiological means (spontaneous EEG or evoked responses) by which to assess anesthetic depth (Bruhn et al., 2006; Mashour et al., 2011; Escallier et al., 2014). Commercial devices are available for intraoperative monitoring of anesthesia depth, based on, for example, spectral information and entropy measures of scalp EEG, and in part EMG (Rampil, 1998; Maksimow et al., 2005; Purdon et al., 2015). However, these measures can provide discrepant results, and therefore even for research purposes the raw EEG signals should be recorded and analyzed by a neurophysiological expert (Aho et al., 2015).

Middle-latency auditory-evoked potentials (see Chapter 13) have also been previously used for monitoring anesthesia depth, but validation of methods should still be improved (Bruhn et al., 2006).

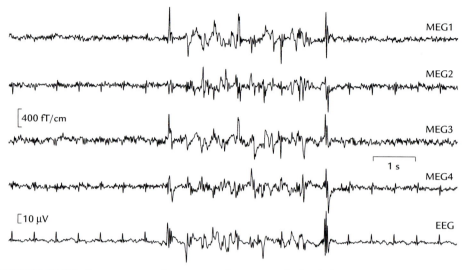

MEG1

MEG2

400 fT/cm

MEG3

1 s

MEG4

10 µV

EEG

FIGURE 11.12. **Burst–suppression pattern in an anesthetized dog.** An enflurane-induced MEG and EEG burst suppression pattern in a beagle. The recording was made with a 122-channel planar MEG sensor helmet, but signals are shown only from four posterior channels; here MEG1 and MEG2 (and MEG3 and MEG4) are orthogonal gradients recorded with a single sensor unit housing two orthogonal figure-of-eight flux transformers. EEG was recorded with two Ag/AgCl disk electrodes between the top of the dog's head and the left ear. A cardiac artifact can be seen in both MEG and EEG recordings. The recording shows one burst (center of traces) in the middle of two periods of suppression (flat signals at the start and end of the traces). Despite the very small (3 × 4 × 5 cm²) brain of the dog, the MEG signals are large—about the same size as typical epileptic discharges. The filter settings were 0.05 to 100 Hz for MEG and 0.3 to 100 Hz for EEG, and the data were digitized at 300 Hz. Adapted and reprinted from Jäntti V, Baer G, Yli-Hankala A, Hämäläinen M, Hari R: MEG burst suppression in an anaesthetized dog. *Acta Anaesthesiol Scand* 1995, 39: 126–128. With permission from John Wiley & Sons.

In Chapters 5 and 7 we discussed the challenges to measuring EEG and evoked responses in the operating room in the presence of various sources of artifacts from power-line and monitoring equipment. During neurosurgery, electrode placement itself may not be optimal due to spatial constraints imposed by the craniotomy site. Additionally, it may be impossible to reach the electrodes during the surgery, for example to add conductive gel, as the patient may be lying on them and everything is also covered by a sterile drape.

As drugs of many types affect MEG and EEG, healthy subjects should refrain from ingesting "uppers" or "downers" (stimulants or sedatives) in the 24-hour period preceding the MEG/EEG recording. A number of drugs and pharmacological agents, for example tobacco (Conrin, 1980), caffeine (Barry et al., 2005), and cocaine (Reid et al., 2008) can affect the EEG/MEG records. However, most of these effects are nonspecific, changing the EEG/MEG signals—spectral, amplitude, and latency measures—via changes of alertness. However, benzodiazepines are known to elicit "drug beta" (see the previous section on beta rhythms), which is rhythmic activity characteristically seen in the EEG over precentral/frontal sites (see Figure 20.1 for an example).

■ REFERENCES

Achermann P, Borbely AA: Low-frequency (< 1 Hz) oscillations in the human sleep electroencephalogram. *Neuroscience* 1997, 81: 213–222.

Adrian ED, Matthews BHC: The Berger rhythm: potential changes from the occipital lobes in man. *Brain* 1934, 57: 355–384.

Aho AJ, Kamata K, Jäntti V, Kulkas A, Hagihira S, Huhtala H, Yli-Hankala A: Comparison of Bispectral Index and Entropy values with electroencephalogram during surgical anaesthesia with sevoflurane. *Br J Anaesth* 2015, 115: 258–266.

Aladjalova NA: Infra-slow rhythmic oscillations of the steady potential of the cerebral cortex. *Nature* 1957, 179: 957–959.

Arnulfo G, Wang SH, Myrov V, Toselli B, Hirvonen J, Fato MM, Nobili L, Cardinale F, Rubino A, Zhigalov A, Palva S, Palva JM: Long-range phase synchronization of high-frequency oscillations in human cortex. *Nat Commun* 2020, 11: 5363.

Aru J, Aru J, Priesemann V, Wibral M, Lana L, Pipa G, Singer W, Vicente R: Untangling cross-frequency coupling in neuroscience. *Curr Opin Neurobiol* 2015, 31: 51–61.

Aserinsky E, Kleitman N: Regularly occurring periods of eye motility, and concomitant phenomena, during sleep. *Science* 1953, 118: 273–274.

Babiloni C, Barry RJ, Basar E, Blinowska KJ, Cichocki A, Drinkenburg W, Klimesch W, Knight RT, Lopes da Silva F, Nunez P, Oostenveld R, Jeong J, Pascual-Marqui R, Valdés-Sosa P, Hallett M: International Federation of Clinical Neurophysiology (IFCN)—EEG research workgroup: recommendations on frequency and topographic analysis of resting state EEG rhythms. Part 1: Applications in clinical research studies. *Clin Neurophysiol* 2020, 131: 285–307.

Baker SN: Oscillatory interactions between sensorimotor cortex and the periphery. *Curr Opin Neurobiol* 2007, 17: 649–655.

Barnett L, Muthukumaraswamy SD, Carhart-Harris RL, Seth AK: Decreased directed functional connectivity in the psychedelic state. *NeuroImage* 2020, 209: 116462.

Barry RJ, Rushby JA, Wallace MJ, Clarke AR, Johnstone SJ, Zlojutro I: Caffeine effects on resting-state arousal. *Clin Neurophysiol* 2005, 116: 2693–2700.

Bastos AM, Lundqvist M, Waite AS, Kopell N, Miller EK: Layer and rhythm specificity for predictive routing. *Proc Natl Acad Sci USA* 2020, 117: 31459–31469.

Bazanova OM, Vernon D: Interpreting EEG alpha activity. *Neurosci Biobehav Rev* 2014, 44: 94–110.

Bente D: *Die Insuffizienz des Vigilitätstonus.* Habilitationsschrift (postdoctoral thesis). University of Erlangen-Nürnberg, 1964.

Bourguignon M, De Tiège X, Op de Beeck M, Ligot N, Paquier P, Van Bogaert P, Goldman S, Hari R, Jousmäki V: The pace of prosodic phrasing couples the reader's voice to the listener's cortex. *Hum Brain Mapp* 2013, 34: 314–326.

Brazier MA, Finesinger JE: Action of barbiturates on the cerebral cortex: electroencephalographic studies. *Arch Neurol Psychiatr* 1945, 53: 51–58.

Brovelli A, Ding M, Ledberg A, Chen Y, Nakamura R, Bressler SL: Beta oscillations in a large-scale sensorimotor cortical network: directional influences revealed by Granger causality. *Proc Natl Acad Sci U S A* 2004, 101: 9849–9854.

Bruhn J, Myles PS, Sneyd R, Struys MM: Depth of anaesthesia monitoring: what's available, what's validated and what's next? *Br J Anaesth* 2006, 97: 85–94.

Buzsáki G, Logothetis N, Singer W: Scaling brain size, keeping timing: evolutionary preservation of brain rhythms. *Neuron* 2013, 80: 751–764.

Buzsáki G, Wang XJ: Mechanisms of gamma oscillations. *Annu Rev Neurosci* 2012, 35: 203–225.

Cannon J, McCarthy MM, Lee S, Lee J, Borgers C, Whittington MA, Kopell N: Neurosystems: brain rhythms and cognitive processing. *Eur J Neurosci* 2014, 39: 705–719.

Canolty RT, Knight RT: The functional role of cross-frequency coupling. *Trends Cogn Sci* 2010, 14: 506–515.

Cavanagh JF, Frank MJ: Frontal theta as a mechanism for cognitive control. *Trends Cogn Sci* 2014, 18: 414–421.

Chandrasekaran C, Trubanova A, Stillittano S, Caplier A, Ghazanfar AA: The natural statistics of audiovisual speech. *PLoS Comput Biol* 2009, 5: e1000436.

Chang BS, Schomer DL, Niedermeyer E: Normal EEG and sleep: Adults and elderly. In: Schomer DL, Lopes da Silva FH, eds. *Niedermeyer's Electroencephalography: Basic Principles, Clinical Applications, and Related Fields*. Philadelphia, PA: Lippincott Williams & Wilkins, 2011: 183–214.

Cohen MX: Where does EEG come from and what does it mean? *Trends Neurosci* 2017, 40: 208–218.

Colgin LL: Mechanisms and functions of theta rhythms. *Annu Rev Neurosci* 2013, 36: 295–312.

Conrin J: The EEG effects of tobacco smoking—a review. *Clin Electroencephalogr* 1980, 11: 180–187.

Damoiseaux JS, Rombouts SA, Barkhof F, Scheltens P, Stam CJ, Smith SM, Beckmann CF: Consistent resting-state networks across healthy subjects. *Proc Natl Acad Sci U S A* 2006, 103: 13848–13853.

Dang-Vu TT, Bonjean M, Schabus M, Boly M, Darsaud A, Desseilles M, Degueldre C, Balteau E, Phillips C, Luxen A, Sejnowski TJ, Maquet P: Interplay between spontaneous and induced brain activity during human non-rapid eye movement sleep. *Proc Natl Acad Sci U S A* 2011, 108: 15438–15443.

Dement W, Kleitman N: Cyclic variations in EEG during sleep and their relation to eye movements, body motility, and dreaming. *Electroencephalogr Clin Neurophysiol* 1957a, 9: 673–690.

Dement W, Kleitman N: The relation of eye movements during sleep to dream activity: an objective method for the study of dreaming. *J Exp Psychol* 1957b, 53: 339–346.

Elliott TM, Theunissen FE: The modulation transfer function for speech intelligibility. *PLoS Comput Biol* 2009, 5: e1000302.

Engel AK, Fries P: Beta-band oscillations—signalling the status quo? *Curr Opin Neurobiol* 2010, 20: 156–165.

Engel AK, Gerloff C, Hilgetag CC, Nolte G: Intrinsic coupling modes: multiscale interactions in ongoing brain activity. *Neuron* 2013, 80: 867–886.

Escallier KE, Nadelson MR, Zhou D, Avidan MS: Monitoring the brain: processed electroencephalogram and peri-operative outcomes. *Anaesthesia* 2014, 69: 899–910.

Fisch B: *Fisch and Spehlmann's EEG Primer*, 3rd ed. Amsterdam: Elsevier, 1999.

Fries P, Nikolic D, Singer W: The gamma cycle. *Trends Neurosci* 2007, 30: 309–316.

Gastaut H: Etude électrocorticographique de la réactivité des rythmes rolandiques. [Electrocorticographic study of the reactivity of rolandic rhythms]. *Rev Neurologique (Paris)* 1952, 87: 176–182.

Gibbs FA, Gibbs EL, Lennox WG: Effect on the electro-encephalogram of certain drugs which influence nervous activity. *Arch Int Med* 1937, 60: 154–166.

Gonzalez C, Jiang X, Gonzalez-Martinez J, Halgren E: Human spindle variability. *J Neurosci* 2022, 42: 4517–4537.

Gray CM, König P, Engel AK, Singer W: Oscillatory responses in cat visual cortex exhibit inter-columnar synchronization which reflects global stimulus properties. *Nature* 1989, 338: 334–337.

Guedel AE: *Inhalational Anaesthesia: A Fundamental Guide*. New York: Macmillan, 1937.

Haegens S, Cousijn H, Wallis G, Harrison PJ, Nobre AC: Inter- and intra-individual variability in alpha peak frequency. *NeuroImage* 2014, 92: 46–55.

Hari R: Magnetoencephalography: methods and applications. In: Schomer DL, Lopes da Silva FH, eds. *Niedermeyer's Electroencephalography: Basic Principles, Clinical Applications, and Related Fields*, 6th ed. Philadelphia, PA: Lippincott Williams & Wilkins, 2011: 865–900.

Hari R, Parkkonen L: The brain timewise: how timing shapes and supports brain function. *Philos Trans R Soc Lond B Biol Sci* 2015, 370: 20140170.

Hari R, Salmelin R, Mäkelä JP, Salenius S, Helle M: Magnetoencephalographic cortical rhythms. *Internat J Psychophysiol* 1997, 26: 51–62.

Hasselmo ME, Stern CE: Theta rhythm and the encoding and retrieval of space and time. *NeuroImage* 2014, 85 Pt 2: 656–666.

Herrmann CS, Fründ I, Lenz D: Human gamma-band activity: a review on cognitive and behavioral correlates and network models. *Neurosci Biobehav Rev* 2010, 34: 981–992.

Hsieh LT, Ranganath C: Frontal midline theta oscillations during working memory maintenance and episodic encoding and retrieval. *NeuroImage* 2014, 85: 721–729.

Hughes SW, Lorincz ML, Parri HR, Crunelli V: Infraslow (< 0.1 Hz) oscillations in thalamic relay nuclei basic mechanisms and significance to health and disease states. *Prog Brain Res* 2011, 193: 145–162.

Hyafil A, Giraud AL, Fontolan L, Gutkin B: Neural cross-frequency coupling: connecting architectures, mechanisms, and functions. *Trends Neurosci* 2015, 38: 725–740.

Ioannides AA, Liu L, Kostopoulos GK: The emergence of spindles and K-complexes and the role of the dorsal caudal part of the anterior cingulate as the generator of K-complexes. *Front Neurosci* 2019, 13, 814.

Jäntti V, Baer G, Yli-Hankala A, Hämäläinen M, Hari R: MEG burst suppression in an anaesthesized dog. *Acta Anaesthes Scand* 1995, 39: 126–128.

Jasper H, Penfield W: Electrocorticograms in man: effect of voluntary movement upon the electrical activity of the precentral gyrus. *Arch Psychiatr Zeitschr Neurol* 1949, 183: 163–174.

Jensen O, Goel P, Kopell N, Pohja M, Hari R, Ermentrout B: On the human sensorimotor-cortex beta rhythm: sources and modeling. *NeuroImage* 2005, 26: 347–355.

Jensen O, Mazaheri A: Shaping functional architecture by oscillatory alpha activity: gating by inhibition. *Front Hum Neurosci* 2010, 4: 186.

Klimesch W: Alpha-band oscillations, attention, and controlled access to stored information. *Trends Cogn Sci* 2012, 16: 606–617.

Knyazev GG, Slobodskoj-Plusnin JY, Bocharov AV, Pylkova LV: The default mode network and EEG alpha oscillations: an independent component analysis. *Brain Res* 2011, 1402: 67–79.

Lehtelä L, Salmelin R, Hari R: Evidence for reactive magnetic 10-Hz rhythm in the human auditory cortex. *Neurosci Lett* 1997, 222: 111–114.

Lisman JE, Jensen O: The theta-gamma neural code. *Neuron* 2013, 77: 1002–1016.

Loomis AL, Harvey EN, Hobart G: Further observations on the potential rhythms of the cerebral cortex during sleep. *Science* 1935a, 82: 198–200.

Loomis AL, Harvey EN, Hobart G: Potential rhythms of the cerebral cortex during sleep. *Science* 1935b, 81: 597–598.

Lopes da Silva F: EEG and MEG: relevance to neuroscience. *Neuron* 2013, 80: 1112–1128.

Lu S-T, Kajola M, Joutsiniemi S-L, Knuutila J, Hari R: Generator sites of spontaneous MEG activity during sleep. *Electroencephalogr Clin Neurophysiol* 1992, 82: 182–196.

Lü Z-L, Wang J-Z, Williamson S: Neuronal sources of human parieto-occipital alpha rhythm. In: Hoke M, Erne S, Okada Y, Romani G, eds. *Biomagnetism: Clinical Aspects.* Amsterdam: Excerpta Medica, 1992: 33–37.

Lutz ND, Admard M, Genzoni E, Born J, Rauss K: Occipital sleep spindles predict sequence learning in a visuo-motor task. *SLEEPJ* 2021, 44: 1–18.

Maksimow A, Kaisti K, Aalto S, Mäenpää M, Jääskeläinen S, Hinkka S, Martens S, Särkelä M, Viertiö-Oja H, Scheinin H: Correlation of EEG spectral entropy with regional cerebral blood flow during sevoflurane and propofol anaesthesia. *Anaesthesia* 2005, 60: 862–869.

Mantini D, Perrucci MG, Del Gratta C, Romani GL, Corbetta M: Electrophysiological signatures of resting state networks in the human brain. *Proc Natl Acad Sci U S A* 2007, 104: 13170–13175.

Marsden JF, Ashby P, Limousin-Dowsey P, Rothwell JC, Brown P: Coherence between cerebellar thalamus, cortex and muscle in man: cerebellar thalamus interactions. *Brain* 2000, 123: 1459–1470.

Marshall L, Cross N, Binder S, Dang-Vu TT: Brain rhythms during sleep and memory consolidation: neuro-biological insights. *Physiology (Bethesda)* 2020, 35: 4–15.

Mashour GA, Orser BA, Avidan MS: Intraoperative awareness: from neurobiology to clinical practice. *Anesthesiology* 2011, 114: 1218–1233.

Michalareas G, Vezoli J, van Pelt S, Schoffelen JM, Kennedy H, Fries P: Alpha-beta and gamma rhythms subserve feedback and feedforward influences among human visual cortical areas. *Neuron* 2016, 89: 384–397.

Monto S, Palva S, Voipio J, Palva JM: Very slow EEG fluctuations predict the dynamics of stimulus detection and oscillation amplitudes in humans. *J Neurosci* 2008, 28: 8268–8272.

National Heart, Lung, and Blood Institute. *Sleep Apnea: Is Your Patient at Risk?* Bethesda, MD: National Heart, Lung and Blood Institute, 1995.

National Institutes of Health. *Working Group Report on Problem Sleepiness, National Heart, Lung, and Blood Institute.* Bethesda, MD: National Institutes of Health, 1997.

Numminen J, Mäkelä J, Hari R: Distribution and sources of magnetoencephalographic K-complexes. *Electroencephalogr Clin Neurophysiol* 1996, 99: 544–555.

Ohara S, Mima T, Baba K, Ikeda A, Kunieda T, Matsumoto R, Yamamoto J, Matsuhashi M, Nagamine T, Hirasawa K, Hori T, Mihara T, Hashimoto N, Salenius S, Shibasaki H: Increased synchronization of cortical oscillatory activities between human supplementary motor and primary sensorimotor areas during voluntary movements. *J Neurosci* 2001, 21: 9377–9386.

Oken BS, Chiappa KH: Short-term variability in EEG frequency analysis. *Electroencephalogr Clin Neurophysiol* 1988, 69: 191–198.

Palva S, Palva JM: New vistas for alpha-frequency band oscillations. *Trends Neurosci* 2007, 30: 150–158.

Peelle JE, Davis MH: Neural oscillations carry speech rhythm through to comprehension. *Front Psychol* 2012, 3: 320.

Peelle JE, Gross J, Davis MH: Phase-locked responses to speech in human auditory cortex are enhanced during comprehension. *Cerebr Cortex* 2013, 23: 1378–1387.

Perez-Borja C, Chatrian GE, Tyce FA, Rivers MH: Electrographic patterns of the occipital lobe in man: a topographic study based on use of implanted electrodes. *Electroencephalogr Clin Neurophysiol* 1962, 14: 171–182.

Pernet P, Garrido M, Gramfort A, Maurits N, Michel C, Pang E, Salmelin R, Schoffelen JM, Valdés-Sosa PA, Puce A: Issues and recommendations from the OHBM COBIDAS MEEG committee for reproducible EEG and MEG research. *Nat Neurosci* 2020, 23: 1473–1483.

Pfurtscheller G, Lopes da Silva FH: Event-related EEG/MEG synchronization and desynchronization: basic principles. *Clin Neurophysiol* 1999, 110: 1842–1857.

Purdon PL, Sampson A, Pavone KJ, Brown EN: Clinical electroencephalography for anesthesiologists: Part I: background and basic signatures. *Anesthesiology* 2015, 123: 937–960.

Raghavachari S, Kahana MJ, Rizzuto DS, Caplan JB, Kirschen MP, Bourgeois B, Madsen JR, Lisman JE: Gating of human theta oscillations by a working memory task. *J Neurosci* 2001, 21: 3175–3183.

Ramkumar P, Parkkonen L, Hari R, Hyvärinen A: Characterization of neuromagnetic brain rhythms over time scales of minutes using spatial independent component analysis. *Hum Brain Mapp* 2012, 33: 1648–1662.

Rampil IJ: A primer for EEG signal processing in anesthesia. *Anesthesiology* 1998, 89: 980–1002.

Reid MS, Flammino F, Howard B, Nilsen D, Prichep LS: Cocaine cue versus cocaine dosing in humans: evidence for distinct neurophysiological response profiles. *Pharmacol Biochem Behav* 2008, 91: 155–164.

Riviello JJ Jr, Nordli DRJ, Niedermeyer E: Normal EEG and sleep: infants to adolescents. In: Schomer DL, Lopes da Silva FH, eds. *Niedermeyer's Electroencephalography: Basic Principles, Clinical Applications, and Related Fields*, 6th ed. Philadelphia, PA: Lippincott Williams & Wilkins, 2011: 163–181.

Roche D, Mahon P: Depth of anesthesia monitoring. *Anesthesiol Clin* 2021, 39: 477–492.

Salenius S, Hari R: Synchronous cortical oscillatory activity during motor action. *Curr Opin Neurobiol* 2003, 13: 678–684.

Salmelin R, Hari R: Characterization of spontaneous MEG rhythms in healthy adults. *Electroencephalogr Clin Neurophysiol* 1994a, 91: 237–248.

Salmelin R, Hari R: Spatiotemporal characteristics of sensorimotor neuromagnetic rhythms related to thumb movement. *Neuroscience* 1994b, 60: 537–550.

Salmelin R, Hämäläinen M, Kajola M, Hari R: Functional segregation of movement-related rhythmic activity in the human brain. *NeuroImage* 1995, 2: 237–243.

Salmelin R, Hari R, Lounasmaa OV, Sams M: Dynamics of brain activation during picture naming. *Nature* 1994, 368: 463–465.

Schönauer M, Pöhlchen D: Sleep spindles. *Curr Biol* 2018, 28: R1129–R1130.

Sedley W, Cunningham MO: Do cortical gamma oscillations promote or suppress perception? An underasked question with an over-assumed answer. *Front Hum Neurosci* 2013, 7: 595.

Singer W: Cortical dynamics revisited. *Trends Cogn Sci* 2013, 17: 616–626.

Sloan TB: Anesthetic effects on electrophysiologic recordings. *J Clin Neurophysiol* 1998, 15: 217–226.

Snow J: *On the Inhalation of the Vapour of Ether in Surgical Operations.* London: John Churchill, 1847.

Srinivasan R, Nunez PL, Tucker DM, Silberstein RB, Cadusch PJ: Spatial sampling and filtering of EEG with spline laplacians to estimate cortical potentials. *Brain Topogr* 1996, 8: 355–366.

Tallon-Baudry C, Bertrand O, Pernier J: A ring-shaped distribution of dipoles as a source model of induced gamma-band activity. *Clin Neurophysiol* 1999, 110: 660–665.

Tiihonen J, Hari R, Kajola M, Karhu J, Ahlfors S, Tissari S: Magnetoencephalographic 10-Hz rhythm from the human auditory cortex. *Neurosci Lett* 1991, 129: 303–305.

Tiihonen J, Kajola M, Hari R: Magnetic mu rhythm in man. *Neuroscience* 1989, 32: 793–800.

Uhlhaas PJ, Pipa G, Neuenschwander S, Wibral M, Singer W: A new look at gamma? High- (>60 Hz) gamma-band activity in cortical networks: function, mechanisms and impairment. *Prog Biophys Mol Biol* 2011, 105: 14–28.

Weisz N, Hartmann T, Muller N, Lorenz I, Obleser J: Alpha rhythms in audition: cognitive and clinical perspectives. *Front Psychol* 2011, 2: 73.

Weng YY, Lei X, Yu J: Sleep spindle abnormalities related to Alzheimer's disease: a systematic mini-review. *Sleep Med* 2020, 75: 37–44.

Wennberg R, Cheyne D: On noninvasive source imaging of the human K-complex. *Clin Neurophysiol* 2013, 124: 941–955.

Whittington MA, Cunningham MO, LeBeau FE, Racca C, Traub RD: Multiple origins of the cortical gamma rhythm. *Dev Neurobiol* 2011, 71: 92–106.

CHAPTER 12

EVOKED AND EVENT-RELATED RESPONSES

It's not what happens to you, but how you react to it that matters.

—EPICTETUS

Our life evokes our character. You find out more about yourself as you go on. That's why it's good to put yourself in situations that will evoke your higher nature rather than your lower.

—JOSEPH CAMPBELL

■ INTRODUCTION

The earliest evoked responses detected from the human brain are auditory-evoked responses generated in the brainstem, displaying multiple deflections within the first 10 ms after stimulus onset. Subsequent cortical responses can continue for many hundreds of milliseconds poststimulus. Quite sustained potentials and fields can be recorded during long-duration stimuli or during tasks involving motor planning, attention, and other cognitive operations. Figure 12.1 shows one example of a long-duration response where MEG was recorded without any high-pass filtering during an auditory task. Altogether 10.5 s of averaged ($N = 60$) MEG signal is shown, including a prestimulus period of 0.5 s, followed by a brief cue sound, an expectation interval of 2 s, and then a neutral sound of 6 s (Yokosawa et al., 2013). The sustained field differing from the zero level persists for almost 10 s, indicating that some long-lasting neural responses are visible with proper filter settings.

It is common to differentiate between *transient* and *steady-state* evoked responses. Transient responses denote activity that is elicited by discrete stimuli that all evoke a complete sequence of early and late deflections. These responses are thus analyzed and interpreted within the time domain, by paying much attention to peak latencies and amplitudes of the main deflections. Steady-state responses (SSRs), in contrast, are elicited by stimuli that are repeated so frequently (say at 3 Hz, or even 10–40 Hz) that successive deflections of the evoked responses overlap. At the same time, long-latency parts

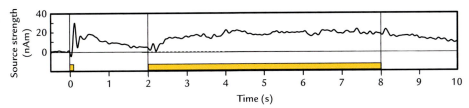

FIGURE 12.1. **Ultraslow activity in a DC-coupled MEG recording.** The trace shows the source strength (in units of nAm; mean of 15 subjects) in the left auditory cortex. The passband is 0 to 8 Hz. A brief cue sound occurred at time 0 s and a neutral 6-s sound started at time 2 s (respective yellow bars at the base of the plot). Clear transient evoked responses follow the onsets of both sounds. Slow activity, clearly exceeding the baseline level, is seen both during the anticipation period after the cue sound and during the long sound, and it decays slowly after the stimulus has ended. Reprinted with permission from Yokosawa K, Pamilo S, Hirvenkari L, Hari R, Pihko E: Activation of auditory cortex by anticipating and hearing emotional sounds: an MEG study. *PLoS One* 2013, 8: e80284.

of the response become suppressed relatively more than the earlier parts. Thus SSRs appear cyclical and correspond closely to the original stimulus repetition rate (and its harmonics) (Regan, 1972). SSRs can be analyzed and interpreted both within frequency and time domains.

Typical evoked responses are small with respect to the ongoing spontaneous MEG/EEG, varying in size from fractions of a microvolt to tens of microvolts for EEG, and from 1 to 200 fT for MEG, depending on the type of activity that is being studied (see Chapters 13–19). From the evoked response point of view, spontaneous MEG/EEG activity can be seen as "noise," and signal averaging has been the mainstream method for improving the signal-to-noise ratio (see Chapter 10).

Peaks of evoked-response deflections are typically quantified relative to a prestimulus baseline. Typical prestimulus baselines are 100 to 250 ms for long-latency evoked responses and can be shorter for earlier responses. However, more extended prestimulus baselines (e.g., 500–600 ms) may be useful for separating and identifying slow evoked responses in patients from abnormally slow background EEG/MEG activity (Puce et al., 1989) or for single-trial analyses (e.g., time–frequency analysis) that are performed in parallel (Rossi et al., 2014) (see Chapter 10). Note that if signals associated with motor events (rather than stimulus events) are sought, then similar epoching is applied around the onset of the motor action, with a suitably long premovement baseline.

For SSRs of all sensory systems, a good signal-to-noise ratio is obtained in a relatively short time; however, the SSR latencies (or phases) are ambiguous because the responses are cyclic, and it is not clear which particular stimulus cycle is associated with a certain part of the SSR. Sometimes multiples of one cycle (2π) may need to be added to (or subtracted from) the measured peak latencies. Thus for SSRs, only "apparent" latencies or phases can be reported (Van der Tweel & Lunel, 1965; Regan, 1966).

SSRs can be used as an effective tool to *frequency-tag* different parts of the visual display or certain auditory or somatosensory inputs, so that each stimulus condition can be associated with a particular tagging frequency that is totally separate from the frequency or other characteristics of the stimulus of interest.

■ AN INITIAL EXAMPLE

The benefit of recording both MEG and EEG evoked responses using the same stimuli and tasks can be appreciated from the following example that demonstrates the relationship between evoked electric potentials and magnetic fields to auditory stimuli.

It has been known since 1939 that abrupt, loud sounds elicit a prominent 100-ms EEG response, with an amplitude maximum at the vertex (Davis, 1939). The source of this "vertex potential" was not known, and because of its wide distribution, it was considered nonspecific with respect to the sensory modality. This interpretation was feasible as visual and somatosensory stimuli also elicit EEG responses that are largest at the vertex, largely resembling the transient vertex responses observed during light sleep (see Figure 11.10).

In 1970, however, Vaughan and Ritter radically claimed that both the 100-ms and 200-ms deflections of the auditory vertex response, as well as some earlier 40- to 60-ms deflections, were generated in, or near, the primary auditory cortex in the superior surface of the temporal lobe. Their reasoning was based on the observation of polarity reversals of all these deflections over the Sylvian fissure when they measured EEG along a coronal line spanning from the midline to the mastoids, with all electrodes referenced to an electrode at the tip of the nose (see Figure 12.2). Comparison of the measurements with predictions from a multishell volume-conductor model supported the view that the likely source was a current dipole in the auditory cortex (Vaughan & Ritter, 1970).

This proposal regarding a modality-specific origin of the middle- and long-latency auditory responses was strongly rebutted in a subsequent study where no polarity reversal was observed in surface EEG recordings using a *noncephalic* reference electrode (Kooi et al., 1971). However, the latter claims were based on an incomplete understanding of the effects of the reference site. The situation was similar to the schematic demonstrated in Figure 5.8, where we had a local source in the middle of the recording area but no polarity reversal was seen when the reference electrode was at one extremum of the potential distribution. These erroneous interpretations of recording with a noncephalic reference electrode continued to confuse the community for many years to come.

The results of Vaughan and Ritter (1970) were soon supported by scalp recordings of three patients who had injured auditory cortex in one hemisphere and in whom the polarity reversal in the coronal electrode array was seen only over the healthy hemisphere (Peronnet et al., 1974). Moreover, intracranial recordings in patients during surgical treatment of partial epilepsy showed a sequence of evoked potentials peaking from 10 to 225 ms in the supratemporal auditory cortex (Celesia, 1976). Meanwhile, support for the generation of auditory-evoked potentials in the auditory cortex had also been obtained in monkey intracranial recordings (Arezzo et al., 1975).

The generation of the long-latency evoked responses peaking around 100 ms and 200 ms was strongly supported also by MEG recordings (Elberling et al., 1980; Hari et al., 1980) that agreed with source currents on the upper surface of the temporal lobes. These recordings, as shown in Figure 12.3 also demonstrated agreement between the direction of the intracellular current flow as deduced separately from the patterns of both MEG and EEG responses.

Only a few years later, with the advent of a spatiotemporal two-dipole model to explain the sources of evoked potentials, the EEG community started to accept the substantial contribution of auditory cortex to long-latency evoked potentials triggered by abrupt sounds (Scherg & von Cramon, 1985).

Still one major contributor to the confusion about the generators of the auditory-evoked responses, besides the poor understanding of the effects of the reference electrode

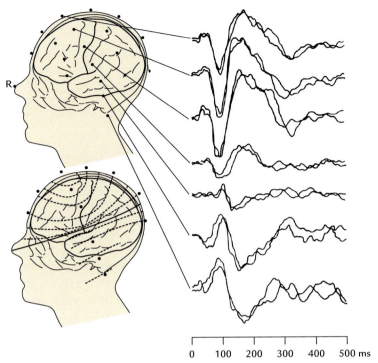

0   100   200   300   400   500 ms

FIGURE 12.2. Auditory-evoked long-latency potentials and polarity reversals in EEG signals. AEPs (right panel) to 100 tone pips (1 kHz, 30 ms duration) presented once every 2 s. The EEG traces were recorded from a linear array of seven electrodes spanning the midline to the left mastoid as shown on the upper schematic head. The 500-ms traces begin at tone onset. All recordings were referenced to the nose tip (R). Note the polarity reversals across the Sylvian fissure in both 100-ms and 200-ms deflections. The lower schematic head shows the approximate potential distribution for the 200-ms deflection, with the zero potential line indicated as a solid line. Adapted and reprinted from Vaughan HG Jr, Ritter W: The sources of auditory evoked responses recorded from the human scalp. *Electroencephalogr Clin Neurophysiol* 1970, 28: 360–367. With permission from Elsevier.

and the differences between electric and magnetic responses, has been the diversity of experimental parameters. In this chapter we show that, for example, the interstimulus interval is an important parameter that can recruit or extinguish some neural sources and thus modify the results.

All evoked responses can be used as tools to probe the functions of their specific generator areas, both in healthy subjects and in patients suffering from disorders of sensory systems and/or the brain.

■ NOMENCLATURE OF EVOKED RESPONSES AND BRAIN RHYTHMS

Any sensory stimulus evokes a sequence of neuronal events that move along the afferent pathways from the peripheral sensory organs to the primary projection cortex in the brain and are then distributed to many other brain areas.

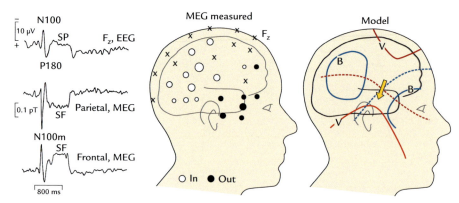

FIGURE 12.3. Auditory-evoked fields and potentials and a putative source model. Left: AEPs (top) and AEFs (middle and bottom) from a single subject to 800-ms tones presented once every 4 s. The AEP is the average of 87 single responses (recording from Fz referred to nose tip) whereas the AEFs show an average of 330 responses (recorded from midline parietal and frontal sites). Display passband is 0.03 to 15 Hz. Middle: Distributions of N100m responses over the right hemisphere of a single subject. The areas of the circles are proportional to N100m peak amplitude at each location; the white circles indicate magnetic flux into the head and black circles flux out of the head. Right: A schematic of the potential distribution (V, red lines) and magnetic field (B, blue lines) associated with a current dipole that is the likely source of the measured N100 and N100m signals; the dashed red and blue lines show the zero lines for EEG and MEG signals, respectively. SP = sustained potential; SF = sustained field. Adapted and reprinted from Hari R, Aittoniemi K, Järvinen ML, Katila T, Varpula T: Auditory evoked transient and sustained magnetic fields of the human brain. localization of neural generators. *Exp Brain Res* 1980, 40: 237–240. With permission of Springer.

Historically, stimulus-driven activity has been called an *evoked potential* in EEG recordings and an *evoked field* in MEG recordings, and the term *evoked response* has been applied to both. In contrast, the terms *event-related potential* (ERP) and *event-related field* (ERF) have been used more generally to describe changes in MEG/EEG signals triggered by either external stimuli or related to internal mental or task-related events. In this book, we use the terms *evoked response* and *event-related response* to collectively refer to brain activity recorded either with MEG or EEG, and we use the abbreviations EP and ERP to refer to EEG responses and the abbreviations EF and ERF to refer to MEG responses. So, for example, the respective auditory, somatosensory, and visual responses would be denoted as AEP and AEF, SEP and SEF, and VEP and VEF.

In the vast EEG and MEG literature, the nomenclature of evoked responses is diverse and confusing. An old naming convention numbered successive deflections separately for scalp-positive (P) and scalp-negative (N) EPs—where the polarities refer to the "active electrode"—resulting in notations such as P1, N1, P2, N2, P3. This convention is, however, highly confusing as the sequence of deflections can vary according to stimulus parameters, reference location, and even subjects, and because similar labels are used for early and later responses, depending on when the first response within the specific experimental setting happens to start. To make matters worse, letters are sometimes added to these labels, such as P3a and P3b. We have previously recommended that this practice be abandoned for new studies (see also Pernet et al., 2020). It is, however, important for those working in the area to be familiar with all the potential forms of nomenclature, so that common findings can be identified across the earlier literature.

A less ambiguous way—first recommended by the International Federation of Clinical Neurophysiology in 1984 and updated in 1999 (http://www.clinph-journal.com/content/guidelinesIFCN)—is to combine the polarity (N or P) of the response peak or trough with the nominal peak latency in milliseconds, for example, P60, N100, and P200 (see Figure 10.2). This convention has been advocated on multiple occasions (Donchin et al., 1977; Pivik et al., 1993; Picton et al., 2000; Duncan et al., 2009). Note that in most cases it is clear enough to use in the response name the approximate (or nominal) latency (and not the measured individual latency). For example, the mean peak latency of the N100 deflection may vary between, say, 90 or 110 ms without causing any confusion in the nomenclature as long as we are speaking about the same prominent response with the same well-defined functional characteristics across different individuals.

However, as an EEG deflection that is scalp-negative at one site can be scalp-positive at another site because of the orientation of the underlying generators (and the reference location), it is critical to add the recording site to this nomenclature. For example, terms such as "vertex N100" or "frontal N20" are much more specific than the terms "N100" and "N20" used in isolation.

In MEG recordings, combining the flux direction (exiting and entering the head) with the signal names would only confuse the researchers because the magnetic field patterns are orthogonal to the potential distribution (see Figure 1.2). Moreover, the signal polarities in the two hemispheres may be difficult to grasp. For example, during the auditory evoked 100-ms response, the flux is directed *into the head* at the posterior end of the *right* Sylvian fissure but *out of the head* at the corresponding location in the *left* hemisphere (see a graphic presentation in Figure 13.6). Hence, the first attempts to combine MEG and EEG data used terms such as N100m and P200m to refer to the magnetic ("m") counterparts of the electric N100 and P200 responses (Hari et al., 1980). Another system of notation for MEG recordings is to indicate just the latency, preceded by "M" to magnetic (e.g., M170 as the face-sensitive evoked response). However, even here it would be good to indicate recording (or source) site as accurately as possible when describing the responses, and one might refer to, for example, the Rolandic N20m response or the Rolandic 20-ms response, or to the auditory-cortex 100-ms response or the auditory-cortex N100m (or M100) response. Note, however, that the exact locations of the maximum MEG signals depend on the configuration of the flux transformer: with a planar gradiometer, the largest signals occur just over the local source but with a magnetometer, or an axial magnetometer, the same site shows zero signal and polarity reversal, with maximum signals several centimeters away (see Figure 5.15).

In addition to this nomenclature, some event-related responses have acquired special names, such as the contingent negative variation, mismatch negativity, and error-related negativity that we discuss later (see Chapter 18).

The literature also makes the distinction between *exogenous* and *endogenous* event-related responses (Picton et al., 2000). Exogenous responses are triggered by external stimuli, and they change as a function of the physical characteristics of the stimuli (bottom-up processes). They reflect activity in sensory pathways and are sometimes called *obligatory*. In contrast, endogenous responses are associated with cognitive or affective (top-down) processing. However, this distinction is often arbitrary, since both types of brain signals can be influenced by bottom-up and top-down processes. Hence we do not recommend this nomenclature.

The successive deflections in averaged MEG/EEG signals, either as peaks or troughs, are sometimes called *components* that should be linked to some functional brain processes with characteristic spatial distributions or generator sites, as well as a clear relationship to some experimental variables (Donchin et al., 1978). One example of an evoked response that has (at least) two functional components is the already-mentioned auditory-evoked 100-ms response N100, with one component generated in the auditory cortex and another close to the vertex, differentiated by their resilience to stimulus repetition (Hari et al., 1982) as we describe in Chapter 13. An additional reason to be cautious with the word *component* (and to use the word *deflection* instead; see below) is that analyses commonly used in the MEG/EEG field also speak about components. For example, in principal component analysis, *components* refer to waveforms that account for some proportion of the variance in the data, without bearing any functional relationship to the measured responses. Moreover, in independent-component analysis (see Chapter 10), *components* display features of the original MEG/EEG recording (such as eye-blink artifacts, alpha activity, etc.).

Altogether, the EEG and MEG literature is so full of various identifying labels that the resulting "bumpology" has been criticized with good reason (Allison et al., 1986). It is now with improved source analyses and functional characterization that we can move toward more functional and brain-activity-related descriptions. Given the earlier discussion that a response peak or trough may not directly correspond to a functional component, if there is uncertainty when describing various parts of MEG/EEG responses, the term *deflection* may be more useful. We use this term throughout this book, as well as the term *response* to refer to the entire averaged MEG/EEG waveform.

One final point regarding nomenclature and conventions: for displaying EEG and evoked response signals, the traditional convention for polarity has been "negative-up," meaning that scalp negativity (at the assumed "active" electrode) is plotted upwards. Clinical EEG still uses this tradition. However, it is becoming more common to plot EEG/ERP data "positive up," to be consistent with other types of scientific data. To avoid confusion, especially in comparisons with earlier EEG/ERP literature, the polarity should be clearly marked on all displays of evoked responses as well as spontaneous EEG data. We note that guidelines put forward by the Organization for Human Brain Mapping's Committee on Best Practices in Data Analysis & Sharing in Neuroimaging using MEEG (COBIDAS MEEG) (see Pernet et al., 2018, 2020) follow the nomenclature and conventions we have advocated (see the first edition of our *Primer* in 2017).

■ EFFECTS OF INTERSTIMULUS INTERVAL AND STIMULUS TIMING

Sometimes it is necessary to make a distinction between parameters describing aspects of stimulus timing. Stimulus onset asynchrony (SOA) refers to the time between two successive stimulus onsets, interstimulus interval (ISI) refers to the time between the offset of one stimulus and the onset of another, and the intertrial interval (ITI) refers to the time between successive trials (during which multiple stimuli may be presented). SOA and ISI can be quite different from each other if the stimulus duration is long (ISI = SOA – stimulus duration). However, if stimulus duration is short relative to SOA, then it does not really matter whether one speaks about ISI or SOA (e.g., if 1 ms clicks are presented once every 4 s).

In general, the longer the latency of the response (and thereby, generally, the more synapses crossed), the more sensitive the response is to stimulus repetition rate, as well as to vigilance, anesthesia, and so on (see also Chapter 11). Therefore, responses closest to the primary projection areas (or even afferent pathways) are the most resilient to stimulus repetition. On the other hand, the same brain region can generate evoked responses that show

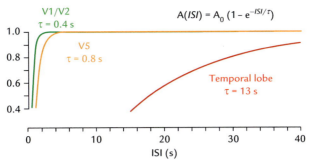

FIGURE 12.4. **Recovery cycles in three visually sensitive cortical areas.** Schematic presentation of the effect of ISI on visual-evoked fields recorded from different brain areas (V1/V2 = early projection cortices in the occipital lobe; V5 = visual-motion-sensitive brain area in the posterior temporal cortex, and temporal lobe = temporal cortex anterior to V5). The lifetimes of the signals (indicated by τ) are longer, the higher the brain area is in the processing stream. The equation at the top gives the signal amplitude A as a function of ISI, compared with the maximum signal A_0. Adapted and reprinted from Hari R, Parkkonen L, Nangini C: The brain in time: insights from neuromagnetic recordings. *Annals NY Acad Sci* 2010, 1191: 89–109. With permission from John Wiley & Sons.

very different recovery cycles, implying existence of several (possibly nested) local temporal scales (Hari & Parkkonen, 2015).

The behavior of an evoked response during repeated stimulation can be characterized by computing a "lifetime," which is the exponent of the exponential decay curve that models the response's recovery cycle (see Figure 12.4). The lifetimes can be considered to index the strength of the trace that previous stimuli have left in the system; they depend on the brain area and are different for successive deflections of the same evoked response. For visual stimuli, for example, the lifetimes vary from 0.2 to 15 s in different visual areas: the shortest lifetimes are in the primary visual cortex, and the longest are in the temporal lobe (Uusitalo et al., 1996). In the auditory system, the 100-ms response reaches its maximum amplitude at ISIs longer than 8 to 10 s (corresponding to lifetimes of about 2 s) (Hari et al., 1982). Similar lifetimes have been demonstrated for somatosensory 100-ms responses at the SII cortex (Hari et al., 1993) and to proprioceptive stimulation elicited by passive movements (Smeds et al., 2017). Similarly, responses to noxious laser stimuli recover in 8 to 16 s (Raij et al., 2003), whereas responses to painful carbon-dioxide stimulation of the nasal mucosa have much longer recovery cycles of the order of 20 to 30 s (Hari et al., 1997).

Note, however, that the situation may not be always as straightforward, because at short ISIs the responses may even be enhanced by preceding stimuli. For example, when noise bursts were presented in pairs with an interpair interval of 1.2 to 1.4 s with a varying SOA from 70 to 500 ms, the responses to the second sound were enhanced compared with the responses to the first sound, most clearly at SOAs of 150 ms (Loveless et al., 1989), as is illustrated in Figure 12.5. One explanation offered by the authors was that the effect of the ISI is a dual process involving one component regulating the number of neural elements reacting to the new stimulus and another component affecting the reactivity of single neurons.

The more responses are averaged, the better the signal-to-noise ratio, provided that the noise is stationary. However, if data collection expands over a long period of time, the subject's attentional state and vigilance will likely change, and the response may decrease because of short-term habituation or even receptor adaptation (as is the case of olfactory

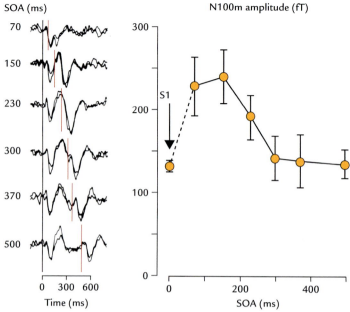

FIGURE 12.5. Effect of short SOA of sounds on N100m amplitudes. Left: Responses of one subject (with replicates) to pairs of 50-ms noise bursts presented once in 1.2 to 1.4 s, with six different SOAs (70, 150, 230, 300, 370, and 500 ms) varying randomly within the sequence. The first sound of a pair always starts at time zero, and the onset of the second sound is indicated by the short vertical red lines. Signals are shown from one axial first-order gradiometer (of a seven-channel device) placed over the posterior end of the right Sylvian fissure. Recording passband 0.05 to 100 Hz, sampling rate 500 Hz; the averaged responses (N of at least 50) have been low-pass filtered at 45 Hz. Right: Mean ± SEM amplitudes of N100m to the second stimuli of the pairs as a function of SOA. The value at time zero is the N100m amplitude to the first stimulus of the pair, averages across all six pairs. Adapted and reprinted from Loveless N, Hari R, Hämäläinen M, Tiihonen J: Evoked responses of human auditory cortex may be enhanced by preceding stimuli. *Electroencephalogr Clin Neurophysiol* 1989, 74: 217–227. With permission from Elsevier.

stimulation, see Chapter 16). Especially demanding are recordings with long interstimulus intervals, because identical runs at either end of the recording session often produce different results. Such potential order effects should be carefully monitored by comparing responses obtained at the beginning and the end of the experiment.

■ EFFECTS OF OTHER STIMULUS PARAMETERS

Offsets of long stimuli can elicit clear evoked responses (see, e.g., almost equal-size 100-ms responses to sound onsets and offset responses when the stimuli and ISIs are of the same duration; Hari et al., 1987), suggesting that any sudden and unexpected changes in the environment may synchronize spontaneous activity and thereby elicit an evoked response. Therefore, the stimuli must either be made to be so brief that no offset responses are elicited or so long that the offset responses do not interfere with onset responses of interest. Optimal stimulus durations will vary across sensory modalities because the latencies of sensory responses vary from tens to hundreds of milliseconds, as will be demonstrated in Chapters 13 through 19.

Stimulus intensity is an important variable in all types of evoked-response studies. When the intensity is increased above the threshold of sensation, the transient evoked responses first increase very strongly but then saturate (i.e., do not show any further augmentation despite increases in stimulus intensity). The most reliable transient responses are obtained at saturated stimulation levels. Steady-state responses tend to contain mainly the fundamental-frequency component that increases as a function of stimulus intensity (modulation depth), whereas the presence and amplitudes of harmonic components depend on many different factors, among them the stimulation frequency; moreover, some harmonic responses may reflect distortions of the stimulus without necessarily indicating nonlinearities in the sensory system under study (Van der Tweel & Lunel, 1965).

Jittering the timing of stimulus presentation (e.g., using a base stimulus presentation rate around which the ISIs vary randomly) can help avoid synchronization of MEG/EEG signals to power-line noise artifacts, decrease the predictability of the stimuli, and minimize entrainment of some brain rhythms to stimulus delivery. The stimulus timing jitter could be described, for example, as 1500 ms ± 25 ms, or as 1475 to 1525 ms (with a note whether the distribution is even across the variation interval and what the increments are). In countries with a 50-Hz line frequency, using SOAs of, for example, 1005 ms instead of 1000 ms can effectively decrease the line noise in the averaged responses because the power-line noise (comprising cycles of 20 ms) is then sampled in different phases in successive responses.

Other important variables specific to the sensory modality under study include visual angle, luminance, contrast, loudness, and intensity of electrical stimuli delivered to a peripheral nerve. We discuss these parameters in each respective evoked-response chapter. Importantly, all stimulus characteristics should be described when presenting or publishing the data to the level of detail that other investigators can reproduce the same experiment. Detailed guidelines are available for performing studies, describing stimulus attributes and other criteria for publishing EEG studies (Picton et al., 2000; Duncan et al., 2009; Keil et al., 2014), MEG studies (Burgess et al., 2011; Gross et al., 2013; Hari et al., 2018), and MEG/EEG studies (Keil et al., 2014; Pernet et al., 2018, 2020).

■ **REFERENCES**

Allison T, Wood CC, McCarthy G: The central nervous system. In: Coles MG, Donchin E, Porges SW, eds. *Psychophysiology*. New York: Guilford Press, 1986: 5–25.

Arezzo J, Pickoff A, Vaughan HG Jr: The sources and intracerebral distribution of auditory evoked potentials in the alert rhesus monkey. *Brain Res* 1975, 90: 57–73.

Burgess RC, Funke ME, Bowyer SM, Lewine JD, Kirsch HE, Bagić AI, ACPG Committee: American Clinical Magnetoencephalography Society Clinical Practice Guideline 2: presurgical functional brain mapping using magnetic evoked fields. *J Clin Neurophysiol* 2011, 28: 355–361.

Celesia GG: Organization of auditory cortical areas in man. *Brain* 1976, 99: 403–414.

Davis PA: Effects of acoustic stimuli on the waking human brain. *J Neurophysiol* 1939, 2: 494–499.

Donchin E, Callaway E, Cooper R, Desmedt JE, Goff WR, Hillyard SA, Sutton S: Publication criteria for studies of evoked potentials (EP) in man: methodology and publication criteria. In: Desmedt JE, ed. *Progress in Clinical Neurophysiology: Vol. 1. Attention, Voluntary Contraction and Event-Related Cerebral Potentials*. Basel, Switzerland: Karger, 1977: 1–11.

Donchin E, Ritter W, McCallum WC: Cognitive physiology: the endogenous components of the ERP. In: Callaway E, Tueting P, Koslow S, eds. *Brain Event-Related Potentials in Man*. New York: Academic Press, 1978: 349–441.

Duncan CC, Barry RJ, Connolly JF, Fischer C, Michie PT, Näätänen R, Polich J, Reinvang I, Van Petten C: Event-related potentials in clinical research: guidelines for eliciting, recording, and quantifying mismatch negativity, P300, and N400. *Clin Neurophysiol* 2009, 120: 1883–1908.

Elberling C, Bak C, Kofoed B, Lebech J, Saermark K: Magnetic auditory responses from the human brain: a preliminary report. *Scand Audiol* 1980, 9: 185–190.

Gross J, Baillet S, Barnes GR, Henson RN, Hillebrand A, Jensen O, Jerbi K, Litvak V, Maess B, Oostenveld R, Parkkonen L, Taylor JR, van Wassenhove V, Wibral M, Schoffelen JM: Good practice for conducting and reporting MEG research. *NeuroImage* 2013, 65: 349–363.

Hari R, Aittoniemi K, Järvinen ML, Katila T, Varpula T: Auditory evoked transient and sustained magnetic fields of the human brain: localization of neural generators. *Exp Brain Res* 1980, 40: 237–240.

Hari R, Kaila K, Katila T, Tuomisto T, Varpula T: Interstimulus-interval dependence of the auditory vertex response and its magnetic counterpart: implications for their neural generation. *Electroencephalogr Clin Neurophysiol* 1982, 54: 561–569.

Hari R, Pelizzone M, Mäkelä JP, Hällström J, Leinonen L, Lounasmaa OV: Neuromagnetic responses of the human auditory cortex to on- and offsets of noise bursts. *Audiology* 1987, 25: 31–43.

Hari R, Karhu J, Hämäläinen M, Knuutila J, Salonen O, Sams M, Vilkman V: Functional organization of the human first and second somatosensory cortices: a neuromagnetic study. *Eur J Neurosci* 1993, 5: 724–734.

Hari R, Portin K, Kettenmann B, Jousmäki V, Kobal G: Right-hemisphere preponderance of responses to painful CO_2 stimulation of the human nasal mucosa. *Pain* 1997, 72: 145–151.

Hari R, Parkkonen L: The brain timewise: how timing shapes and supports brain function. *Philos Trans R Soc Lond B Biol Sci* 2015, 370: 20140170.

Hari R, Baillet S, Barnes G, Burgess R, Forss N, Gross J, Hämäläinen M, Jensen O, Kakigi R, Mauguière F, Nakasato N, Puce A, Romani GL, Schnitzler A, Taulu S: IFCN-endorsed practical guidelines for clinical magnetoencephalography (MEG). *Clin Neurophysiol* 2018, 129: 1720–1747.

Keil A, Debener S, Gratton G, Junghofer M, Kappenman ES, Luck SJ, Luu P, Miller GA, Yee CM: Committee report: publication guidelines and recommendations for studies using electroencephalography and magnetoencephalography. *Psychophysiology* 2014, 51: 1–21.

Kooi KA, Tipton AC, Marshall RE: Polarities and field configurations of the vertex components of the human auditory evoked response: a reinterpretation. *Electroencephalogr Clin Neurophysiol* 1971, 31: 166–169.

Loveless N, Hari R, Hämäläinen M, Tiihonen J: Evoked responses of human auditory cortex may be enhanced by preceding stimuli. *Electroencephalogr Clin Neurophysiol* 1989, 74: 217–227.

Pernet P, Garrido M, Gramfort A, Maurits N, Michel C, Pang E, Salmelin R, Schoffelen JM, Valdés-Sosa PA, Puce A: Best practices in data analysis and sharing in neuroimaging using MEEG. 2018. White paper https://osf.io/a8dhx/

Pernet C, Garrido MI, Gramfort A, Maurits N, Michel CM, Pang E, Salmelin R, Schoffelen JM, Valdés-Sosa PA, Puce A: Issues and recommendations from the OHBM COBIDAS MEEG committee for reproducible EEG and MEG research. *Nat Neurosci* 2020, 23: 1473–1483.

Peronnet F, Michel F, Echallier JF, Girod J: Coronal topography of human auditory evoked responses. *Electroencephalogr Clin Neurophysiol* 1974, 37: 225–230.

Picton TW, Bentin S, Berg P, Donchin E, Hillyard SA, Johnson R Jr, Miller GA, Ritter W, Ruchkin DS, Rugg MD, Taylor MJ: Guidelines for using human event-related potentials to study cognition: recording standards and publication criteria. *Psychophysiology* 2000, 37: 127–152.

Pivik RT, Broughton RJ, Coppola R, Davidson RJ, Fox N, Nuwer MR: Guidelines for the recording and quantitative analysis of electroencephalographic activity in research contexts. *Psychophysiology* 1993, 30: 547–558.

Puce A, Kalnins RM, Berkovic SF, Donnan GA, Bladin PF: Limbic P3 potentials, seizure localization, and surgical pathology in temporal lobe epilepsy. *Ann Neurol* 1989, 26: 377–385.

Raij TT, Vartiainen NV, Jousmäki V, Hari R: Effects of interstimulus interval on cortical responses to painful laser stimulation. *J Clin Neurophysiol* 2003, 20: 73–79.

Regan D: Some characteristics of average steady-state and transient responses evoked by modulated light. *Electroencephalogr Clin Neurophysiol* 1966, 20: 238–248.

Regan D: *Evoked Potentials in Psychology, Sensory Physiology and Clinical Medicine*. London: Chapman and Hall, 1972.

Rossi A, Parada FJ, Kolchinsky A, Puce A: Neural correlates of apparent motion perception of impoverished facial stimuli: a comparison of ERP and ERSP activity. *NeuroImage* 2014, 98: 442–459.

Scherg M, von Cramon D: Two bilateral sources of the late AEP as identified by a spatio-temporal dipole model. *Electroencephalogr Clin Neurophysiol* 1985, 62: 232–244.

Smeds E, Piitulainen H, Bourguignon M, Jousmäki V and Hari R: Effect of interstimulus interval on cortical proprioceptive responses to passive finger movements. *Eur J Neurosci* 2017, 45: 290–298.

Uusitalo M, Williamson S, Seppä M: Dynamical organisation of the human visual system revealed by life-times of activation traces. *Neurosci Lett* 1996, 213: 149–156.

Van der Tweel LH, Lunel HF: Human visual responses to sinusoidally modulated light. *Electroencephalogr Clin Neurophysiol* 1965, 18: 587–598.

Vaughan HG Jr, Ritter W: The sources of auditory evoked responses recorded from the human scalp. *Electroencephalogr Clin Neurophysiol* 1970, 28: 360–367.

Yokosawa K, Pamilo S, Hirvenkari L, Hari R, Pihko E: Activation of auditory cortex by anticipating and hearing emotional sounds: an MEG study. *PLoS One* 2013, 8: e80284.

CHAPTER 13

AUDITORY RESPONSES

No one is as deaf as the man who will not listen.

—PROVERB

I decided it is better to scream. Silence is the real crime against humanity.

—NADEZHDA MANDELSTAM

Neural activity across the various parts of the auditory system can be noninvasively mapped out using MEG and EEG. In this chapter we briefly describe the various types of evoked and event-related responses that can be recorded in response to auditory stimulation. A comprehensive handbook covering the details of recording and analysis of auditory-evoked potentials is available (Hall, 2007), and the early steps of auditory-evoked magnetic fields have been reviewed as well (Hari, 1990).

Auditory-evoked responses are generally grouped into three major categories according to their latencies, as is schematically depicted in Figure 13.1 for electrical responses: (1) brainstem auditory evoked potentials (BAEPs) occur within the first 8–10 ms; here only the most prominent deflection (wave V) is indicated; (2) middle-latency auditory-evoked potentials (MLAEPs) occur within 12 to 50 ms; and (3) long-latency auditory-evoked potentials (LLAEPs) range from about 50 to 250 ms. Due to data-acquisition constraints, brainstem responses are recorded separately from the later evoked responses. Middle-latency and long-latency responses have also frequently been recorded separately, usually because there is interest in one particular part of the response continuum.

Multiple auditory responses are related to change detection (Carbajal & Malmierca, 2018; see Chapter 18) and clinical use is emerging, in addition to auditory-evoked potentials, also for cortical auditory-evoked magnetic fields (Shvarts & Mäkelä, 2020; see Chapter 20).

■ ASPECTS OF AUDITORY STIMULATION

Hearing Threshold

Auditory stimuli are typically presented at fixed levels (in dB) above an individual's hearing threshold. When the aim of the study is not specific to auditory function, it will be enough to first ask the subjects about their hearing and then test their hearing threshold with a single frequency, typically 1 kHz, or with the frequency at which the stimuli are delivered.

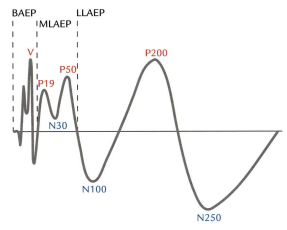

FIGURE 13.1. **Nomenclature of auditory-evoked responses.** A schematic presentation of auditory-evoked potentials. The earliest responses are recorded within 8–10 ms from the brainstem; here only the fifth deflection (wave V) is labeled. The MLAEPs span latencies from about 12 to 50 ms, and the LLAEPs latencies from 50 to 250 ms. The polarities are indicated here with positive up. For MEG, response labels may include an "m" at the end (e.g., N100m).

Even if speech with varying frequencies is delivered, this information is typically satisfactory as it is difficult to adapt the stimulus intensity on-the-fly to match the subject's hearing level at all frequencies.

Testing a subject's hearing thresholds by an audiogram may be necessary in clinical studies, but in these cases a complete audiogram is often already available before the MEG/EEG examination. Once hearing threshold has been determined, the auditory stimuli can be delivered at a constant specified value above the individual's hearing threshold, for example, 70 dB HL (see Chapter 6). Also note that for click stimuli the subjective loudness increases when the click rate is increased, and thus the physical properties of single stimuli as such may not tell the whole story. In some cases, one may ask the participant to subjectively match the intensity of clicks with a continuous tone of known intensity.

Stimulus Type, Duration, Envelope, and Other Characteristics

Commonly used auditory stimuli consist of brief clicks, chirps, and pure-tone stimuli. Clicks (i.e., square-wave pulses of 0.1–1 ms duration) are commonly used to elicit brainstem and middle-latency responses; they contain a broad band of frequencies and thus activate the basilar membrane of the cochlea widely. The shorter the click, the wider the presented frequency spectrum but the lower the loudness; thus compromises have to be made in stimulus selection. Chirps contain an ordered sweep of frequencies, usually from low to high, designed to evenly activate parts of the basilar membrane. In this way, each frequency reaches its sensitive spot on the cochlea at the same time, resulting in synchronous firing in the auditory nerve. Chirps have become the choice stimulus, particularly in clinical BAEP studies testing hearing loss in neonates (Eder et al., 2022).

Tone stimuli are sinusoidal bursts of just one frequency, usually with specific rise and fall times. For example, 30- to 50-ms tone pips are typically shaped with rise and fall times of about 5 ms as abrupt onsets and offsets add the unwanted percept of a click as well as an additional evoked response to the presented tone burst.

Human speech and environmental sounds can also be used as auditory stimuli, but their characteristics are harder to specify, as they have complex spectral content. Frequency spectra or the envelopes of such stimuli are usually included with the published data. However, even natural connected speech can be used as a stimulus in MEG/EEG studies, as we discuss in Chapters 18 and 19.

■ AUDITORY BRAINSTEM RESPONSES

The earliest recordable auditory responses occur within 8 ms from the sound onset in the brainstem within an area a few centimeters in length. The electrical response (the BAEP) was first detected in scalp EEG between the vertex and a reference electrode either on the neck, the earlobe, or the chin (Jewett et al., 1970; Jewett & Williston, 1971). It took time before BAEPs were accepted by the EEG community, partly because the responses were so tiny and also because at that time most researchers working in the field did not really understand volume conduction. Put simply, how could such a small potential change or current be seen so far from its site of origin?

BAEPs are typically elicited by 0.1- to 0.2-ms clicks repeated at about 10 to 20 Hz. Because of the short duration of these stimuli, their intensities, when compared with continuous sounds of the same peak amplitudes (as seen on an oscilloscope), can be as high as 110 to 130 dB SPL (sound pressure level; see Chapter 6). The click can produce an air-pressure wave either *toward* the tympanic membrane in the cochlea (the so-called condensation click) or *away* from the cochlea (rarefaction click), and these two types of clicks elicit BAEPs with slightly different latencies and waveshapes. In clinical settings, the unstimulated ear is commonly masked with white noise during the recording.

Because the BAEPs are only a fraction of a microvolt in size (see Figure 13.2), typically 1,000 to 4,000 artifact-free epochs are collected and averaged to generate reliable waveforms in clinical studies; however, sometimes a few hundred (or just 100) responses are enough to show the main features of the BAEP waveform. (Increasing the number of responses from 100 to 1,000 will improve the signal-to-noise ratio by a factor of $\sqrt{10} = 3.2$). If 4,000 responses are collected, it is preferable to average them in subsets of 1,000 and then super-impose the traces to easily evaluate response replicability.

Clinically, BAEPs are recorded between the vertex and a *unilateral* mastoid/earlobe using amplifier gains of 50,000 to 100,000, bandpass filtering from about 50 to 150 Hz to 2 to 3 kHz, and sampling rates of 8 to 10 kHz. Sometimes clinical BAEPs are recorded to more than one stimulus type, for example to both rarefaction and condensation clicks, or to two stimulus intensities, or to chirps (Eder et al., 2022), to resolve unclear waveforms (Chiappa, 1997).

The successive deflections of brainstem responses are typically identified using Roman numerals from I to VII (or 1 to 7); see Figure 13.2. Each of these seven deflections (conventionally referred to as *waves*) that occur within the first 10 ms after sound delivery have been associated with different brainstem structures, originally identified by clinical lesion data and invasive recordings in animals. For example, wave I reflects the acoustic-nerve action potential and is seen only ipsilateral to the stimulated ear. Wave V is thought to originate in the inferior colliculus/lateral lemniscus (Jewett et al., 1970). BAEP deflections can be useful as a diagnostic test for different brainstem pathologies. For example, in the diagnosis of acoustic neuroma, a tumor of the auditory nerve, abnormalities will be already seen in wave I. Additionally, a very important measure for various brainstem abnormalities is the latency difference between waves I and V (Chiappa, 1997), often called brainstem conduction time.

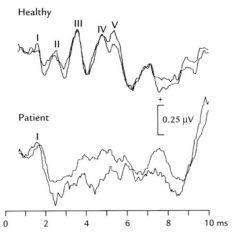

FIGURE 13.2. BAEPs from a healthy person and a patient with brainstem injury. Top: Normal BAEPs from a healthy person to binaurally presented clicks (80 dB SPL, repetition rate 10 Hz) recorded between Fpz and M2. Each trace is the average of about 1,200 single responses. The superimposed traces (that start 0.6 ms after the click onset) indicate good replicability. Bottom: BAEPs from a comatose patient, with an intact wave I and no other visible deflections, suggesting a brainstem lesion. For further details, see the text. Adapted and reprinted from Hari R, Sulkava R, Haltia M: Brainstem auditory evoked responses and alpha-pattern coma. *Ann Neurol* 1982, 11: 187–189. With permission from John Wiley & Sons.

Figure 13.2 (lower traces) shows total abolition of deflections after the acoustic-nerve wave I in a 32-year-old patient who was studied because of unconsciousness of unknown origin. His EEG displayed signs of alpha coma (with unreactive alpha-range oscillations distributed widely across the whole scalp), which is considered to indicate a poor prognosis for recovery. However, alpha coma potentially could be reversible if it was caused by drug intoxication. As no background information was available of the cause of the patient's coma, this recording in the early days of BAEP was diagnostic as it implied a brainstem lesion; a massive pontomesencephalic vascular lesion was confirmed in autopsy (Hari et al., 1982b).

The first brainstem auditory-evoked fields (BAEFs) were demonstrated by averaging 16,000 single responses (Erné et al., 1987) because the magnetic fields from such deep parts of the head are very small outside the head (see Figure 1.4). The simultaneously recorded BAEPs and BAEFs in Figure 13.3 show a correspondence in the timing of the main deflections of the responses but also some differences that indicate that MEG and EEG provide complementary information (Parkkonen et al., 2009). Because of their sources deep in the brainstem, the BAEFs were in this study clearly visible only in magnetometer recordings (see types of flux transformers in Figure 5.15).

It is to be noted that we do not promote BAEFs for clinical use as BAEPs can be collected in a fraction of time. The MEG recordings do demonstrate that it is possible to obtain reliable MEG responses from very deep brain areas.

■ MIDDLE-LATENCY AUDITORY-EVOKED RESPONSES

MLAEPs were first described to click stimuli; the responses peaked at about 30 ms and started to emerge when the stimulus intensity exceeded the sensory threshold (Geisler

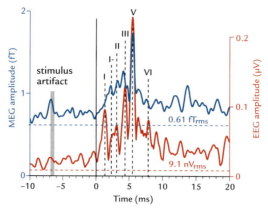

FIGURE 13.3. Simultaneously recorded BAEPs and BAEFs. Grand averages (across seven subjects) of magnetic (blue) and electric (red) auditory brainstem responses. The response latencies have been adjusted so that individual wave V responses overlap. For MEG, root-mean-squared signals are shown across 102 magnetometer channels of a whole-scalp-covering device, and for EEG, the amplitude is in tenths of microvolts recorded at FPz (see Figure 5.6) with respect to M1 (filter setting 180–1000 Hz). Intrinsic noise levels of the respective MEG and EEG systems are indicated by the horizontal lines (generated relative to the same number of averaged responses). Stimulus artifact (grey shading) occurs early as the stimuli were delivered via a 2-m long tube. About 16,000 single responses were averaged. Adapted and reprinted from Parkkonen L, Fujiki N, Mäkelä JP: Sources of auditory brainstem responses revisited: contribution by magnetoencephalography. *Hum Brain Mapp* 2009, 30: 1772–1782. With permission from John Wiley & Sons.

et al., 1958). MLAEPs and their magnetic counterparts (middle-latency auditory-evoked fields [MLAEFs]) occur within the first 50 ms after the delivery of a click or tone (see Figure 13.1 and Figure 13.4, upper panel). The first robust cortical MEG responses appear at 18 to 19 ms (Scherg et al., 1989; Parkkonen et al., 2009) and according to some reports can already be present at 11 ms (Kuriki et al., 1995).

In EEG recordings, MLAEPs are largest at the vertex with respect to an earlobe/mastoid, and they are so resilient to stimulus repetition rate that even 10-Hz click stimulation rates have been used. As already described, MLAEPs peaking at 40 to 60 ms were, on the basis of their scalp topography, suggested to be generated in the primary auditory cortex (Vaughan & Ritter, 1970). To not dampen or abolish the middle-latency responses, the recording band-pass should extend up to 150 Hz, at least (with an appropriate digitization rate, as always; see Chapter 8). A few hundred trials may need to be averaged to visualize good-quality responses.

MLAEPs show similar morphology and timing to MLAEFs. Sequential MLAEP peaks have been named with alphabetic sequences, for example, Pa, Na, Pb, and only in some specific stimulation set-ups the recommended latency-based nomenclature has been used. We recommend using the polarity of the response and its nominal latency, for example, P50 instead of Pb.

◾ LONG-LATENCY AUDITORY-EVOKED RESPONSES

We have already mentioned the LLAEPs that peak about 100 ms after an abrupt sound (Chapter 12). The first recordings of auditory-evoked fields (AEFs) in humans, from only a few locations over the head, showed deflections at 43 to 48 and 98 to 118 ms, in (heavily filtered at 5–15 Hz) responses to click stimuli repeated at 4 Hz but without indication of a source location in the auditory cortex (Reite et al., 1978). Convincing data of the generation of the 100-ms AEFs in the supratemporal auditory were obtained in subsequent MEG recordings (Elberling et al., 1980; Hari et al., 1980).

The P50/P50m, a response that peaks about 50 ms after the stimulus onset, is often considered to be the last middle-latency response (see Figures 13.1 and 13.4) but is sometimes also included in the group of long-latency responses. P50 has been frequently recorded using a "sensory-gating paradigm," where click pairs separated by 500 ms are repeated once every 8 to 10 s. In such a setting, the response to the second stimulus (S2) decreases because the response has not had time to recover (for effects of the ISI on response amplitudes, see Chapter 12), and the amplitude ratio of S2/S1 between responses to the second and first stimulus (S1) has been considered to be an index of sensory gating. Healthy subjects, as a group, have been reported to have lower S2/S1 ratios (indicating stronger suppression of the second response) relative to groups of schizophrenic individuals (Adler et al., 1982; Freedman et al., 1983). This result could be interpreted to reflect stronger inhibition in healthy subjects toward stimuli containing redundant information (Javitt & Sweet, 2015); see also discussion of the role of active inhibition in response suppression (Loveless et al., 1989). However, the reliability of the paired-click findings in various patient populations needs further examination.

The most prominent auditory response, the N100/N100m, peaks around 100 ms after sound onset (Figure 13.4, bottom panel). N100m increases in amplitude, and its peak latency decreases as stimulus duration increases from 5 to 20 ms (Joutsiniemi et al., 1989). Both N100 and N100m are more sensitive to experimental manipulations than are the earlier middle-latency responses, as is usual for long-latency responses. Interestingly, N100/N100m can also be elicited by stimulus offsets (onsets of pauses), and the 100-ms offset response increases in amplitude when the duration of the gap within continuous noise increases (Hari et al., 1987; Joutsiniemi et al., 1989). However, offsets of long stimuli do not trigger the 50-ms response (P50m), indicating that the successive deflections of the auditory-evoked response need not be causally linked.

Although N100 and N100m share many properties, their recovery cycles will differentiate them at longer ISIs. Figure 13.5 (top two panels on left) shows the effect of progressively increasing ISI from 0.5 to 16 s on AEPs recorded from the midline and right temporal scalp relative to a mastoid reference (mast) and show a maximum at the vertex. Up to ISIs of 4 s, the scalp distribution of N100 remains relatively stable in that responses increase to the same extent in all traces. However, at ISIs of 8 and 16 s the increase is clearly strongest in the frontocentral midline (Hari et al., 1982a). The non-similar ISI dependencies at different scalp locations indicate that the electrical N100 cannot be generated by a single fixed source that according to MEG recordings is likely to be in the auditory cortex (or auditory cortices of both hemispheres). Comparison of AEFs and AEPs recorded simultaneously (top right panel) shows an amplitude increase as a function of ISI, but with different rates. Consequently, the amplitude ratio of the electrical N100 and magnetic N100m changes as a function of the ISI (Figure 13.5, lower left panel), which again implies that the two responses cannot—at all ISIs—be explained by the same source(s) (Hari et al., 1982a). Even more support for the rejection of the same-source hypothesis comes from the response latencies (Figure 13.5, lower right panel) that increase by over 20 ms as a function of the ISI for the electrical N100 but remain stable for the magnetic N100m (Tuomisto et al., 1983).

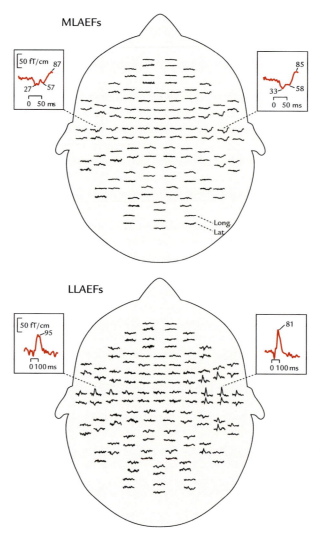

FIGURE 13.4. MLAEFs and LLAEFs. Middle-latency (top) and long-latency (bottom) AEFs of one subject, recorded with the planar gradiometers of a 122-channel whole-scalp-covering device (filter settings 0.03–220 Hz; sampling rate is 723 Hz for MLAEFs and 397 Hz for LLAEFs; averaged MLAEFs have been digitally low-pass filtered at 140 Hz and LLAEFs at 40 Hz). Two traces are shown at each recording location, one from a longitudinal (Long) and the other from a latitudinal (Lat) planar gradiometer. Response amplitudes are largest over temporal areas. The two insets in each figure display magnified examples of MLAEFs and LLAEFs; note their different time scales. Adapted and reprinted from McEvoy L, Mäkelä JP, Hämäläinen M, Hari R: Effect of interaural time differences on middle-latency and late auditory evoked magnetic fields. *Hear Res* 1994, 78: 249–257. With permission from Elsevier.

It can thus be postulated that the electric N100 has at least three sources: modality-specific sources at the supratemporal auditory cortices of both hemispheres and an additional source close to the vertex (Hari et al., 1982a). One likely vertex source could be the supplementary motor area, which is located just anterior to the vertex (Cz electrode

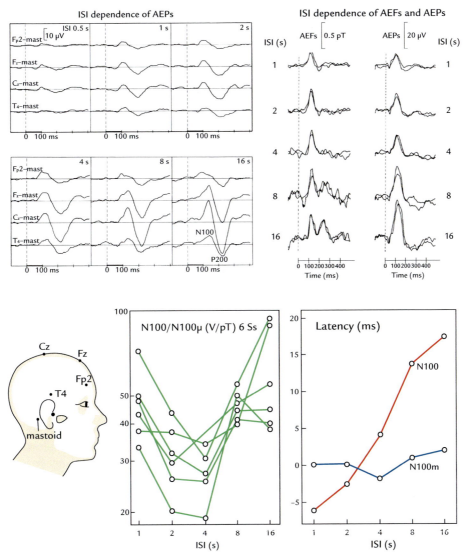

FIGURE 13.5. Effect of ISI on electrical and magnetic long-latency auditory-evoked evoked responses. Top left panels: LLAEPs elicited by 20-ms tone pips at four scalp locations in a single subject (filter passband 0.3–70 Hz; mastoid reference [mast]). The number of averaged responses varied from 128 to 28, depending on the ISI. Top right: Simultaneous recordings of magnetic and electric auditory evoked responses from a single subject at different ISIs. AEFs are from the posterior end of the right Sylvian fissure (first-order axial gradiometer; upward deflections indicate magnetic flux into the skull). AEPs are from a derivation between vertex and right mastoid; negative is up. All top panels adapted and reprinted from Hari R, Kaila K, Katila T, Tuomisto T, Varpula T: Interstimulus-interval dependence of the auditory vertex response and its magnetic counterpart: implications for their neural generation. *Electroencephalogr Clin Neurophysiol* 1982, 54: 561–569. With permission from Elsevier. Bottom left: The 10–20 system electrode locations for the recordings in the top panel are indicated on the schematic head. Bottom middle: The amplitude ratio of the electric N100 and magnetic N100m as a function of ISI for 6 subjects. Adapted and reprinted from Hari

location) and from where long-latency responses to many sensory modalities have been recorded in human intracranial EEG recordings (Libet et al., 1975).

N100/N100m is followed by a deflection of opposite polarity, P200/P200m, and for long (> 500 ms) sound stimuli by a sustained potential/field that MEG recordings imply to be generated at the supratemporal auditory cortex (Hari et al., 1980); see Figure 12.3.

In audition (in contrast to vision and somesthesia), information on stimulus location does not exist at the receptor level, and therefore sound-source locations have to be found centrally from time and intensity differences between the incoming sounds (interaural time and intensity differences, respectively). Quite complex effects can be elicited by varied sounds in a particular experiment. For example, when binaural 600-ms click trains are presented so that in the first half of the recording all clicks were left-ear leading with a time difference of +0.7 ms, and then in the middle of the train (at 300 ms), the interaural difference was changed to +0.4, +0.1, –0.1, –0.4, or –0.7 ms, the amplitude of N100m to the change increases with increasing interaural time differences; the response peaks as late as 130 ms poststimulus, probably due to masking effects introduced by the continued presence of the sound (Sams et al., 1993).

LLAEPs/LLAEFs can be elicited by any abrupt sound onset and even by a change within the stimulus. For example, words that start with a fricative consonant that is followed by a vowel (e.g., /hei/ and /sei/) elicit the normal onset response N100m to sound onset but an additional 100-ms response (which was originally named the N100m') after the transition from consonant to vowel (Kaukoranta et al., 1987) (see Figure 13.6). The occurrence of N100m' can be delayed by prolonging the fricative consonant (e.g., from /hei/ to /hhei/ or /hhhhei/). Although word /ssssei/ evokes a clear N100m', word /eissss/ does not. Similar double responses are elicited by stimuli in which a noise burst is followed by a square-wave sound (Mäkelä et al., 1988). Thus one has to pay attention to the acoustical contents of the stimuli beyond onsets, offsets, and duration.

For long-latency auditory responses, an appropriate recording bandwidth is up to 100 Hz, which can be digitally narrowed to a low-pass of 40 Hz without losing information. Depending on the ISI, averaging 30 to 100 single responses typically gives reliable results.

■ AUDITORY STEADY-STATE RESPONSES

Galambos and colleagues (1981) demonstrated that auditory steady-state responses are largest at stimulus repetition rates of about 40 Hz and likely arise as the superposition of middle-latency responses. The authors thought that these EEG responses are unlikely to be generated in the cerebral cortex mainly because the cortex was thought not to respond to such high frequencies. However, MEG recordings using brief trains of 40-Hz clicks— which elicited the whole sequence of responses at the same time—indicated that even the steady-state responses have a cortical rather than a thalamic origin (Mäkelä & Hari, 1987).

FIGURE 13.5. Continued
R, Kaila K, Katila T, Tuomisto T, Varpula T: Interstimulus-interval dependence of the auditory vertex response and its magnetic counterpart: implications for their neural generation. *Electroencephalogr Clin Neurophysiol* 1982, 54: 561–569. With permission from Elsevier. Bottom right: Relative peak latencies as a function of ISI for N100 (red line) and N100m (blue line) for the same subjects. Adapted and reprinted from Tuomisto T, Hari R, Katila T, Poutanen T, Varpula T: Studies of auditory evoked magnetic and electric responses: modality specificity and modelling. *Il Nuovo Cimento* 1983, 2D: 471–494. With permission of Springer.

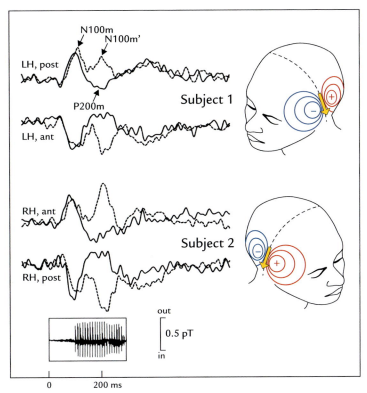

FIGURE 13.6. Auditory-evoked fields to sound onsets and to changes within the sound. AEFs of two subjects to /hei/ words (dashed lines) where a 100-ms fricative consonant /h/ preceded the vowels /ei/ (the acoustic waveform is shown beneath the traces) and to equal-duration noise bursts (solid lines). Recording passband 0.05 to 100 Hz, sampling rate 500 Hz; the averaged responses (N = 120) have been low-pass filtered at 50 Hz. For Subject 1 (top panel), the recordings are from the left hemisphere (LH) where the magnetic flux during N100m and N100m' emerges from the skull (red isocontour lines) at the posterior (post) end of the Sylvian fissure and enters the skull (blue isocontour lines) at the anterior (ant) end. For Subject 2 (bottom panel), the recordings are from the right hemisphere (RH); note that now the flux emerges from the skull anteriorly and enters at the posterior end of the Sylvian fissure. Thus the magnetic field patterns follow—in both hemispheres—the right-hand rule on the basis of the currents (indicated by yellow arrows) in the supratemporal auditory cortex. A first-order axial gradiometer was used. Adapted and reprinted from Kaukoranta E, Hari R, Lounasmaa OV: Responses of the human auditory cortex to vowel onset after fricative consonants. *Exp Brain Res* 1987, 69: 19–23. With permission of Springer.

Of course this claim does not rule out the likely possibility that, at about the same time, considerable activity also exists in the thalamus.

Because the largest amplitudes of the steady-state responses occur at 40 Hz, 40 Hz has often been noted to be a type of "resonant frequency" in the brain. However, one can build up a large 40-Hz response just by linearly summing up cumulative responses to 10 Hz stimulation (Hari et al., 1989) (Figure 13.7, right lower panels). Thus one does not need to necessarily propose the existence of any *resonance* as we explained in Chapter 11; however,

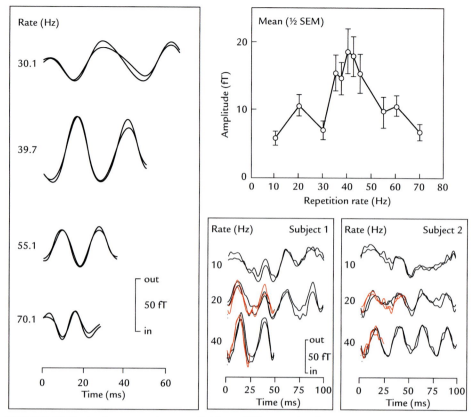

FIGURE 13.7. Auditory steady-state fields at different stimulus repetition rates. Left: SSFs (averages of about 1,000 single traces of two cycles each) in one subject to 0.5-ms clicks presented at four repetition rates. The passband was 0.05 to 100 Hz. Top right: Mean ± SEM (standard errors of the mean) SSF amplitudes from 10 subjects as a function of stimulus repetition rate. Bottom right: Averaged responses of two subjects with a wider passband of 0.05 to 250 Hz and a larger number (1,500–1,800) of averaged responses. The black traces show measured SSFs at repetition rates of 10.1, 20.1, and 40.1 Hz, with replications superimposed. The superimposed red traces show synthetic responses computed by assuming that each click in the 20.1-Hz and 40.1-Hz rates elicits identical responses to those obtained at the 10.1-Hz rate. In other words, the 10.1-Hz responses were shifted by times corresponding to the stimulation rates at 20.1 and 40.1 Hz (i.e., by about 40 ms and by 25 ms) and averaged. The high similarity of the measured and synthetized responses indicates that the amplitudes of the single responses remained the same irrespective of stimulus repetition rate (from 10 to 40 Hz). Thus the amplitude enhancement cannot be considered as a sign of resonance as understood in physics. Reproduced from Hari R, Hämäläinen M, Joutsiniemi SL: Neuromagnetic steady-state responses to auditory stimuli. *J Acoust Soc Am* 1989, 86: 1033–1039, with the permission of Acoustical Society of America.

it seems likely that the characteristics of brain structure and function may favor the development of activity at certain frequencies. Simulations using slightly different waveforms for the single responses demonstrated that the amplitude of the steady-state response at a 40 Hz stimulation rate strongly depends on the waveforms of the single responses (Hari et al., 1989). These same considerations are relevant for visual steady-state responses (see Chapter 14).

■ FREQUENCY TAGGING

From each ear, the auditory pathways project to the auditory cortices of both hemispheres. During simultaneous binaural stimulation, it is thus not possible to determine which part of the response derives from the left or the right ear. One solution to this problem is to "tag" the input sounds with amplitude modulations that have different frequencies at both ears.

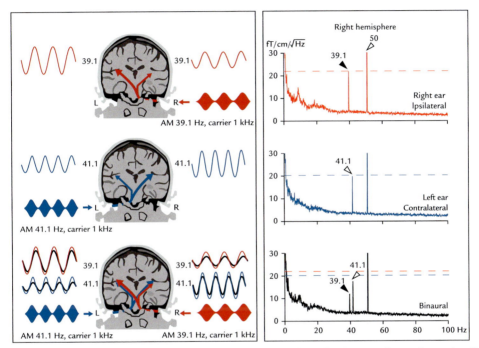

FIGURE 13.8. Frequency tagging used to study binaural mechanisms. Left: A schematic of the recording setup and stimulated auditory pathways. Continuous 1-kHz carrier tones are amplitude modulated (AM) at different frequencies (39.1 Hz for the right ear, 41.1 Hz for the left ear) so that the elicited responses are "frequency tagged". Because auditory pathways project more strongly to the contralateral than the ipsilateral hemisphere, the SSFs are larger for contralateral than ipsilateral stimuli. During binaural stimulation (lowest panel), the responses (black lines) are far below to the sum of left- and right-ear responses (blue and red lines); in fact, they are smaller than any unilateral response. We thank Dr. Ken-ichi Kaneko for originally drafting this figure. Right: Frequency-domain responses over the right hemisphere to the stimuli presented in the left panel. Both unilateral stimuli produce sharp peaks at the tagging frequency; line artifact is visible at 50 Hz (top two plots). During binaural stimulation (bottom plot), both peaks are suppressed, the ipsilateral response (at 39.1 Hz) considerably more than the contralateral one (at 41.1 Hz); the horizontal dashed lines give the amplitude levels of responses to unilateral contralateral (red) and ipsilateral (blue) stimuli. Adapted and reprinted from Kaneko K-I, Fujiki N, Hari R: Binaural interaction in the human auditory cortex revealed by neuromagnetic frequency tagging: no effect of stimulus intensity. *Hear Res* 2003, 183: 1–6. With permission from Elsevier.

One can then record steady-state responses at two respective frequencies from each auditory cortex.

Figure 13.8 shows such a situation schematically, following a real experimental set-up (Kaneko et al., 2003). During unilateral stimulation, a 1-kHz carrier tone is amplitude-modulated at 39.1 Hz in the right ear and at 41.1 Hz in the left ear. The resulting steady-state responses are clearly stronger in the contralateral than the ipsilateral hemisphere (two top left panels). During binaural stimulation, the responses (black traces) are much smaller than the sum of responses to unilateral stimulation and even smaller than responses to con-tralateral stimulation. Moreover, compared with unilateral stimulation, during binaural stimulation the responses to ipsilateral stimulation are suppressed more than the responses to contralateral stimulation in both hemispheres; this effect can be seen very clearly in the frequency spectra of Figure 13.8 (right). The functional consequences of this suppression could be that during binaural stimulation each hemisphere becomes more tuned to the contralateral auditory space (Fujiki et al., 2002; Kaneko et al., 2003). Such an interaural interaction agrees with findings of responses to brief tones as the 100-ms MEG responses to binaural tones are not sums of responses to unilateral left- and right-ear stimulations but rather much smaller, even smaller than the responses to contralateral sounds presented alone (Tiihonen et al., 1989).

The tagging frequencies should not be multiples of one another or have common multiples or divisors with the line frequency (50 or 60 Hz). For example, Fujiki and collaborators (2002) used modulation frequencies of 20.1 and 26.1 Hz and Kaneko et al. (2003) used 39.1 and 41.1 Hz (as in Figure 13.8).

One example of the power of frequency tagging is the demonstration of impaired interaural interaction in a group of dyslexic subjects with weak expression of the ROBO1 gene, which regulates midline crossing of major nerve tracts (Lamminmäki et al., 2012). The weakened midline crossing of auditory pathways was not visible in structural diffusion tensor imaging.

Note that this kind of frequency tagging works best when the elicited responses are large, as it would be for 100% amplitude modulations of continuous tones or noise. In music and speech, as well as in other natural sounds, the amplitude varies constantly, and the responses to amplitude modulations are smaller although in many cases still recordable (Lamminmäki et al., 2014).

■ REFERENCES

Adler LE, Pachtman E, Franks RD, Pecevich M, Waldo MC, Freedman R: Neurophysiological evidence for a defect in neuronal mechanisms involved in sensory gating in schizophrenia. *Biol Psychiatry* 1982, 17: 639–654.

Carbajal GV, Malmierca MS: The neuronal basis of predictive coding along the auditory pathway: from the subcortical roots to cortical deviance detection. *Trends Hear* 2018, 22: 2331216518784822.

Chiappa KH: *Evoked Potentials in Clinical Medicine*, 3rd ed. Philadelphia, PA: Lippincott Williams & Wilkins, 1997.

Eder K, Polterauer D, Semmelbauer S, Schuster M, Rader T, Hoster E, Flatz W: Comparison of ABR and ASSR using narrow-band-chirp-stimuli in children with cochlear malformation and/or cochlear nerve hypo-plasia suffering from severe/profound hearing loss. *Eur Arch Otorhinolaryngol* 2022, 279: 2845–2855.

Elberling C, Bak C, Kofoed B, Lebech J, Saermark K: Magnetic auditory responses from the human brain: a preliminary report. *Scand Audiol* 1980, 9: 185–190.

Erné SN, Scheer HJ, Hoke M, Pantew C, Lütkenhöner B: Brainstem auditory evoked magnetic fields in response to stimulation with brief tone pulses. *Int J Neurosci* 1987, 37: 115–125.

Freedman R, Adler LE, Waldo MC, Pachtman E, Franks RD: Neurophysiological evidence for a defect in inhibitory pathways in schizophrenia: comparison of medicated and drug-free patients. *Biol Psychiatry* 1983, 18: 537–551.

Fujiki N, Jousmäki V, Hari R: Neuromagnetic responses to frequency-tagged sounds: a new method to follow inputs from each ear to the human auditory cortex during binaural hearing. *J Neurosci* 2002, 22, RC205: 1–4.

Galambos R, Makeig S, Talmachoff PJ: A 40-Hz auditory potential recorded from the human scalp. *Proc Natl Acad Sci U S A* 1981, 78: 2643–2647.

Geisler CD, Frishkopf LS, Rosenblith WA: Extracranial responses to acoustic clicks in man. *Science* 1958, 128: 1210–1211.

Hall JWI: *New Handbook of Auditory Evoked Responses*. Boston: Pearson, 2007.

Hari R, Aittoniemi K, Järvinen ML, Katila T, Varpula T: Auditory evoked transient and sustained magnetic fields of the human brain: localization of neural generators. *Exp Brain Res* 1980, 40: 237–240.

Hari R, Kaila K, Katila T, Tuomisto T, Varpula T: Interstimulus-interval dependence of the auditory vertex response and its magnetic counterpart: implications for their neural generation. *Electroencephalogr Clin Neurophysiol* 1982a, 54: 561–569.

Hari R, Sulkava R, Haltia M: Brainstem auditory evoked responses and alpha-pattern coma. *Ann Neurol* 1982b, 11: 187–189.

Hari R, Pelizzone M, Mäkelä JP, Hällström J, Leinonen L, Lounasmaa OV: Neuromagnetic responses of the human auditory cortex to on- and offsets of noise bursts. *Audiology* 1987, 25: 31–43.

Hari R, Hämäläinen M, Joutsiniemi SL: Neuromagnetic steady-state responses to auditory stimuli. *J Acoust Soc Am* 1989, 86: 1033–1039.

Hari R: The neuromagnetic method in the study of the human auditory cortex. In: Grandori F, Hoke M, Romani G, eds. Auditory Evoked Magnetic Fields and Potentials. *Advances in Audiology*, Vol 6, 1st ed. Basel, Switzerland: Karger, 1990: 222–282.

Javitt DC, Sweet RA: Auditory dysfunction in schizophrenia: integrating clinical and basic features. *Nat Rev Neurosci* 2015, 16: 535–550.

Jewett D, Romano M, Williston J: Human auditory evoked potentials: possible brain stem components detected on the scalp. *Science* 1970, 167: 1517–1518.

Jewett DL, Williston JS: Auditory-evoked far fields averaged from the scalp of humans. *Brain* 1971, 94: 681–696.

Joutsiniemi SL, Hari R, Vilkman V: Cerebral magnetic responses to noise bursts and pauses of different durations. *Audiology* 1989, 28: 325–333.

Kaneko K-I, Fujiki N, Hari R: Binaural interaction in the human auditory cortex revealed by neuromagnetic frequency tagging: no effect of stimulus intensity. *Hear Res* 2003, 183: 1–6.

Kaukoranta E, Hari R, Lounasmaa OV: Responses of the human auditory cortex to vowel onset after fricative consonants. *Exp Brain Res* 1987, 69: 19–23.

Kuriki S, Nogai T, Hirata Y: Cortical sources of middle latency responses of auditory evoked magnetic field. *Hear Res* 1995, 92: 47–51.

Lamminmäki S, Massinen S, Nopola-Hemmi J, Kere J, Hari R: Human ROBO1 regulates interaural interaction in auditory pathways. *J Neurosci* 2012, 32: 966–971.

Lamminmäki S, Parkkonen L, Hari R: Human neuromagnetic steady-state responses to amplitude-modulated tones, speech, and music. *Ear Hear* 2014, 35: 461–467.

Libet B, Alberts W, Wright EJ, Lewis M, Feinstein B: Cortical representation of evoked potentials relative to conscious sensory responses, and of somatosensory qualities – in man. In: Albe-Fessard D, Kornhuber HH, eds. *The Somatosensory System*. Stuttgart: Thieme, 1975: 291–307.

Loveless N, Hari R, Hämäläinen M, Tiihonen J: Evoked responses of human auditory cortex may be enhanced by preceding stimuli. *Electroencephalogr Clin Neurophysiol* 1989, 74: 217–227.

Mäkelä J, Hari R: Evidence for cortical origin of the 40-Hz auditory evoked response in man. *Electroencephalogr Clin Neurophysiol* 1987, 66: 539–546.

Mäkelä JP, Hari R, Leinonen L: Magnetic responses of the human auditory cortex to noise/tone-transitions. *Electroencephalogr Clin Neurophysiol* 1988, 69: 423–430.

Parkkonen L, Fujiki N, Mäkelä JP: Sources of auditory brainstem responses revisited: contribution by magnetoencephalography. *Hum Brain Mapp* 2009, 30: 1772–1782.

Reite M, Edrich J, Zimmerman JT, Zimmerman JE: Human magnetic auditory evoked fields. *Electroencephalogr Clin Neurophysiol* 1978, 45: 114–117.

Sams M, Hämäläinen M, Hari R, McEvoy L: Human auditory cortical mechanisms of sound lateralization: I. Interaural time differences within sound. *Hear Res* 1993, 67: 89–97.

Scherg M, Hari R, Hämäläinen M: Frequency-specific sources of the auditory N19–P30 detected by a multiple source analysis of evoked magnetic fields and potentials. In: Williamson SJ, Hoke M, Stroink G, Kotani M, eds. *Advances in Biomagnetism*. New York: Plenum Press, 1989: 97–100.

Shvarts V, Mäkelä JP: Auditory mapping with MEG: an update on the current state of clinical research and practice with considerations for clinical practice guidelines. *J Clin Neurophysiol* 2020, 37: 574–584.

Tiihonen J, Hari R, Kaukoranta E, Kajola M: Interaural interaction on the human auditory cortex. *Audiology* 1989, 28: 37–48.

Tuomisto T, Hari R, Katila T, Poutanen T, Varpula T: Studies of auditory evoked magnetic and electric responses: modality specificity and modelling. *Il Nuovo Cimento* 1983, 2D: 471–494.

Vaughan HG Jr., Ritter W: The sources of auditory evoked responses recorded from the human scalp. *Electroencephalogr Clin Neurophysiol* 1970, 28: 360–367.

VISUAL RESPONSES

Gracias a la vida que me ha dado tanto
Me dio dos luceros que cuando los abro
Perfecto distingo lo negro del blanco
Y en el alto cielo su fondo estrellado
Y en las multitudes el hombre que yo amo.

VIOLETA PARRA

The only thing worse than being blind is having sight but no vision.

HELEN KELLER

■ INTRODUCTION

In Chapter 14, we described the twentieth-century beginnings of noninvasive measurements of electrical brain activity via EEG and MEG. Figure 4.1 featured a recording from the eye of a water beetle, showing alpha-like rhythms that were indistinguishable from human brain electrical activity recorded by Lord Adrian in the 1930s. At that time, it was already known that it is possible to record electrical activity to light stimuli from both the brain and the retina.

After Dawson's demonstration of evoked-response averaging in 1947, several researchers (Mary Brazier, Horace Barlow, Will Cobb, and Dawson himself [Regan, 1989]) demonstrated visual evoked potentials (VEPs) in human scalp EEG. Because of some debate regarding the origin of these responses in the brain or in the retina, Cobb and Dawson (1960) recorded both the electroretinogram (ERG) and VEPs simultaneously to flash stimuli. Their observation of longer VEP than ERG latencies supported the cerebral origin of the VEPs. Later work began to use pattern-reversing checkerboard stimuli that elicit robust VEPs over the posterior scalp. These responses consist of three main deflections—N75, P100, and N135—with the exact latencies varying as a function of stimulus characteristics. Among others, P100 has been used to assess the integrity of the optic nerve, as prolonged latencies from one eye typically indicate optic neuritis, which is commonly associated with multiple sclerosis.

Magnetic visual evoked fields (VEFs) were first reported in 1975 by two groups. Teyler and collaborators (1975) recorded transient evoked responses, with main peaks around 100 ms, to flash stimuli of different intensities repeated at 1 Hz 100 times. The recordings were obtained with a magnetometer in the Massachusetts Institute of Technology magnetically shielded room. Brenner and colleagues (1975), on the other hand, used a second-order axial gradiometer that allowed them to make the recordings without shielding in the middle of New York's Manhattan; to improve the signal-to-noise ratio, they averaged 1,000 steady-state responses (SSRs) to black-and-white grating presented at 10 Hz. In both studies, the signals implied clear connections to visual processing without any further physiological implications.

Here we start our visual neurophysiological tour by discussing visual stimuli, their attributes, and ways of presentation. We next turn to electrical and magnetic activity generated by the retina and then to activity arising from the brain. We describe various types of visual evoked responses triggered by simple visual stimuli, such as light flashes and gratings/checkerboards, and by higher-level stimuli, such as objects, faces, and words. The responses to moving and naturalistic visual stimuli round out this chapter.

■ VISUAL STIMULI

The VEPs/VEFs can be elicited by myriad stimuli, such as flashing lights, pattern onsets/offsets, pattern reversals, and natural images. The responses are affected by the physical attributes of the stimuli, such as the overall stimulus luminance and contrast, size and eccentricity, spatial and temporal frequency, stimulus complexity, and type of display device. Hence, stimulus standardization is essential for clinical VEP/VEF studies (for reviews, see Chiappa, 1997; Odom et al., 2016).

Visual Acuity

Subjects who require visual correction in daily life should participate in MEG/EEG studies with the same visual correction. If the visual stimuli appear blurred, the VEPs/VEFs will be dampened and delayed. Moreover, poor fixation will increase spontaneous alpha activity in the posterior brain areas and potentially compromise the evoked responses' signal-to-noise ratio.

Distance and Visual Angle of the Stimulus

The distance to the screen/image is measured from the level of the subject's eyes. The horizontal and vertical visual angles subtended by the visual stimulus can be calculated using basic trigonometric principles, as shown in Figure 14.1.

Foveal, Parafoveal, and Extrafoveal Stimulation

VEPs/VEFs will differ from stimuli presented in various parts of the visual field. The fovea (also called the central fovea, with its exact center often called the foveola) contains only cones and is responsible for high-resolution vision. It subtends about 2° of visual angle, which is 1° either side of the visual fixation point. (One degree of visual angle is approximately the size of a thumbnail when the arm is held fully extended.) Stimuli presented within the 2° of visual angle are called foveal, those within 5° are parafoveal, and extrafoveal stimuli extend beyond 5° of eccentricity. Together, these areas of sharp vision make up the macula, with a diameter of about 17°. It is also common to differentiate central and peripheral vision, but there can be variations in how this is specified. Sometimes the border is drawn at 30° eccentricity, assuming a 60° diameter for central vision (Strasburger et al., 2011), but peripheral vision can also be considered to cover over 99% of the visual field (Rosenholtz, 2016).

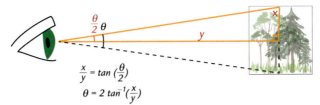

$$\frac{x}{y} = \tan\left(\frac{\theta}{2}\right)$$

$$\theta = 2 \tan^{-1}\left(\frac{x}{y}\right)$$

FIGURE 14.1. **Calculation of visual angle.** To calculate horizontal and vertical angles subtended by a visual stimulus, one must measure the distance of the visual display to the subject's eyes and the respective horizontal and vertical sizes of the stimulus on the display. In the example, visual angle is calculated for the vertical extension of the stimulus. In the right-angled triangle, the opposite x equals half the height of the stimulus, and the adjacent y equals the distance from the subject's eyes to the display; the angle in this triangle is $\theta/2$. The visual angle θ for the total height $2x$ of the stimulus is then, according to basic trigonometry, $2 \tan^{-1}(x/y)$ as is indicated in the figure ($\tan^{-1}$ is inverse tangent); the visual angles are typically expressed in degrees. Once measured at the start of the study, landmarks drawn or stuck on the floor in the lab (for subject chair and visual display) can ensure a constant visual angle during the course of the entire study.

Receptive field (RF) size and cortical magnification factor (CMF) need to be mentioned here. RF refers to the visual space that is commonly coded by a single neuron or group of neurons in a particular brain region, and CMF indicates how many millimeters on the surface of the cortex are devoted to 1° of visual angle (or skin area in the somatosensory system). Both RF and CMF change as a function of visual eccentricity. In the primary visual cortex, RFs are small and CMFs are large, whereas in extrastriate visual regions, RFs are large and the CMFs small. The CMF is 10 to 100 times higher for foveal than for peripheral vision.

Luminance and Contrast

Luminance of a stimulus can be measured with a well-calibrated photometer directly from the visual display, separately for the white area and black area of a black-and-white stimulus, such as a grating or checkerboard pattern. For complex stimuli, such as faces and landscapes, however, this procedure is not feasible. Instead, one may (a) use a visual display that has been calibrated using specific color test stimuli with a photometer and (b) measure and compute the mean and standard deviations of the pixel values of brightness and contrast over the entire stimulus image using image-processing software. For complex images, this latter measurement procedure has to be performed on every stimulus exemplar. For color stimuli, additional quantification of overall red–green–blue (RGB) values may also be helpful. If stimuli have a regular structure, such as checkerboards or gratings, their visibility (Michelson contrast) can be calculated by dividing the difference of the two luminance extrema by their sum. The luminance values can be measured with a photometer.

Another important feature to measure and specify is the background on which the stimuli are presented. Variations in background color and contrast relative to presented stimuli can modify the VEPs/VEFs. It is preferable that the stimuli arise from a background that has the mean luminance of all stimuli so that large nonspecific responses to luminance changes at stimulus onsets can be minimized. For color stimuli, the mean RGB value for the entire stimulus set can serve as a background if a uniform background is required.

Spatial Frequency

For periodic stimuli, such as gratings and checkerboard patterns, the spatial frequency is most typically expressed as cycles/degree of visual angle. For more complex stimuli, such as, for example, faces and landscapes, the spatial frequency must be approximated for example by calculating a range of spatial frequencies (in two dimensions) in units such as cycles/face, cycles/image, or cycles/degree of visual angle (Jeantet et al., 2018).

The effects of the higher-frequency details, such as facial wrinkles and eyelashes, can be eliminated by spatial low-pass filtering (e.g., at four cycles/degree), and these details can be highlighted by spatial high-pass filtering (Figure 14.2; Obayashi et al., 2009). The image is typically filtered in two dimensions using a 2D Fourier transform.

VEPs to faces filtered through 6.7–22.6 cycles/face do not differ from those elicited to unfiltered faces (Collin et al., 2012). The spatial frequency of faces, objects, and complex

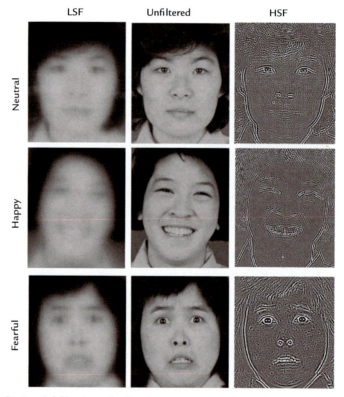

FIGURE 14.2. **Spatial filtering of a face image.** Images of a neutral, happy, and fearful face (top, middle, and bottom rows, respectively) are shown in the original (unfiltered) form in the middle column. The left column shows a blurred face that has been spatially low-pass filtered keeping only the low spatial frequencies (LSF) < 4.0 cycles/face. Fine details such as any wrinkles or facial creases are lost. The right column displays the high spatial frequencies (HSF) > 30.0 cycles/face. Only the fine details such as facial creases and outlines of the eyes, mouth, and teeth are seen. Adapted and reproduced from Obayashi C, Nakashima T, Onitsuka T, Maekawa T, Hirano Y, Hirano S, Oribe N, Kaneko K, Kanba S, Tobimatsu S: Decreased spatial frequency sensitivities for processing faces in male patients with chronic schizophrenia. *Clin Neurophysiol* 2009, 120: 1525–1533. With permission from Elsevier.

scenes can be manipulated also by pixelation and noise masking. However, the spatial-frequency problem is a thorny one in practice because of the retina's nonuniform sensitivity to spatial frequencies (see discussion on multifocal responses below). Additionally, in naturalistic viewing conditions, biases may arise in spatial frequencies as people tend to gaze at important objects, such as faces, in central vision, whereas other less relevant details in a scene tend to remain in the periphery (Levy et al., 2001). For the effects of spatial frequency of complex stimuli on brain activity, see recent reviews (Groen et al., 2017; Jeantet et al., 2018).

■ ELECTRORETINOGRAM AND MAGNETORETINOGRAM

The term *Elektroretinogramm* was first coined by Kahn and Löwenstein in 1924 to describe electrical potentials that occurred in the retina due to changes in visual input (for a review, see Kantola et al., 2019). The first recordings of retinal potentials date to the latter part of the nineteenth century, when the Swedish physiologist Frithiof Holmgren presented evidence in 1866 that light falling on the retina could produce electrical potentials. However, due to the anglocentric nature of science of the day, and because Holmgren had published his findings in Swedish, the credit for the discovery of the ERG is often given to the 1873 publications of Dewar and McKendrick (1873a, 1873b), working in the United Kingdom.

The ERG is typically recorded from electrodes that have been embedded in corneal contact lenses (for a recent review, see Creel, 2019) or less often with EEG electrodes located near the eyes, for example, between the eye and the nose.

In addition to the ERG, it is possible to record the associated magnetic fields, known as a magnetoretinogram (MRG). The first MRG recordings were made with an axial gradiometer close to the eye (Aittoniemi et al., 1979; Katila et al., 1981), similar to the recording in Figure 9.5d, and very recently MRG has been also recorded with optically pumped magnetometers (Westner et al., 2021). The main deflections of both MRG and ERG responses occur at poststimulus latencies shorter than 60 ms, with some slower deflections around 150 ms. Ambient light level can largely affect the amplitudes and latencies of both MRGs and ERGs. Thus, two types of responses can be recorded: one related to photopic (regular daylight) and the other to scotopic (low-light or night) vision. Glial cells (specifically Müller cells) contribute to the longer-latency ERG deflections (Galambos & Juhasz, 1997).

■ VISUAL EVOKED POTENTIALS AND FIELDS

The main deflections of VEPs and VEFs display a characteristic topography, where the VEF pattern is rotated by 90º relative to VEP distribution, thus both agreeing partially with the same current sources in the visual cortices. Figure 14.3 shows this kind of orthogonal VEP and VEF pattern in response to quadrantic checkerboard stimulation, with activation in the right visual cortex to left visual field (LVF) stimuli and in the left visual cortex to right visual field (RVF) stimuli, as expected due to the crossing of the visual pathways.

Invasive recordings in human medial striate and peristriate cortex show polarity reversed P100/N100 to checkerboard pattern reversals, with P100 in the more dorsal and N100 in the more ventral occipital pole (Allison et al., 1999). Source modeling of scalp VEPs, using fMRI data as seeds to constrain source locations, agrees with these intracranially specified source sites (Di Russo et al., 2007).

Complex stimuli, such as faces and objects, elicit multiphasic evoked responses that in intracranial recordings can be seen in widespread areas of lateral and ventral visually sensitive cortex (Allison et al., 1994; Puce et al., 1999), as we discuss below. Still, various

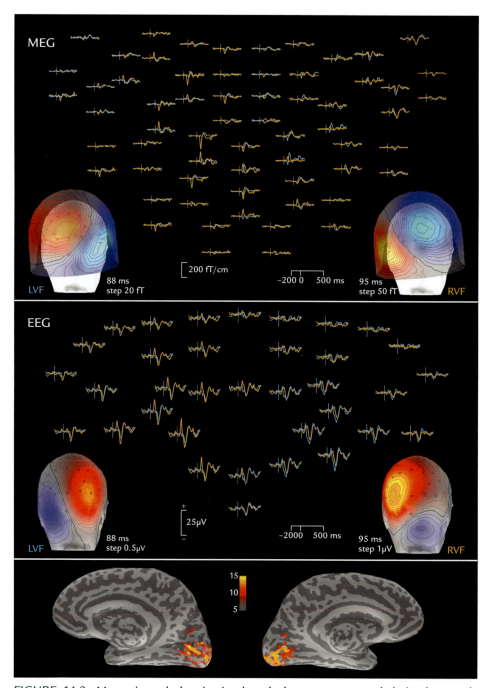

FIGURE 14.3. Magnetic and electric visual evoked responses recorded simultaneously from a single subject. Upper panel: VEFs recorded with a 306-channel neuromagnetometer, shown for planar gradiometers over the posterior part of the head in pairs where the upper and lower traces display two orthogonal gradients fields. Left and right lower-quadrantic checkerboard stimuli were presented to left (LVF) and right (RVF) visual fields (LVF, blue traces; RVF, orange traces) once every 600–800 ms, and ~60 single responses were averaged; passband = 0.1 to 40 Hz. The heads displayed from the back show the field patterns at the

stimuli preferentially evoke responses in different brain regions: edges in early visual cortices V1/V2 and faces/objects in higher-order visual regions in temporal and lateral occipital cortex, converging with functional magnetic resonance imaging (fMRI) and positron emission tomographic (PET) findings. The complex anatomy of the occipital visual cortex and the closeness of several active areas poses a real challenge for source modeling, as has been demonstrated by simulations including realistic source areas in the visual cortices (Stenbacka et al., 2002).

The main principle of cortical activation by stimuli applied to different parts of the visual field (in so-called retinotopic mapping) can be understood by considering the cruciform model of the primary visual (striate) cortex (Jeffreys & Axford, 1972). Figure 14.4 (left) shows the model schematically, as seen from an oblique coronal slice through V1 and V2 cortices. Briefly, this model assumes that (a) the left visual field is mapped to the right hemisphere (striate cortex) and vice versa, and (b) the upper visual field is mapped to the lower part of the striate cortex and vice versa. The arrows in the figure illustrate the locations of the most likely neural sources for quadrantic visual stimuli.

In general, retinotopic MEG recordings are in reasonably good agreement with the cruciform model, although they can show considerable interindividual variation (Ahlfors et al., 1992; Aine et al., 1996). The cruciform model also helps to clarify the reported "paradoxical lateralization" of VEPs: hemifield visual stimuli that activate the contralateral visual cortex, much of which is in the mesial surface of the hemisphere, typically elicit the largest VEP amplitudes on the scalp *ipsilateral* to the stimulus. The reason is that the source currents in the active mesial cortex point in the direction of the recording electrode on the contralateral occipital scalp (Barett et al., 1976) (Figure 14.4, right). Note, however, that if sources of the scalp EEG signals are modeled, the currents will be correctly located in the contralateral hemisphere. A similar paradoxical lateralization occurs after somatosensory stimulation of the foot, which activates the contralateral primary somatosensory cortex in the mesial wall of the parietal cortex and elicits larger potentials on the ipsilateral than the contralateral scalp (Cruse et al., 1982) (see Chapter 15).

Importantly, visual responses whose polarities change as predicted by the cruciform model do not necessarily reflect activity of V1 cortex (only) because similar contributions may be obtained from V2 as well (Ales et al., 2010). During natural viewing when the gaze is not constrained, different parts of the cruciform visual cortex are activated at the same time, leading to very complex VEP/VEF distributions. In general, it is easier to interpret the VEF than the VEP patterns because the radial currents are largely invisible in MEG recordings. Similarly, with regard to the cruciform model, MEG recordings have been easier to interpret, as Figure 14.5 illustrates.

FIGURE 14.3. Continued
peaks of the responses (at 88 ms and 95 ms, respectively). Middle panel: VEPs from the back of the head. Other details as for the VEFs but the heads display potential distributions. Lower panel: Statistically significant source current estimates, derived from dynamic statistical parametric mapping (dSPM; see Dale AM, Liu AK, Fischl BR, Buckner RL, Belliveau JW, Lewine JD, Halgren E: Dynamic statistical parametric mapping: combining fMRI and MEG for high-resolution imaging of cortical activity. *Neuron* 2000, 26: 55–67). Courtesy of Seppo Ahlfors and Matti Hämäläinen, Athinoula A. Martinos Center for Biomedical Imaging, Massachusetts General Hospital, Charlestown, MA, USA.

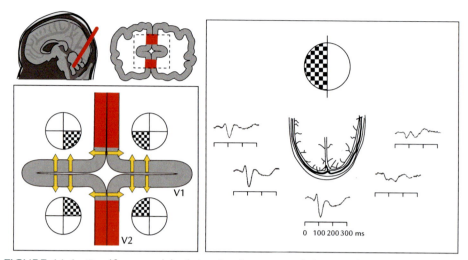

FIGURE 14.4. Cruciform model of the visual cortex and the paradoxical localization of visual evoked potentials. Left: An oblique coronal slice through the posterior aspect of the brain (top left) and its schematic cross section is displayed at top right, with the broken-lined box expanded on bottom left. In this cruciform model (viewed from back), the striate (calcarine) cortex (V1) is represented with gray shading, and extrastriate cortex (V2) with red shading. Maximum sensitivity to checkerboard stimulation in different quadrants is depicted. Left V1 responds to right visual field and right V1 to left visual field stimulation. Similarly, inferior calcarine cortex responds to upper visual field and the superior V1 to lower visual field. The yellow arrows represent current flow from the surface to the depth of cortex in brain areas responding to quadrantic visual stimulation according to this cruciform model. Right: Paradoxical localization of visual evoked potentials to left-hemifield checkerboard stimulation. Recordings are from five electrodes (spaced at 5 cm distances) over the posterior scalp relative to an anterior midline scalp reference; the horizontal brain slice is viewed from above. The largest VEP occurs over the left scalp, because source currents in the right mesial occipital cortex point up, toward the left posterior scalp. VEPs are averages of 200 single responses. Adapted and reprinted from Barett G, Blumhardt L, Halliday AM, Halliday E, Kriss A: A paradox in the lateralization of the visual evoked response. *Nature* 1976, 261: 253–255. With permission from Macmillan Publishers Ltd.

■ MULTIFOCAL VISUAL EVOKED RESPONSES

EEG and MEG can detect reliable neural responses to very subtle and fine-grained visual stimulation, as we discuss explicitly in this section.

The human visual system has two broad divisions that start in the retina. The magnocellular (M) system is important for detection of low-brightness/low-contrast and moving stimuli, with its receptors (rods) distributed across the peripheral retina. The parvocellular (P) system responds preferentially to high-brightness/high-contrast, high-spatial frequencies and color information, and its receptors (cones) are concentrated in the foveal and parafoveal regions. We thus have high sensitivity for detail and color in the central visual field and a preference for motion (and high temporal frequencies but low spatial frequencies) in the peripheral visual field. This segregated M and P information travels from the retina to separate layers of the lateral geniculate nucleus (LGN), and then finally reaches

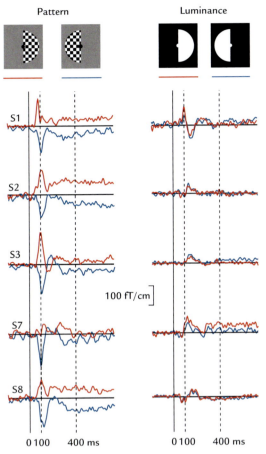

FIGURE 14.5. VEFs to hemifield pattern (left) versus luminance (right) stimulation. Averaged VEFs from a midline occipital planar gradiometer from five subjects to stimulation of the right and left visual fields (red and blue traces, respectively) with checkerboard patterns (left column) and luminance stimuli (right column). Pattern stimulation elicits clear VEFs in all subjects, with opposite polarities to stimulation of the left and right hemifields. Luminance stimulation also elicits VEFs in all subjects, but the responses are smaller and of same polarity to stimulation of both hemifields. Passband 0.03–90 Hz, sampling rate 300 Hz. Adapted and reprinted from Portin K, Salenius S, Salmelin R, Hari R: Activation of the human occipital and parietal cortex by pattern and luminance stimuli: neuromagnetic measurements. *Cereb Cortex* 1998, 8: 253–260. With permission from Oxford University Press.

V1 (striate cortex). M-related information is also channeled to the superior colliculus and pulvinar nucleus of the thalamus and then onto extrastriate cortex.

Although the division is not strict, we can roughly equate signals emerging from the peripheral retina with the M pathway and signals coming from the fovea with the P pathway. Intracellular recordings in monkey retina indicated that signaling from the periphery is considerably faster (by about 30 ms) than signaling from the fovea, thereby suggesting a clear timing difference between the M and P pathways (Masland, 2017; Sinha et al., 2017). ERG recordings of stimulation of selective parts of the visual field also revealed differences between these two visual subsystems, and the latency

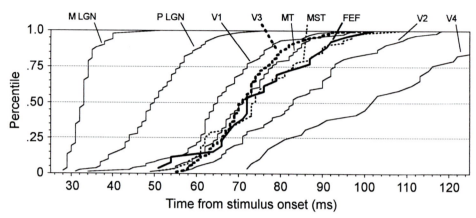

FIGURE 14.6. Cumulative distributions of the onset latencies of single-unit responses flashing light stimuli in selected areas of the macaque visual system. The percentile of cells that have begun to respond are plotted as a function of time from stimulus onset. Visual areas include magnocellular (M) and parvocellular (P) layers of the lateral geniculate nucleus (LGN), striate visual cortex (V1), various extrastriate areas (V3, middle temporal visual area [MT that is also known as V5], medial superior temporal area (MST), V2, V4) and the frontal eye field (FEF). Note that the V4 plot is truncated to improve visibility of the other curves; the V4 range extends to 159 ms. Adapted and reprinted from Schmolesky MT, Wang Y, Hanes DP, Thompson KG, Leutgeb S, Schall JD, Leventhal AG: Signal timing across the macaque visual system. *J Neurophysiol* 1998, 79: 3272–3278. Reproduced with permission from the American Physiological Society.

difference in the M and P responses persisted throughout the visual system. A comprehensive investigation of the macaque visual system indicated that across the alternate layers of M and P cells in the LGN, P-cell responses lagged those of M cells by about 20 ms, and that at the level of the cortex, response onset latencies varied widely both within a cortical region and between different regions (Figure 14.6; Schmolesky et al., 1998). The dorsal pathway and the frontal eye fields typically reacted faster than the ventral regions.

It is also possible to examine selective M and P contributions to human VEFs and VEPs. An efficient way to explore the reactivity of the whole visual field is to use "multifocal" stimulation, which is flashing stimuli in rapid succession to different retinal locations in a pseudorandom order ("m-sequence") (Srebro, 1992; Chen et al., 1996). Figure 14.7a illustrates such a stimulus pattern, with a hexagonal grid comprising illuminated and unilluminated parts that flash on and off as a function of time.

This pseudorandom stimulation sequence elicits "multifocal (mf)" responses in both retina and cortex (mfMRG/ERG and mfVEF/VEP, respectively). In Figure 14.7b, mfVEPs recorded from Oz with Fz reference are shown for multiple stimulus locations. The responses are larger for stimulation of the lower than the upper central portion of the display, consistent with psychophysiological findings of the advantage of the lower visual field in complex visual processing as well as with MEG recordings of stronger VEFs for lower than upper visual field stimulation (Portin et al., 1999; Sutter & Tran, 1992; Klistorner et al., 1997; Crewther et al., 2002).

During rapid mf stimulation, the multifocal evoked responses overlap in both space and time. Therefore, a special analysis is needed to extract linear and nonlinear responses, as

(a)　　　　　　　　　　　(b)

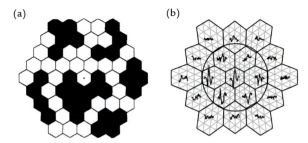

FIGURE 14.7. Multifocal visual evoked responses. (a) Example of a retina-centered hexagonal display where individual hexagons (4 deg of visual field vertex-to-vertex) can be independently turned on or off, and the size of the stimulus can be increased to correspond to larger receptive fields in the peripheral retina. White versus black hexagons show illuminated versus unilluminated parts of the display at an instant in time. (b) Schematic of a hexagonal visual display with superimposed VEPs elicited to stimulation of a particular hexagon in the display. In this case red (not shown here) hexagons were displayed on a gray background. The black circle delineates an area where an "off" central annulus can be implemented. Part (a) is adapted and reprinted from Klistorner A, Crewther DP, Crewther SG: Separate magnocellular and parvocellular contributions from temporal analysis of the multifocal VEP. *Vision Res* 1997, 37: 2161–2169. With permission from Elsevier. Part (b) is reproduced from Crewther DP, Luu CD, Crewther SG: Separation of contour and area dependent components in the first and second order kernels of the multifocal pattern appearance evoked potential. *Clin Exp Ophthalmol* 2002, 30: 231–234. With permission from Elsevier.

well as the M- and P-related responses. For details of the analysis procedure, see Sutter and Tran (1992) and Klistorner et al. (1997).

Other types of finer-grain stimulation of the visual system can be performed by varying the check size in high-contrast checkerboard stimuli that are routinely used in research and clinical laboratories. Increasing the check size leads to larger and earlier VEPs and VEFs (Nakamura et al., 2000). Responses to such fine-grain visual stimuli presented across the visual field allow the estimation of CMFs that concur with magnification factors estimated by psychophysics, invasive cortical stimulation/electrocorticography (ECoG)/stereoencephalography EEG (SEEG), and fMRI (see Slotnick et al., 2001).

In sum, cortical activity peaks earlier to M-biased than P-biased stimuli, preserving the M-pathway advantage seen already in the retina. Additionally, in agreement with the different M and P contributions from the peripheral and foveal retina, the ratio of P/M contributions to evoked responses decreases as a function of eccentricity (Baseler & Sutter, 1997).

According to analyses of effective connectivity (see Chapter 10), P-biased information follows the usual bottom-up route from retina via LGN to occipital cortex and extrastriate cortex (fusiform gyrus), whereas M-biased information tends to flow to extrastriate visual cortex. Somewhat surprisingly, latencies as short as 130 ms for M-biased stimuli can occur in orbitofrontal cortex (OFC), whereas higher-level, visual category-selective responses occur in extrastriate cortex (fusiform gyrus) 40 ms later (Kveraga et al., 2007). These results are consistent with top-down gist processing that facilitates the prediction and recognition of objects (Bar et al., 2006).

It is evident that we need to keep in mind the *multiplicity of visual routes*—as well as the bidirectionality of sensory information flow in most parts of the brain. We next discuss ventral and dorsal visual streams.

■ ASSESSING THE VENTRAL VISUAL STREAM

The human brain has been suggested to have two distinct visual streams: a ventral stream (the "what" pathway) mainly for face and object perception and a dorsal stream (the "where" pathway) for spatial location (Ungerleider & Mishkin, 1982), which is critical for action (Goodale & Milner, 1992). The ventral stream is predominantly active in the recognition, identification, and detailed processing of objects, including faces. More recently, a third visual stream has been proposed, where information from V1 is brought directly to the superior temporal sulcus (STS) for social perception (Pitcher & Ungerleider, 2021; discussed further in Chapter 19).

Given that two of these three visual pathways respond vigorously to faces, the spatial distribution of the MEG/EEG responses can be rather complex in both sensor and source space. The original finding of a vertex-positive scalp potential (VPP) at 150 to 200 ms to line drawings of faces (Jeffreys, 1989) initiated a strong interest in studies of brain responses to faces. The VPP differed from the classic checkerboard VEP in that it did *not* change its polarity or scalp distribution as a function of the retinal site of stimulation (Jeffreys, 1989). Soon, with a more extensive array of scalp electrodes, a prominent bilateral temporoparietal scalp N170 response, much larger in size than the VPP, was reported to be elicited by faces and particularly by eyes (Bentin et al., 1996) (see Figure 14.8, left panel). The electrical N170 tends to be largest over the right temporal scalp (Rossion & Jacques, 2008; Itier &

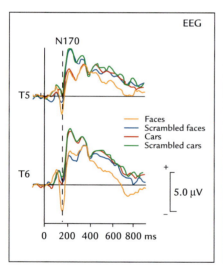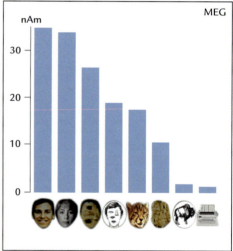

FIGURE 14.8. **Visual evoked responses to faces.** Left: Grand-average VEPs (*N* = 12) from scalp EEG sites T5 and T6 in response to various stimulus categories. The largest scalp-negative potential (N170) is elicited by faces. Passband 0.1–100 Hz, sampling rate 250 Hz. Adapted and modified with permission from Bentin S, Allison R, Puce A, Perez A, McCarthy G: Electrophysiological studies of face perception in humans. *J Cogn Neurosci* 1996, 8: 551–565. © 1996 by the Massachusetts Institute of Technology, published by the MIT Press. Right: Mean source strengths (in nAm; *N* = 10) of the magnetic M170 response in the putative fusiform gyrus to different visual stimulus categories; the colored intact whole faces elicited the largest responses. Passband 0.03–90 Hz, sampling rate 297 Hz. Adapted and reprinted from Halgren E, Raij T, Marinkovic K, Jousmäki V, Hari R: Cognitive response profile of the human fusiform face area as determined by MEG. *Cereb Cortex* 2000, 10: 69–81. With permission from Oxford University Press.

Batty, 2009), and the magnetic 170-ms response M170 has a right-hemisphere dominance as well (Lu et al., 1991; Sams et al., 1997). Figure 14.8 also indicates that both N170 (left panel) and M170 (right panel) can be elicited to stimuli other than faces, however with significantly smaller amplitudes (Bentin et al., 1996; Halgren et al., 2000). Therefore, it is more appropriate to say that the N170/M170 response is sensitive, rather than specific, to faces.

An intracranial potential N200 to faces has been recorded from epilepsy surgery patients from two separate sites—one in the ventral occipitotemporal cortex and another in the lateral temporal cortex (Allison et al., 1994; Puce et al., 1999), consistent with the idea that face stimuli can activate multiple visual pathways. When recorded from the same patients, scalp VPP and ventral occipitotemporal intracranial N200 have identical latencies (Rosburg et al., 2010). In depth recordings, N200/N170 reverses its polarity within the fusiform gyrus, consistent with a local generator in this region (Jonas et al., 2012).

Figure 14.9 shows the two separate brain loci that generate the intracranial N200/N170, and it is likely that these respective areas give rise to the lateral temporal scalp N170

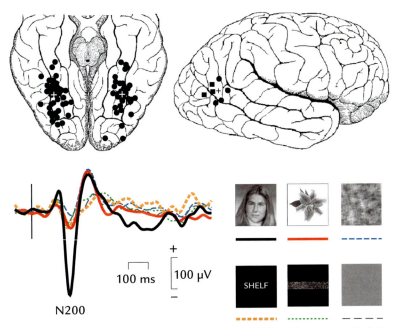

FIGURE 14.9. Intracranial visual responses to faces. Left: Schematic of inferior surface of the brain showing intracranial recording locations of face-sensitive N200 in 97 surgical patients. White crosses depict the centers of mass for the N200 in each hemisphere. Right: Schematic of the right lateral surface of the brain (top) showing sites of face-sensitive N200 in the same patients. Data from left and right hemispheres are displayed as black squares and circles, respectively. Black cross depicts the N200 center of mass. Example potentials (bottom) show prominent responses to faces and very small amplitudes to other stimulus categories. Passband 0.1–100 Hz, sampling rate 250 Hz. Adapted and reprinted from Allison T, Puce A, Spencer DD, McCarthy G: Electrophysiological studies of human face perception: I. Potentials generated in occipitotemporal cortex by face and non-face stimuli. *Cereb Cortex* 1999, 9: 415–430. With permission from Oxford University Press.

and the vertex-centered VPP. The equivalent source currents of VPP point upward in the fusiform, toward the occipitoparietal cortex, as can be deduced from the surface negativity at the lower surface of the fusiform gyrus (see Figure 14.9) as well as from the direction of the current dipole during M170 (Lu et al., 1991; Sams et al., 1997; Halgren et al., 2000). The scalp N170 could receive an additional contribution from a source in the lateral temporal cortex.

Stimulus rise times vary depending on the presentation device (e.g., an abrupt camera shutter or a computer screen) and consequently can affect the response latencies, which in part explains why the N170/N170m peak latencies have ranged from 140 ms to beyond 170 ms across different studies.

■ ASSESSING THE DORSAL VISUAL STREAM

It is also possible to measure strong visual responses from the parieto-occipital sulcus (human POS), which is an important part of the dorsal visual stream driven mainly by the magnocellular pathway and thus especially by peripheral vision. Accordingly, the human POS is more strongly activated by luminance than pattern stimuli, and activation does not depend on the stimulated visual field (left vs. right) or on foveal versus nonfoveal stimulus location (Portin & Hari, 1999; Portin et al., 1999). The same POS area seems to be the main generator of the human parieto-occipital alpha rhythm (Hari & Salmelin, 1997), as well as of the prominent responses at 220 to 280 ms after voluntary blinks (Hari et al., 1994) and about 170 ms after self-paced horizontal saccades (Jousmäki et al., 1996).

VEPs and VEFs originating from the visual-motion-sensitive area V5 can be elicited by dynamic stimuli, including complex motion patterns, such as kinematic random-dot displays (Niedeggen & Wist, 1998) and optic flow (van der Meer et al., 2008). Figure 14.10 illustrates VEFs from the human V5 region in response to 1-s presentation of a patterned stimulus that either stays steady (blue traces) or is rotating (red traces). While both stimuli elicit a robust transient response to stimulus onset, the response to the rotating pattern is larger and also includes a prominent sustained field, which, after the offset response, decays slowly, potentially related to a movement aftereffect during which subjects perceive the already stopped wheel to rotate in the opposite direction (Uusitalo et al., 1997).

Robust VEPs/VEFs can be elicited also using apparent-motion stimuli by presenting two static images in succession. Indeed, even a checkerboard reversal stimulus produces a strong illusion of check motion (Spekreijse et al., 1985). Examples of more complex apparent motion are facial images with eyes open, closed, and then open to simulate an eye blink (Brefczynski-Lewis et al., 2011), eyes with direct gaze and averted gaze to simulate a gaze change, or mouth opening and closing movements generated from static facial images (Puce et al., 2000) (see Chapter 19).

■ VISUAL STEADY-STATE RESPONSES

Since the 1960s, sinusoidally modulated light has been known to elicit visual SSRs that vary as a function of stimulus frequency (Spekreijse, 1965). SSRs are strongest at around 10, 20, and 40 Hz (Regan, 1972), resembling the stimulus-rate dependence of auditory SSRs (see Figure 13.7). The phase of the visual SSR plotted as a function of increasing frequency shows three linear segments, whose slopes (in milliseconds) are comparable with the latencies of the three main components of the transient VEPs (Van der Tweel & Lunel, 1965; Regan, 1966).

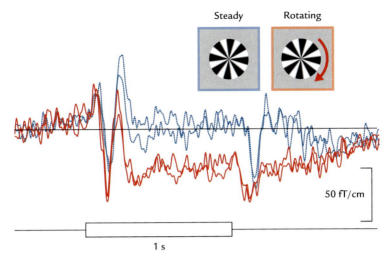

FIGURE 14.10. **VEF from area V5 elicited to visual motion.** VEFs of a single subject to 1-s steady (blue) or rotating (red) circular gratings in replicated recordings. Onsets of both stimuli elicit transient VEFs, whereas the rotating stimulus additionally induces a clear sustained field, which gradually returns to baseline following stimulus offset; the subject reported a strong motion aftereffect. Passband 0.03–90 Hz, sampling rate 300 Hz. Adapted and reprinted from Uusitalo MA, Virsu V, Salenius S, Näsänen R, Hari R: Activation of human V5 complex and Rolandic regions in association with moving visual stimuli. *NeuroImage* 1997, 5: 241–250. With permission from Elsevier.

Figure 14.11 shows the buildup of visual SSRs when the presentation rate of checkerboard patterns is increased. The top red trace shows the typical transient VEP with full recovery before the next stimulus arrives. As the presentation rate increases in the subsequent traces, the responses start to overlap, and the system reaches a steady state, with the responses becoming increasingly sinusoidal. Importantly, the black lines show synthetic responses computed by shifting the single transient responses at each stimulus presentation and then summing up the responses. Here, as for the auditory SSRs (see Figure 13.7), the SSR can be explained as a linear summation of the transient responses.

Visual SSRs, due to their good signal-to-noise ratio even to quite small stimuli, can be used for frequency tagging (again, compare with auditory frequency tagging [Figure 13.8]). Figure 14.12 shows an example of visual frequency tagging aimed to study brain activations related to the change of percept in the well-known ambiguous Rubin's face–vase figure. Dynamic noise was superimposed on the image so that it was updated at 12 Hz on the vase and at 15 Hz on the faces making the image appear slightly smoothed; importantly, the subjects did not notice the differences in noise frequencies in the two areas. Their MEG frequency spectra over the posterior brain (Figure 14.12, top right) displayed sharp peaks at both tag frequencies, with the relative strengths covarying with the change of percept (between vase and faces) that the subject indicated by a button press. Activation of the early visual cortices covaried with percepts, most likely because of top-down influences. Eye tracking indicated that the subject fixated at the center of the screen at all times, meaning that the changes of the MEG signals were not due to gaze deviations (Parkkonen et al., 2008).

Frequency tagging provides an effective tool for designing increasingly complicated sensory tasks for MEG/EEG recordings (e.g., Fujiki et al., 2002, for audition; Parkkonen

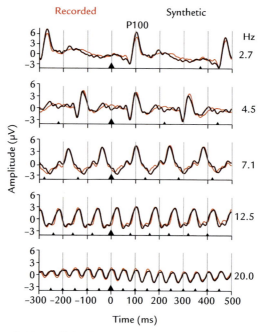

FIGURE 14.11. Visual SSRs elicited at multiple repetition rates. Grand-average VEPs (across 24 subjects) to checkerboard reversals presented at 2.7–20 Hz; the reversals are marked on the horizontal axes with black triangles. At 2.7 Hz (top), the main response is a prominent P100, preceded and followed by deflections of opposite polarities at around 75 ms and 135 ms. As stimulation frequency increases, the VEPs gradually merge with one another to produce a sinusoidal SSRs at the 20 Hz stimulation rate. The red traces depict the recorded responses, whereas the black traces indicate synthetic responses obtained by using templates formed on the basis of transient responses. Passband 0.5–100 Hz with a 50-Hz notch filter, sampling rate 1000 Hz. Adapted and reprinted with permission from Capilla A, Pazo-Alvarez P, Darriba A, Campo P, Gross J: Steady-state visual evoked potentials can be explained by temporal superposition of transient event-related responses. *PLoS One* 2011, 6: e14543.

et al., 2008, and Jonas et al., 2016, for vision), and a frequency-tagging toolbox is now available (Figueira et al., 2022). If multiple tagging frequencies are used within the same stimulus sequence, one has to be careful to select frequencies that do not interact with each other and do not contain harmonics with the line frequency or have other intermodulation effects (Gordon et al., 2019).

■ DECODING OF VISUAL CATEGORIES

Machine learning (ML) methods (Chapter 10) have already benefited the analysis of neurophysiological data in systems and cognitive/social neuroscience. In the area of visual object recognition, some interesting findings related to natural image statistics and brain function have emerged (reviewed by Contini et al., 2017). Early ML work used fMRI activation to show that visual categorization in the human brain relies on not only category-selective visual brain regions but also a mosaic of coactivated distributed brain regions (Haxby et al., 2001).

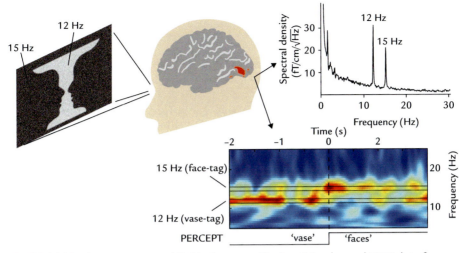

FIGURE 14.12. Frequency-tagged Rubin face–vase illusion. Stimulus and MEG data from one subject in the study of the ambiguous faces-versus-vase percept, with the subject indicating by button press the change of the percept. Left: The visual stimulus consists of a static Rubin face–vase image upon which dynamic noise with 15 Hz and 12 Hz update frequencies was superimposed on the face and vase areas, respectively. Right: The frequency spectrum (top) from one occipital planar gradiometer in a single subject shows clear peaks at both tag frequencies. The time–frequency plot of the occipital MEG signal (bottom), averaged across 31 perceptual flips, shows perception-related shift of signal power from 12 Hz to 15 Hz (corresponding to a change from vase to face tag frequency). Time zero indicates the change in percept. Passband 0.1–170 Hz, sampling rate 600 Hz. Adapted and reprinted from Parkkonen L, Andersson J, Hämäläinen M, Hari R: Early visual brain areas reflect the percept of an ambiguous scene. *Proc Natl Acad Sci USA* 2008, 105: 20500–20504. ©2008 National Academy of Sciences, USA.

Building on that early work, representational similarity analysis (RSA)—as one versatile version of multivariate pattern analysis—examined if category-specific visual responses to real-world images could be differentiated on the basis of human fMRI signals or primate single-unit neurophysiological data. The idea was to see if the *characteristics of the brain activity itself*, without anchoring it to any specific brain area, could differentiate between faces, bodies, natural objects, and man-made objects. Using RSA, pairwise response-pattern dissimilarities were created to individual stimuli for all brain regions, and from these data dissimilarity matrices clear differentiation emerged between animate/inanimate, face/body, natural/man-made dimensions in both human and primate inferior temporal cortex (Kriegeskorte et al., 2008). RSA also enables comparison between MEG and fMRI results (see e.g., Henriksson et al., 2019).

The high temporal resolution of MEG/EEG offers advantages for RSA and other brain "decoding" methods. For example, pattern-classification analysis of MEG data discriminated signals that evolved over different time intervals for the different stimulus categories in an object recognition task (Carlson et al., 2013)—a result that cannot be obtained with temporally sparse methods, such as fMRI. Other studies have shown the importance of perceptual similarity in low-level visual areas between items within a natural object category, thereby providing a context for resolving the underlying functional neuroanatomy of face- and objective-selective visual cortex (Wardle et al., 2016).

■ REFERENCES

Ahlfors S, Ilmoniemi R, Hämäläinen M: Estimates of visually evoked cortical currents. *Electroencephalogr Clin Neurophysiol* 1992, 82: 225–236.

Aine C, Supek S, George J, Ranken D, Lewine J, Sanders J, Best E, Tiee W, Flynn E, Wood C: Retinotopic organization of human visual cortex: departures from the classical model. *Cereb Cortex* 1996, 6: 354–361.

Aittoniemi K, Katila T, Kuusela M-L, Varpula T: Magnetoretinography. Detection of the transient magnetic field of the eye. In: *Proc 12th Int Conf Med Biol Eng* 1979, 96: 4. Israel: Petah Tikva.

Ales JM, Yates JL, Norcia AM: V1 is not uniquely identified by polarity reversals of responses to upper and lower visual field stimuli. *NeuroImage* 2010, 52: 1401–1409.

Allison T, Ginter H, McCarthy G, Nobre AC, Puce A, Luby M, Spencer DD: Face recognition in human extrastriate cortex. *J Neurophysiol* 1994, 71: 821–825.

Allison T, Puce A, Spencer DD, McCarthy G: Electrophysiological studies of human face perception: I. Potentials generated in occipitotemporal cortex by face and non-face stimuli. *Cereb Cortex* 1999, 9: 415–430.

Bar M, Kassam KS, Ghuman AS, Boshyan J, Schmid AM, Dale AM, Hämäläinen MS, Marinkovic K, Schacter DL, Rosen BR, Halgren E: Top-down facilitation of visual recognition. *Proc Natl Acad Sci U S A* 2006, 103: 449–454.

Barett G, Blumhardt L, Halliday AM, Halliday E, Kriss A: A paradox in the lateralisation of the visual evoked response. *Nature* 1976, 261: 253–255.

Baseler HA, Sutter EE: M and P components of the VEP and their visual field distribution. *Vision Res* 1997, 37: 675–690.

Bentin S, Allison T, Puce A, Perez A, McCarthy G: Electrophysiological studies of face perception in humans. *J Cogn Neurosci* 1996, 8: 551–565.

Brefczynski-Lewis JA, Berrebi ME, McNeely ME, Prostko AL, Puce A: In the blink of an eye: neural responses elicited to viewing the eye blinks of another individual. *Front Hum Neurosci* 2011, 5: 68.

Brenner D, Williamson SJ, Kaufman L: Visually evoked magnetic fields of the human brain. *Science* 1975, 190: 480–481.

Carlson T, Tovar DA, Alink A, Kriegeskorte N: Representational dynamics of object vision: the first 1000 ms. *J Vision* 2013, 13: 1–19.

Chen HW, Aine CJ, Best E, Ranken D, Harrison RR, Flynn ER, Wood CC: Nonlinear analysis of biological systems using short M-sequences and sparse-stimulation techniques. *Ann Biomed Eng* 1996, 24: 513–536.

Chiappa KH: *Evoked Potentials in Clinical Medicine*, 3rd ed. Philadelphia: Lippincott Williams & Wilkins, 1997.

Cobb WA, Dawson GD: The latency and form in man of the occipital potentials evoked by bright flashes. *J Physiol* 1960, 152: 108–121.

Collin CA, Therrien ME, Campbell KB: Effects of band-pass spatial frequency filtering of face and object images on the amplitude of N170. *Perception* 2012, 41: 717–732.

Contini EW, Wardle SG, Carlson TA: Decoding the time-course of object recognition in the human brain: from visual features to categorical decisions. *Neuropsychologia* 2017, 105: 165–176.

Creel DJ: Electroretinograms. In: Levin KH, Chauvel P, eds. *Handbook of Clinical Neurology*, Vol. 160 (3rd series). *Clinical Neurophysiology: Basis and Technical Aspects*. Amsterdam: Elsevier, 2019: 481–493.

Crewther DP, Luu CD, Crewther SG: Separation of contour and area dependent components in the first and second order kernels of the multifocal pattern appearance evoked potential. *Clin Exp Ophthalmol* 2002, 30: 231–234.

Cruse R, Klem G, Lesser RP, Leuders H: Paradoxical lateralization of cortical potentials evoked by stimulation of posterior tibial nerve. *Arch Neurol* 1982, 39: 222–225.

Dewar J, McKendrick JG: On the physiological action of light: No. I. *J Anat Physiol* 1873a, 7: 275–278.

Dewar J, McKendrick JG: On the physiological action of light: No. II. *J Anat Physiol* 1873b, 7: 278–282.

Di Russo F, Pitzalis S, Aprile T, Spitoni G, Patria F, Stella A, Spinelli D, Hillyard SA: Spatiotemporal analysis of the cortical sources of the steady-state visual evoked potential. *Hum Brain Mapp* 2007, 28: 323–334.

Figueira JSB, Kutlu E, Scott LS, Keil A: The FreqTag toolbox: a principled approach to analyzing electrophysiological time series in frequency tagging paradigms. *Dev Cogn Neurosci* 2022, 54: 101066.

Fujiki N, Jousmäki V, Hari R: Neuromagnetic responses to frequency-tagged sounds: a new method to follow inputs from each ear to the human auditory cortex during binaural hearing. *J Neurosci* 2002, 22, RC205.

Galambos R, Juhasz G: The contribution of glial cells to spontaneous and evoked potentials. *Int J Psychophysiol* 1997, 26: 229–236.

Goodale MA, Milner AD: Separate visual pathways for perception and action. *Trends Neurosci* 1992, 15: 20–25.

Gordon N, Hohwy J, Davidson MJ, van Boxtel JJA, Tsuchiya N: From intermodulation components to visual perception and cognition—a review. *NeuroImage* 2019, 199: 480–494.

Groen A II, Silson EH, Baker CI: Contributions of low- and high-level properties to neural processing of visual scenes in the human brain. *Philos Trans R Soc Lond B Biol Sci* 2017, 372: 20160102.

Halgren E, Raij T, Marinkovic K, Jousmäki V, Hari R: Cognitive response profile of the human fusiform face area as determined by MEG. *Cereb Cortex* 2000, 10: 69–81.

Hari R, Salmelin R, Tissari S, Kajola M, Virsu V: Visual stability during eyeblinks. *Nature* 1994, 367: 121–122.

Hari R, Salmelin R: Human cortical oscillations: a neuromagnetic view through the skull. *Trends Neurosci* 1997, 20: 44–49.

Haxby JV, Gobbini MI, Furey ML, Ishai A, Schouten JL, Pietrini P: Distributed and overlapping representations of faces and objects in ventral temporal cortex. *Science* 2001, 293: 2425–2430.

Henriksson L, Mur M, Kriegeskorte N: Rapid invariant encoding of scene layout in human OPA. *Neuron* 2019, 103: 161–171 e163.

Holmgren F: Metod att objektiverafs effecten af ljusintryck på retina. *Upsala Läkareförenings Förhandlingar* 1866, 1: 177–191.

Itier RJ, Batty M: Neural bases of eye and gaze processing: the core of social cognition. *Neurosci Biobehav Rev* 2009, 33: 843–863.

Jeantet C, Caharel S, Schwan R, Lighezzolo-Alnot J, Laprevote V: Factors influencing spatial frequency extraction in faces: a review. *Neurosci Biobehav Rev* 2018, 93: 123–138.

Jeffreys DA, Axford JG: Source locations of pattern-specific components of human visual evoked potentials: I. Component of striate cortical origin. *Exp Brain Res* 1972, 16: 1–21.

Jeffreys DA: A face-responsive potential recorded from the human scalp. *Exp Brain Res* 1989, 78: 193–202.

Jonas J, Descoins M, Koessler L, Colnat-Coulbois S, Sauvee M, Guye M, Vignal JP, Vespignani H, Rossion B, Maillard L: Focal electrical intracerebral stimulation of a face-sensitive area causes transient prosopagnosia. *Neuroscience* 2012, 222: 281–288.

Jonas J, Jacques C, Liu-Shuang J, Brissart H, Colnat-Coulbois S, Maillard L, Rossion B: A face-selective ventral occipito-temporal map of the human brain with intracerebral potentials. *Proc Natl Acad Sci U S A* 2016, 113: E4088–E4097.

Jousmäki V, Hämäläinen M, Hari R: Magnetic source imaging during a visually guided task. *Neuroreport* 1996, 7: 2961–2964.

Kahn R, Löwenstein A: Das Elektroretinogramm. *Arch klin exp Ophthalmol* 1924, 114: 304–331.

Kantola L, Piccolino M, Wade N: The action of light on the retina: translation and commentary of Holmgren (1866). *J Hist Neurosci* 2019, 28: 399–415.

Katila T, Maniewski R, Poutanen T, Varpula T: Magnetic fields produced by the human eye. *J Appl Phys* 1981, 52: 2565–2571.

Klistorner A, Crewther DP, Crewther SG: Separate magnocellular and parvocellular contributions from temporal analysis of the multifocal VEP. *Vision Res* 1997, 37: 2161–2169.

Kriegeskorte N, Mur M, Ruff DA, Kiani R, Bodurka J, Esteky H, Tanaka K, Bandettini P: Matching categorical object representations in inferior temporal cortex of man and monkey. *Neuron* 2008, 60: 1126–1141.

Kveraga K, Boshyan J, Bar M: Magnocellular projections as the trigger of top-down facilitation in recognition. *J Neurosci* 2007, 27: 13232–13240.

Levy I, Hasson U, Avidan G, Hendler T, Malach R: Center-periphery organization of human object areas. *Nat Neurosci* 2001, 4: 533–539.

Lu S, Hämäläinen M, Hari R, Ilmoniemi R, Lounasmaa OV, Sams M, Vilkman V: Seeing faces activates three brain areas outside the occipital visual cortex in man. *Neuroscience* 1991, 43: 287–290.

Masland RH: Vision: Two speeds in the retina. *Curr Biol* 2017, 27: R294–R317.

Nakamura M, Kakigi R, Okusa T, Hoshiyama M, Watanabe K: Effects of check size on pattern reversal visual evoked magnetic field and potential. *Brain Res* 2000, 872: 77–86.

Niedeggen M, Wist ER: Motion evoked brain potentials parallel the consistency of coherent motion perception in humans. *Neurosci Lett* 1998, 246: 61–64.

Obayashi C, Nakashima T, Onitsuka T, Maekawa T, Hirano Y, Hirano S, Oribe N, Kaneko K, Kanba S, Tobimatsu S: Decreased spatial frequency sensitivities for processing faces in male patients with chronic schizophrenia. *Clin Neurophysiol* 2009, 120: 1525–1533.

Odom JV, Bach M, Brigell M, Holder GE, McCulloch DL, Mizota A, Tormene AP, International Society for Clinical Electrophysiology of V. ISCEV standard for clinical visual evoked potentials: (2016 update). *Doc Ophthalmol* 2016, 133: 1–9.

Parkkonen L, Andersson J, Hämäläinen M, Hari R: Early visual brain areas reflect the percept of an ambiguous scene. *Proc Natl Acad Sci U S A* 2008, 105: 20500–20504.

Pitcher D, Ungerleider LG: Evidence for a third visual pathway specialized for social perception. *Trends Cogn Sci* 2021, 25: 100–110.

Portin K, Hari R: Human parieto-occipital visual cortex: lack of retinotopy and foveal magnification. *Proc Biol Sci* 1999, 266: 981–985.

Portin K, Vanni S, Virsu V, Hari R: Stronger occipital cortical activation to lower than upper visual field stimuli: neuromagnetic recordings. *Exp Brain Res* 1999, 124: 287–294.

Puce A, Allison T, McCarthy G: Electrophysiological studies of human face perception: III. Effects of top-down processing on face-specific potentials. *Cereb Cortex* 1999, 9: 445–458.

Puce A, Smith A, Allison T: ERPs evoked by viewing facial movements. *Cogn Neuropsychol* 2000, 17: 221–239.

Regan D: Some characteristics of average steady-state and transient responses evoked by modulated light. *Electroencephalogr Clin Neurophysiol* 1966, 20: 238–248.

Regan D: *Evoked Potentials in Psychology, Sensory Physiology and Clinical Medicine*. London: Chapman and Hall, 1972.

Regan D: *Human Brain Electrophysiology: Evoked Potentials and Evoked Magnetic Fields in Science and Medicine*. New York: Elsevier Science, 1989.

Rosburg T, Ludowig E, Dumpelmann M, Alba-Ferrara L, Urbach H, Elger CE: The effect of face inversion on intracranial and scalp recordings of event-related potentials. *Psychophysiology* 2010, 47: 147–157.

Rosenholtz R: Capabilities and limitations of peripheral vision. *Annu Rev Vis Sci* 2016, 2: 437–457.

Rossion B, Jacques C: Does physical interstimulus variance account for early electrophysiological face sensitive responses in the human brain? Ten lessons on the N170. *NeuroImage* 2008, 39: 1959–1979.

Sams M, Hietanen JK, Hari R, Ilmoniemi RJ, Lounasmaa OV: Face-specific responses from the human inferior occipito-temporal cortex. *Neuroscience* 1997, 77: 49–55.

Schmolesky MT, Wang Y, Hanes DP, Thompson KG: Signal timing across the macaque visual system. *J Neurophysiol* 1998, 79: 3272–3278.

Sinha R, Hoon M, Baudin J, Okawa H, Wong ROL, Rieke F: Cellular and circuit mechanisms shaping the perceptual properties of the primate fovea. *Cell* 2017, 168: 413–426 e412.

Slotnick SD, Klein SA, Carney T, Sutter EE: Electrophysiological estimate of human cortical magnification. *Clin Neurophysiol* 2001, 112: 1349–1356.

Spekreijse H: Linearisation of evoked responses to sinusoidally modulated light by noise. *Nature* 1965, 205: 913.

Spekreijse H, Dagnelie G, Maier J, Regan D: Flicker and movement constituents of the pattern reversal response. *Vision Res* 1985, 25: 1297–1304.

Srebro R: An analysis of the VEP to luminance modulation and of its nonlinearity. *Vision Res* 1992, 32: 1395–1404.

Stenbacka L, Vanni S, Uutela K, Hari R: Comparison of minimum current estimate and dipole modeling in the analysis of simulated activity in the human visual cortices. *NeuroImage* 2002, 16: 936–943.

Strasburger H, Rentschler I, Juttner M: Peripheral vision and pattern recognition: a review. *J Vis* 2011, 11: 13.

Sutter EE, Tran D: The field topography of ERG components in man—I. The photopic luminance response. *Vision Res* 1992, 32: 433–446.

Teyler TJ, Cuffin BN, Cohen D: The visual magnetoencephalogram. *Life Sci* 1975, 17: 683–692.

Ungerleider LG, Mishkin M: Two cortical visual systems. In: Ingle DJ, Goodale MA, Mansfield RJW, eds. *Analysis of Visual Behavior*. Cambridge, MA: MIT Press, 1982: 549–586.

Uusitalo M, Virsu V, Salenius S, Näsänen R, Hari R: Human cortical activation related to perception of visual motion and movement after-effect. *NeuroImage* 1997, 5: 241–250.

van der Meer AL, Fallet G, van der Weel FR: Perception of structured optic flow and random visual motion in infants and adults: a high-density EEG study. *Exp Brain Res* 2008, 186: 493–502.

Van der Tweel LH, Lunel HF: Human visual responses to sinusoidally modulated light. *Electroencephalogr Clin Neurophysiol* 1965, 18: 587–598.

Wardle SG, Kriegeskorte N, Grootswagers T, Khaligh-Razavi S-M, Thomas A, Carlson TA: Perceptual similarity of visual patterns predicts dynamic neural activation patterns measured with MEG. *NeuroImage* 2016, 132: 59–70.

Westner BU, Lubell JI, Jensen M, Hokland S, Dalal SS: Contactless measurements of retinal activity using optically pumped magnetometers. *NeuroImage* 2021, 243: 118528.

CHAPTER 15

SOMATOSENSORY RESPONSES

The great art of life is sensation, to feel that we exist, even in pain.

—LORD BYRON

I touch the future. I teach.

—CHRISTA MCAULIFFE

■ COMPOUND ACTION POTENTIALS AND FIELDS OF PERIPHERAL NERVES

After a peripheral somatosensory stimulus, such as a touch to the finger, an action potential volley begins to travel along the peripheral nerve, first to the spinal cord, and then onward to the thalamus and somatosensory cortex. Peripheral nerves comprise bundles of fibers of different diameters. Mixed nerves, such as the median and ulnar nerves (that can be stimulated at the wrist and cubita/elbow), contain both sensory and motor fibers. Some nerves (such as the distal part of the radial nerve in the hand dorsum and the sural nerve in the ankle and calf of the leg) are only sensory.

If one stimulates the trunk of a peripheral nerve electrically or mechanically, action potentials start to travel in both directions until they reach a synapse that serves as a rectifier and lets impulses pass only in one direction.

The first recordings of an action potential were obtained from a squid giant axon, which can be up to 1 mm in diameter (Hodgkin & Huxley, 1939). Compound action potentials (CAPs), the sum of all action potentials in a nerve trunk, are dominated by the fastest-conducting (and largest) fibers of the nerve. In humans, they can be recorded with electrodes placed on the skin above the nerve trunk.

CAPs are routinely measured as a part of a clinical electroneuromyographic examination where conduction velocities of sensory pathways need to be determined. Figure 15.1 shows CAPs to median-nerve stimulation at the wrist with electrodes placed over the skin at the cubita (the volar side of the elbow) and brachial plexus (Erb's point); additional electrodes can be placed over the vertebral processes (e.g., at the level of C4/C5). The latencies of the propagating surface-negative CAPs depend on the properties of the nerve under study, the subject's limb length, and skin temperature. (Normal CAP values are typically given for skin temperatures of 33 °C, so cooler limbs should be warmed before the measurement.)

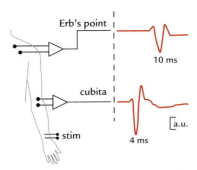

FIGURE 15.1. Schematics of CAPs to median-nerve stimulation (stim). Median nerve is assumed to be stimulated at the wrist, and CAPs are measured at the cubita (lower trace) and Erb's point (brachial plexus; upper trace). During the progression of the CAP, its latency increases, amplitude slightly decreases, and the waveform broadens because of dispersion of conduction times of different fibers.

The conduction velocity can be computed by dividing the response latency by the distance from the stimulation electrode to the recording site.

For the motor fibers of the mixed median nerve, the conduction velocity is typically measured by placing the recording electrode over the muscles of the thenar eminence (located between the wrist and the base of thumb) and by stimulating the nerve trunk over the wrist as well as over the cubita. The stimulation will evoke twitches in the thenar muscles, with an associated large electrical response on the skin. The motor conduction velocity is then obtained by subtracting the latencies of these two responses and dividing the difference by the distance between the two stimulation sites. Thus the distal conduction delay from the stimulation site to the muscle itself does not alter the measurement. (Note that a prolonged distal latency from wrist to thenar is a typical finding in carpal tunnel syndrome, where the median nerve is compressed by the transverse ligament in the wrist.)

The first measurements of the magnetic field associated with the action potential were made from a frog sciatic-nerve bundle that was threaded through a toroid in a conducting saline bath (Wikswo et al., 1980), an experimental setting very similar to the lowest panel in Figure 3.6. These measurements, made with an induction-coil magnetometer at room temperature (recording passband from 0.01 Hz to 5 kHz), showed a monophasic electric potential but a biphasic compound action field (CAF) of the order of 0.1 nT. The result agrees with the description of Figure 2.2 of two opposite intracellular current dipoles, one at the leading and another at the trailing end of the action potential, thereby forming a current quadrupole.

The conduction velocity of the nerve determines how far away these two dipoles of opposite directions are from each other. In a healthy median nerve, the conduction velocity exceeds 50 m/s, and thus an AP will progress at least 5 cm during 1 ms. Hence the two dipoles associated with the depolarization and repolarization fronts of the AP will be separated by $\geq$ 5 cm.

Thus it seems likely that in a peripheral nerve the intracellular current dipoles associated with the leading and trailing ends of the propagating AP volley could be seen in magnetic measurements at a distance. Accordingly, CAFs have been noninvasively recorded from human peripheral nerves (Erné et al., 1988; Hari et al., 1989). (Note that in the cerebral cortex the conduction is so slow that the two dipoles are just a few millimeters apart, meaning that the resulting quadrupole cannot be seen far away from the source.)

Figure 15.2 shows noninvasively recorded CAFs at the elbow after stimulation of the right median nerve, with clear signals at 6 to 7 ms poststimulus. The signal is monophasic at most locations, with opposite polarities on the two sides of the nerve in recordings performed with axial gradiometers. The lack of clear repolarization-related signals may reflect larger temporal dispersion of the repolarization than depolarization front (top left panel). The panel at the top right shows magnetic recordings from the cubita, plexus, and cortex (over primary sensory cortex [SI]), with the plexal and cortical signals showing increasingly longer latencies.

An electrical stimulus to the peripheral nerve will induce a stimulus artifact in both CAP and CAF recordings. For this reason, some commercially produced amplifiers will either null out, or dampen, the signals that are recorded in the first few milliseconds after the

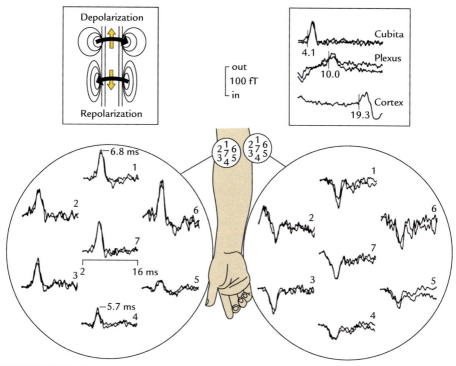

FIGURE 15.2. CAFs recorded from the right median nerve. Main figure: CAFs recorded from the right cubita to 0.3-ms median-nerve stimuli applied at the wrist. The array of seven axial gradiometers was positioned on either side of the nerve in a single subject. Passband 0.05 Hz–2 kHz, sampling rate 8 kHz. Each trace shows an average of 1,000 single responses. Left insert: Schematic of intracellular currents (yellow arrows) in the median nerve during the upward propagating action potential; the associated magnetic flux around the nerve is indicated by black curved arrows. The repolarization currents (lower part of the nerve) are distributed along a wider area than the denser depolarization currents (upper part of the nerve). Right insert: Responses of the same subject to median-nerve stimulation at the cubita, plexus, and somatosensory cortex, with response onset latencies indicated on a time scale from 2–27 ms. Adapted and reprinted from Hari R, Hällström J, Tiihonen J, Joutsiniemi S: Multichannel detection of magnetic compound action fields of median and ulnar nerves. *Electroencephalogr Clin Neurophysiol* 1989, 72: 277–280. With permission from Elsevier.

stimulus is delivered. The stimulus artifact can be minimized in CAP recordings by siting a ground electrode between the stimulating and recording electrodes. It is important to keep the filter passband as wide as possible during the recording, so that the artifact does not spread too broadly over time.

Note that not all deflections observed in a CAP or a somatosensory-evoked potential (SEP) recording reflect propagation of the neural action-potential currents. Instead, some consistent deflections with a fixed latency, amplitude, and waveform may be observed in recordings performed from any part of the body, for example, with reference electrodes on the knee or nose. The latency of such *stationary* deflections can correspond, for example, to the arrival of the action-potential volley from the (cylindrical) upper limb to the much wider trunk of the body. It is thus the *change of the volume conductor* that causes this "far-field" potential, the generation mechanism of which should be clearly separated from far-away recordings of time-varying neuronal activation in a fixed location (such as the brainstem auditory responses that we discussed in Chapter 13). This kind of effect would not occur if the volume conductor were homogeneous and infinite (Stegeman et al., 1997).

■ RESPONSES FROM THE SI CORTEX

Compared with hearing and vision, natural stimuli related to touch and other somatosensory senses are very difficult to reproduce in a laboratory setting (see Chapter 6 for a description of tactile and vibratory stimulation of local skin areas). Thus electric stimulation of peripheral nerves is commonly used to elicit robust somatosensory responses. The intensities of the electrical stimuli are, besides the exact values in milliamperes, reported with respect to either the sensory or motor threshold. Electrical median-nerve stimulation at the wrist below the motor but above the sensory threshold typically produces tingling sensations in the thumb, index finger, middle finger, and the thumb-side of the ring finger, and ulnar-nerve stimulation produces sensations in the little finger and the lateral half of the ring finger. Above the motor threshold, median-nerve stimuli elicit thumb twitches and ulnar-nerve stimulation may produce movements in all fingers (due to stimulation of the interosseus muscles that bring the fingers closer to each other during contraction). Anomalous innervation of the hand, however, is not uncommon, and thus one may not always be able to elicit, for example, thumb twitches by stimulating the thumb side of the volar (palm side) wrist.

Dawson was the first to noninvasively record human SEPs; the stimuli were electrical pulses applied at 1 Hz to the ulnar nerve at the wrist (Dawson, 1947). Since then, the early SEPs peaking at about 20 to 30 ms (and later) over the Rolandic cortex have become widely used experimental and clinical tools to assess the afferent somatosensory pathways and early cortical processing (for a review, see Mauguière, 2011).

In general, when an N20–P30 complex occurs in the Rolandic cortex posterior to the central sulcus, a P20–N30 complex can be recorded anterior to the central sulcus. However, the anterior and posterior SEPs are not just mirror images, and their peak latencies can differ. These findings have led to strong arguments that both the anterior and posterior SEPs would be generated by their own radial source currents just under the electrodes (as schematically presented in Figure 15.3, right top).

In contrast, the emerging MEG data, starting from recordings of steady-state somatosensory-evoked fields (SEFs) to 13-Hz electrical stimulation of the little finger or thumb (Brenner et al., 1978), suggested tangential sources in the central sulcus. Similar evidence of tangential sources in the wall of the central sulcus, especially in cytoarchitectonic area 3b, were obtained with recordings of transient somatosensory evoked fields from the

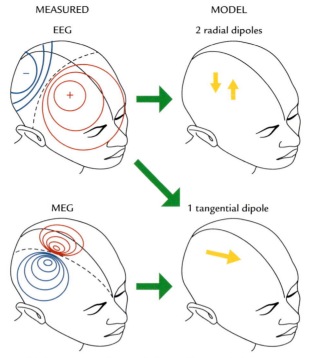

MEASURED   MODEL

EEG   2 radial dipoles

MEG   1 tangential dipole

FIGURE 15.3. Combining EEG and MEG information to deduce source configuration of the 20-ms somatosensory response. The measured EEG pattern (top left) could be equally well explained by either two radial dipoles or a single tangential dipole. The existence of a dipolar MEG pattern (bottom left) suggests that the source is a tangential dipole because radial dipoles would not be visible in MEG. Therefore, combined information from EEG and MEG recordings strongly supports tangential source currents in the posterior wall of the central sulcus.

Rolandic cortex (Kaufman et al., 1981; Hari et al., 1984b; Wood et al., 1985). As the EEG recordings could equally well be explained by models containing either two radial dipoles and one tangential dipole, the combined information from EEG and MEG recordings was decisive as it supported one tangential dipole in the posterior wall of the central sulcus (see Figure 15.3).

Strong support for the tangential area 3b source in the primary somatosensory cortex was obtained from the comparison of 20- to 30-ms MEG and EEG responses that showed dipolar patterns rotated by 90º with respect to each other, as expected for MEG and EEG signals generated by the same tangential sources (Wood et al., 1985) (see also Figure 15.3); the electric and magnetic responses were similar but not identical in their time courses, meaning that additional contributions from some other sources were plausible. Moreover, in agreement with the tangential generators in the posterior wall of the central sulcus, intracranial SEP recordings showed a N20–P30 complex in the postcentral gyrus and P20–N30 on the precentral gyrus (Allison et al., 1989a, 1991).

But if one tangential dipole is the main source of the 20 to 30-ms complex, how can we sometimes record N20 posterior to the central sulcus but P22 anterior to it? Figure 15.4 gives one possible explanation, assuming that, in addition to the tangential source, a radial source with slightly longer latency is activated anterior to the central sulcus. As the

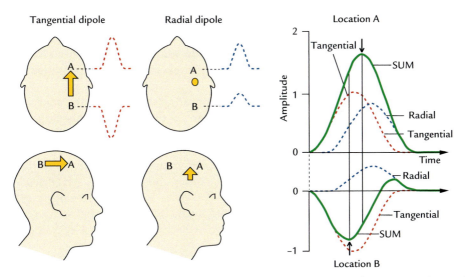

FIGURE 15.4. A potential explanation for latency differences in early SEPs anterior and posterior to the central sulcus. Left panel: A tangential dipole in the central sulcus, in the middle of electrode positions A and B, produces at A and B potentials of opposite polarities but identical time courses, serving as the model for the source of the N20–P20 SEP (negative posterior to the central sulcus). An additional radial dipole beneath electrode A is depicted with a slightly longer latency; it produces potentials of same polarity and time course at both electrodes but with larger amplitude at A than B. Right: The summed potential (SUM, green solid line) at locations A (top) and B (bottom). Note that the peak latencies of the summed potentials differ at locations A and B, as indicated by the arrows. Adapted and reprinted from Hari R: On brain's magnetic responses to sensory stimuli. *J Clin Neurophysiol* 1991, 8: 157–169. With permission from Wolters Kluwer Health, Inc.

contributions from all sources sum up linearly, latency differences will necessarily appear, as is schematically presented in Figure 15.4.

Both MEG measurements and intracranial EEG recordings have suggested that the intracellular current flows during the 20-ms response from the depth toward superficial layers in area 3b of the SI cortex, and thus in a postero-anterior direction. Such a net current direction agrees with excitation in the deep cortical layers, as would be expected on the basis of intracortical recordings in animals (Towe, 1966).

The next deflection in hand area SEPs/SEFs to electrical median nerve stimulation peaks around 30 to 35 ms (P30/P30m) with a polarity opposite to N20/N20m. N20m is more resilient than P30m to fast stimulus repetition rates, implying that the generation of the P30/P30m involves more synapses (Tiihonen et al., 1989). The peak latency of the P30m deflection shortens when the interstimulus interval decreases (Wikström et al., 1996), which could result from stronger rate effects on one component of the generator.

In the SI hand area, MEG recordings provide millimeter resolution for the differentiation of the origin of signals to stimulation of different fingers in the area of the "hand knob" (for anatomical description, see Figure 20.4); altogether, the fingers occupy a 15- to 20-mm strip along the SI cortex (Hari et al., 1993). Activation of the hand knob is somatotopically ordered, and, because of the curved cortical surface, the orientations of sources related to different fingers can be rotated with respect to each other. Consequently, if the whole hand knob was activated at once, the equivalent current dipole would be mislocalized to be in the center of the volume surrounded by the curved cortex. This kind of mislocalization likely happened when vibrotactile stimuli were applied to the whole palm, resulting in a more anterior source location than stimulation of the median nerve in the same subjects (Jousmäki & Forss, 1998).

In the first SEF recordings, carried out with a steady-state approach, the dipolar field patterns were about 2 cm more lateral for stimulation of the thumb than the little finger, consistent with the known somatotopy of the SI cortex (Brenner et al., 1978). The subsequent MEG recordings (Hari et al., 1984a; Okada et al., 1984; Narici et al., 1991) further provided noninvasive information about the well-known "homuncular" organization documented by both direct cortical stimulation (Horsley, 1909; Foerster, 1931; Penfield & Boldrey, 1937) and intracranial recordings from the cortical surface, with medial-to-lateral representation of the foot, trunk, hand, lips, and tongue across the lateral surface of the Rolandic cortex and foot and genitalia represented in the mesial wall (Woolsey & Erickson, 1950; Jasper et al., 1960; Hirsch et al., 1961; Allison et al., 1989a,1996).

Because of the insensitivity of MEG to radial currents, responses to upper limb stimulation seem to arise mainly from the walls of the central sulcus (where currents are tangential with respect to head surface) and with negligible contribution from the convexial cortex. For stimulation of the lower limb, however, one may expect to see signals from more widely spread areas. The reason is that, for most subjects, the foot *representation* area in SI cortex is on the mesial wall of the hemisphere. Therefore, all source currents there should be tangential with respect to the skull. Accordingly, sequential activation of orthogonal cytoarchitectonic areas should be visible as *rotating* magnetic field patterns. This is exactly what happens after tibial, peroneal, and sural nerve stimulation (Huttunen et al., 1987; Fujita et al., 1995; Kakigi et al., 1995b; Hari et al., 1996).

Figure 15.5 shows an example of such a field-pattern rotation after stimulation of the right tibial nerve at the ankle. The first cortical response peaks at 38 ms, which is—due to the longer traveling distance of the action potentials—about 20 ms later than the corresponding responses after upper-limb stimulation. The field patterns are dipolar at several latencies, and they seem to rotate counterclockwise, indicating that the source configuration changes as a function of time. The patterns can be explained by two approximately orthogonal current dipoles with fixed locations and orientations (corresponding to activations of two orthogonal walls of the mesial cortex) but with varying relative strengths as a function of time. Examining the behavior of the dipole moments as a function of time (top right insert) indicated that sources separated by only 3 ms in time can be easily differentiated if their orientations clearly differ (Hari et al., 1996).

One important class of responses from the SI cortex are those triggered by passive movements (see experimental set-ups in Figure 6.3). We discuss these signals in association with corticokinematic coherence (CKC) in Chapter 17 but mention here that the responses peak in SI cortex 70 to 90 ms after passive finger movements (Smeds et al., 2017). These responses predominantly reflect the activity from proprioceptive afferents for two main reasons. First, the responses to passive and active movements are very similar (Piitulainen et al., 2013). Second, analysis of partial directed coherence implies that CKC is considerably (2.7–15.5 times) stronger in the afferent than efferent direction (Bourguignon et al., 2015). Although concomitant tactile stimulation (by letting the moving forefinger touch the table) can increase the afferent coherence by up to 40% (Bourguignon et al., 2015), even in that case, the proprioceptive signaling is the leading contributor to the cortical responses. One may envision that the possibility to quantify and monitor proprioceptive afferents will open new avenues to clinical testing of several patient populations.

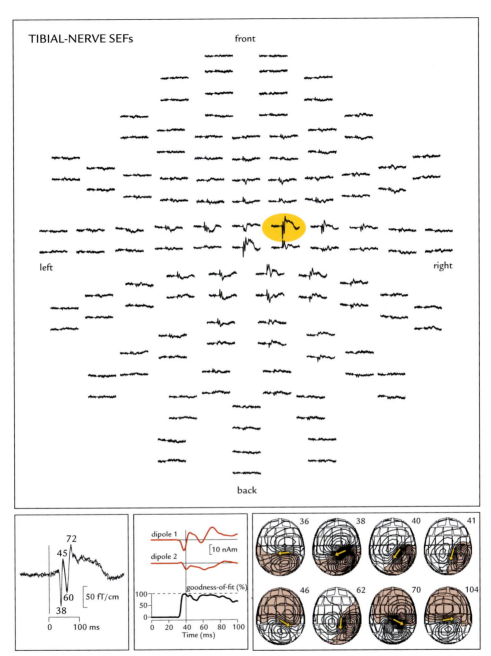

FIGURE 15.5. Posterior tibial nerve SEFs and rotation of the associated field patterns. Top: Spatial distribution of SEFs to electrical stimulation of the left posterior tibial nerve; responses are shown from 122 planar gradiometers; two orthogonal gradients from each sensor locations are grouped together; the head is viewed from above, nose pointing upward in the figure. Passband 0.03–275 Hz, sampling rate 973 Hz, and 800 single responses were averaged. The largest SEF over the right foot area is highlighted by yellow shading. Bottom left: Two averaged SEFs superimposed (from the location highlighted in the left part of the figure), with peak response latencies indicated. Bottom middle: Time courses of dipole

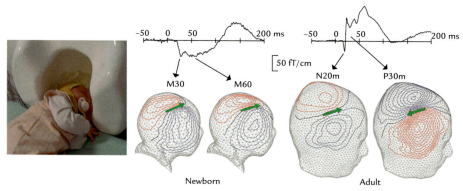

FIGURE 15.6. SEFs in an infant versus an adult. Left: A newborn lies asleep within an adult-sized MEG system so that one side of head is as close to the detectors as possible. Hence recordings were conducted from one hemisphere at a time. Photograph courtesy of Dr. Elina Pihko. Middle: SEFs from a single planar gradiometer over the right somatosensory cortex and the whole field patterns to left-sided median-nerve stimulation in a healthy newborn subject. The earliest deflections peak at 30 and 60 ms, both with the same polarities. Right: SEFs and field patterns in a healthy adult subject to stimulation of the left median nerve. The earliest deflections peak at 20 and 30 ms, with opposite polarities, showing the normal N20m–P30m response. The 306-channel MEG recording was obtained with a passband of 0.03 to 220 Hz and a sampling rate of 987 Hz. Adapted and reprinted from Lauronen L, Nevalainen P, Wikström H, Parkkonen L, Okada Y, Pihko E: Immaturity of somatosensory cortical processing in human newborns. *NeuroImage* 2006, 33: 195–203. With permission from Elsevier.

Figure 15.6 indicates that SEFs reflect activation of the SI cortex also in newborns, but the latencies, polarities, and relative amplitudes of successive deflections differ compared with adult waveforms (Lauronen et al., 2006). These differences likely reflect combined effects of changing myelination that affects conduction velocity, increasing connectivity between brain areas, and the age-dependent changes in the effects of transmitters. A follow-up study in extremely preterm children showed that absence of the SII response at the term-equivalent age predicted impaired motor outcome at the age of 6 years (Lönnberg et al., 2021).

FIGURE 15.5. Continued

moments (in nAm) for two current dipoles used to model the SEFs. These dipoles deviate by 68° in their orientation, identified at 36 and at 41 ms, respectively. The goodness-of-fit of the model is shown on the lowest trace. Bottom right: Field patterns of SEFs presented in the left panel at eight time points. The patterns and the equivalent current dipoles (yellow arrows) rotate counterclockwise as a function of time. Adapted and reprinted from Hari R, Nagamine T, Nishitani N, Mikuni N, Sato T, Tarkiainen A, Shibasaki H: Time-varying activation of different cytoarchitectonic areas of the human SI cortex after tibial nerve stimulation. *Neuroimage* 1996, 4: 111–118. With permission from Elsevier.

■ RESPONSES FROM THE POSTERIOR PARIETAL CORTEX

The posterior parietal cortex (PPC), just posterior to SI, integrates sensory and motor processing and combines tactile and proprioceptive information with other sensory modalities. In MEG recordings, current-dipole sources, with peak activity at 70 to 110 ms, have been identified to airpuff and median-nerve stimuli in PPC medial and posterior to the SI hand area. Airpuffs activate the right PPC irrespective of the laterality of stimulation (Forss et al., 1994), suggesting dominance of the right parietal associative cortex in the processing of complex tactile stimuli that occur in the real world (at least in the six right-handed subjects of this small study). Other sources to electrical stimulation of peripheral nerves have been observed in the mesial cortex in the paracentral lobule (Forss et al., 1996) and bilaterally in the middle and inferior frontal gyri (Mauguière et al., 1997).

Given the importance of the posterior parietal cortex for integration of multisensory sensory inputs (Chapter 16) and cognitive functions—well established in clinical, anatomical, and neurophysiological studies (for reviews, see, e.g., Berlucchi & Vallar, 2018; Freedman & Ibos, 2018)—it is quite surprising how many "blank spots" this brain region with multiple clearly defined subdivisions still contains from the MEG/EEG point of view. Future studies are thus warranted to add noninvasive temporal information on parietal-lobe functions, although one challenge for MEG/EEG recordings is the decreasing synchrony of neuronal firing at the higher levels of the processing hierarchy.

■ RESPONSES FROM THE SII CORTEX

Tactile input from the periphery activates several cortical areas, including the second somatosensory cortex (SII) that is buried deep within the Sylvian fissure. Signals from the human SI and SII cortices were differentiated for the first time by means of MEG almost 40 years ago (Hari et al., 1983a; Teszner et al., 1983; Hari et al., 1984b), before both direct cortical recordings (Allison et al., 1989a) and indirect neuroimaging with PET (Burton et al., 1993); fMRI studies of the SII cortex emerged even later. The sources of SEFs in the SII cortex peak at 90 to 125 ms, with slightly longer latencies to ipsilateral than contralateral stimulation. Interestingly, the SII SEFs are very similar in waveform to intracranial SEPs recorded directly from the cortical surface during neurosurgery (Allison et al., 1989b).

Figure 15.7 shows SEFs to median-nerve stimulation from a healthy control and a patient with progressive myoclonic epilepsy. In the healthy person (left traces), SEFs are elicited in the contralateral, but not ipsilateral, SI cortex as well as bilaterally in the SII cortices. In the patient (right traces), "giant" SEFs are seen in the contralateral SI cortex and are also clearly evident (but delayed) in the ipsilateral SI. Despite these huge SI responses, the SII responses are abolished (Forss et al., 2001). This example illustrates the usefulness of evoked-response recordings in single subjects to unravel the functions of the cortical somatosensory network in health and disease.

We have already compared (see Figure 10.9) the potential and field patterns simulated in a four-layer spherical model to clarify data obtained to peroneal nerve stimulation at the foot dorsum (Kaukoranta et al., 1986). In MEG, distinct activation patterns occur over contralateral primary projection cortex at the top of the head (where the primary representation area of the foot is) and over the SII cortices bilaterally, indicating that these field patterns reflect three distinct sources. The simulation further demonstrates that these sources would produce the maximum EEG response over the contralateral scalp, clearly lateral to

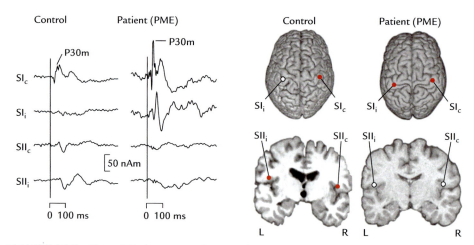

FIGURE 15.7. Giant SEFs in progressive myoclonus epilepsy (PME). Left: Time courses of source strengths of SEFs from contra- and ipsilateral SI (SI$_c$ and SI$_i$) and from the contra- and ipsilateral SII (SII$_c$ and SII$_i$) in a healthy control subject and a patient with PME to stimulation of the left median nerve. Right: Source locations for the healthy control subject and patient superimposed on the individual three-dimensional brain renderings viewed from top and on coronal MRI slices (L = left; R = right). Source locations found on the basis of the MEG data are indicated by red dots whereas the white dots refer to likely source areas that could not be inferred from the measured signals. Adapted and reproduced with permission from Forss N, Silén T, Karjalainen T: Lack of activation of human secondary somatosensory cortex in Unverricht-Lundborg type of progressive myoclonus epilepsy. *Ann Neurol* 2001, 49: 90–97. With permission from John Wiley & Sons.

foot SI and medial to foot SII, and the most likely (but erroneous) interpretation of these data would be thus a radial source just under the potential maximum. It was this clear-cut separation of magnetic field patterns generated by SI and SII activations to lower-limb stimulation that originally allowed the sources in the SII cortex to be identified (Teszner et al., 1983).

◼ SOMATOSENSORY STEADY-STATE RESPONSES

As already mentioned, SSRs, with their robust signal-to-noise ratio, were the first MEG signals recorded from the somatosensory system. Somatosensory SSRs can be elicited, for example, by a vibrator (Franzen & Offenloch, 1969) or by repetitive electrical stimulation of the fingers. However, strong electrical stimuli applied on a motor nerve or directly on the muscle belly and repeated at > 20 Hz can cause painful tetanic contraction of the muscles. As in other sensory modalities, several stimuli with different repetition rates can be presented at the same time and differentiated (cf. auditory frequency tagging in Chapter 13 and visual frequency tagging in Chapter 14). One potential application for somatosensory SSRs, recorded with mobile EEG devices, is for BCIs for people with motor disabilities, as the somatosensory stimulation does not involve the person's vision or hearing that may be needed for other purposes, for example, when driving a motorized wheelchair (Petit et al., 2021).

■ HIGH-FREQUENCY OSCILLATIONS IN THE SI CORTEX

Using MEG with a very wide recording passband and a high number of averaged responses, it is possible to pick up 600-Hz oscillatory bursts (HFOs) from the human SI cortex after stimulation of different sensory nerves (Curio et al., 1994, 1997; Hashimoto et al., 1996), as shown in Figure 15.8, left. Upper-limb stimulation HFOs are superimposed on the 20-ms response and are generated close to its source; furthermore, both responses show similar somatotopy (Curio et al., 1997). Interestingly, the HFOs are suppressed during sleep, whereas the 20-ms response is not (Hashimoto et al., 1996), which is a rare exception to the general rule that the higher the dominant frequency of a response, the more resilient it is to stimulus repetition and changes of vigilance. Consequently it was suggested (Curio et al., 1994) that the 20-ms response and the HFOs reflect different cortical currents: Whereas the 20-ms response results from postsynaptic currents, HFOs may arise from cortical action potential bursts, possibly in cortical inhibitory interneurons (see also Hashimoto et al., 1996).

Expanding these lines of thought, it was suggested that high-frequency EEG, recorded from the scalp using advanced amplifier technology and sophisticated signal analysis, could provide a new, noninvasive window to monitoring cortical spiking in behaving humans in the future (Telenczuk et al., 2011). Now, 10 years later, a recent study with an ultra-low noise single-channel magnetometer (Waterstraat et al., 2021) demonstrated that it really is possible to record single-trial HFOs, as seen in the bottom panel of Figure 15.8. The "noise floor" (see Chapter 10) of the first-order axial gradiometer (baseline 120 mm, pickup-coil diameter of 45 mm) was as low as $0.18\,fT/\sqrt{Hz}$ around 600 Hz, and thus lower by a factor of 10 compared with conventional MEG devices. At this noise level, the limiting factor of the recordings was the thermal body noise.

An interesting functional dissociation between the HFOs and N20m is that the occurrence of weak versus strong HFOs does not correlate with N20m amplitude, suggesting that HFOs do not directly depend on thalamocortical input but rather reflect local networks (Waterstraat et al., 2021). These results show how important it is to invest in improving the sensitivity of measurement instruments, and not only focus on extending spatial coverage.

■ PAIN AND NOCICEPTIVE RESPONSES

MEG recordings have provided the first evidence in humans that noxious input reaches the SII region in the parietal operculum. MEG responses were recorded to (painful) electric stimulation of dental pulp (Hari et al., 1983b) and later to carbon dioxide stimulation of the nasal mucosa (Huttunen et al., 1986; Hari et al., 1997), as well as to CO_2-laser and thulium-laser stimulation of the skin (Kakigi et al., 1995a; Forss et al., 2005b). All these stimuli activated the upper bank of the Sylvian fissure.

The intensity of noxious stimuli is differentially represented in the SI and SII cortices, with a possible role for the bilateral SII cortex in the detection and recognition of the noxious nature of stimuli (Timmermann et al., 2001).

The laser pulses can activate both Aδ- and C-fibers in the skin, but interestingly one can manipulate the stimulus to be rather selective to either fiber type. The method is based on findings that C-fiber endings are more dense in the skin than are the Aδ-fibers, and their activation threshold is lower (Bragard et al., 1996). Thus C-fibers can be activated rather selectively by restricting low-intensity laser pulses to a tiny skin area (e.g., by directing the laser beam through a plate that contains small holes and is attached to the skin).

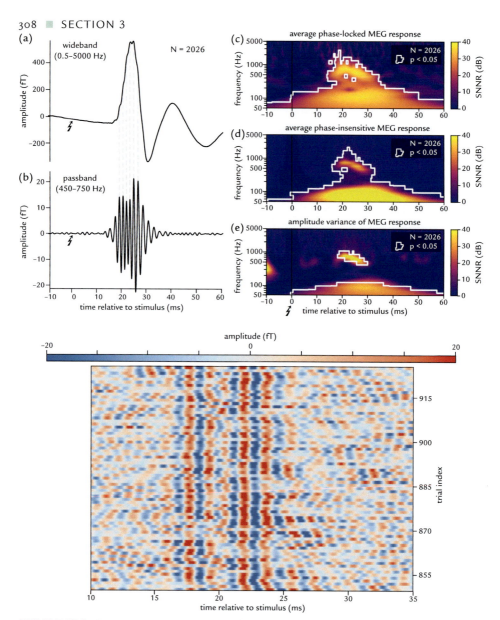

FIGURE 15.8. Human somatosensory cortical 600-Hz HFOs. Upper half of the figure, panels (a) and (b): SEFs and HFOs (averaged across about 2,000 trials) from a healthy human to electrical stimulation of the left median nerve at 3.27 Hz; an axial gradiometer picked up activity from the right SI hand area. Trace (a) shows a typical wideband SEF (passband 0.5–5000 Hz) with a prominent N20m deflection, whereas trace (b) shows HFOs after bandpass filtering through 450–750 Hz. HFO peaks are visible as small bumps on the rising and falling slopes of the N20m SEF. (c) to (e): Time–frequency plots of the averaged full-band responses phase-locked to the stimulus (panel (c)) or without paying attention to phase locking (panel (d)). Panel (e) displays amplitude variance of the responses. SNNR refers to signal-plus-noise-to-noise ratio. Lower half of the figure: Amplitudes of successive (from bottom to top) single-trial responses (passband 450–750 Hz), with color-coded amplitude. Despite intertrial variability, the main features of the single-trial HFOs are clearly visible. Adapted and reprinted from Waterstraat G, Korber R, Storm JH, Curio G: Noninvasive neuromagnetic single-trial analysis of human neocortical population spikes. *Proc Natl Acad Sci U S A* 2021, 118: e2017401118. With permission from the Proceedings of the National Academy of Sciences U S A.

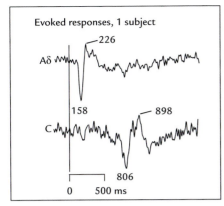
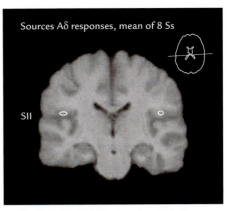

FIGURE 15.9. Responses to painful laser stimulation of the left hand in a healthy human subject. Left: MEG responses recorded with a planar gradiometer over the right (contralateral) SII region to selective laser stimulation of Aδ- (top) and C-fibers (bottom) in a single subject. Peak latencies are indicated. About 100 single responses were averaged; passband 0.03–200 Hz, sampling rate 600 Hz. Right: A coronal brain slice was generated by averaging elastically transformed MR images of eight subjects (Ss); the white ovals show the same eight individuals' mean (± standard error of mean) source locations in the SII cortex to Aδ-stimuli. Adapted and reprinted from Forss N, Raij TT, Seppä M, Hari R: Common cortical network for first and second pain. *NeuroImage* 2005, 24: 132–142. With permission from Elsevier.

Figure 15.9 shows responses of a single subject to thulium-laser pulses aimed to preferentially activate either the Aδ-fibers (with strong ~520 mJ pulses on a 10-mm^2 area of skin) or the C-fibers (with weak 50 mJ pulses on an area of 0.2–0.3 mm^2). The SII responses peak at about 160 ms to Aδ-fiber stimulation and at about 800 ms to C-fiber stimuli (Forss et al., 2005b). (For the experimental setup, see Figure 6.2 and the associated text.)

Despite these selective stimulation methods and distinct neurophysiological evoked responses, detailed studies of chronic pain syndromes with MEG/EEG are still rare, whereas fMRI-based assessment strategies are commonly applied (Mayer et al., 2015).

Measures relying on modified power ratios between (MEG) rhythms of different frequency bands show potential for differentiating chronic pain patients from healthy persons (e.g., Witjes et al., 2021), but they do not provide specificity regarding other brain disorders. Similarly, (EEG) responses elicited by nociceptive stimulation can differentiate patients with neuropathic pain from healthy control subjects but cannot distinguish between pain syndromes of different etiologies (Lenoir et al., 2020).

Chronic pain often affects the motor system, and thus—in addition to studies of the somatosensory cortex (Juottonen et al., 2002)—the reactivity of motor-cortex rhythms might offer a new tool in the future to study chronic pain of different etiologies (Kirveskari et al., 2010). MEG has been used to monitor how chronic regional pain syndrome (CRPS), a serious pain disorder, might develop and spread to involve different parts of the brain and body (Forss et al., 2005a; Iwatsuki et al., 2021).

Hartley and Slater (2014, p 238) wisely concluded, while discussing nociceptive brain activity in newborns: "Simultaneously measuring the changes that are evoked in behaviour, physiology and the cortex following noxious events will provide the best approach to understanding the neonate's experience of pain." The same is certainly true for adults as well.

■ REFERENCES

Allison T, McCarthy G, Wood CC, Darcey TM, Spencer DD, Williamson PD: Human cortical potentials evoked by stimulation of the median nerve: I. Cytoarchitectonic areas generating short-latency activity. *J Neurophysiol* 1989a, 62: 694–710.

Allison T, McCarthy G, Wood C, Williamson P, Spencer D: Human cortical potentials evoked by stimulation of the median nerve: II. Cytoarchitectonic areas generating long-latency activity. *J Neurophysiol* 1989b, 62: 711–722.

Allison T, McCarthy G, Wood CC, Jones SJ: Potentials evoked in human and monkey cerebral cortex by stimulation of the median nerve: a review of scalp and intracranial recordings. *Brain* 1991, 114: 2465–2503.

Allison T, McCarthy G, Luby M, Puce A, Spencer DD: Localization of functional regions of human mesial cortex by somatosensory evoked potential recording and by cortical stimulation. *Electroencephalogr Clin Neurophysiol* 1996, 100: 126–140.

Berlucchi G, Vallar G: The history of the neurophysiology and neurology of the parietal lobe. In: Vallar G, Coslett HB, eds. *Handbook of Clinical Neurology, Vol. 151, The Parietal Lobe*, 2018: 3–30.

Bourguignon M, Piitulainen H, De Tiège X, Jousmäki V, Hari R: Corticokinematic coherence mainly reflects movement-induced proprioceptive feedback. *NeuroImage* 2015, 106: 382–390.

Bragard D, Chen AC, Plaghki L: Direct isolation of ultra-late (C-fibre) evoked brain potentials by CO_2 laser stimulation of tiny cutaneous surface areas in man. *Neurosci Lett* 1996, 209: 81–84.

Brenner D, Lipton J, Kaufman L, Williamson SJ: Somatically evoked magnetic fields of the human brain. *Science* 1978, 199: 81–83.

Burton H, Videen T, Raichle M: Tactile-vibration-activated foci in insular and parietal-opercular cortex studied with positron emission tomography: mapping the second somatosensory area in humans. *Somatos Mot Res* 1993, 10: 297–308.

Curio G, Mackert BM, Burghoff M, Koetitz R, Abraham-Fuchs K, Harer W: Localization of evoked neuromagnetic 600 Hz activity in the cerebral somatosensory system. *Electroencephalogr Clin Neurophysiol* 1994, 91: 483–487.

Curio G, Mackert B-M, Burghoff M, Neumann J, Nolte G, Scherg M, Marx P: Somatotopic source arrangement of 600 Hz oscillatory magnetic fields at the human primary somatosensory hand cortex. *Neurosci Lett* 1997, 234: 131–134.

Dawson GD: Cerebral responses to electrical stimulation of peripheral nerve in man. *J Neurol Neurosurg Psychiatry* 1947, 10: 134–140.

Erné S, Curio G, Trahms L, Trontelj Z, Aust P: Magnetic activity of a single peripheral nerve in man. In: Atsumi K, Kotani M, Ueno S, Katila T, Williamson S, eds. *Biomagnetism '87.* Tokyo: Tokyo Denki University Press, 1988: 166–169.

Foerster O: The cerebral cortex of man. *Lancet* 1931, 218: 309–312.

Forss N, Salmelin R, Hari R: Comparison of somatosensory evoked fields to airpuff and electric stimuli. *Electroencephalogr Clin Neurophysiol* 1994, 92: 510–517.

Forss N, Merlet I, Vanni S, Hämäläinen M, Mauguière F, Hari R: Activation of human mesial cortex during somatosensory attention task. *Brain Res* 1996, 734: 229–235.

Forss N, Silén T, Karjalainen T: Lack of activation of human secondary somatosensory cortex in Unverricht-Lundborg type of progressive myoclonus epilepsy. *Ann Neurol* 2001, 49: 90–97.

Forss N, Kirveskari E, Gockel M: Mirror-like spread of chronic pain. *Neurology* 2005a, 65: 748–750.

Forss N, Raij TT, Seppä M, Hari R: Common cortical network for first and second pain. *NeuroImage* 2005b, 24: 132–142.

Franzen O, Offenloch K: Evoked response correlates of psychophysical magnitude estimates for tactile stimulation in man. *Exp Brain Res* 1969, 8: 1–18.

Freedman DJ, Ibos G: An integrative framework for sensory, motor, and cognitive functions of the posterior parietal cortex. *Neuron* 2018, 97: 1219–1234.

Fujita S, Nakasato N, Matani A, Tamura I, Yoshimoto T: Short latency somatosensory evoked field for tibial nerve stimulation: rotation of dipole pattern over the whole head. In: Baumgartner C, Deecke

L, Stroink G, Williamson SJ, eds. *Biomagnetism: Fundamental Research and Clinical Applications*. Amsterdam: Elsevier, 1995: 95–98.

Hari R, Hämäläinen M, Kaukoranta E, Reinikainen K, Teszner D: Neuromagnetic responses from the second somatosensory cortex in man. *Acta Neurol Scand* 1983a, 68: 207–212.

Hari R, Kaukoranta E, Reinikainen K, Huopaniemi T, Mauno J: Neuromagnetic localization of cortical activity evoked by painful dental stimulation in man. *Neurosci Lett* 1983b, 42: 77–82.

Hari R, Hämäläinen M, Ilmoniemi R, Kaukoranta E, Reinikainen K, Salminen J, Alho K, Näätänen R, Sams M: Responses of the primary auditory cortex to pitch changes in a sequence of tone pips: neuromagnetic recordings in man. *Neurosci Lett* 1984a, 50: 127–132.

Hari R, Reinikainen K, Kaukoranta E, Hämäläinen M, Ilmoniemi R, Penttinen A, Salminen J, Teszner D: Somatosensory evoked cerebral magnetic fields from SI and SII in man. *Electroencephalogr Clin Neurophysiol* 1984b, 57: 254–263.

Hari R, Hällström J, Tiihonen J, Joutsiniemi S: Multichannel detection of magnetic compound action fields of median and ulnar nerves. *Electroencephalogr Clin Neurophysiol* 1989, 72: 277–280.

Hari R, Karhu J, Hämäläinen M, Knuutila J, Salonen O, Sams M, Vilkman V: Functional organization of the human first and second somatosensory cortices: a neuromagnetic study. *Eur J Neurosci* 1993, 5: 724–734.

Hari R, Nagamine T, Nishitani N, Mikuni N, Sato T, Tarkiainen A, Shibasaki H: Time-varying activation of different cytoarchitectonic areas of the human SI cortex after tibial nerve stimulation. *NeuroImage* 1996, 4: 111–118.

Hari R, Portin K, Kettenmann B, Jousmäki V, Kobal G: Right-hemisphere preponderance of responses to painful CO_2 stimulation of the human nasal mucosa. *Pain* 1997, 72: 145–151.

Hartley C, Slater R: Neurophysiological measures of nociceptive brain activity in the newborn infant—the next steps. *Acta Paediatr* 2014, 103: 238–242.

Hashimoto I, Mashiko T, Imada T: Somatic evoked high-frequency magnetic oscillations reflect activity of inhibitory interneurons in the human somatosensory cortex. *Electroencephalogr Clin Neurophysiol* 1996, 100: 189–203.

Hirsch JF, Pertuiset B, Calvet J, Buisson-Ferey J, Fischgold H, Scherrer J: Etude des responses electrocorticales obtenues chez l'homme par des stimulations somesthesiques et visuelles [Study of electrocortical responses obtained in man by somesthetic and visual responses]. *Electroencephalogr Clin Neurophysiol* 1961, 13: 411–424.

Hodgkin AL, Huxley AF: Action potentials recorded from inside a nerve fibre. *Nature* 1939, 144: 710–711.

Horsley V: The function of the so-called motor area of the brain (Linacre Lecture). *Br Med J* 1909, 11: 125–132.

Huttunen J, Kobal G, Kaukoranta E, Hari R: Cortical responses to painful CO_2 stimulation of the nasal mucosa. *Electroencephalogr Clin Neurophysiol* 1986, 64: 347–349.

Huttunen J, Kaukoranta E, Hari R: Cerebral magnetic responses to stimulation of tibial and sural nerves. *J Neurol Sci* 1987, 79: 43–54.

Iwatsuki K, Hoshiyama M, Yoshida A, Uemura JI, Hoshino A, Morikawa I, Nakagawa Y, Hirata H: Chronic pain-related cortical neural activity in patients with complex regional pain syndrome. *IBRO Neurosci Rep* 2021, 10: 208–215.

Jasper H, Lende R, Rasmussen T: Evoked potentials from the exposed somatosensory cortex in man. *J Nerv Ment Dis* 1960, 130: 526–537.

Jousmäki V, Forss N: Effects of stimulus intensity on signals from human somatosensory cortices. *Neuroreport* 1998, 9: 3427–3431.

Juottonen K, MG, Silén T, Hurri H, Hari R, Forss N: Altered central sensorimotor processing in patients with complex regional pain syndrome. *Pain* 2002, 98: 315–323.

Kakigi R, Koyama S, Hoshiyama M, Kitamura Y, Shimojo M, Watanabe S: Pain-related magnetic fields following painful CO_2 laser stimulation in man. *Neurosci Lett* 1995a, 192: 45–48.

Kakigi R, Koyama S, Hoshiyama M, Shimojo M, Kitamura Y, Watanabe S: Topography of somatosensory evoked magnetic fields following posterior tibial nerve stimulation. *Electroencephalogr Clin Neurophysiol* 1995b, 95: 127–134.

Kaufman L, Okada Y, Brenner D, Williamson S: On the relation between somatic evoked potentials and fields. *Int J Neurosci* 1981, 15: 223–239.

Kaukoranta E, Hari R, Hämäläinen M, Huttunen J: Cerebral magnetic fields evoked by peroneal nerve stimulation. *Somatosens Res* 1986, 3: 309–321.

Kirveskari E, Vartiainen NV, Gockel M, Forss N: Motor cortex dysfunction in complex regional pain syndrome. *Clin Neurophysiol* 2010, 121: 1085–1091.

Lauronen L, Nevalainen P, Wikström H, Parkkonen L, Okada Y, Pihko E: Immaturity of somatosensory cortical processing in human newborns. *NeuroImage* 2006, 33: 195–203.

Lenoir D, Willaert W, Coppieters I, Malfliet A, Ickmans K, Nijs J, Vonck K, Meeus M, Cagnie B: Electroencephalography during nociceptive stimulation in chronic pain patients: a systematic review. *Pain Med* 2020, 21: 3413–3427.

Lönnberg P, Pihko E, Lauronen L, Nurminen J, Andersson S, Metsäranta M, Lano A, Nevalainen P: Secondary somatosensory cortex evoked responses and 6-year neurodevelopmental outcome in extremely preterm children. *Clin Neurophysiol* 2021, 132: 1572–1583.

Mauguière F, Merlet I, Forss N, Vanni S, Jousmäki V, Adeleine P, Hari R: Activation of a distributed somatosensory cortical network in the human brain: a dipole modelling study of magnetic fields evoked by median nerve stimulation. Part I: location and activation timing of SEF sources. *Electroencephalogr Clin Neurophysiol* 1997, 104: 281–289.

Mauguière F: Somatosensory-evoked potentials: normal responses, abnormal waveforms, and clinical applications in neurological disease In: Schomer DL, Lopes da Silva FH, eds. *Niedermeyer's Electroencephalography: Basic Principles, Clinical Applications, and Related Fields.* Philadelphia, PA: Lippincott Williams & Wilkins, 2011: 1003–1056.

Mayer EA, Gupta A, Kilpatrick LA, Hong JY: Imaging brain mechanisms in chronic visceral pain. *Pain* 2015, 156 Suppl 1: S50–S63.

Narici L, Modena I, Opsomer RJ, Pizzella V, Romani GL, Torrioli G, Traversa R, Rossini PM: Neuromagnetic somatosensory homunculus: a non-invasive approach in humans. *Neurosci Lett* 1991, 121: 51–54.

Okada YC, Tanenbaum R, Williamson SJ, Kaufman L: Somatotopic organization of the human somatosensory cortex revealed by neuromagnetic measurements. *Exp Brain Res* 1984, 56: 197–205.

Penfield W, Boldrey E: Somatic motor and sensory representation in the cerebral cortex of man as studied by electrical stimulation. *Brain* 1937, 60: 389–443.

Petit J, Rouillard J, Cabestaing F: EEG-based brain-computer interfaces exploiting steady-state somatosensory-evoked potentials: a literature review. *J Neural Eng* 2021, 18: 051003.

Piitulainen H, Bourguignon M, De Tiege X, Hari R, Jousmäki V: Corticokinematic coherence during active and passive finger movements. *Neuroscience* 2013, 238: 361–370.

Smeds E, Piitulainen H, Bourguignon M, Jousmäki V, Hari R: Effect of interstimulus interval on cortical proprioceptive responses to passive finger movements. *Eur J Neurosci* 2017, 45: 290–298.

Stegeman DF, Dumitru D, King JC, Roeleveld K: Near- and far-fields: source characteristics and the conducting medium in neurophysiology. *J Clin Neurophysiol* 1997, 14: 429–442.

Telenczuk B, Baker SN, Herz AV, Curio G: High-frequency EEG covaries with spike burst patterns detected in cortical neurons. *J Neurophysiol* 2011, 105: 2951–2959.

Teszner D, Hari R, Nicolas P, Varpula T: Somatosensory evoked magnetic fields: mapping and the influence of stimulus repetition rate. *Nuovo Cimento* 1983, 2D: 429–437.

Tiihonen J, Hari R, Hämäläinen M: Early deflections of cerebral magnetic responses to median nerve stimulation. *Electroencephalogr Clin Neurophysiol* 1989, 74: 290–296.

Timmermann L, Ploner M, Haucke K, Schmitz F, Baltissen R, Schnitzler A: Differential coding of pain intensity in the human primary and secondary somatosensory cortex. *J Neurophysiol* 2001, 86: 1499–1503.

Towe AL: On the nature of the primary evoked response. *Exp Neurol* 1966, 15: 113–139.

Waterstraat G, Korber R, Storm JH, Curio G: Noninvasive neuromagnetic single-trial analysis of human neocortical population spikes. *Proc Natl Acad Sci U S A* 2021, 118: e2017401118

Wikström H, Huttunen J, Korvenoja A, Viranen J, Salonen O, Aronen H, Ilmoniemi R: Effects of interstimulus interval on somatosensory evoked magnetic fields (SEFs): a hypothesis concerning SEF generation at the primary sensorimotor cortex. *Electroencephalogr Clin Neurophysiol* 1996, 100: 479–487.

Wikswo JP, Barach JP, Freeman JA: Magnetic field of a nerve impulse: first measurements. *Science* 1980, 208: 53–55.

Witjes B, Baillet S, Roy M, Oostenveld R, Huygen FJPM, de Vos CC: Magnetoencephalography reveals increased slow-to-fast alpha power ratios in patients with chronic pain. *Pain Rep* 2021, 6: e928.

Wood CC, Cohen D, Cuffin BN, Yarita M, Allison T: Electric sources in the human somatosensory cortex: identification by combined magnetic and potential field recordings. *Science* 1985, 227: 1051–1053.

Woolsey CN, Erickson TC: Study of the postcentral gyrus of man by the evoked potential technique. *Trans Am Neurol Assoc* 1950, 51: 50–52.

CHAPTER 16

OTHER SENSORY RESPONSES, MULTISENSORY INTERACTION, AND INTEROCEPTION

The senses deceive from time to time, and it is prudent never to trust wholly those who have deceived us even once.

RENÉ DESCARTES

Tears come from the heart and not from the brain.

LEONARDO DA VINCI

After having discussed in the previous chapters the most extensively studied three exteroceptive senses—audition, vision, and somatosensation—in this chapter we first turn to smell and taste and then consider multisensory interactions. We then take a brief tour through the rapidly expanding research area of interoception that is related to sensations from the inner body.

■ OLFACTORY AND GUSTATORY RESPONSES

Our ability to enjoy a fine haute cuisine dinner paired with a vintage wine relies on the ability of our brains to blend olfactory and gustatory information—one highly appreciated multisensory interaction. Olfactory sensations depend on context, and some odors trigger autobiographic memories that take us back to childhood (Willander & Larsson, 2006). For an excellent source about olfaction's historical scientific and philosophical connections, see Barwich (2020).

In 2004, the Nobel Prize in Physiology or Medicine was awarded to Richard Axel and Linda B. Buck "for their discoveries of odorant receptors and the organization of the olfactory system." The coupling between specific odors and olfactory receptors is a very complex one, and the brain mechanisms of olfaction remain insufficiently understood, especially in humans and compared with our overall understanding of hearing, vision, and touch. Some important evidence on the functional neuroanatomy of human olfaction and gustation comes from epilepsy patients in whom direct electrical stimulation of insular cortex during surgery has elicited infrequent gustatory and olfactory hallucinations described mainly as "unpleasant" or "nasty" or sometimes unidentifiable sensations (Iannilli & Gudziol, 2019;

Yih et al., 2019). The unpleasant smells included chlorine, ether, and something with a "metallic quality."

In Chapter 6, we introduced the equipment for olfactory and gustatory stimulation and the related experimental setups. Here we present some EEG/MEG findings, although the field is still developing, mainly because of technological challenges and relatively few researchers in these areas.

Olfactory Responses

In the 1950s, olfactory stimulation was observed to elicit evoked responses and prolonged sinusoidal oscillations in rabbit olfactory bulb (Adrian, 1950; Ottoson, 1954), and detailed high-density electrical mapping of the responses in cat olfactory cortex started in the early 1960s (Freeman, 1975). In humans, the first olfaction-evoked EEG responses were recorded almost 60 years ago (Finkenzeller, 1966).

A point regarding nomenclature and some ambiguities in the literature needs to be made. Some investigators refer to OERPs or olfactory event-related potentials. However, others use the term chemosensory evoked potentials (CSEPs) or sometimes chemosensory event-related potentials to denote *both* olfactory and gustatory evoked responses; thus the terms oCSEPs and gCSEPs can appear in the literature to specify olfactory and gustatory responses, respectively. Here we use the terms olfactory CSEP/CSEF and gustatory CSEP/CSEF to denote electric potentials (P) and magnetic fields (F) elicited by smell and taste, respectively.

Reliable olfactory CSEPs can be recorded by averaging as few as 10 to 30 single responses (Kobal & Hummel, 1988; Rombaux et al., 2006), but the ISIs have to be on the order of 30 to 40 s to prevent response decrements (which result in part from adaptation of the receptors). The reliability of the responses increases if subjects breathe through their mouth during stimulus delivery. Traditionally, olfactory CSEPs have been recorded from midline sites (Fz, Cz, Pz).

Noxious CO_2 stimulation applied to the nostril evokes a clear peripheral receptor potential in the nasal mucosa, as is shown in Figure 16.1 (left), where brief painful carbon dioxide pulses are presented at very long interstimulus intervals (ISIs), once every 2 min. The eight superimposed single traces show excellent replicability of this nasal mucosa potential (NMP) that begins about 30 ms after stimulus onset and last for about 1 s (Kobal, 1985b); in some cases, these NMPs can last up to 8 s (Lötsch et al., 1997).

In many studies, typically cortical olfactory EEG responses show a prominent widespread scalp-negative deflection peaking between 300 and 480 ms (see Kobal, 1981; Kobal & Hummel, 1988), followed by a scalp-positive deflection at 350 to 455 ms or even later (Rombaux et al., 2012). The peak latencies do strongly depend on the odor, its concentration, and the applied ISI; shorter ISIs elicit later (and smaller) responses (reviewed by Gudziol & Guntinas-Lichius, 2019). Moreover, the peak latencies differ considerably in EEG and MEG recordings (see Figure 16.1), as a clear indication of the sensitivity of these two methods to potentially different source configurations.

Figure 16.1 (right) shows simultaneously recorded magnetic and electric olfactory responses to three odorants: 2-phenylethyl alcohol (producing a rose-like smell), hydrogen sulfide (H_2S), and vanillin. The stimuli were applied nonsynchronously to breathing once every 40 s within a continuous, temperature- and humidity-controlled airflow (with a presentation similar to the CO_2 pulses in the left panel of the figure). The MEG responses peaked at 770 ± 30, 820 ± 30, and 700 ± 50 ms (mean ± SEM) for phenylethyl alcohol, hydrogen sulfide, and vanillin, respectively. Interestingly, the peaks of the EEG vertex responses (at

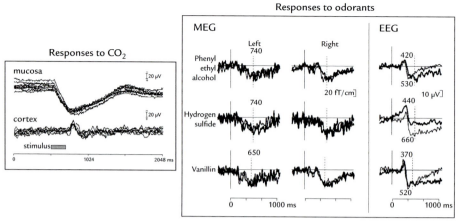

FIGURE 16.1. Responses to CO_2 and odorant stimulation of the nasal mucosa. Left panel: Eight single responses are superimposed from the nasal mucosa (top traces) and cortex, as recorded from vertex (bottom traces; EEG referenced to A1), indicating good response reproducibility. Filter setting was DC–100 Hz. The stimulus was 200-ms bolus of 54% CO_2 delivered once every 120 s to the nostril ipsilateral to the peripheral recording (grey bar). The peripheral response starts at ~30 ms and the main deflection of the cerebral response peaks at ~290 ms. Adapted and reproduced with permission from Kobal G: Pain-related electrical potentials of the human nasal mucosa elicited by chemical stimulation. *Pain* 1985, 22: 151–163. Right panel: Magnetic responses from the left and right temporal lobes and electric responses from the vertex in a single subject to three odorants. The superimposed thick and thin traces refer to stimulation of the right and left nostrils, respectively. Adapted and reproduced with permission from Kettenmann B, Jousmäki V, Portin K, Salmelin R, Kobal G, Hari R: Odorants activate the human superior temporal sulcus. *Neurosci Lett* 1996, 203: 143–145.

610 ± 20, 710 ± 30, and 580 ± 50 ms, respectively) did not coincide with those from MEG (Kettenmann et al., 1996), suggesting that the sources of the MEG and EEG responses may differ, at least in part. The sources from the Kettenmann et al. (1996) study were suggested to be in the region of the posterior STS; however, subsequent combined MEG and EEG recordings have implicated putative source areas in the anterior-central insula and parainsular cortex (Kettenmann et al., 1997; Gudziol & Guntinas-Lichius, 2019).

Olfactory evoked responses are technically difficult to record because of the complexity of stimulation equipment as well as the necessity to use a long ISI to avoid receptor adaptation. Unfortunately, the latter adds noise to the responses because the subject's vigilance will likely vary during a long experiment unless extremely engaged participants can be found. It is thus understandable that because of their large interindividual variability and complicated collection procedure, olfactory CSEPs have not been clinically used for studying olfactory impairments (Lötsch & Hummel, 2006; Rombaux et al., 2012), although they have been reported to be abolished in anosmic individuals (see Huart et al., 2013; Güdücü et al., 2019). Current diagnostics and follow-up of anosmias relies on validated psychophysical smell tests.

One extra challenge for olfactory studies is the possibility of concomitant tactile stimulation of the nasal mucosa, which produces a somatosensory-evoked response of its own and thereby confounds the recording. In Chapter 6 we described how to avoid this problem by embedding stimuli within a continuous humidified and warmed airflow. Still other experimental parameters, such as airflow and odorant concentration, affect the results. For example, the odor-induced changes in the brain's 1- to 3-Hz and 5- to 9-Hz rhythms depend on odorant concentration (Han et al., 2018). Perhaps the lack of parametric standardization across laboratories in the past may be responsible, in part, for the variability in observed findings?

Gustatory Responses

Taste stimuli can be delivered via a "gustometer" on the tongue as pulsed boluses of salt and sugar solutions interspersed with boluses of a tasteless saliva-like ionic solution, with the option of incorporated recording electrodes on the dorsal surface of the tongue (see Chapter 6). Similar to the olfactory NMP, a peripheral electrotastegram (ETG)—reflecting summed potentials from the lingual fungiform papillae—can be recorded directly from the tongue (Feldman et al., 2003). Similar to somatosensory responses, the temperature of the tissue is important for reliable responses, and the modern gustometer thus allows the temperature of the tongue to be maintained at 36 °C as the mouth must be kept open during this stimulation (Iannilli et al., 2014).

Similar to olfactory CSEPs, the gustatory CSEPs have been traditionally recorded from scalp midline using long ISIs—typically around 30 s—to avoid adaptation at the receptor level (Kobal, 1985a). In the experiment illustrated in Figure 16.2 (Iannilli & Gudziol, 2019), about 80 trials were collected per one average, which means that the experiment lasted as long as 48 min; thus the changes in subject's vigilance—as noted above—are a potential issue.

Figure 16.2 shows simultaneously recorded electric and magnetic responses to salty (200 mM NaCl) liquid pulses (Iannilli et al., 2014). The EEG responses show a spatially diffuse negativity ~250 ms after stimulus onset (maximal at the temporal scalp and with a likely source in the middle insula), followed by centroparietal positivity peaking at ~650 ms (with sources in the posterior insula and parietal operculum).

Although reliable gustatory MEG and EEG responses can be readily obtained, currently these remain largely limited to research laboratories because of the associated technical challenges.

▪ MULTISENSORY INTERACTION

Overview

Our everyday experiences involve inputs from multiple senses, and their temporal coincidence helps to perceive and recognize objects and events. Multisensory processing occurs even when we think that we rely on just one sense—tasting our favorite food is one very florid example of this, as is entering a spacious cathedral where the immediately perceivable ambiance is the result of visual, auditory, and olfactory inputs, also affected by the space's temperature. Despite this obvious multisensory integration in human perception, the bulk of the neurophysiological and neuroimaging literature has been devoted to examining neural responses to stimuli presented in a single sensory modality. One likely reason is that studies of multisensory interaction pose technical challenges for not only stimulus delivery and triggering but also data interpretation because the integration (fusion) of information from different senses can be complex and depends on the stimulus types and their relative intensities (Stein et al., 2009). The fusion of multisensory stimuli to a unified percept occurs within a temporal integration window that can be asymmetric, as has been demonstrated by subjects viewing a film where a man was reading prose or a hammer was

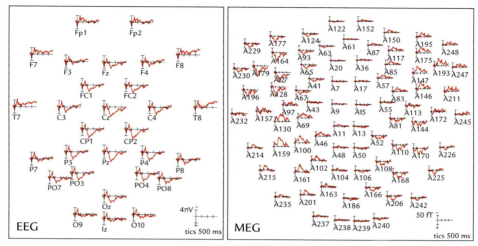

FIGURE 16.2. Simultaneously measured electric and magnetic gustatory responses to salty solution stimuli (NaCl 200 mM) presented as boluses once every 28 to 33 s. Group results are shown from 14 subjects, each receiving about 80 stimuli. Left panel: EEG scalp distribution, with selected 10–10 system measurement locations indicated. Right panel: MEG responses from magnetometer sensors; the letter A refers to device-specific sensor notations (BTI Magnes 3600 WH). Both EEG and MEG responses start at 170–180 ms, with EEG responses peaking at about 250 ms and MEG responses at about 300 ms. Note the polarity reversals of the main MEG responses between the anterior and posterior locations on each hemisphere and the opposite polarities at corresponding areas on the two hemispheres. Recording passband DC–50 Hz. Adapted and reproduced with permission from Iannilli E, Noennig N, Hummel T, Schoenfeld AM: Spatio-temporal correlates of taste processing in the human primary gustatory cortex. *Neuroscience* 2014, 273: 92–99.

hitting a peg (Dixon & Spitz, 1980) or by testing the simultaneity window of the auditory and visual syllables fused during the McGurk illusion (van Wassenhove et al., 2007).

Figure 16.3 demonstrates temporal integration windows for different types of auditory and visual stimuli. All curves are asymmetric so that—in agreement with the earlier results (Dixon & Spitz, 1980; van Wassenhove et al., 2007)—the integration window is *shorter if the auditory stimulus leads rather than lags the visual stimulus* (Wallace & Stevenson, 2014). The wide temporal integration window, on the order of hundreds of milliseconds, is advantageous in natural conditions, especially for human speech (see right panel in Figure 16.3). Imagine watching an outdoor concert far away from the orchestra, where the audiovisual event is perceived as a unified entity despite the clear delay from the seen actions of the conductor and musicians to the heard music.

In any study of multisensory interaction, each unisensory and multisensory condition needs to be presented in the same experiment so that the individual responses to unisensory and multisensory stimuli can be compared with each other, and the multisensory responses can be compared with the computed sum of the two unisensory responses. If these last two measures differ, some type of multisensory interaction has likely occurred. Care must also be taken with stimulus delivery to ensure that timing of stimuli in the two sensory modalities is accurate (see Chapter 6).

Naturally occurring multisensory stimuli are rather difficult to mimic in a well-controlled laboratory experiment. For this reason, many studies of audiovisual integration have used

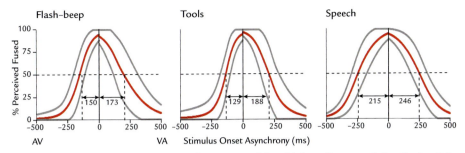

FIGURE 16.3. Temporal binding windows (TBWs) in which auditory and visual stimuli fuse to create audiovisual percepts. TBW width depends on stimulus type: for the three examples of audiovisual stimuli, simple flashes and beeps have the narrowest TBW, tools and their sounds a broader TBW, and seen and heard human speech the broadest TBW. The x-axis presents the stimulus onset asynchrony between the audiovisual stimuli, with negative values corresponding to the auditory stimulus being presented first (i.e., AV) and positive values indicating that the visual stimulus occurs first (i.e., VA). The y-axis indicates the percentage of percepts of audiovisual fusion. The red curves depict the mean and the grey curves the standard deviations of the mean for 39 subjects. The horizontal broken line identifies the 50% fusion point, and the arrows show the corresponding left and right sides of the window (for AV versus VA binding, respectively). Adapted and reprinted from Wallace MT, Stevenson RA: The construct of the multisensory temporal binding window and its dysregulation in developmental disabilities. *Neuropsychologia* 2014, 64: 105–123. With permission from Elsevier.

simple stimuli that do not occur together in real life but that subjects learn to associate during the experiment (e.g., a red square with a high-pitched tone vs. a yellow sphere with a low-pitched tone). For example, when two "objects" were differentiated visually by two shapes and auditorily by two pitches, the quite complex response waveforms observed in the multisensory condition contained, in addition to somewhat modulated visual and auditory responses, activity at around 140 to 165 ms related to multisensory integration (Giard & Peronnet, 1999). Similar early event-related potentials (ERPs) were elicited with more complex audiovisual stimuli, involving dynamic faces associated with nonverbal vocalizations; however, later potentials exhibited complex interactions but tended to be larger for combined audiovisual stimulation (Brefczynski-Lewis et al., 2009). These findings are encouraging for future experimentation using naturalistic stimuli.

Interestingly, other categorical stimuli, such as the letters of the alphabet and their matching auditory (phonemic) and visual (graphemic) forms, evoke similar early MEG responses and show *suppressive* audiovisual integration at 380 to 540 ms in the STS regions of both hemispheres (Raij et al., 2000), interpreted as reflecting the integration of the graphemic and phonemic forms of the letters. Results such as these demonstrate how complex multisensory interactions can be in brain regions that are part of a larger neuronal network of multisensory interaction. Below, we examine other types of multisensory interactions and discuss seemingly anomalous findings in their MEG correlates.

Audiotactile Interaction

In systems neuroscience, the most commonly studied multisensory interaction is between hearing and seeing, whereas audiotactile interactions have been largely neglected. Concomitant sound, however, can affect the percept from hands rubbed together (the so-called parchment-skin illusion in which accentuating the high sound frequencies makes the subjects think that the skin of their hands has become dry; Jousmäki & Hari, 1998). Furthermore, sinusoidal sounds delivered at the same time to the palms via a vibrating tube lower the hearing threshold and thereby improve the ability to hear the faint sounds (Schürmann et al., 2004). This strong audiotactile interaction is understandable given the physical similarity of sounds and vibratory somatosensory stimuli; this likeness was often emphasized by Georg von Békésy—the recipient of the Nobel Prize in Physiology or Medicine 1961—who used the skin to study cochlear mechanisms (Békésy, 1960). Thus, it should not come as a surprise that vibration has access to the auditory cortex, as has been demonstrated in both monkeys (Kayser et al., 2005) and humans (Levänen et al., 1998; Schürmann et al., 2004).

Deaf children often enjoy vibrations caused by music, feeling them by touching the instrument or by putting the face above a vibrating balloon close to a loudspeaker. Another interesting manifestation of audiotactile interaction is the perception of the crispness of food as a combined result of hardness from somatosensory input from the mouth coupled with biting sounds—a phenomenon with obvious applications in the food industry. For a review of audiotactile interactions, see Soto-Faraco and Deco (2009).

An MEG Case Study

Figure 16.4 gives an example of an audiotactile MEG study where hasty data interpretation could lead to erroneous conclusions (Gobbelé et al., 2003). Whole-scalp MEG responses were recorded to auditory stimuli presented alone (A; 50-ms, 1-kHz tone pips); tactile stimuli presented alone (T; electrical median-nerve stimuli); and audiotactile stimuli (AT; both stimuli simultaneously). The figure also displays the computed A + T waveform with which the AT condition should be compared to identify any signs of audiotactile interaction.

The depicted responses are from a single planar gradiometer over the right Sylvian fissure. To A, a typical auditory long-latency response is recorded, with the source in the supratemporal auditory cortex in the lower lip of the Sylvian fissure (red trace and red arrow on the schematic brain). The response to T shows short-latency transients that likely arose in the primary somatosensory cortex, a few centimeters from the recording site, and a clear long-latency response arising from the second somatosensory cortex in the upper lip of the Sylvian fissure. The lowest traces show the measured response to AT stimuli (green line) and the computed A + T waveform (black dotted line). It is the comparison between AT and A + T traces on which we should base our inference of the possible occurrence of audiotactile interaction.

In this kind of interaction, various outcomes are possible (Stein et al., 2009): (a) if AT ≈ A + T (i.e., the responses do not differ statistically significantly), we have no signs of audiotactile interaction in the area under study; (b) if AT > A + T, we have enhancement (or facilitation or superadditive interaction); and (c) if AT < A + T, we have suppression (or depression or underadditive interaction). The last two situations would indicate the presence of nonlinear multisensory interactions that would occur, for example, if the integration varies depending on stimulus intensity, with the largest multisensory enhancement for weak multimodal stimuli, or if the less effective stimulus would suppress the response of the highly effective stimulus from the other modality (Meredith & Stein, 1996).

Figure 16.4 (lowest traces) indicates that the main deflection of the measured AT response is clearly enhanced compared with the synthetic A + T response. Thus, at the first glance, we seem to have evidence for nonlinear audiotactile enhancement. However, before jumping to this conclusion, it is necessary to take a closer look at the signals and the sources. Importantly, the sources of A and T responses are in *opposite walls of the Sylvian*

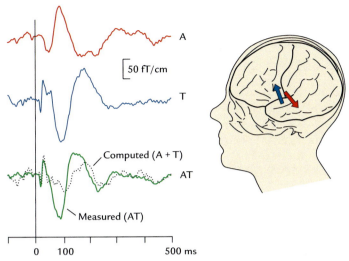

FIGURE 16.4. **Audiotactile interactions in MEG data.** Left: Averaged evoked fields to right-sided auditory stimuli presented alone (A, red trace), tactile (median-nerve) stimuli presented alone (T, blue trace), and simultaneous AT stimuli (green trace) in a single subject. The computed (expected) response (black broken line) is the sum of the unisensory conditions (A + T). The recording was made with a 306-channel neuromagnetometer, and responses are shown for one planar gradiometer over the left Sylvian fissure. The interstimulus interval was 1.5 s, passband 0.1–70 Hz, and sampling rate 600 Hz. Right: The arrows in the schematic head show the equivalent current dipoles for the auditory (red) and tactile (blue) stimuli. Adapted and reprinted from Gobbelé R, Schürmann M, Forss N, Juottonen K, Buchner H, Hari R: Activation of the human posterior parietal and temporoparietal cortices during audiotactile interaction. *NeuroImage* 2003, 20: 503–511. With permission from Elsevier.

fissure so that the current has opposite direction during the main response (that coincides in time). A relatively flat AT response (like the synthetic A + T response) would be expected if the A and T responses were independent during simultaneous AT presentation. Thus the clear deviance of the measured AT response from the expected A + T responses indicates that multisensory interaction has taken place. However, the significantly larger AT response does not necessarily indicate multisensory *enhancement*. In fact, the AT response shows a peculiar similarity in wave shape to the T response. What has likely happened is that the auditory response has been strongly *suppressed* in the AT condition! Thus, looking at both the signals *and* sources (and source-current directions) has turned the physiological interpretation of the obtained results upside down.

Multisensory Integration During Human Communication

Human-generated communicative stimuli, be they verbal or nonverbal, are temporally complex, and thus EEG and MEG recordings could help resolve the temporal processes driving multisensory integration. For example, when a dynamic avatar face and nonverbal vocalizations, such as sneezes, coughs, and other utterances that are not typically associated with affect, were shown either alone or in audiovisual combinations, the early (< 80 ms) EEG responses showed superadditivity at occipitotemporal sites and the later (100–250 ms) responses underadditivity at occipitotemporal and vertex sites (Brefczynski-Lewis et al., 2009).

We have already noted that stimulus type can greatly influence multisensory integration. Figure 16.5 shows results from an EEG study where *only* audiovisual stimuli were presented, but done so that their auditory and visual components were either congruent or incongruent. A human or monkey face and a house image were presented in an apparent-motion paradigm where either the mouth opened or the front door opened, during which a human burp, a monkey screech, or a creaking door was heard. The type of visual stimulus influenced the auditory N100, which was significantly larger to the congruent *primate* face/vocalizations relative to the congruent *inanimate* image/sound stimuli (Figure 16.5, top panel). Additionally, the congruent *human* face/voice stimuli elicited larger auditory N100 than any incongruent pairings of the human face with the other sound stimuli. This effect did not occur with either the monkey face or the house (Figure 16.5, bottom panel), suggesting that the human brain is more sensitive to human faces associated with vocal signals than to other categories of audiovisual stimuli (Puce et al., 2007).

Face-to-face encounters form a special case of audiovisual integration where seen *articulatory* movements of the speaker affect speech perception. In the well-known McGurk effect, discordant auditory and visual input from a speaker result in the illusion of hearing a sound that was not actually uttered (McGurk & MacDonald, 1976). For example, visually articulated /ka/ associated with auditory syllable /pa/ typically results in auditory perception of /ta/. MEG recordings during a McGurk illusion have indicated that visual input from articulatory movements can affect auditory processing in the supratemporal auditory cortex about 170 ms after the voice onset (Sams et al., 1991).

Similar effects were obtained in a more naturalistic condition, using the MEG setup of Figure 1.1, where the subject was seeing two side-by-side faces on the screen, one articulating congruently (with /apa/) and the other incongruently (with /aka/) with respect to the auditorily presented /apa/; all these stimuli were presented synchronously. The subject's percept changed depending on which of these two faces the subject chose to gaze on. Eye gaze tracked with an infrared camera determined how MEG responses were selectively averaged and depended on which face was viewed. Percept-related modulation of the auditory responses were seen in the right auditory cortex (Hirvenkari et al., 2010).

The complex waveforms elicited by multisensory stimuli and the possible caveats in the interpretation of the interactions emphasize the importance of a good understanding of the waveforms, stimulus dependencies, and generator sites of responses to unimodal stimuli. It is advisable to examine multisensory interactions based in MEG/EEG responses in source space, or at least consider the likely source areas and current directions whenever possible.

Other Types of Multisensory Evoked Responses

One rarely studied visuotactile interaction occurs when people in their everyday life touch and manipulate visible objects (e.g., Brozzoli et al., 2012). Visuotactile interaction involving haptic input is especially important in disambiguating objects that by vision alone could be either 2D or 3D; with hands, one may perceive even the unseen sides of the objects.

As we mentioned previously in this chapter, olfaction and taste form a natural pair during eating and drinking. However, olfaction can also influence seemingly unrelated visual input. For example, viewing faces during the presence of unpleasant odors leads to more negative behavioral ratings and larger long-latency, event-related activity than when the face is seen in the presence of a pleasant odor, consistent with associations of danger or unwanted social interactions (Cook et al., 2018).

congruent audiovisual stimulus

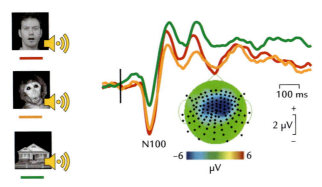

congruent vs incongruent audiovisual stimuli

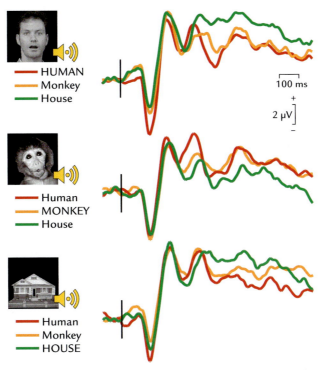

FIGURE 16.5. Audiovisual stimulus type and evoked potentials. Top: Auditory N100 (peak latency 140 ms) recorded from a six-electrode cluster at the vertex to congruent audiovisual stimuli (nose reference electrode. The largest responses occur to human face–human voice (red trace) and monkey face–monkey sound (orange trace) pairs relative to the house image–environmental sound pairing (green trace). Bottom: Comparison of congruent and incongruent audiovisual stimulation shows a significantly larger auditory N100 to the human face/sound pairing (top set of traces, red trace); no such difference is seen for either the monkey face or house images when they are paired with their congruent sound. Passband 0.1–100 Hz, sampling rate 250 Hz. Adapted and reprinted from Puce A, Epling JA, Thompson JC, Carrick OK: Neural responses elicited to face motion and vocalization pairings. *Neuropsychologia* 2007, 45: 93–106. With permission from Elsevier.

The interactions between auditory verbal and olfactory inputs were studied in an experiment where epilepsy surgery patients were asked to match spoken cues (mint or rose) to odors presented a few seconds later, their iEEG recordings displayed phase-locking of 1- to 7-Hz and 36- to 200-Hz activity between the auditory cortex and the primary olfactory (piriform) cortex but only when the odor matched the cue (Zhou et al., 2019). Activity related to auditory cues appeared first in the auditory cortex and about 300 ms later in the piriform cortex. These observations are consistent with the idea that olfactory processing is heavily driven by context (see Barwich, 2020). Zhou and colleagues (2019) interpreted these results in the predictive-coding framework, assuming that the sound cue informs the future presentation of a certain odor by readying olfactory processing via an increase in piriform cortex activity prior to the odor being presented. Predictive coding has also been postulated for audiovisual interactions, where concordant visual speech is reported to speed up auditory speech processing, as indexed by decreased latencies of neurophysiological responses (van Wassenhove et al., 2005).

Models of Multisensory Interaction

Multisensory integration is flexible and dynamic, potentially involving interactions between different neural processes in both early sensory and higher-order brain regions (for reviews, see Stevenson et al., 2014; Keil & Senkowski, 2018). The existing models of multisensory integration have benefited from advances in animal research. For example, one influential model that emphasizes inverse effectiveness is based on extensive research on the feline superior colliculus (Stein et al., 2009). The principle of inverse effectiveness says that stimuli that produce strong unimodal responses produce only small multisensory enhancements, whereas the situation is opposite for multisensory depression, where stimuli that produce the smallest unimodal responses result in the strongest depressive multisensory interactions.

Another model assumes that the multisensory integration relies on two canonical brain operations: (1) phase resetting of internally or externally generated rhythmic phenomena and (2) divisive normalization (van Atteveldt et al., 2014). Phase resetting of internal phenomena can be related to, for example, active sensing (and the associated motor actions) or allocation of selective attention, whereas external stimuli, such as audiovisual speech, can entrain the brain and thus be associated with externally driven phase resetting. The divisive normalization refers to normalization of the output of a neuron or a neuronal population by surrounding neurons. In low-level sensory cortices, such as primary auditory cortex, the likely mechanism could be oscillatory phase resetting triggered by incoming audiovisual inputs. However, in higher-order brain regions, such as the STS, divisive normalization could result from converging excitatory multisensory inputs.

Neural oscillations in different frequency bands are a central feature of another model for multisensory integration (Keil & Senkowski, 2018). Figure 16.6 presents a framework for such multisensory processing with three key mechanisms that can act in parallel in brain regions ranging from primary sensory cortices, to connecting multisensory regions (e.g., the superior temporal or angular gyri), and to higher-order cortical areas (e.g., frontal cortical areas). The framework includes feedforward/feedback interactions, attention modulation, and predictive coding. Local and network oscillatory signals in different canonical frequency bands are depicted.

The putative multiple mechanisms of multisensory integration proposed in Figure 16.6 could be tested in hypothesis-driven experiments examining interactions between different MEG/EEG frequency bands across these brain regions.

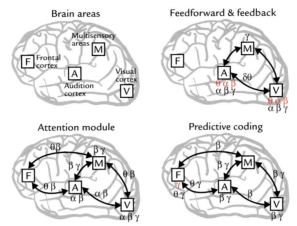

FIGURE 16.6. A framework for multisensory processing with three key parallel mechanisms. Top left: candidate brain regions include primary sensory cortices (A and V); connecting multisensory regions (M, e.g., the superior temporal or angular gyri) and higher-order cortical areas (F, e.g., frontal cortical areas). The framework includes feedforward/feedback interactions (top right); attention modulation (bottom left) and predictive coding (bottom right). Local (red lettering) and long-range or network (black lettering) oscillatory signals in the canonical frequency bands are depicted. Adapted from Keil J, Senkowski D: Neural oscillations orchestrate multisensory processing. *The Neuroscientist* 2018, 24: 609–626. Reproduced with permission by Sage Publications Inc.

In the next section we turn our gaze inward, to our internal organs and to our abilities to receive sensations from within the body itself.

■ INTEROCEPTION

Overview

Interoception refers to "the bidirectional signal processing between the brain and the internal organs that generates a representation of the internal state of an organism" (Chen et al., 2021, p. 4). Sensations arising from the body affect and modulate various physiological functions and are registered via interoceptive mechanisms. Interoception is also tightly bound to emotions and body awareness (Park & Blanke, 2019), and its dysfunction could be involved in anxiety (Tumati et al., 2021) and other clinical disorders. As interoception affects how we "feel" (well or ill), interoceptive dysfunction has been suggested as a good target for treatment (Chen et al., 2021).

The intrinsic monitoring of inner organs, such as the heart or the gut, might contribute significantly to the subject-centered reference frame and "the first-person perspective" (Tallon-Baudry et al., 2018). Similar to work in exteroception, interoception research is being increasingly drawn into the predictive-coding framework, as is motor action and proprioceptive feedback (Seth & Friston, 2016). We discuss predictive coding in more detail in Chapter 18.

Related to the previous chapter section, we note that multisensory interactions can also occur between exteroceptive and interoceptive signals, as will be evident below.

We begin this section with an overview of the neural pathways and brain areas involved in interoception. Some specialized interoreceptive sensors react to changes in chemical states of the body. For example, chemoreceptors sense carbon dioxide pressure and pH, glucoreceptors sense glucose levels, and osmoreceptors sense osmotic balance. Other receptors assess other bodily changes: mechanoreceptors sense mechanical pressure and stretch, thermoreceptors sense temperature, and baroreceptors sense (blood) pressure. For appetite-related signaling, humoral receptors sense substances such as leptin for satiation and ghrelin for hunger, and, of course, free nerve endings sense pain (Berntson & Khalsa, 2021).

The main afferent pathway for interoception is the *vagus nerve*, the main parasympathetic pathway in the body, containing both motor (efferent; ~20%) and sensory (~80%) fibers (see Figure 16.7; Prescott & Liberles, 2022).

Two important concepts in the interoception literature are homeostasis and allostasis (Schulkin & Sterling, 2019). According to the classical model of homeostasis, the body regulates its internal milieu within preset limits. In contrast, allostasis continually adjusts the internal milieu to promote survival and reproduction (Sterling, 2012). Allostasis thus works according to predictive-coding principles (Chapter 18), adjusting the body as the environment changes (e.g., temperature and humidity).

Visceral Responses

The term *viscera* refers to the internal organs of the body. The hollow inner organs (e.g., stomach, intestines, bladder, blood vessels) are lined by smooth muscles. Compared with skeletal muscles, which shorten at the command of action potentials arriving at neuromuscular junctions (end plates), the visceral smooth muscles are very different. First, they cannot be voluntarily controlled. Second, smooth muscle cells are organized in layers, with a quite distributed innervation, allowing contraction in multiple dimensions. Such a contraction mechanism is important during peristalsis, which arises when food in the intestine causes pressure on the wall of the gut or stomach and the contracting muscle layer propels the food forward through the gastrointestinal system.

Some examples of electrical responses from viscera are examined next.

Evoked Responses to Distension of Esophagus, Urethra, and Rectum
Electrical stimulation of the esophagus evokes EEG responses that peak around 90 to 380 ms when recorded between the vertex and a frontal site. Similarly, balloon distension and deflation at 2 Hz of the esophagus produces evoked potentials in the centroparietal midline (relative to a midline frontal reference), with a series of deflections around 200 to 400 ms following balloon distention (Castell et al., 1990). At the other end of the body, it is also possible to use balloon distention via a catheter to stimulate the vesicourethral junction (Sarica & Karacan, 1986) and the rectosigmoid colon (Frieling et al., 1989), resulting in scalp evoked potentials at 55 to 150 ms poststimulus.

Spontaneous Contractions of the Stomach and Upper Gut
The brain–gut axis, in both health and disease, is attracting increasing attention among neuroscientists and clinicians (Jones et al., 2006; Cryan & Dinan, 2012; Farmer et al., 2014), and this relationship is now accessible also by electrophysiological means.

In our digestive system, a slow peristaltic wave of progressive contraction and relaxation aids the stomach and upper gastrointestinal tract to break down food and facilitates its passage to the lower gut and ultimately for excretion. These involuntary contractions of the gut wall can be monitored with the electrogastrogram (EGG) as measured with surface electrodes on the upper central regions of the abdomen, as shown in Figure 16.8. The EGG signals typically fluctuate at 0.05–0.1 Hz, depending on phases of feeding and fasting (for

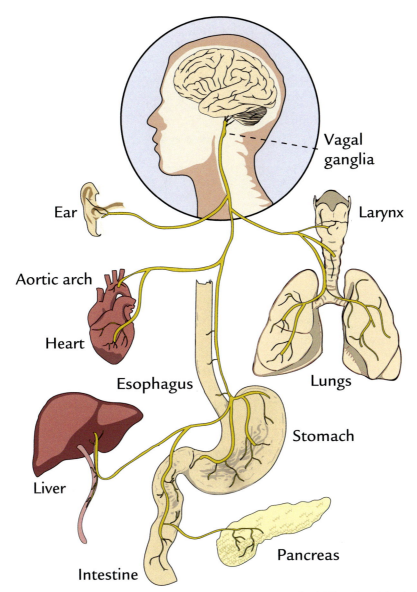

FIGURE 16.7. **Anatomy of the vagus nerve contributing to the bidirectional brain–body connection.** The cell bodies of vagal sensory neurons reside in the vagal ganglia at the base of the neck. Vagal neurons target numerous organs within the body as depicted in the figure. Adapted and reprinted from Prescott SL, Liberles SD: Internal senses of the vagus nerve. *Neuron* 2022, 110: 579–599. With permission from Elsevier.

tutorial reviews, see Yin & Chen, 2013; Wolpert et al., 2020). Figure 16.8 illustrates the complexity of EGG signals in the time and frequency domains. The EGG trace is normally contaminated by ECG and respiratory signals. In this case, these physiological signals are artifacts that can be separated from the EGG on the basis of their power spectral signatures: ECG signals have the highest frequencies, respiration lies in the midrange, and gastric activity has the slowest frequencies (Wolpert et al., 2020).

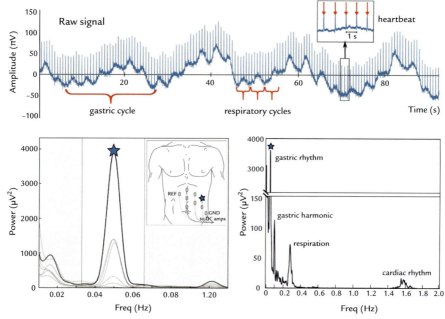

FIGURE 16.8. Electrogastrogram (EGG). Top panel: Single subject's raw EGG displays cycles of ~20 s length (in a DC recording). Faster fluctuations superimposed on the trace are due to respiration and heartbeats, as indicated. The inset shows individual heartbeat with the R wave highlighted by red arrows. Bottom left panel: Positions of seven recording electrodes and a power spectrum from seven recording electrodes. Maximum response at a peak frequency of 0.05 Hz and the site of recording is indicated by the blue star. The white band in the power spectral plot corresponds to the normal frequency range of the EGG ("normo-gastria, 2–4 cycles per minute or 0.033–0.066 Hz). The body inset shows surface electrode siting on the left abdomen, with the location of the electrode displaying the largest spectral power (blue star). Reference (REF) and ground (GND) electrodes are also shown. DC-coupled amplifiers were used to record the signals. Bottom right panel: Power spectrum over a wider frequency range at the selected channel, displaying respiratory (~0.3 Hz) and cardiac rhythms (~1.5 Hz) separated from the lower-frequency gastric rhythm and its harmonic. Adapted and reproduced from Wolpert N, Rebollo I, Tallon-Baudry C: Electrogastrography for psychophysiological research: practical considerations, analysis pipeline, and normative data in a large sample. *Psychophysiology* 2020, 57: e13599. With permission from John Wiley & Sons.

In addition to the spectral separation of the signals, the cardiac and respiratory contamination can be minimized in EGG recordings by calculating the Laplacian (second spatial derivative) of these potentials (Hjorth, 1975): one can use five surface electrodes on the body in the shape of a cross (Prats-Boluda et al., 2007) or a special flexible tripolar surface electrode comprising three concentric ring electrodes (Garcia-Casado et al., 2014). In the literature, these recordings are also called the electroenterogram (EEnG) (Prats-Boluda et al., 2007) or the electrointestinogram (EIG) (Hashimoto et al., 2015).

The corresponding biomagnetic gastrointestinal signal (MGG, magnetogastrogram) was first recorded by asking the subject to ingest a small, magnetized marker pill and then recording activity over the stomach with a magnetometer housed in a flat-bottom dewar

(Di Luzio et al., 1989); recent studies have suggested that such recordings are capable of indicating some pathophysiologies of gastric function (Bradshaw et al., 2016).

Some recent studies have found coupling of the infra-slow gastric rhythm and the amplitude modulation of alpha-range EEG oscillations in bilateral occipitoparietal cortex and in right insula, with indications that the effects are due to ascending influence from the stomach (Richter et al., 2017). Functional MRI data combined with EGG recordings have further suggested a "resting-state gastric network" (Rebollo et al., 2018), with the insula playing a central role in this relationship (Hashimoto et al., 2015). In general, the communication between brain and viscera, and in fact the whole body, deserves much more attention than it has had until now, with relevant scientific questions ranging from cognition and emotion to subjectivity and even consciousness (Azzalini et al., 2019; Chen et al., 2021; Criscuolo et al., 2022).

Data analysis of brain–organ coupling relies on many of the principles and methods that we introduced in Chapter 10. For a recent review that is specific to this area of research and statistical analysis, see Wolpert and Tallon-Baudry (2021).

Contractions of the Uterus

During a regular pregnancy, uterine contractions are normal as the fetus comes closer to term. Uterine activity, combined with cardiac function of the fetus, is routinely monitored during hospital deliveries to assess fetal well-being. Unfortunately, the widely available cardiotocography (CTG) recordings, comprising simultaneous monitoring of fetal heartbeats and uterine contractions (with devices that have been on the commercial market over 50 years), suffer from many technical problems, in both recording and interpretation. More detailed analysis of CTG traces can, however, be informative of early signs of fetal hypoxia and thus of the risk of neurological complications (Tarvonen et al., 2021).

CTG monitors uterus contractions indirectly, with an elastic belt that senses changes in belly shape. Thus, CTG can only indicate the frequency and duration of the uterine contractions without informing about their intensity or efficiency, despite the importance of these factors for proper labor management (Huber et al., 2021). Consequently, an intrauterine pressure catheter may need to be inserted to monitor uterine activity and the progression of labor more directly.

Electrohysterography (EHG), which is the noninvasive monitoring of the electric activity associated with uterine contractions with surface electrodes positioned over the belly of the mother, has been proposed as an alternative for this invasive procedure. The idea of EHG emerged in the late 1940s (for a review, see Huber et al., 2021), but the method is still considered experimental. However, EHG is a technically straightforward, low-cost, and noninvasive way to monitor uterine contractions that also might be attractive to neuroscientists from the brain–body connection point of view. An open-source database of 16-electrode EHG recordings from 45 Icelandic women is available (Alexandersson et al., 2015).

The Brain–Heart Axis: Evoked Activity to One's Own Heartbeat

The systolic part of the cardiac cycle produces a pressure pulse throughout the body. (If you sit cross-legged you might notice small periodic movements of the foot with every cardiac pulsation. The stiffer your arteries are and the higher your blood pressure is, the greater the movement.) Interestingly, the pulsation and the associated modified proprioceptive afference due to stretching of muscles and tendons can cause small modulations in the ~3-Hz feedback from proprioceptors to cortex during motor action, as seen in studies of cortico-muscular coherence (see Chapter 17) (Bourguignon et al., 2017).

Some individuals deemed to be "good perceivers" can readily attend to and sense the beating of their own heart. Therefore, it should not be surprising that one's own heartbeat can cause evoked responses in the EEG or MEG, as has been known since the 1960s. The heartbeat-evoked potential (HEP) consists of a scalp-negative deflection peaking 200–300 ms after the Q wave of the ECG (see Figure 9.16) (Callaway & Layne, 1964). Subsequent studies have repeatedly confirmed that HEPs can be seen most clearly in good perceivers (Schandry et al., 1986; Montoya et al., 1993). Corresponding MEG heart-evoked responses can also be recorded (e.g., Babo-Rebelo et al., 2016).

However, as we have explained in Chapter 9, the electrical activity of the heart may cause strong artifacts in EEG and MEG recordings, and ballistocardiographic artifact may also be visible. Thus, the artifact issue needs careful attention in all studies focusing on brain responses to heartbeats.

Interesting evidence of brain-generated HEPs comes from ECoG recordings in epilepsy surgery patients, where a biphasic response was observed in the primary somatosensory cortex 280–360 ms after the ECG-R wave (Figure 16.9; Kern et al., 2013). However, somewhat puzzlingly, simultaneously recorded scalp EEG did not show HEPs, which leaves the origin of the signals still somewhat open.

The phase of the cardiac cycle has also been shown to affect sensory and motor actions. Successful localization and detection of subtle touch stimuli varies inversely by HEP component amplitude and is better if the stimuli are presented during diastole, after the (systolic) ventricular contraction has occurred (Al et al., 2020). Elite target shooters,

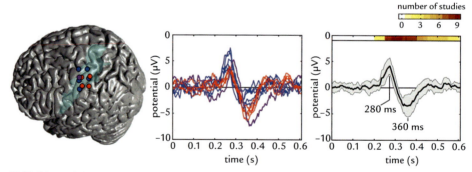

FIGURE 16.9. Heartbeat-evoked potentials (HEPs) recorded using ECoG. Left panel: Electrode contacts (colored circles) from 3 patients showing an HEP superimposed on a standard brain surface. Blue and red circles denote left hemisphere sites. Purple circle denotes a right hemisphere site mirrored to the left side for comparison. The left somatosensory cortex is highlighted in light blue. Middle panel: HEPs at the electrode contacts indicated with identical color coding, time-locked to R-peak of the ECG. Right panel: Grand-average HEP (black curve) over all selected intracranial sites; the gray band displays standard deviations. The color bars at the top of the plot indicate corresponding HEP latencies from 12 existing EEG studies in the literature, indicating agreement if the HEP latencies between non-invasive and ECoG recordings. Adapted and reprinted from Kern M, Aertsen A, Schulze-Bonhage A, Ball T: Heart cycle-related effects on event-related potentials, spectral power changes, and connectivity patterns in the human ECoG. *NeuroImage* 2013, 81:178–190. With permission from Elsevier.

such as biathletes, benefit from sensing their own heartbeat, as target shooting is most accurate during the "quiet part" of the cardiac cycle, just at the end of diastole (Helin et al., 1987). During systole, accuracy is diminished because of small jerks that occur in the body due to the blood pressure pulse. According to transcranial magnetic stimulation data, the excitability of motor cortex also varies as a function of the cardiac cycle (Al et al., 2022).

Evoked Activity to One's Own Respiration

We breathe spontaneously yet can modulate our respiration rate when required. Multiple methods allow easy and accurate monitoring of the spontaneous respiration rate based, for example, on airflow from the nostrils, movements of the chest and abdomen recorded with a "respiration belt" (see Al-Khalidi et al., 2011), or whole-body movement detection recorded with static-charge-sensitive material covering a bed or a chair.

An indirect way to extract information on respiration rate only needs heart rate monitoring (ECG-derived respiration, or EDR) as it exploits the idea of heart-rate variability (HRV), where during inspiration the heart rate increases, whereas during expiration the heart rate decreases; this method is implemented in an open-source software package (Karlen et al., 2013). However, one has to note that this "respiratory sinus arrythmia" is most prominent in children and young adults, and thus the modeling of respiration rate on the basis of heart rate signals is strongly age dependent. Hence, direct (and relatively easy) measurement of the respiration might be preferred.

The respiratory cycle is known to affect tactile perception (Grund et al., 2022), and this effect is also visible in evoked responses (Al et al., 2020). For respiration-linked evoked responses in somatosensory areas, see a review article describing the technical aspects of the technique (Chan & Davenport, 2010).

■ REFERENCES

Adrian ED: The electrical activity of the mammalian olfactory bulb. *Electroencephalogr Clin Neurophysiol* 1950, 2: 377–388.

Al E, Iliopoulos F, Forschack N, Nierhaus T, Grund M, Motyka P, Gaebler M, Nikulin VV, Villringer A: Heart–brain interactions shape somatosensory perception and evoked potentials. *Proc Natl Acad Sci U S A* 2020, 117: 10575–10584.

Al E, Stephani T, Engelhardt M, Villringer A, Nikulin V: Cardiac activity impacts cortical motor excitability. Preprint 2022. https://doi.org/10.21203/rs.3.rs-1023617/v1.

Alexandersson A, Steingrimsdottir T, Terrien J, Marque C, Karlsson B: The Icelandic 16-electrode electrohysterogram database. *Sci Data* 2015, 2: 150017.

Al-Khalidi FQ, Saatchi R, Burke D, Elphick H, Tan S: Respiration rate monitoring methods: a review. *Pediatr Pulmonol* 2011, 46: 523–529.

Azzalini D, Rebollo I, Tallon-Baudry C: Visceral signals shape brain dynamics and cognition. *Trends Cogn Sci* 2019, 23: 488–509.

Babo-Rebelo M, Richter CG, Tallon-Baudry C: Neural responses to heartbeats in the default network encode the self in spontaneous thoughts. *J Neurosci* 2016, 36: 7829–7840.

Barwich AS: *Smellosophy: What the Nose Tells the Mind*. Cambridge, MA: Harvard University Press, 2020.

Békésy G: *Experiments in Hearing*. New York: McGraw-Hill, 1960.

Berntson GG, Khalsa SS: Neural circuits of interoception. *Trends Neurosci* 2021, 44: 17–28.

Bourguignon M, Piitulainen H, Smeds E, Zhou G, Jousmäki V, Hari R: MEG insight into the spectral dynamics underlying steady isometric muscle contraction. *J Neurosci* 2017, 37: 10421–10437.

Bradshaw LA, Cheng LK, Chung E, Obioha CB, Erickson JC, Gorman BL, Somarajan S, Richards WO: Diabetic gastroparesis alters the biomagnetic signature of the gastric slow wave. *Neurogastroenterol Motil* 2016, 28: 837–848.

Brefczynski-Lewis J, Lowitszch S, Parsons M, Lemieux S, Puce A: Audiovisual non-verbal dynamic faces elicit converging fMRI and ERP responses. *Brain Topogr* 2009, 21: 193–206.

Brozzoli C, Makin TR, Cardinali L, Holmes NP, Farnè A: Peripersonal space: a multisensory interface for body–object interactions. In: Murray MM, Wallace MT, eds. *The Neural Bases of Multisensory Processes*. Boca Raton, FL: CRC Press/Taylor & Francis, 2012: 449–466.

Callaway E 3rd, Layne RS: Interaction between the visual evoked response and two spontaneous biological rhythms: the EEG alpha cycle and the cardiac arousal cycle. *Ann N Y Acad Sci* 1964, 112:421–431.

Castell DO, Wood JD, Frieling T, Wright FS, Vieth RF: Cerebral electrical potentials evoked by balloon distention of the human esophagus. *Gastroenterology* 1990, 98: 662–666.

Chan PY, Davenport PW: Respiratory related evoked potential measures of cerebral cortical respiratory information processing. *Biol Psychol* 2010, 84: 4–12.

Chen WG, Schloesser D, Arensdorf AM, Simmons JM, Cui C, Valentino R, Gnadt JW, Nielsen L, St Hillaire-Clarke C, Spruance V, Horowitz TS, Vallejo YF, Langevin HM: The emerging science of interoception: sensing, integrating, interpreting, and regulating signals within the self. *Trends Neurosci* 2021, 44: 3–16.

Cook S, Kokmotou K, Soto V, Wright H, Fallon N, Thomas A, Giesbrecht T, Field M, Stancak A: Simultaneous odour-face presentation strengthens hedonic evaluations and event-related potential responses influenced by unpleasant odour. *Neurosci Lett* 2018, 672: 22–27.

Criscuolo A, Schwartze M, Kotz SA: Cognition through the lens of a body–brain dynamic system. *Trends Neurosci* 2022, 45: 667–677.

Cryan JF, Dinan TG: Mind-altering microorganisms: the impact of the gut microbiota on brain and behaviour. *Nat Rev Neurosci* 2012, 13: 701–712.

Di Luzio S, Comani S, Romani GL, Basile M, Del Gratta C, Pizzella V: A biomagnetic method for studying gastro-intestinal activity. *Nuovo Cimento* 1989, 11: 1853–1859.

Dixon NF, Spitz L: The detection of auditory visual desynchrony. *Perception* 1980, 9: 719–721.

Farmer AD, Randall HA, Aziz Q: It's a gut feeling: how the gut microbiota affects the state of mind. *J Physiol* 2014, 592: 2981–2988.

Feldman GM, Mogyorosi A, Heck GL, DeSimone JA, Santos CR, Clary RA, Lyall V: Salt-evoked lingual surface potential in humans. *J Neurophysiol* 2003, 90: 2060–2064.

Finkenzeller P: Gemittelte EEG-Potentiale bei olfactorischer Reizung. *Pflügers Arch ges Physiol* 1966, 292: 76–80.

Freeman WJ: *Mass Action in the Nervous System*. New York: Academic Press, 1975.

Frieling T, Enck P, Wienbeck M: Cerebral responses evoked by electrical stimulation of the esophagus in normal subjects. *Gastroenterology* 1989, 97: 475–478.

Garcia-Casado J, Zena-Gimenez V, Prats-Boluda G, Ye-Lin Y: Enhancement of non-invasive recording of electroenterogram by means of a flexible array of concentric ring electrodes. *Ann Biomed Eng* 2014, 42: 651–660.

Giard MH, Peronnet F: Auditory-visual integration during multimodal object recognition in humans: a behavioral and electrophysiological study. *J Cogn Neurosci* 1999, 11: 473–490.

Gobbelé R, Schürmann M, Forss N, Juottonen K, Buchner H, Hari R: Activation of the human posterior parietal and temporoparietal cortices during audiotactile interaction. *NeuroImage* 2003, 20: 503–511.

Grund M, Al E, Pabst M, Dabbagh A, Stephani T, Nierhaus T, Gaebler M, Villringer A: Respiration, heartbeat, and conscious tactile perception. *J Neurosci* 2022, 42: 643–656.

Güdücü C, Olcay BO, Schäfer L, Aziz M, Schriever VA, Özgören M, Hummel T: Separating normosmic and anosmic patients based on entropy evaluation of olfactory event-related potentials. *Brain Res* 2019, 1708: 78–83.

Gudziol H, Guntinas-Lichius O: Electrophysiologic assessment of olfactory and gustatory function. *Handb Clin Neurol* 2019, 164: 247–262.

Han P, Schriever VA, Peters P, Olze H, Uecker FC, Hummel T: Influence of airflow rate and stimulus concentration on olfactory event-related potentials (OERP) in humans. *Chem Senses* 2018, 43: 89–96.

Hashimoto T, Kitajo K, Kajihara T, Ueno K, Suzuki C, Asamizuya T, Iriki A: Neural correlates of electrointestinography: insular activity modulated by signals recorded from the abdominal surface. *Neuroscience* 2015, 289: 1–8.

Helin P, Sihvonen T, Hänninen O: Timing of the triggering action of shooting in relation to the cardiac cycle. *Br J Sports Med* 1987, 21: 33–36.

Hirvenkari L, Jousmäki V, Lamminmäki S, Saarinen VM, Sams ME, Hari R: Gaze-direction-based MEG averaging during audiovisual speech perception. *Front Hum Neurosci* 2010, 4: 17.

Huart C, Rombaux P, Hummel T, Mouraux A: Clinical usefulness and feasibility of time-frequency analysis of chemosensory event-related potentials. *Rhinology* 2013, 51: 210–221.

Huber C, Shazly SA, Ruano R: Potential use of electrohysterography in obstetrics: a review article. *J Matern Fetal Neonatal Med* 2021, 34: 1666–1672.

Hjorth B: An on-line transformation of EEG scalp potentials into orthogonal source derivations. *Electroencephalogr Clin Neurophysiol* 1975, 39: 526–530.

Iannilli E, Gudziol H: Gustatory pathway in humans: a review of models of taste perception and their potential lateralization. *J Neuro Res* 2019, 97: 230–240.

Iannilli E, Noennig N, Hummel T, Schoenfeld AM: Spatio-temporal correlates of taste processing in the human primary gustatory cortex. *Neuroscience* 2014, 273: 92–99.

Jones MP, Dilley JB, Drossman D, Crowell MD: Brain–gut connections in functional GI disorders: anatomic and physiologic relationships. *Neurogastroenterol Motil* 2006, 18: 91–103.

Jousmäki V, Hari R: Parchment-skin illusion: sound-biased touch. *Curr Biol* 1998, 8: 190.

Karlen W, Raman S, Ansermino JM, Dumont GA: Multiparameter respiratory rate estimation from the photoplethysmogram. *IEEE Trans Biomed Eng* 2013, 60: 1946–1953.

Kayser C, Petkov CI, Augath M, Logothetis NK: Integration of touch and sound in auditory cortex. *Neuron* 2005, 48: 373–384.

Keil J, Senkowski D: Neural oscillations orchestrate multisensory processing. *Neuroscientist* 2018, 24: 609–626.

Kern M, Aertsen A, Schulze-Bonhage A, Ball T: Heart cycle-related effects on event-related potentials, spectral power changes, and connectivity patterns in the human ECoG. *NeuroImage* 2013, 81:178–190.

Kettenmann B, Jousmäki V, Portin K, Salmelin R, Kobal G, Hari R: Odorants activate the human superior temporal sulcus. *Neurosci Lett* 1996, 203: 143–145.

Kettenmann B, Hummel C, Stefan H, Kobal G: Multiple olfactory activity in the human neocortex identified by magnetic source imaging. *Chem Senses* 1997, 22: 493–502.

Kobal G: *Electrophysiologische Untersuchungen des menschlichen Geruchssinnes*. Stuttgart: Thieme, 1981.

Kobal G: Gustatory evoked potentials in man. *Electroencephalogr Clin Neurophysiol* 1985a, 62: 449–454.

Kobal G: Pain-related electrical potentials of the human nasal mucosa elicited by chemical stimulation. *Pain* 1985b, 22: 151–163.

Kobal G, Hummel C: Cerebral chemosensory evoked potentials elicited by chemical stimulation of the human olfactory and respiratory nasal mucosa. *Electroencephalogr Clin Neurophysiol* 1988, 71: 241–250.

Levänen S, Jousmäki V, Hari R: Vibration-induced auditory-cortex activation in a congenitally deaf adult. *Curr Biol* 1998, 8: 869–872.

Lötsch J, Hummel T: The clinical significance of electrophysiological measures of olfactory function. *Behav Brain Res* 2006, 170: 78–83.

Lötsch J, Hummel T, Kraetsch H, Kobal G: The negative mucosal potential: separating central and peripheral effects of NSAIDs in man. *Eur J Clin Pharmacol* 1997, 52: 359–364.

McGurk H, MacDonald J: Hearing lips and seeing voices. *Science* 1976, 264: 746–748.

Meredith MA, Stein BE: Spatial determinants of multisensory integration in cat superior colliculus neurons. *J Neurophysiol* 1996, 75: 1843–1857.

Montoya P, Schandry R, Müller A: Heartbeat evoked potentials (HEP): topography and influence of cardiac awareness and focus of attention. *Electroencephalogr Clin Neurophysiol* 1993, 88: 163–172.

Ottoson D: Sustained potentials evoked by olfactory stimulation. *Electroencephalogr Clin Neurophysiol* 1954, 32: 384–386.

Park H-D, Blanke O: Coupling inner and outer body for self-consciousness. *Trends Cogn Sci* 2019, 23: 377–388.

Prats-Boluda G, Garcia-Casado J, Martinez-de-Juan JL, Ponce JL: Identification of the slow wave component of the electroenterogram from Laplacian abdominal surface recordings in humans. *Physiol Meas* 2007, 28: 1115–1133.

Prescott SL, Liberles SD: Internal senses of the vagus nerve. *Neuron* 2022, 110: 579–599.

Puce A, Epling JA, Thompson JC, Carrick OK: Neural responses elicited to face motion and vocalization pairings. *Neuropsychologia* 2007, 45: 93–106.

Raij T, Uutela K, Hari R: Audiovisual integration of letters in the human brain. *Neuron* 2000, 28: 617–625.

Rebollo I, Devauchelle A-D, Béranger B, Tallon-Baudry C: Stomach-brain synchrony reveals a novel, delayed-connectivity resting-state network in humans. *eLife* 2018, 7: e33321.

Richter CG, Babo-Rebelo M, Schwartz D, Tallon-Baudry C: Phase-amplitude coupling at the organism level: the amplitude of spontaneous alpha rhythm fluctuations varies with the phase of the infra-slow gastric basal rhythm. *NeuroImage* 2017, 146: 951–958.

Rombaux P, Mouraux A, Bertrand B, Guerit JM, Hummel T: Assessment of olfactory and trigeminal function using chemosensory event-related potentials. *Neurophysiol Clin* 2006, 36: 53–62.

Rombaux P, Huart C, Mouraux A: Assessment of chemosensory function using electroencephalographic techniques. *Rhinology* 2012, 50: 13–21.

Sams M, Aulanko R, Hämäläinen M, Hari R, Lounasmaa OV, Lu S-T, Simola J: Seeing speech: visual information from lip movements modifies activity in the human auditory cortex. *Neurosci Lett* 1991, 127: 141–145.

Sarica Y, Karacan I: Cerebral responses evoked by stimulation of the vesico-urethral junction in normal subjects. *Electroencephalogr Clin Neurophysiol* 1986, 65: 440–446.

Schandry R, Sparrer B, Weitkunat R: From the heart to the brain: a study of heartbeat contingent scalp potentials. *Int Neurosci* 1986, 30: 261–275.

Schulkin J, Sterling P: Allostasis: A brain-centered, predictive mode of physiological regulation. *Trends Neurosci* 2019, 42: 740–752.

Schürmann M, Caetano G, Jousmäki V, Hari R: Hands help hearing: facilitatory audiotactile interaction at low sound-intensity levels. *J Acoust Soc Am* 2004, 115: 830–832.

Seth AK, Friston KJ: Active interoceptive inference and the emotional brain. *Philos Trans R Soc Lond B Biol Sci* 2016, 371: 20160007.

Soto-Faraco S, Deco G: Multisensory contributions to the perception of vibrotactile events. *Behav Brain Res* 2009, 196: 145–154.

Stein BE, Stanford TR, Ramachandran R, Perrault TJ Jr, Rowland BA: Challenges in quantifying multisensory integration: alternative criteria, models, and inverse effectiveness. *Exp Brain Res* 2009, 198: 113–126.

Sterling P: Allostasis: a model of predictive regulation. *Physiol Behav* 2012, 106: 5–15.

Stevenson RA, Ghose D, Fister JK, Sarko DK, Altieri NA, Nidiffer AR, Kurela LR, Siemann JK, James TW, Wallace MT: Identifying and quantifying multisensory integration: a tutorial review. *Brain Topogr* 2014, 27: 707–730.

Tallon-Baudry C, Campana F, Park H-D, Babo-Rebelo M: The neural monitoring of visceral inputs, rather than attention, accounts for first-person perspective in conscious vision. *Cortex* 2018, 102: 139–149.

Tarvonen M, Hovi P, Sainio S, Vuorela P, Andersson S, Teramo K: Intrapartum zigzag pattern of fetal heart rate is an early sign of fetal hypoxia: a large obstetric retrospective cohort study. *Acta Obstet Gynecol Scand* 2021, 100: 252–262.

Tumati S, Paulus MP, Northoff G: Out-of-step: brain-heart desynchronization in anxiety disorders. *Mol Psychiatry* 2021, 26: 1726–1737.

van Atteveldt N, Murray MM, Thut G, Schroeder CE: Multisensory integration: flexible use of general operations. *Neuron* 2014, 81: 1240–1253.

van Wassenhove V, Grant KW, Poeppel D: Visual speech speeds up the neural processing of auditory speech. *Proc Natl Acad Sci U S A* 2005, 102: 1181–1186.

van Wassenhove V, Grant KW, Poeppel D: Temporal window of integration in auditory-visual speech perception. *Neuropsychologia* 2007, 45: 598–607.

Wallace MT, Stevenson RA: The construct of the multisensory temporal binding window and its dysregulation in developmental disabilities. *Neuropsychologia* 2014, 64: 105–123.

Willander J, Larsson M: Smell your way back to childhood: autobiographical odor memory. *Psychon Bull Rev* 2006, 13: 240–244.

Wolpert N, Rebollo I, Tallon-Baudry C: Electrogastrography for psychophysiological research: practical considerations, analysis pipeline, and normative data in a large sample. *Psychophysiology* 2020, 57: e13599.

Wolpert N, Tallon-Baudry C: Coupling between the phase of a neural oscillation or bodily rhythm with behavior: evaluation of different statistical procedures. *NeuroImage* 2021, 236: 118050.

Yih J, Beam DE, Fox KCR, Parvizi J: Intensity of affective experience is modulated by magnitude of intracranial electrical stimulation in human orbitofrontal, cingulate and insular cortices. *Soc Cogn Affect Neurosci* 2019, 14: 339–351.

Yin J, Chen JD: Electrogastrography: methodology, validation and applications. *J Neurogastroenterol Motil* 2013, 19: 5–17.

Zhou G, Lane G, Noto T, Arabkheradmand G, Gottfried JA, Schuele SU, Rosenow JM, Olofsson JK, Wilson DA, Zelano C: Human olfactory-auditory integration requires phase synchrony between sensory cortices. *Nat Commun* 2019, 10: 1168.

CHAPTER 17

MOTOR FUNCTION

The body is the instrument of our hold on the world.

—SIMONE DE BEAUVOIR

Those who can't dance say the music is no good.

—JAMAICAN PROVERB

■ MOVEMENT-RELATED READINESS POTENTIALS AND FIELDS

Voluntary movements are preceded by slow neural activity that was called the Bereitschaftspotential (BP) by its discoverers (Kornhuber & Deecke, 1965). Later, the BP became known as the readiness potential (RP) and its magnetic counterpart as the readiness field (RF). RPs and RFs can begin a few seconds before movement onset and they depend strongly on the movement's parameters, such as the speed of onset.

RPs and RFs are averaged with respect to either changes in electromyographic (EMG) signals recorded from the moving muscle or the timing of a button press or similar accurate indicator of movement onset. In the early days before modern computing, EEG signals were recorded on magnetic tape and played back in reverse order, to average the signals that had preceded the trigger. To record reliable RP/RFs, one should not filter out the slow frequencies of the signals, and thus a high-pass filter setting at 0.03 Hz or even lower is recommended. Typically, 30 to 60 responses are adequate to generate a clear averaged RP/RF, but the onset and size of the response depend critically on the timing of the performed movements. If some of the movements are brisk and others sluggish, the averaged premotor shifts are distorted and dampened.

Figure 17.1 compares the time courses of the electrical RP and magnetic RF recorded in association with finger movements (Nagamine et al., 1996). In these specific recording locations, the RP culminates in a steeper slope (movement potential), and the RF ends with a prominent movement-evoked field that peaks about 100 ms after movement onset and likely reflects proprioceptive afference to the somatosensory cortex.

In general, the RF is contralaterally dominant, whereas the simultaneously recorded RP is rather symmetric, especially during its early phases. Thus the RP may receive contribution from the early bilateral activation of the premotor cortex in the medial walls of both hemispheres (Deecke, 1996) in addition to the primary motor cortex, whereas the RF

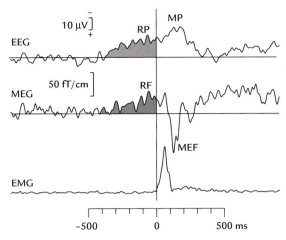

FIGURE 17.1. Simultaneously recorded RP (EEG) and RF (MEG) in association with finger movements in a single subject. The subject made self-paced brisk right index finger abductions at intervals exceeding 6 s. Passband 0.03–100 Hz for MEG and 0.01–100 Hz for EEG; sampling rate 397 Hz. A button positioned against the finger generated a trigger pulse at the beginning of each movement. The traces (lowpass filtered at 40 Hz) start 1 s before and end 1 s after the button press (black vertical line); movement onset is also evident as the clear rise in the rectified EMG signal. The RP was recorded from a 10–10 electrode site C1 relative to M2, whereas the RF trace comes from a planar gradiometer placed over left sensorimotor cortex. The slow RP and RF become evident around 400 ms prior to the movement (gray shading). As only single locations are shown for both traces, the waveforms show some clear differences. For example, the RP continues to rise after the movement, culminating into a so-called movement potential (MP), whereas the RF is followed by a large movement-evoked field (MEF) likely reflecting proprioceptive afference to the cortex. Note the negative-up display for EEG on this figure. Adapted and reprinted from Grafton S, Hari R and Salenius S: The human motor system. In: Toga AW, Mazziotta JC, eds. *Brain Mapping: The Systems.* New York: Academic Press, 2000: 331–363 (based on data of Nagamine T, Kajola M, Salmelin R, Shibasaki H, Hari R: Movement-related slow cortical magnetic fields and changes of spontaneous MEG- and EEG-brain rhythms. *Electroencephalogr Clin Neurophysiol* 1996, 99: 274–286).

mainly reflects activity of the fissural primary motor cortex. Intracranial recordings have demonstrated RP components in the supplementary motor cortex during the initiation of the movement and in the primary motor cortex both before and after the execution of the movement (Ikeda & Shibasaki, 1992; Ikeda et al., 1993). Shibasaki and Hallett (2006), in summarizing the cumulative EEG, MEG, and intracranial data gathered over the years, suggested that the early part of the RP reflects a slowly increasing cortical excitability that may signal subconscious preparation for the forthcoming movement, whereas the later parts likely reflect conscious preparation for movement.

Figure 17.2 (right) shows the first MEG recordings of readiness fields preceding foot movements; the recordings were made with a single-channel first-order axial gradiometer from 12 sites along a diagonal line, shown in red over the left lower head. The RFs preceding plantar flexion of the right foot reverse in polarity over the midline, suggesting a source in the foot motor cortex in the mesial wall of the left hemisphere. The corresponding pattern for the left-foot movements (traces not shown) indicated activation in the right-hemisphere motor cortex. Although these field patterns were mapped quite sparsely, they suggest that the sources were tilted with respect to the scalp midline (in Figure 17.2 see also the enlarged piece of cortex in the inset, with the small arrows indicating local activations in two orthogonal walls of the Rolandic mesial cortex in the left hemisphere) (Hari et al., 1983). For these kinds of tilted sources, the polarities of electric RPs (upper two schematic heads) are mirror-symmetric with respect to the head midline, whereas the magnetic RFs (lower two heads) are symmetric with respect to the coronal line connecting the two ears. These characteristics are in line with our earlier considerations of the generation of topographic MEG and EEG patterns, but they are emphasized here because they are often misinterpreted by EEG-trained scientists (see also left- vs right-hemisphere field patterns for auditory stimulation in Figure 13.6).

Because the sources of RP/RFs for foot movement are typically located in the mesial surface of the hemisphere, bilateral foot movements produce considerable cancellation, even abolition, of the RFs when both feet are moved at once because the opposite sides

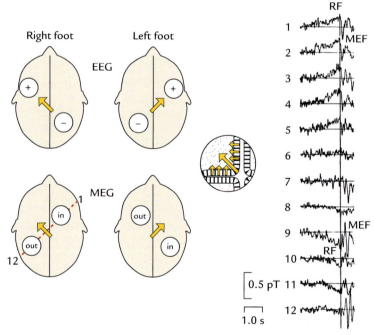

FIGURE 17.2. **RFs recorded to foot movements.** Recordings were made with a first-order axial gradiometer successively from 12 locations (1–12) along a diagonal line (broken red line on lower left head). The MEG traces (averages for about 60 single movements) show a polarity reversal between recording sites 5 and 9 in the RF as well as the subsequent MEF. Polarity reversals occur in the corresponding EEG data (not shown) as well; however, the pattern was rotated by 90° relative to the MEG pattern as shown schematically on the heads on the left panel. Movement onset is indicated by the vertical line. Passband 0.03–30 Hz. The inset shows the net current dipole (large arrow) and currents in the active cortex assumed to expand both the mesial wall and the wall of the central sulcus. See text for further explanation. Adapted and reprinted from Hari R, Antervo A, Katila T, Poutanen T, Seppänen M, Tuomisto T, Varpula T: Cerebral magnetic fields associated with voluntary movements in man. *Il Nuovo Cimento* 1983, 2D: 484–494. With permission from Springer.

of the mesial wall (a large fissure) are simultaneously active (Hari et al., 1983). A similar cancellation probably explains the difficulty of picking up MEG signals from bilaterally activated supplementary motor area of healthy subjects although intracranial EEG recordings, as mentioned earlier, show strong premovement shifts in the supplementary motor cortex in the mesial wall (Ikeda et al., 1993).

The time courses of RPs and RFs resemble, but are not identical to, the time course of corticospinal excitability, as determined by transcranial magnetic stimulation (Chen et al., 1998). Interestingly, RPs and RFs also resemble the time courses of the suppression of 10-Hz and 20-Hz Rolandic (mu) oscillations that occur both while a subject is executing actions and while she or he is observing another person's actions (see Figure 17.3), indicating excitation of the primary motor cortex (Caetano et al., 2007).

The existence of RPs/RFs and their emergence long before the subjects become conscious of their own intentions to move have led to a heated debate about the existence of free will (see, e.g., Libet, 1985; Gomes, 1998; Libet, 2002; Rigoni et al., 2011). Recent studies have brought up interesting experimental results suggesting that the subjects tend to move when the premovement buildup of slow spontaneous cortical fluctuations has reached a certain level (Schurger et al., 2012; Schmidt et al., 2016). These fluctuations have been suggested to drive arbitrary decisions and actions that are not purposeful and do not have any real implication, whereas real-life deliberate actions that matter are not preceded by such fluctuations (Maoz et al., 2019). Consequently, the relationship between readiness potential and volition is under reassessment (Schurger et al., 2021).

■ COHERENCE BETWEEN BRAIN ACTIVITY AND MOVEMENTS/MUSCLES

Overview

As we have previously noted, it is helpful for both the analysis and interpretation of brain data to include some peripheral signals as triggers or regressors. The peripheral signals (e.g., EMG, ECG) provide a context for the occurrence of the brain activity, picking up information that is otherwise difficult to extract from MEG/EEG signals. Indeed, brain activity should not be studied in isolation, as we also emphasized in Chapter 16 on interoception. Here we briefly introduce cortex–muscle coherence (CMC), corticokinematic coherence (CKC), and corticovocal coherence (CVC)—measures that all reveal the intricate relationships between the brain and body.

Cortex–Muscle Coherence

CMC refers to the coupling of MEG/EEG signals to surface EMG activity of a steadily contracted muscle (for reviews, see, e.g., Mima & Hallett, 1999; Salenius & Hari, 2003). Figure 17.4 illustrates CMC between MEG signals and left and right upper- and lower-limb muscles during isometric contraction. CMC peaks at about 20 Hz for intermediate-strength contractions, and the brain sites showing maximum coherence agree with the known somatotopy of the motor cortex: for right-sided contractions in the left hemisphere and vice versa, and for feet close to the midline and for hands in the hand representation cortex some 5 cm lateral from the midline (Salenius et al., 1997). The cortex leads in time, with a difference corresponding to the conduction time of the muscle: the latency is about 20 ms for upper-limb muscles and about 40 ms for lower-limb muscles (Salenius et al., 1997; Gross et al., 2002).

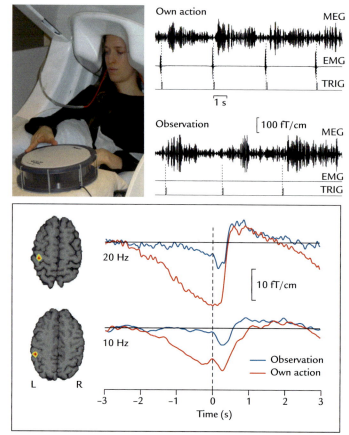

FIGURE 17.3. Suppression of brain rhythms during own finger-tapping movements and during observation of those of another person. Top left: The subject taps a nonmagnetic drum with the right index finger and sees her own action during an MEG recording. Top right: MEG (from one planar gradiometer over the left motor cortex) and EMG (from the first interosseous muscle) displayed relative to a trigger signal (TRIG) indicating when the drum was struck. Data are shown both during Own Action and Observation. In the latter condition the subject observed the experimenter strike the drum—as is evident by the lack of any EMG signal. Bottom: Density plots of the current dipoles (left) for the 20 Hz and 10 Hz Rolandic rhythms depicted on horizontal MRI slices. Red refers to the highest density. The time courses for the mean amplitudes of the 20-Hz and 10-Hz oscillations are shown during Own Action (red traces) and Observation (blue traces). Adapted and reprinted from Caetano G, Jousmäki V, Hari R: Actor's and observer's primary motor cortices stabilize similarly after seen or heard motor actions. *Proc Natl Acad Sci USA* 2007, 104: 9058–9062. ©2007 National Academy of Sciences, USA.

During stronger muscle contractions, the frequency of CMC does not increase progressively but jumps from around 20 Hz to around 40 Hz (Brown et al., 1998). The 40-Hz CMC corresponds to the muscular "Piper rhythm," named after Hans Piper who detected it by listening to the contracted thenar muscles with a stethoscope (Piper, 1907).

The CMC studies suggest that the motor cortex drives the spinal motoneuron pool with a *rhythmic output*. It is, however, obvious that the observed cortical frequencies are

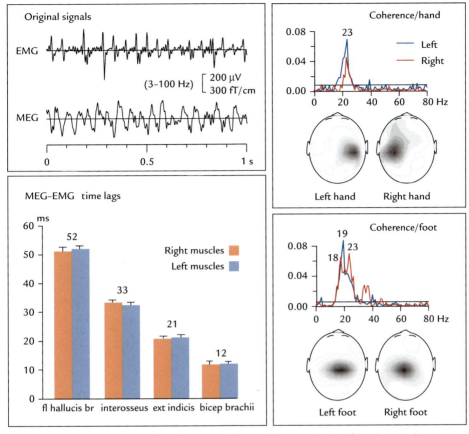

FIGURE 17.4. Cortex–muscle coherence. One subject maintained an isometric contraction of one upper- or lower-limb muscle at a time while whole-scalp MEG and surface EMG signals were recorded with passbands of 0.03 to 330 Hz and 3 to 300 Hz, respectively; sampling rate was 1 kHz. Left: Examples of original EMG and MEG signals (top). The motor-unit potentials in the EMG from left flexor hallucis brevis muscle in the foot appear to be synchronized with oscillatory MEG activity recorded with a planar gradiometer over the right-hemisphere foot area. The histograms (bottom) display mean (± SEM of six subjects) time lags in ms between MEG and EMG activity for three upper-limb muscles (first dorsal interosseous, extensor [ext] indicis, and bicep brachii) and one lower-limb muscle (flexor hallucis brevis [fl hallucis br]). The delays do not differ between right- (red) and left-sided (blue) contractions but reflect the distance from the brain to the respective muscle. Right: Coherence spectra between MEG and EMG signals for isometric contraction of the left (blue) and right (red) hand muscles (interosseus; top box) and foot muscles (flexor halluces brevis; bottom box). The spatial distributions show the amplitudes of the coherence spectra, with maxima located over the respective motor cortices in all four conditions. Adapted and reprinted from Salenius S, Portin K, Kajola M, Salmelin R, Hari R: Cortical control of human motoneuron firing during isometric contraction. *J Neurophysiol* 1997, 77: 3401–3405. American Physiological Society.

too high for driving the firing of individual motor units, and they thus rather modulate the firing at population level.

CMC is typically abolished during strong contractions and ramp movements (e.g., rapid changes of finger position from one location to another while the subject is keeping a pinch against a manipulandum), as is illustrated in Figure 17.5.

Corticokinematic Coherence

CKC refers to coherence of MEG/EEG signals with respect to the *acceleration or velocity* of the moving limb, finger, and so on. Acceleration can be measured by attaching an accelerometer to the moving body part (see Figure 6.3). Maximum coherence between limb/finger acceleration and MEG signals occurs at the fundamental frequency (F0) of a repetitive movement and at its harmonics, often most clearly at the first harmonic (F1). The first robust recordings of CKC between MEG signals with respect to 2- to 5-Hz track-ball movements of the hand (Jerbi et al., 2007) and self-paced flexion–extensions of the fingers repeated at 3 Hz (Bourguignon et al., 2011) were interpreted by emphasizing the prominent role of slow fluctuations in M1 cortex in encoding the parameters of voluntary movements. However, more recent work has clearly indicated that the CKC is mainly driven by proprioceptive afferent input so that CKC can be regarded a kind of a steady-state response to proprioceptive input.

Support for the proprioceptive-driving interpretation derives from the similarity of the CKC signals during active and passive movements (Figure 17.6) (Piitulainen et al., 2013), as well by the findings that the directed coherence is always larger in the afferent than the efferent direction (Bourguignon et al., 2015).

Slow movements are not smooth but are interrupted by discontinuities at 8–10 Hz. These rhythmic variations in contraction force are distinct from physiological tremor and likely reflect periodic output to the motor system (Vallbo & Wessberg, 1993). Even during isometric contraction, accelerometer measurements indicate force fluctuations that—combined with measurements of corticomotor and corticokinetic coherence—suggest that the cortex sends population-level motor commands modulated at ~20 Hz (i.e., at the pace of the cortical sensorimotor rhythm) and dynamically adapted to the < 3-Hz proprioceptive feedback from the periphery (Bourguignon et al., 2017). Such a bidirectional control mechanism would be quintessential, for example, when we are holding something slippery, such as an icy drinking glass. A recent review discussed the analysis, findings, limitations, and future perspectives of the coupling between brain's electrophysiological signals and motor activity (Bourguignon et al., 2019).

Corticovocal Coherence

One special case of the CKC is corticovocal coherence, CVC, the coherence between brain signals and the fundamental frequency of own or another person's voice. If an accelerometer is placed on an individual's throat (Figure 17.7), it will pick up vibrations related to the fundamental frequency, F0, of that person's voice (nicely without contamination by any other sound or voice in the environment). Coherence of MEG signals with respect to the voice F0 of another person who is reading a text was most prominent at 0.5 Hz, likely due to sentence rhythm, and 4 to 6 Hz, likely due to syllable rhythm (Bourguignon et al., 2013). Figure 17.7 presents an example of this relationship. The robustness of CVC indicates that it would be feasible, in the future, to compute coherence between the MEG/EEG signals and many other peripheral signals, as well.

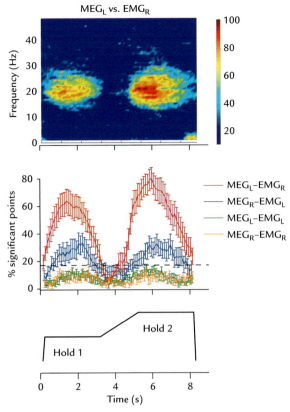

FIGURE 17.5. Abolition of cortex–muscle coherence during ramp movements. Top plot: Time–frequency map (pooled across six subjects and three muscles) for contralateral MEG–EMG coherence while subjects held a lever for 3 s with the right fingers (Hold 1), then linearly increased their force from 1.3 N to 1.6 N over a 2-s period, then again maintained a steady contraction (Hold 2) for 3 s, and finally released the lever (see bottom schematic). The coherence is largest during each hold period and disappears during the ramp. The color scale on the right shows the percentage of significant coherence points (see explanation of the middle plot). Middle plot: The percentage of significant points in 15 to 30 Hz coherence for different MEG–EMG combinations (averages across trials, muscles, and subjects; error bars indicate standard error of the mean) replicates the same time course, with abolition of coherence during the ramp movement. The dashed horizontal line shows the $p = 0.05$ significance level. Adapted and reprinted from Kilner JM, Salenius S, Baker SN, Jackson A, Hari R, Lemon RN: Task-dependent modulations of cortical oscillatory activity in human subjects during a bimanual precision grip task. *NeuroImage* 2003, 18: 67–73. With permission from Elsevier.

■ MORE COMPLEX MOTOR ACTIONS

In this chapter, we have discussed simple motor acts, such as button presses and repetitive finger movements, associated with MEG/EEG signals picked up from the primary sensorimotor cortex. These traditional neurophysiological approaches are well suited for clinical assessment of movement disorders (Hallett et al., 2021), but they fall short in covering the whole complexity of motor functions, for example, how muscular activation patterns change smoothly during walking and running (Cappellini et al., 2006). Although the motor

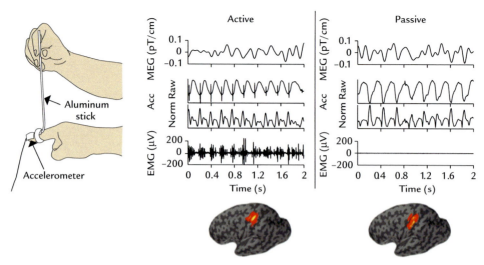

FIGURE 17.6. **Corticokinematic coherence.** Left: Experimental setup for the passive condition, where the experimenter moved the subject's finger up and down. The accelerometer on the finger is shown. Center and middle: Single-subject MEG (top traces), accelerometer (Acc; middle two traces), and EMG (bottom traces) signals in two conditions: Active (left) and Passive (right) movements of the right index finger. The MEG traces, from a gradiometer sited over contralateral primary sensorimotor cortex, originally recorded with a passband of 0.1 to 330 Hz and sampled at 1 kHz, are displayed from 1 to 10 Hz. Accelerometer and EMG (flexor carpi radialis muscle) were recorded time-locked to the MEG signals and filtered and sampled at the same rate. For acceleration, both the raw signal and Euclidian norm (Norm) of three orthogonal components are presented. On the bottom of the figure, group-level left-hemisphere CKC maps (across 15 subjects) show great similarity between the two conditions, with the maximum CKC values at the hand cortex. Adapted and reprinted from Piitulainen H, Bourguignon M, De Tiège X, Hari R, Jousmäki V: Corticokinematic coherence during active and passive finger movements. *Neuroscience* 2013, 238: 361–370. With permission from Elsevier.

system is often considered a rather uninteresting output of more important cognitive brain activity, its centrality in even higher cognitive functions is well established and is evident from, for example, mirroring that supports understanding of actions of other persons (see Chapter 19).

From an evolutionary point of view, the brain's main role is to guide the organism toward food and mates and away from dangers, such as predators. In that sense, motor action can be considered primary, with the senses serving the action. Movements of the eyes, head, and body provide slightly different viewpoints, thereby improving perception (Dipoppa et al., 2018; Guitchounts et al., 2020). Infants' own movements support development of normal visual perception, implying that perception and action are tightly interwoven. Accordingly, the primary motor cortex also responds to somatosensory stimuli (Hatsopoulos & Suminski, 2011).

Motor control is hierarchical, contains much feedback, and works according to the principles of predictive coding (see Chapter 18). Much motor coordination takes place at subcortical levels, including at the spinal cord. Proprioceptors (see Chapter 15) provide detailed information about limb and body position, and haptical processing—which is motor

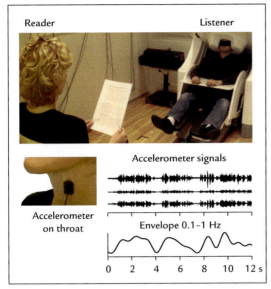
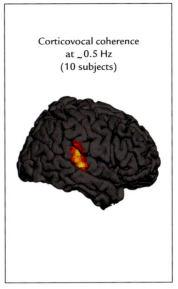

FIGURE 17.7. Corticovocal coherence. Left: Experimental setup during MEG recording when a subject listens to a female reader. An accelerometer is placed on the reader's throat to record the speech's fundamental frequency along three orthogonal axes (Accelerometer signals) and to compute their combined envelope (here filtered from 0.1 to 1 Hz); corticovocal coherence is computed between this envelope of the reader and the MEG signals of the listener. Right: Group-level corticovocal coherence map across 15 subjects depicted at the 0.5 Hz peak of the coherence. Adapted and reprinted from Bourguignon M, De Tiège X, Op de Beeck M, Ligot N, Paquier P, Van Bogaert P, Goldman S, Hari R, Jousmäki V: The pace of prosodic phrasing couples the reader's voice to the listener's cortex. *Hum Brain Mapp* 2013, 34: 314–326. With permission from John Wiley & Sons.

action coupled with proprioceptive feedback—is involved in all active touching, grasping, and manipulating. Consequently, proprioception improves in parallel with motor-skill learning (Mirdamadi & Block, 2020) and is also central for the sense of the bodily self. Cerebellum (see Chapters 2 and 22) and basal ganglia contribute strongly to shaping, initiating, and stopping the movements on the basis of sensory information.

The motor cortex in the frontal lobe contains a mosaic of cytoarchitectonically distinct subareas, all with distinct functional properties and characteristic connections with postcentral parietal areas (Luppino & Rizzolatti, 2000). This network is consistent with the omnipresent sensorimotor interactions during movements, with different frontoparietal circuits for motor planning, visually guided movements, goal-directed movements, hand reaching and grasping, and encoding peripersonal space.

The natural world is full of action choices (Cisek & Kalaska, 2010), and movements are selected on the basis of the goal and optimal environmental and biomechanical possibilities, constrained by initial conditions, such as hand position with respect to the body, and the body position and posture. The multitude of possible action sequences to reach an end point is called *motor equivalence*; for example, one can write with one's hand, foot, or nose. To recruit the best motor sequence at a given time, other possible action sequences must be suppressed. Consequently, *inhibition* is extremely powerful and common in the motor system. Specifically, the output from the basal ganglia is kept under tonic inhibition by

GABAergic neurons until called into action, and here both the pallidum and striatum play an important role (Grillner et al., 2005). The high number of degrees of freedom of reaching and grasping movements guarantees adaptability and flexibility in infants who learn to master motor skills. During increasing sensorimotor experience and training, initial uncoordinated movements become progressively more organized and evolve into goal-directed actions.

Important information, such as movement direction, can be decoded from population activity of motor-cortex neurons (Georgopoulos & Carpenter, 2015), which can be used for controlling brain–computer interfaces (BCIs). Importantly, a motor-cortex lesion by, for example, stroke (see Chapter 20) does not paralyze single muscles but rather impairs movements that involve synergic actions of many muscles.

The complexity of the motor system underscores the need to better characterize motor function in high-temporal-resolution MEG/EEG studies in a much more detailed manner than just recording brain activity related to button presses. Sequencing movements via video monitoring and computational analysis, as has been done in differentiating subsecond structure in mouse behavior (Wiltschko et al., 2015), could be combined with EEG/MEG recordings as well.

■ REFERENCES

Bourguignon M, De Tiège X, Op de Beeck M, Pirotte B, Van Bogaert P, Goldman S, Hari R, Jousmäki V: Functional motor-cortex mapping using corticokinematic coherence. *NeuroImage* 2011, 55: 1475–1479.

Bourguignon M, De Tiège X, Op de Beeck M, Ligot N, Paquier P, Van Bogaert P, Goldman S, Hari R, Jousmäki V: The pace of prosodic phrasing couples the reader's voice to the listener's cortex. *Hum Brain Mapp* 2013, 34: 314–326.

Bourguignon M, Piitulainen H, De Tiège X, Jousmäki V, Hari R: Corticokinematic coherence mainly reflects movement-induced proprioceptive feedback. *NeuroImage* 2015, 106: 382–390.

Bourguignon M, Piitulainen H, Smeds E, Zhou G, Jousmäki V, Hari R: MEG insight into the spectral dynamics underlying steady isometric muscle contraction. *J Neurosci* 2017, 37: 10421–10437.

Bourguignon M, Jousmäki V, Dalal SS, Jerbi K, De Tiège X: Coupling between human brain activity and body movements: insights from non-invasive electromagnetic recordings. *NeuroImage* 2019, 203: 116177.

Brown P, Salenius S, Rothwell JC, Hari R: The cortical correlate of the Piper rhythm in man. *J Neurophysiol* 1998, 80: 2911–2917.

Caetano G, Jousmäki V, Hari R: Actor's and observer's primary motor cortices stabilize similarly after seen or heard motor actions. *Proc Natl Acad Sci U S A* 2007, 104: 9058–9062.

Cappellini G, Ivanenko YP, Poppele RE, Lacquaniti F: Motor patterns in human walking and running. *J Neurophysiol* 2006, 95: 3426–3437.

Chen R, Yaseen Z, Cohen L, Hallett M: Time course of corticospinal excitability in reaction time and self-paced movements. *Ann Neurol* 1998, 44: 317–325.

Cisek P, Kalaska JF: Neural mechanisms for interacting with a world full of action choices. *Annu Rev Neurosci* 2010, 33: 269–298.

Deecke L: Planning, preparation, execution, and imagery of volitional action. *Brain Res Cogn Brain Res* 1996, 3: 59–64.

Dipoppa M, Ranson A, Krumin M, Pachitariu M, Carandini M, Harris KD: Vision and locomotion shape the interactions between neuron types in mouse visual cortex. *Neuron* 2018, 98: 602–615.

Georgopoulos AP, Carpenter AF: Coding of movements in the motor cortex. *Curr Opin Neurobiol* 2015, 33: 34–39.

Gomes G: The timing of conscious experience: a critical review and reinterpretation of Libet's research. *Conscious Cogn* 1998, 7: 559–595.

Grillner S, Hellgren J, Menard A, Saitoh K, Wikström MA: Mechanisms for selection of basic motor programs—roles for the striatum and pallidum. *Trends Neurosci* 2005, 28: 364–370.

Gross J, Timmermann L, Kujala J, Dirks M, Schmitz F, Salmelin R, Schnitzler A: The neural basis of intermittent motor control in humans. *Proc Natl Acad Sci U S A* 2002, 99: 2299–2302.

Guitchounts G, Masis J, Wolff SBE, Cox D: Encoding of 3D head orienting movements in the primary visual cortex. *Neuron* 2020, 108: 512–525 e4.

Hallett M, DelRosso LM, Elble R, Ferri R, Horak FB, Lehericy S, Mancini M, Matsuhashi M, Matsumoto R, Muthuraman M, Raethjen J, Shibasaki H: Evaluation of movement and brain activity. *Clin Neurophysiol* 2021, 132: 2608–2638.

Hari R, Antervo A, Katila T, Poutanen T, Seppänen M, Tuomisto T, Varpula T: Cerebral magnetic fields associated with voluntary movements in man. *Nuovo Cimento* 1983, 2D: 484–494.

Hatsopoulos NG, Suminski AJ: Sensing with the motor cortex. *Neuron* 2011, 72: 477–487.

Ikeda A, Shibasaki H: Invasive recording of movement-related cortical potentials in humans. *J Clin Neurophysiol* 1992, 9: 509–520.

Ikeda A, Lüders HO, Burgess RC, Shibasaki H: Movement-related potentials associated with single and repetitive movements recorded from human supplementary motor area. *Electroencephalogr Clin Neurophysiol* 1993, 89: 269–277.

Jerbi K, Lachaux JP, N'Diaye K, Pantazis D, Leahy RM, Garnero L, Baillet S: Coherent neural representation of hand speed in humans revealed by MEG imaging. *Proc Natl Acad Sci U S A* 2007, 104: 7676–7681.

Kornhuber HH, Deecke L: Hirnpotentialänderungen bei Willkürbewegungen und passiven Bewegungen des Menschen: Bereitschaftspotential and reafferent Potentiale. *Pflügers Archiv* 1965, 284: 1–17.

Libet B: Unconscious cerebral initiative and the role of conscious will in voluntary action. *Behav Brain Sci* 1985, 8: 529–566.

Libet B: The timing of mental events: Libet's experimental findings and their implications. *Conscious Cogn* 2002, 11: 291–299.

Luppino G, Rizzolatti G: The organization of the frontal motor cortex. *News Physiol Sci* 2000, 15: 219–224.

Maoz U, Yaffe G, Koch C, Mudrik L: Neural precursors of decisions that matter—an ERP study of deliberate and arbitrary choice. *eLife* 2019, 8: e39787.

Mima T, Hallett M: Corticomuscular coherence: a review. *J Clin Neurophysiol* 1999, 16: 501–511.

Mirdamadi JL, Block HJ: Somatosensory changes associated with motor skill learning. *J Neurophysiol* 2020, 123: 1052–1062.

Nagamine T, Kajola M, Salmelin R, Shibasaki H, Hari R: Movement-related slow cortical magnetic fields and changes of spontaneous MEG- and EEG-brain rhythms. *Electroencephalogr Clin Neurophysiol* 1996, 99: 274–286.

Piitulainen H, Bourguignon M, De Tiège X, Hari R, Jousmäki V: Corticokinematic coherence during active and passive finger movements. *Neuroscience* 2013, 238: 361–370.

Piper H: Über den willkürlichen Muskeltetanus. *Pflügers Archiv* 1907, 119: 301–338.

Rigoni D, Kuhn S, Sartori G, Brass M: Inducing disbelief in free will alters brain correlates of preconscious motor preparation: the brain minds whether we believe in free will or not. *Psychol Sci* 2011, 22: 613–618.

Salenius S, Portin K, Kajola M, Salmelin R, Hari R: Cortical control of human motoneuron firing during isometric contraction. *J Neurophysiol* 1997, 77: 3401–3405.

Salenius S, Hari R: Synchronous cortical oscillatory activity during motor action. *Curr Opin Neurobiol* 2003, 13: 678–684.

Schmidt S, Jo HG, Wittmann M, Hinterberger T: "Catching the waves"—Slow cortical potentials as moderator of voluntary action. *Neurosci Biobehav Rev* 2016, 68: 639–650.

Schurger A, Sitt JD, Dehaene S: An accumulator model for spontaneous neural activity prior to self-initiated movement. *Proc Natl Acad Sci U S A* 2012, 109: E2904–2913.

Schurger A, Hu P, Pak J, Roskies AL: What is the readiness potential? *Trends Cogn Sci* 2021, 25: 558–570.

Shibasaki H, Hallett M: What is the Bereitschaftspotential? *Clin Neurophysiol* 2006, 117: 2341–2356.

Vallbo AB, Wessberg J: Organization of motor output in slow finger movements in man. *J Physiol* 1993, 469: 673–691.

Wiltschko AB, Johnson MJ, Iurilli G, Peterson RE, Katon JM, Pashkovski SL, Abraira VE, Adams RP, Datta SR: Mapping sub-second structure in mouse behavior. *Neuron* 2015, 88: 1121–1135.

CHAPTER 18

BRAIN SIGNALS RELATED TO CHANGE DETECTION

All things are so very uncertain, and that's exactly what makes me feel reassured.

—TOVE JANSSON

The desire to discover and to experience something new is responsible for growth and development in the individual, progress in civilization. And so it seems to me that the labor which results in something created, to add to the sum total of the world, is infinitely more valuable than the labor devoted to the reproduction of something already familiar.

—MAYA DEREN

■ INTRODUCTION

Over the years, a multitude of evoked responses have been described and discussed within a relatively narrow cognitive context, with the focus mainly on the responses themselves and their attributes, rather than on the brain functions to which they might be related. Because such correlative approaches are slow to advance science, here we try to present evoked responses elicited by various types of *change* in the environment in the context of the predictive-coding framework, describing how the responses are related to variations in stimulus probability and the subject's expectations.

The human nervous system has evolved for predicting the future. Relatively recently an overarching framework—predictive coding and Bayesian probabilistic modeling—has been proposed as a general principle of brain function. It has been especially useful for describing a number of sensory, motor, and cognitive processes (Friston, 2005; Kilner et al., 2007; Koster-Hale & Saxe, 2013). The predictive-coding framework assumes that the brain forms, on the basis of statistical regularities of the environment, probabilistic models of the world. Such models help the individual to act as optimally as possible, even in uncertain conditions.

Predictive coding is assumed to be implemented at several nested and hierarchically organized levels in the central nervous system, involving both feedforward and feedback connections. The higher levels of the system are assumed to generate predictions of the outcomes of lower-level processing. If the predictions are not met, the lower levels create error signals that occur as the result of discrepancies between the expected result (informed by efference copies to other brain areas) and sensory feedback. The prediction error signals can then be used to adjust the internal model to better predict forthcoming events.

To react to changes, the brain first has to adapt to the regularities of the environment. In fact, the effects of stimulation rate (see, e.g., Figure 13.5) reflect such adaptation. In Chapters 13 through 16, we discussed how humans deal with incoming sensory input and how they generate deliberate motor output (Chapter 17). Purposeful actions require some sort of associative learning (conditioning) between input and actions, for example between stimuli of different types (for multisensory interactions, see Chapter 16).

Several widely studied evoked responses to changes in sensory inflow might be related to error signals that arise when predictions and available information do not match. Violations of an otherwise regular sensory inflow, be they minor deviations of the physical stimulus features or totally novel stimuli or even omissions of some stimuli, automatically orient and alert the individual. The associated evoked responses have typically been studied using "odd-ball" paradigms, where low-probability deviant stimuli ("targets" if attention is required) are presented among regularly repeated "standard" stimuli.

In this chapter we discuss four well-known responses elicited by stimulus deviances: (a) the mismatch negativity (MMN) and mismatch field (MMF) peaking at 100 to 250 ms and elicited by changes in stimulus attributes, even if they are not attended to, (b) the P300 response peaking at around 300 ms and typically elicited by attended low-probability stimuli, (c) the N400 peaking at around 400 ms and typically elicited by semantic violations in verbal material, and (d) the error-related negativity (ERN) that arises when the subject makes an error. These slow responses can be badly distorted, or even eliminated, in waveform morphology, amplitude, and latency if an inappropriately high high-pass filter (say, above 0.1 Hz) is applied. The interested reader can consult guidelines for eliciting, recording, and reporting these slow responses (Duncan et al., 2009).

We start the chapter by describing the contingent negative variation, CNV, a response that occurs in the time period during the anticipation of a stimulus in a task requiring a behavioral response.

■ CONTINGENT NEGATIVE VARIATION

The contingent negative variation (CNV), first described by Grey Walter and colleagues in 1964, was a milestone in evoked-response research because it revealed a brain signal that was not only related to the physical attributes of the incoming stimuli but to the *cognitive processes* associating them.

Figure 18.1 shows the original recording of Grey Walter and coworkers from the vertex, averaged across 12 presentations of a single click presented alone, a train of visual light flashes presented alone, or a click followed after 1 s by a train of flashes that the subject either just ignored or had to terminate by a button press; these three types of stimuli were presented at irregular intervals of 3 to 10 s. When a warning stimulus (S1; here, a click) was followed by an imperative stimulus (S2; here, flashes) to which the subject had to respond, a slow surface-negative shift, CNV, appeared during the foreperiod of the trial. For the CNV to be visible, the amplifiers must have long time constants or, even better, be DC-coupled.

The CNV was elicited by different stimulus pairings (e.g., click–flash; flash–click), and it was considered to reflect the mental state of a subject who was making an *association* between the warning and imperative stimulus. After the initial enthusiasm had subsided, however, the applicability of CNV in various cognitive studies has remained relatively

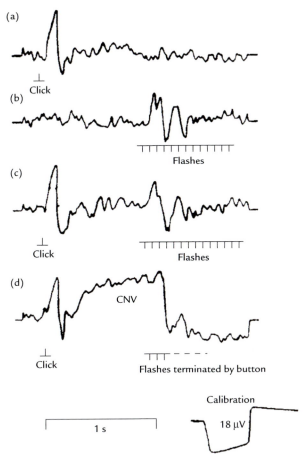

FIGURE 18.1. Contingent negative variation. (a) An auditory EEG response (N100) to a click stimulus (negative is up). (b) A visual response to a set of light flashes. (c) Response to the click followed by light flashes when the subject had no task. (d) Response to the click followed by light flashes when the subject had to terminate the flashes with a button press. A slow scalp-negative CNV is marked in the figure. All recordings were made between vertex (Cz) and mastoid and depict averages of 12 single responses. Note that negative is up. Reprinted from Walter WG, Cooper R, Aldridge VJ, McCallum WC, Winter AL: Contingent negative variation: an electric sign of sensorimotor association and expectancy in the human brain. *Nature* 1964, 203: 380–384. With permission from Macmillan Publishers Ltd. ©1964.

limited. The main reason is that CNV is not a unitary phenomenon but rather an admixture of (at least) two separate processes, with distinct topographies and stimulus relationships. Specifically, an early O (orienting) wave and a late E (expectation) wave became evident when the S1–S2 interval was prolonged (Loveless, 1973; Rohrbaugh et al., 1976; Kok, 1978). The O wave is largest over the frontal cortex and typically peaks 1 s after the onset of the warning stimulus; it likely reflects orientation by S1 and possibly its evaluation. The E wave, appearing toward the end of the S1–S2 interval, is largest over the precentral scalp and is tied more to the generation of the motor response, with contributions from the generators of readiness potentials (see Chapter 17) in precentral motor cortex and lateral prefrontal cortex (Rosahl & Knight, 1995).

Overall, although the CNV clearly has predictive attributes, its formation as an overlap of several EEG (or MEG; see Hultin et al., 1996) phenomena implies that the underlying brain processes are better studied by scrutinizing the relationships of the O- and E-wave components of CNV with sensory and motor processing and behavior. In the change-detection and predictive-coding framework, the O-wave appears a strong (orienting) response to an abrupt stimulus breaking the status quo, whereas the E-wave could reflect predictions that arise from the learned stimulus associations.

■ MISMATCH NEGATIVITY AND MISMATCH FIELD

The mismatch negativity, MMN, was first described by Näätänen and colleagues in 1978 using a dichotic listening task, with attention directed to one ear at the time, and deviant tones (differing from the standard tones either in intensity or pitch) intermingled among the standard tones in both ears. The MMN, which is best visible in a *difference waveform* between responses to deviants minus responses to standards, is a negative potential that is maximal in the frontocentral and temporal scalp (Näätänen et al., 2007). The MMN latency varies across a wide time range within 150 to 250 ms depending on experimental parameters, especially the size of the physical difference between standard and deviant sounds: MMN latency decreases (and the amplitude increases) as the frequency difference between the standard and deviant tones increases. For very large stimulus differences, MMN directly overlaps the auditory N100 vertex response to the standards, and then it is not clear whether any MMN has been elicited. Figure 18.2 depicts the MMN and its simultaneously recorded magnetic counterpart, the mismatch field, MMF (1000-Hz tones as standards and 1050-Hz tones as deviants). The similarity of the MMN and MMF waveforms is striking.

Because MMN and MMF can be elicited when the subject *ignores* the stimuli, for example, by reading a book or viewing a movie, they can be readily used to assess auditory-cortex function in uncooperative individuals, such as small children or comatose patients. For example, the amplitude of the MMN is related to the discrimination threshold of pitch, and the reactivity to sound deviances (generation of MMN) has been suggested as a sign of good prognosis in comatose patients (for a review, see Näätänen et al., 2007). Despite these various advantages, the large interindividual variability of MMN and MMF has largely prevented their diagnostic use at the level of individual patients.

MMN-type responses have also been reported to visual (Alho et al., 1992) and somatosensory (Kekoni et al., 1997) stimuli. It is important to always rule out other causes for these responses. For example, MEG recordings have shown large responses in the second somatosensory cortex to somatosensory stimulation on deviant finger locations, but these responses turned out to be fully explained by stimulus-rate effects (Hari et al., 1990).

MEG recordings have pinpointed MMF/MMN sources in supratemporal auditory cortex, close to the source of N100m (Hari et al., 1984). Additional sources for the MMN/MMF have been proposed in the frontal lobe (Giard et al., 1990; Näätänen & Alho, 1995; Levänen et al., 1996). Despite these other generators, the MMN/MMF has mostly been used as an index of central auditory processing. For example, in dyslexic adults, who have difficulties in processing rapidly repeated sounds, MMFs to small changes in pitch are attenuated in the left hemisphere (Renvall & Hari, 2003).

Figure 18.3 shows how the auditory cortex of a congenitally deaf adult reacts differentially to vibratory stimulation of the palms at frequencies of 180 Hz (standard) versus

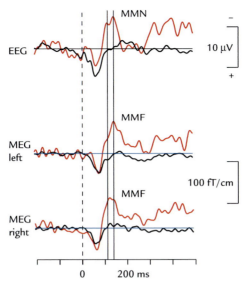

FIGURE 18.2. Simultaneously recorded MMN and MMF. Tone pips of 50 ms duration were repeated once every 505 ms; 90% of them were standards (1000 Hz) and 10% were deviants (1050 Hz). Altogether 200 responses to standards (black traces) and 20 to deviants (red traces) were averaged. The EEG recording (top trace) is from the vertex and the MEG recordings from planar gradiometers over the left (middle trace) and right (lower trace) auditory cortices; the polarities of the MEG signals have been reversed in the plot to facilitate comparison of waveforms. Passband 0.03–330 Hz, sampling rate 1 kHz. The averaged responses have been low-pass filtered at 40 Hz. The peak latencies for the two shoulders in the MMN waveform are highlighted by the solid vertical lines. Note that negative is up. Data recorded at the MEG Core of Aalto NeuroImaging, Aalto University, Finland.

250 Hz (deviant), although it does not react to sounds at all (Levänen et al., 1998). Here the MMF recordings indicate that vibratory somatosensory input can reach the human auditory cortex, as has been also shown in fMRI studies (Schürmann et al., 2006), and that auditory cortical areas can reorganize (or become sensitized) to accommodate information from tactile input. This interpretation makes sense given that both auditory receptors in the cochlea and somatosensory receptors in the skin are driven by vibratory inputs.

A number of hypotheses have been presented about the functional significance of the MMN/MMF. The sensory memory hypothesis posits that the MMN/MMF indexes the deviation in the properties of an incoming sound relative to those of a neural "memory trace" that is created by the preceding standard sounds (Näätänen et al., 2007). Instead, the "fresh afferents" or "neural adaptation" hypothesis assumes that standard stimuli adapt feature-specific neurons and deviant sounds activate fresh, nonadapted neurons so that the MMN/MMF in fact is an (obligatory) N100/N100m response elicited by these fresh afferents (May & Tiitinen, 2010); this hypothesis has been (tentatively) supported by direct recordings from monkey auditory cortex (Fishman, 2014), although additional affirmative evidence is lacking. If either of these hypotheses were true, there would be no need to interpret the mismatch responses in terms of predictive coding that has been proposed to account for MMN generation (Friston, 2005).

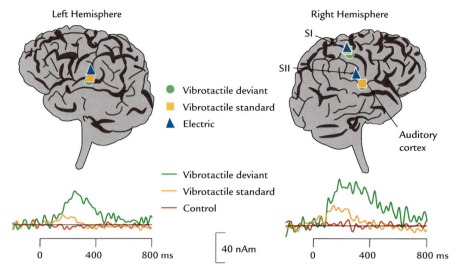

FIGURE 18.3. MMFs from the auditory cortex of a deaf individual. A profoundly deaf individual received 100-ms vibration bursts once every second to his left palm; 85% of them standards (250 Hz; yellow traces) and 15% deviants (180 Hz: green traces). The vibrotactile stimuli activated (in contrast to normally hearing individuals) the auditory cortices of both hemispheres, as shown in the schematic surface renderings based on the individual brain anatomy. The traces at bottom depict time courses of response strengths (in nAm) in the auditory cortices of both hemispheres. Prominent responses are elicited by both vibrotactile stimuli, and in addition a clear mismatch field is seen to the deviant stimuli (green traces), indicating that the auditory cortex was able to differentiate between the vibration frequencies. During the control condition (red trace) the subject did not keep his hand on the device delivering the vibration, and no response was elicited. Source locations are shown also for electrical stimulation of the left median nerve (blue triangles) to pinpoint the locations of SI and SII cortices (SI was activated by the vibratory stimuli as well). This subject's auditory cortex did not react to sounds. Adapted and reprinted from Levänen S, Jousmäki V, Hari R: Vibration-induced auditory-cortex activation in a congenitally deaf adult. *Curr Biol* 1998, 8: 869–872. With permission from Elsevier.

The predictive-coding hypothesis is, however, gaining more support (for a recent review, see Carbajal & Malmierca, 2018). For example, Wacongne and coworkers provided computational evidence that predictive coding implemented in a neuronal circuitry model of the auditory cortex explains the critical features of the MMN, whereas the neuronal adaptation mechanism does not (Wacongne et al., 2011, 2012). Importantly, higher-order predictions were produced at multiple brain areas beyond auditory cortex (Wacongne et al., 2011).

An *omission* of one or more sounds from a monotonous and regular tone sequence is a dramatic violation of expectation. For example, if a small percentage of tones are omitted *and the omissions are attended to*, broad responses peaking 150 to 200 ms after the predicted time of stimulus occurrence peak in the supratemporal auditory cortex (Raij et al., 1997). Thus the auditory cortex keeps track of the regularities of the environment, reacting even to the absence of sounds. This phenomenon can be explained in the predictive-coding framework without the need to assume neuronal adaptation or release from adaptation (Wacongne et al., 2012). Attended omissions are associated with curious temporally distinct percepts of "nothingness" around the time of the expected sound occurrence (see also the subsequent section on P300).

■ P300 RESPONSES

During the 1960s, after Grey Walter's discovery of the CNV, interest quickly grew in "objective" EEG measures of cognitive processes. For example, Chapman and Bragdon (1964) had subjects view numerical stimuli and perform cognitive operations on them, while occasionally infrequent "blank" stimuli appeared that the subjects could not evaluate. Interestingly, the task-relevant numerical stimuli elicited large EEG potentials spanning the midline of the parietal and occipital scalp. Because only one experimental manipulation was used, it was difficult to make sense of the functional significance of the response; nor could topography of the response be determined as only a single two-electrode montage was used. However, it was very clear that brain activity could be modulated by the *meaning of the stimulus* and not just by the physical stimulus features.

Shortly after this study, Sutton et al. (1965) demonstrated neural responses to visual stimuli that also had a specific meaning for the task and to cued auditory and visual stimuli when the subject was uncertain of the type of the incoming stimulus. The response amplitude was large when the probability of receiving the uncertain stimulus was low. This response, which was originally called the "late positive component" and became known as the P300, is a prominent positive scalp potential peaking at the centroparietal midline at 300 to 350 ms; it is characteristically elicited by attended low-probability target stimuli.

Since that time, the literature on P300-type responses has become so extensive that for an interested newcomer it may be better to start by reading a few reviews (Polich, 2007; Duncan et al., 2009). This initial familiarization could be followed with some test recordings that would give an idea of how the responses look and behave. Only at that point would it be advisable to dig deeper into the extensive P300 literature.

P300 can be classically elicited by attended infrequent stimuli in auditory, visual, and somatosensory streams (Snyder et al., 1980; Polich, 2007; Duncan et al., 2009), with larger amplitudes and about 100 ms longer latencies for visual and somatosensory P300s relative to auditory P300s. Stimulus omission can also elicit a P300—an entity that has been called the "emitted P300" (Picton & Hillyard, 1974; Weinberg et al., 1974).

Figure 18.4 depicts a classical visual P300 elicited by an infrequent target in a stream of other visual stimuli. Averaged waveforms from a single subject, shown for a 256-channel EEG recording, display a large positivity centered over the centroparietal midline about 340 ms poststimulus, with a polarity reversal (scalp-negativity) on the face and neck (for a nose reference). Topographic scalp maps (2D on a flat surface and 3D over the head surface) clearly illustrate the amplitude maximum of P300 over the centroparietal scalp.

Sometimes a P300-like response, peaking already at 250 ms and with a more anterior scalp topography, is elicited by infrequent task-irrelevant stimuli that the subject does not actively attend to (Squires et al., 1975; Polich, 2007; Duncan et al., 2009). This response has been typically labeled as the P3a (to differentiate it from the "typical P300," which has also been called the P3b).

In invasive intracranial recordings, large local amplitude gradients and polarity reversals are seen in the human hippocampus (Halgren et al., 1980; Squires et al., 1981; Wood et al., 1984), with abolition in hippocampal sclerosis (Puce et al., 1989b). The curved anatomy of the hippocampus makes it quite a difficult target for scalp EEG and MEG recordings, although hippocampal sources have been suggested on the basis of the MEG field patterns (Okada et al., 1983). Other sources, in addition to the hippocampus, may exist in the

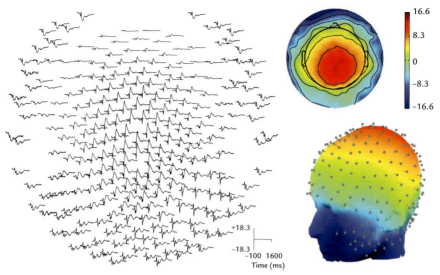

FIGURE 18.4. A visual P300. Left: Evoked responses from a 256-channel EEG recording relative to a nose reference in a single subject to infrequent targets (17% of stimuli) among frequent facial stimuli depicting happy, proud, or neutral expressions; the targets consisted of the same faces but with a "freckle" between the eye and mouth region. Passband 0.1–200 Hz, sampling rate 500 Hz; the responses were low-pass filtered at 40 Hz. Right: 2D (top) and 3D (bottom) scalp topographic maps plotted at the time point of largest P300 (at 342 ms; the calibration bar depicts amplitudes in μV). In the 3D plot, electrode positions are displayed as gray pins. Generated from the dataset of daSilva EB, Crager K, Geisler D, Newbern P, Orem B, Puce A: On dissociating the neural time course of the processing of positive emotions. *NeuroImage* 2016, 127: 227–241.

thalamus (Yingling & Hosobuchi, 1984; Katayama et al., 1985), the frontal lobe (McCarthy & Wood, 1987), and the temporoparietal junction (Soltani & Knight, 2000).

Given the multiple generators for P300, it is difficult to make solid inferences on the basis of P300 amplitude and latency about the functional significance of a certain brain area (or even circuitry). However, the response has been associated with various behavioral phenomena, such as stimulus evaluation independently of response selection (Kutas et al., 1977; McCarthy & Donchin, 1981), mental workload (Kok, 2001), context updating (Donchin & Coles, 1988), and template matching in attention and working memory systems (Chao et al., 1995; Soltani & Knight, 2000; Polich, 2007). In contrast, P3a (which arises without voluntary attention) may be more like an orienting response linked to stimulus-driven attentional mechanisms in the frontal lobe (Polich, 2007).

In terms of the predictive-coding framework, the classic P300 is likely generated because the brain has formed a probabilistic model of the incoming sensory stream—P300 amplitude increases when the stimulus probabilities decrease, and the stimuli thus have a higher surprise value. The multitude of generator areas could imply that similar types of neural responses are instantiated at multiple brain levels and brain regions to update the internal models.

One important source of variance for P300 (and potentially for other cognitive-evoked responses) is the age of the subject: P300 amplitude decreases about 0.2 μV/year and latency increases by 1 to 1.3 ms/year over 15 to 80 years of age across studies (Puce et al.,

1989a). In subjects younger than 15 years, P300 latency is shorter and amplitude larger (Goodin et al., 1978). The negativity preceding P300 is also affected by the age (Goodin et al., 1978), and age should thus be used as a regressor in the analysis of cognitive and affective evoked responses.

■ N400 RESPONSES

A prominent N400 response, a scalp-negative potential peaking over the centroparietal scalp about 400 ms, was first described by Kutas and Hillyard (1980) as a response to semantically incongruous endings of visually presented sentences, such as "I take my coffee with milk and *mud*." In fact, N400 is elicited in multiple experimental set-ups where a semantic evaluation of the stimulus is required (for reviews, see Kutas & Federmeier, 2000; Kutas & Federmeier, 2011).

N400 amplitude is proportional to the degree of the semantic incongruity and can be elicited by both visual and auditory unexpected words (Kutas & Hillyard, 1983), as is shown in Figure 18.5. Data from four midline sites spanning frontal to occipital cortex show a clear N400 potential for sentences with semantically incongruous endings relative to congruous sentences.

N400 is especially large in semantic violations, but it could, in principle, be a normal brain response to any word (Kutas & Federmeier, 2000), although such responses are very difficult to detect for words of continuous speech or written language without using some additional information of the word's predictability.

The magnetic counterpart of N400 is prominent in various reading tasks. For example, Figure 18.6 depicts a summary of MEG recordings during silent reading. The first activation

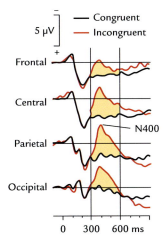

FIGURE 18.5. The N400 semantic incongruity. Grand-average event-related potential across 17 subjects at the frontal (Fz), central (Cz), parietal (Pz), and occipital (Oz) midline (referenced to linked mastoids) in response to viewing sentences with semantically congruent (black line) and incongruent (red line) final words. Low-pass filter at 40 Hz, time constant 8 s, sampling rate 256 Hz. Note that negative is up. The main difference (N400) occurs between 300 and 600 ms (yellow shaded area). Adapted and reprinted from Kutas M, Hillyard SA: Event-related brain potentials to grammatical errors and semantic anomalies. *Memory Cognit* 1983, 11: 539–550. With permission from Springer.

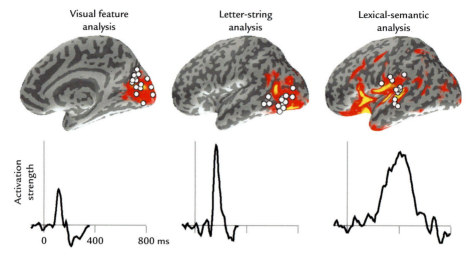

FIGURE 18.6. Time course of cortical activation during silent reading as revealed by MEG. Top: Activations on an MRI surface rendering during visual feature analysis (left; display of the mesial wall of the right hemisphere), letter-string analysis (middle; lateral surface of left hemisphere), and lexical-semantic analysis (right; lateral surface of left hemisphere). The colored patches show group-level anatomically constrained minimum-norm estimates and the dots show the locations of individual current-dipole models. Bottom: The mean time courses of activation strengths corresponding to each activation area. The peak latencies progressively lengthen from visual feature analysis to letter-string analysis and finally to lexical-semantic processing. See text for further details. Adapted and reprinted from Hari R, Salmelin R: Magnetoencephalography: from SQUIDs to neuroscience. *NeuroImage* 2012, 61: 386–396. With permission from Elsevier.

peaks at ~100 ms in the occipital mesial cortex and is related to visual feature analysis, and the next activation peak at 150 ms in the left inferior occipitotemporal region is related to letter-string analysis. Activation peaking around 400 ms in the left superior temporal cortex is thought to reflect lexical–semantic processing and also phonological and syntactic processing (Salmelin et al., 2000; Vartiainen et al., 2009).

The sources of the magnetic M400 to semantic violations and errors have been located to the posterior middle temporal gyrus (Simos et al., 1997), along the perisylvian cortex (Helenius et al., 1998) and in the superior temporal lobe (Service et al., 2007), whereas intracranial EEG recordings have shown bilateral N400 in the anterior mesial temporal lobe (McCarthy et al., 1995). One reason for this discrepancy in source areas could be the difficulty of picking up MEG and scalp EEG signals from the mesial temporal lobe (epileptic discharges are an exception because of their large amplitude). An alternate possibility is these methods pick up signals from different sources.

In an MEG experiment eliciting N400-type responses, visual sentences were presented one word at a time to neurotypical and dyslexic readers. The beginning of each sentence created a high expectation for a certain final word. The brain areas recruited for the semantic processing of the final word included the left superior temporal cortex, with delayed activation in dyslexic subjects. The results were interpreted to suggest that the dyslexic individuals have problems in presemantic analysis and that smaller or less synchronized neuronal populations are activated in their temporal cortex during reading comprehension (Helenius et al., 1999).

Like the P300, the N400 can be elicited to multiple cognitive manipulations beyond semantic violations, such as word repetition, semantic priming, and lexical decision, as is described in the very substantial literature on these instances. The N400 typically co-occurs with a subsequent P600 potential, thereby forming an N400/P600 complex. Typically, new items and semantic primes elicit larger N400s, whereas old items and semantic targets produce larger P600s (Bentin et al., 1985; Rugg, 1985).

In general, N400 is elicited in various tasks that require access to stored representations relevant to the incoming stimuli. It has been postulated that "prior context stimulates the retrieval of knowledge from semantic memory and this information is rapidly integrated with (even partial) perceptual input" and that "words are actively predicted such that reduced N400 amplitudes reflect the benefits of confirmed predictions" (Van Petten & Luka, 2012, p 178). An alternative view posits that an N400 response reflects a binding process that forms a multimodal representation of the stimuli (Kutas & Federmeier, 2011). Altogether, N400 seems to index activation of a distributed brain network related to extraction and addressing meaning to sensory inflow.

As a postscript to the topic on incongruity: physical incongruities between stimuli (e.g., presenting a word in a sentence in a different font, or having a different speaker utter a word) will typically induce a scalp-positive potential, known as the P560 or the physical-incongruity response (McCallum et al., 1984). Similar responses can also be elicited by physical incongruities that occur between *multisensory* stimuli (Puce et al., 2007).

▪ ERROR-RELATED NEGATIVITY

People need to continuously monitor their errors to adjust their actions. Figure 18.7 shows a typical error-related response, the so-called error-related negativity (ERN; also called Ne), which typically peaks less than 100 ms after an error in a choice reaction-time task and thus 300 to 500 ms after the stimulus onset (Falkenstein et al., 1991; Gehring et al., 1993; Falkenstein et al., 2000). In the example shown in Figure 18.7, the ERN peaks 61 ms after the error. A positive slow shift over the parietal cortex follows ERN/Ne at 500 to 700 ms and is called Pe (also visible in Figure 18.7). Both the ERN and its magnetic counterpart (Keil et al., 2010; Charles et al., 2013) are larger when the subjects are aware of their errors and attempt to correct their behavior. Note that ERN analysis requires averaging time-locked to the *response* rather than to the stimulus.

ERN/Ne and Pe are best elicited in subjects who respond to all incoming stimuli *rapidly*, within a designated time interval, thus increasing the likelihood of committing errors. ERN seems to be generated in the anterior cingulate cortex (Dehaene et al., 1994; Luu et al., 2000; Keil et al., 2010) and Pe in the cingulate cortex slightly posterior to the sources of ERN (Vocat et al., 2008).

Multiple functional roles have been proposed for the ERN, such as an error-detection response, an error signal, a conflict-monitoring or comparator response, an error-inhibition response, or an emotional/motivational response to the commission of the error (Falkenstein et al., 2000; Olvet & Hajcak, 2008; Keil et al., 2010; Charles et al., 2013). Interpretations of the Pe have included a resetting of the ERN/Ne error response, or additional processing related to the committed error that is independent of ERN/Ne (Falkenstein et al., 2000).

From a predictive coding point of view, the ERN occurs in a part of the processing hierarchy (i.e., beyond sensory cortices) that supports conscious comparison between a noticed error and the generated response.

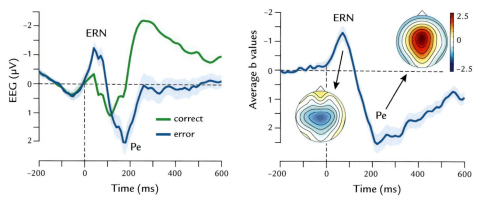

FIGURE 18.7. The error-related negativity (ERN). Left panel: Deflections with negative polarity, ERN, also known as Ne, and subsequent positivity, called Pe, are evoked at the vertex by motor commission errors in simple speeded response tasks (blue waveform), but not in correct trials (green waveform). These averaged ERNs are thought to reflect phase-locked theta activity generated in the midsection of cingulate cortex. The horizontal and vertical gray dotted lines indicate zero voltage and time. Right panel: Topographic maps and waveform showing the results of a single-trial robust regression analysis of the ERN, displaying the time courses of the weights of a response-locked error regressor. The topographic maps of the regressor are shown at the peaks of the ERN and Pe. Adapted and reprinted from Kirschner H, Klein TA: Beyond a blunted ERN—Biobehavioral correlates of performance monitoring in schizophrenia. *Neurosci Biobehav Rev* 2022, 133: 104504. With permission from Elsevier.

■ REFERENCES

Alho K, Woods DL, Algazi A, Näätänen R: Intermodal selective attention: II. Effects of attentional load on processing of auditory and visual stimuli in central space. *Electroencephalogr Clin Neurophysiol* 1992, 82: 356–368.

Bentin S, McCarthy G, Wood CC: Event-related potentials, lexical decision and semantic priming. *Electroencephalogr Clin Neurophysiol* 1985, 60: 343–355.

Carbajal GV, Malmierca MS: The neuronal basis of predictive coding along the auditory pathway: from the subcortical roots to cortical deviance detection. *Trends Hear* 2018, 22: 1–33.

Chao LL, Nielsen-Bohlman L, Knight RT: Auditory event-related potentials dissociate early and late memory processes. *Electroencephalogr Clin Neurophysiol* 1995, 96: 157–168.

Chapman RM, Bragdon HR: Evoked responses to numerical and non-numerical visual stimuli while problem solving. *Nature* 1964, 203: 1155–1157.

Charles L, Van Opstal F, Marti S, Dehaene S: Distinct brain mechanisms for conscious versus subliminal error detection. *NeuroImage* 2013, 73: 80–94.

Dehaene S, Posner, MI, Tucker, DM: Localization of a neural system for error detection and compensation. *Psychol Sci* 1994, 5: 303–305.

Donchin E, Coles MGH: Is the P300 component a manifestation of context updating? *Behav Brain Sci* 1988, 11: 357–374.

Duncan CC, Barry RJ, Connolly JF, Fischer C, Michie PT, Näätänen R, Polich J, Reinvang I, Van Petten C: Event-related potentials in clinical research: guidelines for eliciting, recording, and quantifying mismatch negativity, P300, and N400. *Clin Neurophysiol* 2009, 120: 1883–1908.

Falkenstein M, Hohnsbein J, Hoormann J, Blanke L: Effects of crossmodal divided attention on late ERP components: II. Error processing in choice reaction tasks. *Electroencephalogr Clin Neurophysiol* 1991, 78: 447–455.

Falkenstein M, Hoormann J, Christ S, Hohnsbein J: ERP components on reaction errors and their functional significance: a tutorial. *Biol Psychol* 2000, 51: 87–107.

Fishman YI: The mechanisms and meaning of the mismatch negativity. *Brain Topogr* 2014, 27: 500–526.

Friston K: A theory of cortical responses. *Philos Trans R Soc Lond B Biol Sci* 2005, 360: 815–836.

Gehring WJ, Goss B, Coles MGH, Meyer DE, Donchin E: A neural system for error detection and compensation. *Psychol Sci* 1993, 4: 385–390.

Giard MH, Perrin F, Pernier J, Bouchet P: Brain generators implicated in the processing of auditory stimulus deviance: a topographic event-related potential study. *Psychophysiology* 1990, 27: 627–640.

Goodin DS, Squires KC, Henderson BH, Starr A: Age-related variations in evoked potentials to auditory stimuli in normal human subjects. *Electroencephalogr Clin Neurophysiol* 1978, 44: 447–458.

Halgren E, Squires NK, Wilson CL, Rohrbaugh JW, Babb TL, Crandall PH: Endogenous potentials generated in the human hippocampal formation and amygdala by infrequent events. *Science* 1980, 210: 803–805.

Hari R, Hämäläinen M, Ilmoniemi R, Kaukoranta E, Reinikainen K, Salminen J, Alho K, Näätänen R, Sams M: Responses of the primary auditory cortex to pitch changes in a sequence of tone pips: neuromagnetic recordings in man. *Neurosci Lett* 1984, 50: 127–132.

Hari R, Hämäläinen H, Tiihonen J, Kekoni J, Sams M, Hämäläinen M: Separate finger representations at the human second somatosensory cortex. *Neuroscience* 1990, 37: 245–249.

Helenius P, Salmelin R, Service E, Connolly JF: Distinct time courses of word and context comprehension in the left temporal cortex. *Brain* 1998, 121: 1133–1142.

Helenius P, Salmelin R, Service E, Connolly JF: Semantic cortical activation in dyslexic readers. *J Cogn Neurosci* 1999, 11: 535–550.

Hultin L, Rossini P, Romani GL, Hogstedt P, Tecchio F, Pizzella V: Neuromagnetic localization of the late component of the contingent negative variation. *Electroencephalogr Clin Neurophysiol* 1996, 98: 435–448.

Katayama Y, Tsukiyama T, Tsubokawa T: Thalamic negativity associated with the endogenous late positive component of cerebral evoked potentials (P300): recordings using discriminative aversive conditioning in humans and cats. *Brain Res Bull* 1985, 14: 223–226.

Keil J, Weisz N, Paul-Jordanov I, Wienbruch C: Localization of the magnetic equivalent of the ERN and induced oscillatory brain activity. *NeuroImage* 2010, 51: 404–411.

Kekoni J, Hämäläinen H, Saarinen M, Grohn J, Reinikainen K, Lehtokoski A, Näätänen R: Rate effect and mismatch responses in the somatosensory system: ERP-recordings in humans. *Biol Psychol* 1997, 46: 125–142.

Kilner JM, Friston KJ, Frith CD: Predictive coding: an account of the mirror neuron system. *Cogn Process* 2007, 8: 159–166.

Kok A: The effect of warning stimulus novelty on the P300 and components of the contingent negative variation. *Biol Psychol* 1978, 6: 219–233.

Kok A: On the utility of P3 amplitude as a measure of processing capacity. *Psychophysiology* 2001, 38: 557–577.

Koster-Hale J, Saxe R: Theory of mind: a neural prediction problem. *Neuron* 2013, 79: 836–848.

Kutas M, McCarthy G, Donchin E: Augmenting mental chronometry: the P300 as a measure of stimulus evaluation time. *Science* 1977, 197: 792–795.

Kutas M, Hillyard SA: Reading senseless sentences: brain potentials reflect semantic incongruity. *Science* 1980, 207: 203–205.

Kutas M, Hillyard SA: Event-related brain potentials to grammatical errors and semantic anomalies. *Mem Cognit* 1983, 11: 539–550.

Kutas M, Federmeier KD: Electrophysiology reveals semantic memory use in language comprehension. *Trends Cogn Sci* 2000, 4: 463–470.

Kutas M, Federmeier KD: Thirty years and counting: finding meaning in the N400 component of the event-related brain potential (ERP). *Annu Rev Psychol* 2011, 62: 621–647.

Levänen S, Ahonen A, Hari R, McEvoy L, Sams M: Deviant auditory stimuli activate human left and right auditory cortex differently. *Cereb Cortex* 1996, 6: 288–296.

Levänen S, Jousmäki V, Hari R: Vibration-induced auditory-cortex activation in a congenitally deaf adult. *Curr Biol* 1998, 8: 869–872.

Loveless NE: The contingent negative variation related to preparatory set in a reaction time situation with variable foreperiod. *Electroencephalogr Clin Neurophysiol* 1973, 35: 369–374.

Luu P, Flaisch T, Tucker DM: Medial frontal cortex in action monitoring. *J Neurosci* 2000, 20: 464–469.

May P, Tiitinen H: Mismatch negativity (MMN), the deviance-elicited auditory deflection, explained. *Psychophysiology* 2010, 47: 66–122.

McCallum WC, Farmer SF, Pocock PV: The effects of physical and semantic incongruities on auditory event-related potentials. *Electroencephalogr Clin Neurophysiol* 1984, 59: 477–488.

McCarthy G, Donchin E: A metric for thought: a comparison of P300 latency and reaction time. *Science* 1981, 211: 77–80.

McCarthy G, Wood CC: Intracranial recordings of endogenous ERPs in humans. *EEG Clin Neurophysiol Suppl* 1987, 39: 331–337.

McCarthy G, Nobre AC, Bentin S, Spencer DD: Language-related field potentials in the anterior-medial temporal lobe: I. Intracranial distribution and neural generators. *J Neurosci* 1995, 15: 1080–1089.

Näätänen R, Gaillard AWK, Mäntysalo S: Early selective attention effect reinterpreted. *Acta Psychol* 1978, 42: 313–329.

Näätänen R, Alho K: Generators of electrical and magnetic mismatch responses in humans. *Brain Topogr* 1995, 7: 315–320.

Näätänen R, Paavilainen P, Rinne T, Alho K: The mismatch negativity (MMN) in basic research of central auditory processing: a review. *Clin Neurophysiol* 2007, 118: 2544–2590.

Okada Y, Kaufman L, Williamson S: The hippocampal formation as a source of the slow endogenous potentials. *Electroencephalogr Clin Neurophysiol* 1983, 55: 417–426.

Olvet DM, Hajcak G: The error-related negativity (ERN) and psychopathology: toward an endophenotype. *Clin Psychol Rev* 2008, 28: 1343–1354.

Picton TW, Hillyard SA: Human auditory evoked potentials: II. Effects of attention. *Electroencephalogr Clin Neurophysiol* 1974, 36: 191–199.

Polich J: Updating P300: an integrative theory of P3a and P3b. *Clin Neurophysiol* 2007, 118: 2128–2148.

Puce A, Donnan GA, Bladin PF: Comparative effects of age on limbic and scalp P3. *Electroencephalogr Clin Neurophysiol* 1989a, 74: 385–393.

Puce A, Kalnins RM, Berkovic SF, Donnan GA, Bladin PF: Limbic P3 potentials, seizure localization, and surgical pathology in temporal lobe epilepsy. *Ann Neurol* 1989b, 26: 377–385.

Puce A, Epling JA, Thompson JC, Carrick OK: Neural responses elicited to face motion and vocalization pairings. *Neuropsychology* 2007, 45: 93–106.

Raij T, McEvoy L, Mäkelä J, Hari R: Human auditory cortex is activated by omissions of auditory stimuli. *Brain Res* 1997, 745: 134–143.

Renvall H, Hari R: Diminished auditory mismatch fields in dyslexic adults. *Ann Neurol* 2003, 53: 551–557.

Rohrbaugh JW, Syndulko K, Lindsley DB: Brain wave components of the contingent negative variation in humans. *Science* 1976, 191: 1055–1057.

Rosahl SK, Knight RT: Role of prefrontal cortex in generation of the contingent negative variation. *Cereb Cortex* 1995, 5: 123–134.

Rugg MD: The effects of semantic priming and work repetition on event-related potentials. *Psychophysiology* 1985, 22: 642–647.

Salmelin R, Helenius P, Service E: Neurophysiology of fluent and impaired reading: a magnetoencephalographic approach. *J Clin Neurophysiol* 2000, 17: 163–174.

Schürmann M, Caetano G, Hlushchuk Y, Jousmäki V, Hari R: Touch activates human auditory cortex. *NeuroImage* 2006, 30: 1325–1331.

Service E, Helenius P, Maury S, Salmelin R: Localization of syntactic and semantic brain responses using magnetoencephalography. *J Cogn Neurosci* 2007, 19: 1193–1205.

Simos PG, Basile LF, Papanicolaou AC: Source localization of the N400 response in a sentence-reading paradigm using evoked magnetic fields and magnetic resonance imaging. *Brain Res* 1997, 762: 29–39.

Snyder E, Hillyard SA, Galambos R: Similarities and differences among the P3 waves to detected signals in three modalities. *Psychophysiology* 1980, 17: 112–122.

Soltani M, Knight RT: Neural origins of the P300. *Crit Rev Neurobiol* 2000, 14: 199–224.

Squires NK, Squires KC, Hillyard SA: Two varieties of long-latency positive waves evoked by unpredictable auditory stimuli in man. *Electroencephalogr Clin Neurophysiol* 1975, 38: 387–401.

Squires NK, Halgren E, Wilson CL, Crandall PH: Human endogenous limbic potentials: cross-modality and depth-surface comparisons in epileptic subjects. In: Gaillard AWK, Ritter W, eds. *Biophysical Communications, Quarterly Progress Report, Research Laboratory for Electronics.* Cambridge, MA: MIT Press, 1981: 58–170.

Sutton S, Braren M, Zubin J, John ER: Evoked-potential correlates of stimulus uncertainty. *Science* 1965, 150: 1187–1188.

Van Petten C, Luka BJ: Prediction during language comprehension: benefits, costs, and ERP components. *Int J Psychophysiol* 2012, 83: 176–190.

Vartiainen J, Parviainen T, Salmelin R: Spatiotemporal convergence of semantic processing in reading and speech perception. *J Neurosci* 2009, 29: 9271–9280.

Vocat R, Pourtois G, Vuilleumier P: Unavoidable errors: a spatio-temporal analysis of time-course and neural sources of evoked potentials associated with error processing in a speeded task. *Neuropsychology* 2008, 46: 2545–2555.

Wacongne C, Labyt E, van Wassenhove V, Bekinschtein T, Naccache L, Dehaene S: Evidence for a hierarchy of predictions and prediction errors in human cortex. *Proc Natl Acad Sci U S A* 2011, 108: 20754–20759.

Wacongne C, Changeux JP, Dehaene S: A neuronal model of predictive coding accounting for the mismatch negativity. *J Neurosci* 2012, 32: 3665–3678.

Walter WG, Cooper R, Aldridge VJ, McCallum WC, Winter AL: Contingent negative variation: an electric sign of sensorimotor association and expectancy in the human brain. *Nature* 1964, 203: 380–384.

Weinberg H, Walter WG, Cooper R, Aldridge VJ: Emitted cerebral events. *Electroencephalogr Clin Neurophysiol* 1974, 36: 449–456.

Wood CC, McCarthy G, Squires NK, Vaughan HG, Woods DL, McCallum WC: Anatomical and physiological substrates of event-related potentials: two case studies. *Ann N Y Acad Sci* 1984, 425: 681–721.

Yingling CD, Hosobuchi Y: A subcortical correlate of P300 in man. *Electroencephalogr Clin Neurophysiol* 1984, 59: 72–76.

CHAPTER 19

THE SOCIAL BRAIN

Anyone who either cannot lead the common life or is so self-sufficient as not to need to, and therefore does not partake of society, is either a beast or a god.

—ARISTOTLE

He thought in other heads, and in his own, others besides himself thought.

—BERTOLT BRECHT

■ THEORETICAL FRAMEWORK

Much of what we know about how humans process social information detected from others' faces, utterances, and body postures comes from twentieth-century experiments using isolated face or verbal stimuli in highly controlled laboratory environments. However, our everyday social interaction and decision-making occurs in a complex, unpredicted, and dynamic environment where people can smoothly adapt and synchronize their behaviors to those of their social partners. The disconnection between laboratory data and real-life conditions imposes huge constraints on the theoretical framework, experiments, and analysis of data in social neuroscience. More recently, these limitations have led to the development of "naturalistic" or more ecologically valid setups to study brain–behavior relationships, thereby building on and expanding the rich knowledge acquired in previous well-controlled laboratory studies (Hari & Kujala, 2009; Dumas et al., 2011; Berthenthal & Puce, 2015; Nasiopoulos et al., 2015).

Figure 19.1 divides the experimental set-ups of human neuroimaging to settings of one-person neuroscience (1PN; upper panel) and two-person neuroscience (2PN; lower panel). This division reflects a progression from simple, well-controlled artificial stimuli to real-life-like interactive social interactions (Hari & Kujala, 2009; Schilbach et al., 2013; Hari et al., 2015). Note that 1PN and 2PN only refer to the experimental setups (whether brain functions of one or two persons are studied at the same time). Thus these terms have to be separated from first-person and second-person neuroscience that refer to the perspectives taken by the (single) subjects under study. In classical 1PN studies, the stimuli have been well controlled but artificial, such as checkerboards, sinusoidal sounds, electric stimulation of peripheral nerves, and simple multisensory stimuli (Figure 19.1, upper panel, left; Chapters 13–18). Clearly more complex static social stimuli (upper panel, middle), such

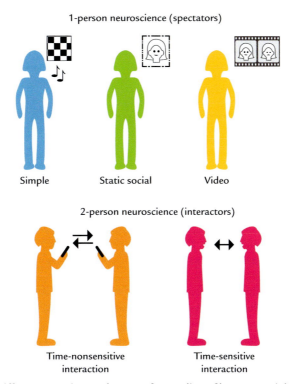

1-person neuroscience (spectators)

Simple   Static social   Video

2-person neuroscience (interactors)

Time-nonsensitive   Time-sensitive
interaction   interaction

FIGURE 19.1. **Different experimental setups for studies of human social neuroscience.** Top panel: The bulk of experiments reported in the literature use 1-person neuroscience (top panel), where the subject is effectively a passive spectator who is not engaged in the portrayed social situations (most typically simple nonsocial stimuli, static social images, or videos are viewed). Bottom panel: Subjects are engaged interactors in social situations, which calls for experimental setups of 2-person neuroscience. Interactions may take place in a non-time-sensitive way, as in sending text and emails (left) or as a face-to-face interaction or conversation via audio or audiovisual links (right). Adapted and reprinted from Hari R, Henriksson L, Malinen S, Parkkonen L: Centrality of social interaction in human brain function. *Neuron* 2015, 88: 181–193. With permission from Elsevier.

as snapshots of faces, activate the fusiform gyrus and lateral temporal cortex, and human vocalizations activate the superior temporal cortices. The next step in the progression toward more natural setups is the presentation of dynamic stimuli, such as movies (right panel) with or without sound. While these complex stimuli challenge and expose the limitations in our current data-analysis methods (Lankinen et al., 2014; Adolphs et al., 2016), subjects typically enjoy them more than the less-engaging artificial stimuli. Other persons' motor actions are important dynamic stimuli for action-observation studies (see discussion later in this chapter).

Despite all the valuable information the 1PN settings have provided about human brain function, they consider the subject as a passive spectator rather than an engaged interactor (Hari et al., 2015). In other words, one would assume, for example, that by presenting affective stimuli (that are randomized to avoid systematic biases), one can extract brain responses that are purely related to the stimuli, assuming that the subject's state has remained the same the entire time despite intervening stimuli. This kind of "spectator science" comprises most current brain-imaging literature, whereas in real life people are engaged in interactions rather than being passive spectators. In other words, their mental and bodily states change as a consequence of incoming dynamic multisensory input and their own actions. Thus subjects do not stay "the same" during the whole experiment. One could defend these typical social neuroscience experiments by saying that the stimuli and tasks will rarely evoke very strong changes in the subject's state. This, however, is hard to ascertain without detailed monitoring of the background MEG/EEG activity, the subject's behavior, and/or other physiological variables, such as pupil dilation and heart-rate variability (see Chapter 16).

The lower panel of Figure 19.1 presents 2PN settings in which two subjects are in a face-to-face social interaction (right). It is conceptually important to differentiate between situations where the two persons are involved in a relatively slow-paced interaction of the order of seconds or longer, such as sending text messages or emails to each other, or in economical decision games via the Internet (left). Although these cases can definitely be considered real social interactions, the experimental set-ups can be replaced by cleverly designed 1PN setups, measuring just one person's brain function at one time, and then swapping the roles.

Much more demanding 2PN setups are called for when one aims to study two persons in a dynamic, 3D embodied interaction, such as during a conversation or joint motor tasks requiring some concrete endpoint. Such interactions occur at a fast pace of the order of 100 ms or less, with preparation and actual responses often overlapping in time; yet the interaction is typically smooth and effortless (for a review, see Hari et al., 2016). Here our estimate of timescale (of 50–100 ms) derives from the typical duration of a phoneme and associated articulatory facial movements; even emotional facial movements that color verbal interactions can change within a 100-ms period, which is the duration of just a single phoneme (Peräkylä & Ruusuvuori, 2006). This kind of dynamic interaction is unique and cannot be exactly repeated in a subsequent experiment or reduced to sequential single-person measurements. It therefore must be captured in real time with "hyperscanning" methods where data are collected from multiple individuals simultaneously while they engage in a 3D interpersonal interaction (see later discussion).

Thus it is the *temporal structure* of the interactive behavior that defines when a 2PN setup would be the most efficient and informative, as the modulations of brain signals would have to be sampled at least at 50-ms intervals, corresponding to about 20 Hz, to properly cover at least 100-ms time scales. Note that micro-expressions (concealed facial expressions) may last only 40 to 70 ms (Porter & ten Brinke, 2008), which further emphasizes the importance of time-resolved (single-millisecond) brain-imaging by means of MEG or EEG to track brain activity supporting face-to-face social interaction.

Figure 19.2 illustrates an action–perception loop between two persons involved in a face-to-face interaction. Whereas each single subject must adjust her or his own (motor) output and (sensory) input, during the interaction one person's output is the other (very similar) person's input, and thus the action–perception loop transforms to an action–perception figure-of-eight loop (Hari & Kujala, 2009). These loops are influenced by the individuals' current emotional and cognitive states and emotional self-regulation, and they are modulated by the individuals' unique set of life experiences and stored memories.

A critical element in any successful social interaction is prediction of the other person's behavior. For example, listeners will automatically anticipate a speaker's output, as well as steer the direction that a conversation or social interaction might take. During a social interaction, two Bayesian brains (and minds) thus will continually try to predict one another's thought stream (Friston & Frith, 2015).

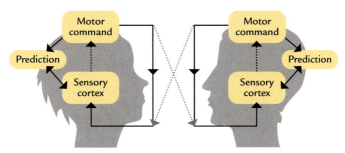

FIGURE 19.2. Action–perception figure-of-eight loop during face-to-face interaction. During social interaction, the individual's action–perception loop (combining motor output with sensory input and the predicted outcome; here shown by the solid lines) will extend to a figure-of-eight loop involving both subjects (solid and dashed lines). One individual's vocal output or other actions will form the interacting partner's sensory input that must be evaluated and compared with predictions so that the two persons can jointly perform this common task (e.g., conversation). See text for additional discussion. Figure based on the ideas expressed in Hari R, Kujala MV: Brain basis of human social interaction: from concepts to brain imaging. *Physiol Rev* 2009, 89: 453–479.

Given the interactive experimental framework presented here, we next briefly discuss some areas of social neuroscience where we believe that MEG/EEG with their excellent temporal resolutions can provide a unique perspective and where initial efforts toward naturalistic experimentation have already been taken.

■ RESPONSES TO EMOTIONS DEPICTED BY FACES AND BODIES

Emotions are evolutionarily essential states that involve both brain and body. They can be observed by others from various nonverbal cues, such as facial expressions, hand and body postures, voice, and even pupil dilation and skin color. We respond to the facial and bodily movements of others reflexively or unintentionally, even when they are not directed at us (Puce, 2013). From just one quick glance, we may recognize (although errors occur, of course) an individual's overall emotional state, irrespective of whether or not we know the person.

Despite the large literature on the subject, we still lack a sufficient understanding of the brain processes that take place while we engage in such social activities. One wonders how limited the view is that we have obtained from only measuring brain activity to static images of faces, bodies, and hands. In fact, it is known that the face-sensitive response N170/M170 (see also Figure 14.8) is larger to (static) real people relative to mannequins or images of faces (Ponkanen et al., 2011) and that dynamic stimuli elicit substantially larger hemodynamic responses than their static counterparts in brain areas such as the superior temporal sulcus (STS; Pitcher et al., 2011).

While extensive information is already available about brain processing of the low-level aspects of social stimuli, such as faces, it is not clear how the main visual cues that characterize an emotion actually drive emotion recognition in the observer's brain (daSilva et al., 2016a). Currently, the general consensus is that a visual stimulus has been recognized as a face by 170 ms (Rossion, 2014) and that the N170 and the subsequent P250 (and their magnetic counterparts) are modulated by happy, angry, and fearful expressions (Hinojosa et al., 2015). However, the effects are variable, potentially reflecting effects of task and the intensity of the emotion (Rellecke et al., 2012; daSilva et al., 2016b). Even low-level visual features, such as the presence of teeth (daSilva et al., 2016a) or changes in the amount of visible eye white (Rossi et al., 2015) will strongly modulate brain responses, as we discuss next.

Figure 19.3 displays the effects of seen teeth on behavioral and neurophysiological responses to mouth expressions. The predominantly sensory responses P100 and N170 are significantly larger to mouth expressions that depict teeth, begging the question of whether the reported ERP enhancements to happy faces are actually driven by the presence of teeth in the image and *not the emotion of happiness* per se. Teeth seen relative to the mouth form a high local luminance-contrast stimulus, which can easily be seen at a distance. However, this is not the complete story when it comes to mouth expressions because mouth movements also affect N170, with significantly larger amplitudes for mouth-opening than mouth-closing movements (Puce et al., 2000), possibly related to detection of biological motion (Rossi et al., 2014). Hence, while dynamic emotions are viewed over several seconds, a number of low-level visual mechanisms can provide information to higher-order brain regions to aid identification of a particular emotion on the basis of characteristic mouth motion and configuration.

The human eye (iris/sclera complex) also displays a high contrast for local luminance, serving as a low-level visual cue for identifying emotions (narrow eyes for happiness or anger and wide eyes for fear or surprise). Changes in gaze direction (signaling changed social attention) can provide additional low-level information but are also context dependent (Latinus et al., 2015). Recent intracranial EEG studies demonstrate that the human STS is particularly sensitive to changes in gaze, with the largest evoked responses occurring to averted gaze. In contrast, activity in the fusiform gyrus depends less on gaze direction but varies more according to facial emotion type (Babo-Rebelo et al., 2022). Future studies need to explore the respective low- and high-level visual effects *and their interactions* during the viewing of natural dynamic faces in social interactions.

Consistent with the more recent intracranial data, scalp N170 is known to occur to observed lateral gaze changes and eye blinks, be they presented as real or apparent motion (Puce et al., 2000; Brefczynski-Lewis et al., 2011). The N170 amplitudes are *larger for gaze aversion* relative to direct gaze, thereby paralleling intracranial findings (Babo-Rebelo et al., 2022), but *only* when subjects make nonsocial judgments about the face (Latinus et al., 2015).

Figure 19.4 shows a whole-head analysis (see Chapter 10) of 256-channel ERPs as a function of task (social vs. nonsocial) and gaze condition (averted vs. direct gaze). Later (> 300 ms) ERP effects typically occur across a large part of the scalp, whereas interaction effects between task and gaze condition are more confined to the anterior scalp. This example indicates how complex brain activity can be in viewers of even simple and discrete facial movements.

Gaze changes and blinks also serve as social signals. When another individual's blinks are viewed, clear MEG signals arise in the viewer's occipital cortex, peaking at ~200 ms (Mandel et al., 2014). Similar responses also occur when the viewed person is narrating a story to which (and not to the narrator's blinks) the subject attends. Thus prominent responses to another person's blinks can be elicited in the absence of attention and despite abundant audiovisual distractors (Mandel et al., 2015). Interestingly, the more empathic the observer (measured via the Interpersonal Reactivity Index questionnaire), the larger the brain responses to the storyteller's blinks are. These studies highlight the richness of social cues that we often are unaware of, or that we think we are disregarding.

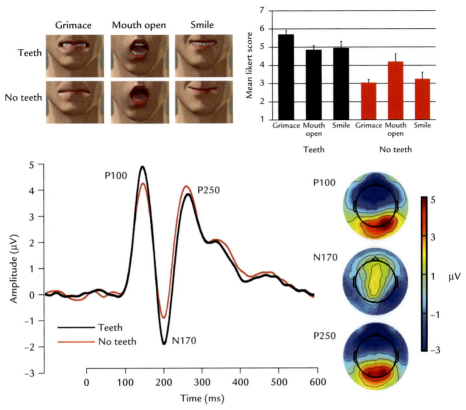

FIGURE 19.3. Low-level visual effects and their likely influence on emotion recognition. Top left: Stimuli were static mouth expressions consisting of a grimace, open mouth, and a smile, shown with (upper row) and without visible teeth (lower row). Expressions were generated from an avatar's face so that the stimuli could be equated for luminance, contrast, and number of pixels for featured teeth. Top right: Mean ± SEM ratings of 20 subjects of the arousal elicited by the stimuli (7-point Likert scale; 1 = least arousing, 7 = most arousing). Stimuli with visible teeth (black bars) were rated as significantly more arousing than stimuli without teeth (red bars). Bottom left: Grand-average ERPs from the same 20 subjects to stimuli with and without teeth visible, showing larger P100 and N170 to stimuli with teeth. For each individual subject, responses were first averaged across a cluster of six electrodes overlying the right occipitotemporal scalp. Bottom right: Scalp voltage maps of P100, N170, and P250 to the stimuli with teeth show the typical topography for face and face-part stimuli. Passband 0.01–200 Hz, sampling rate 500 Hz. Adapted and reprinted from daSilva EB, Crager K, Geisler D, Newbern P, Orem B, Puce A: Something to sink your teeth into: the presence of teeth augments ERPs to mouth expressions. *NeuroImage* 2016, 127: 227–241. With permission from Elsevier.

In general, body postures and movements are highly effective stimuli, likely activating perceptual mechanisms related to biological motion and emotion recognition, particularly when viewing individuals at a distance (de Gelder, 2006). Brain responses to body movements also differentiate between movements of approach and withdrawal (Wheaton et al., 2001). In a recent discussion on the processing of dynamic emotions, the brain was proposed as dealing with important affective information from the face and body in an array of

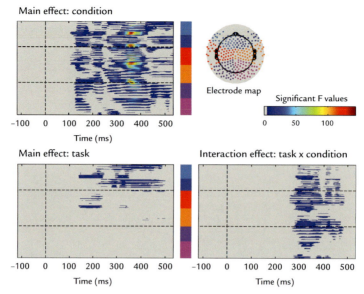

Main effect: condition

Electrode map

Significant F values

0   50   100

Time (ms)

Main effect: task

Interaction effect: task x condition

Time (ms)   Time (ms)

FIGURE 19.4. Neurophysiological changes during social judgments. Averaged 256-channel EEG responses were collected from 22 healthy subjects who were viewing gaze changes (direct versus averted gaze) in two tasks: subjects either decided whether the gaze moved toward or away from them (social task) or whether the gaze went left or right (non-social task). The electrode map at right top shows electrode groups that are color coded by their scalp location (e.g., light and dark blue show left and right frontal sensors, etc.) The plots reflect the results of a whole-head analysis of data using the GLM (see Chapter 10). The main effect of gaze (condition; upper left panel) begins prior to the N170 and persists throughout the epoch and encompasses a large area of the scalp, peaking at around 370 ms post-gaze change. The main effect of task (left bottom panel) is confined to the frontal scalp and extends for a similar time interval. The interaction effect, while relatively widespread, is confined to the post-300 ms time period. Passband 0.01–200 Hz, sampling rate 500 Hz. Adapted and reprinted from Latinus M, Love SA, Rossi A, Parada FJ, Huang L, Conty L, George N, James K, Puce A: Social decisions affect neural activity to perceived dynamic gaze. *Soc Cogn Affect Neurosci* 2015, 10: 1557–1567. With permission from Elsevier.

midlevel visually sensitive brain regions, with a major cortical branch point at the inferior occipital gyrus (IOG) (see Figure 19.5; de Gelder & Poyo Solanas, 2021). This branching of information flow at the IOG is consistent with intracranial recordings as well as the entry and exit points of the associated local white matter pathways (Babo-Rebelo et al., 2022). Notably, this schematic of cortical interactions for processing bodily expressions concurs well with a recently proposed third visual pathway for social information between early visual areas and the STS (Pitcher & Ungerleider, 2021).

Processing of social cues can also be studied with sensory adaptation setups that are commonly used in sensory physiology: one stimulus exemplar is repeated rapidly to dampen neuronal responses to it, so that selective responses can be recorded to interspersing deviant stimuli (see discussion on "fresh afferents" in Chapter 18). For example, sensitivity to faces was studied by presenting a train of visual stimuli (including faces) at 6 Hz so that faces appeared at 1.2-Hz during intracranial recordings that identified responses in wide areas of ventral occipitotemporal cortex, with the largest face-preferential responses

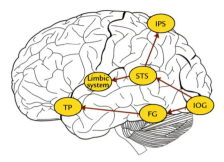

FIGURE 19.5. **Cortical regions implicated in the perception of bodily expressions.** A schematic view of the lateral brain surface shows a potential flow of information related to bodily expression, with a critical branch point at the inferior occipital gyrus and another at the STS. Abbreviations: FG, fusiform gyrus; IOG, inferior occipital gyrus; IPS, intraparietal sulcus; STS, superior temporal sulcus; TP, temporal pole. Adapted and reprinted from de Gelder B, Poyo Solanas M: A computational neuroethology perspective on body and expression perception. *Trends Cogn Sci* 2021, 25: 744–756. With permission from Elsevier.

in the lateral section of the right middle fusiform gyrus (Jonas et al., 2016). These data agree with source modeling of face-sensitive MEG responses (as discussed in Chapter 14). Indeed, results obtained with these rapid stimulus-presentation methods have led to the proposal that visual categorization of faces works in an all-or-none fashion so that when stimuli are categorized as faces, the associated brain responses are of full size even if the stimulus has only been just very briefly flashed (Retter et al., 2020). This type of rapid sensory stimulation might be suited for testing other types of social and emotional stimuli as well.

Patterns of brain activity clearly differ between overt social and emotion judgments relative to other judgments of the same stimuli (Latinus et al., 2015; daSilva et al., 2016b), begging the question as to what the brain does in real life when people interact with other people and objects without necessarily being aware of their social judgments. In fact, we might even work in two "modes" (Puce et al., 2016). In everyday life (and in the laboratory, where the subject performs implicit tasks involving social or affective stimuli), the brain operates in a "default mode" (which is different from the default mode of resting-state brain networks, commonly discussed in fMRI studies) where people may or may not be aware of the social information mainly sent by the low-level cues as we discussed above. In contrast, when subjects make explicit social judgments (in the lab and in real life), the brain operates in a "socially aware mode," where activity in sensory pathways is augmented for optimal processing by higher-level brain regions. These processing modes are predicted to rapidly switch—a supposition that could be easily tested in the laboratory.

■ ACTION VIEWING AND MIRRORING

It is now well known that the monkey premotor cortex contains neurons that discharge during action execution as well as during observation of the same action made by other monkeys or the experimenter (for a review, see Rizzolatti & Craighero, 2004). This "motor mirroring" is assumed to match action observation and execution and to play an important role in action imitation. However, its exact role in understanding the goals of the other individual's actions remains to be determined.

Human brain-imaging studies have demonstrated a similar macroscopic mirroring system (for a recent review of MEG in action observation, see Hari, 2015). The first MEG action-observation study used the 20-Hz rebound, elicited by median-nerve stimuli, as an indicator of the functional state of the primary motor cortex (Hari et al., 1998), as shown in Figure 19.6. The left and right median nerves were stimulated alternatingly at the wrist, and the 20-Hz rebounds were monitored. During rest, the rebounds were prominent in the Rolandic cortex contralateral to the applied median-nerve stimuli, but they were abolished totally when the subject herself manipulated a small object with her fingers, as a sign of motor-cortex activation. When the subject viewed, immobile and without any other task, the experimenter manipulating the object, the rebound was clearly but not totally suppressed, indicating partial activation of the motor cortex by the observed actions.

The effect of viewed actions agrees with the early EEG findings on subjects viewing a movie of a boxing match: their "rhythms en arceau" were blocked whenever the spectators identified themselves with one of the active figures in the movie (Gastaut and Bert, 1954). However, at that time the sources of the EEG mu rhythm were not known. Thus, subsequent work on MEG mu rhythm, showing well-identified sources, allowed more direct conclusions to be made about the underlying brain activity, especially the primary motor and somatosensory cortices that are the main generators of the mu rhythm (Hari & Salmelin, 1997; see Chapter 4).

In Figure 17.3 we showed that the level of the mu rhythm starts to decrease already some 2 s before the subject taps a drum and that during observation of another person's drum-membrane tapping the sequence is similar, but the suppression is weaker and starts less than 1 s before the tap (Caetano et al., 2007). As the suppression and rebound of the

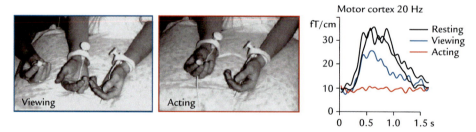

FIGURE 19.6. Effect of action viewing on the primary motor cortex. Left and middle: The experimenter is manipulating a small object while the subject (with median-nerve stimulation electrodes on both wrists) watches the actions (left) or the subject performs similar actions (middle) while being able to see them in the visual periphery. During all conditions, the left and right median nerves were stimulated alternatingly once every 1.5 s to elicit rebounds of the 20-Hz motor-cortex activity. Right: The rebound (increased level as is visible in the amplitude envelope) of the ~20 Hz (15–27 Hz) Rolandic rhythm in response to median nerve stimulation in different experimental conditions in a single subject. The rebound is largest during rest (two separate recordings indicated by black traces) and is totally abolished during own actions (acting; red trace); during action observation, the rebound is dampened but not abolished. Adapted and reprinted from Hari R, Forss N, Avikainen S, Kirveskari E, Salenius S, Rizzolatti G: Activation of human primary motor cortex during action observation: a neuromagnetic study. *Proc Natl Acad Sci U S A* 1998, 95: 15061–15065. ©1998 National Academy of Sciences, USA.

20-Hz rhythm likely reflect excitation and inhibition of the motor cortex, respectively, the findings imply that the motor cortex was activated before and during the viewed action and stabilized afterward, similar to during one's own actions.

One important attribute of neurophysiological methods is the ability to follow cortical activation sequences during various tasks. For example, when a live actor performed hand actions that the subject either only viewed or imitated online, reliable activation sequences with a particular temporal structure were seen (Nishitani & Hari, 2000). Specifically, during one's own action (Execution; leftmost histogram of Figure 19.7), an MEG signal in the left inferior frontal gyrus (IFG; orange bar) was followed by a signal in the left primary motor cortex (M1; yellow bar) by 100 ms. Again, 100 ms later, when the subject saw her own extending hand, activation was seen in the visual cortex (green bar). This sequence of activation was different during observation of the other person's actions (middle histogram): The activation now began in the visual cortex (as a response to the seen experimenter's moving hand), then progressed to the left inferior frontal gyrus (IFG) and left M1. In both cases, the final activation occurred in the right M1.

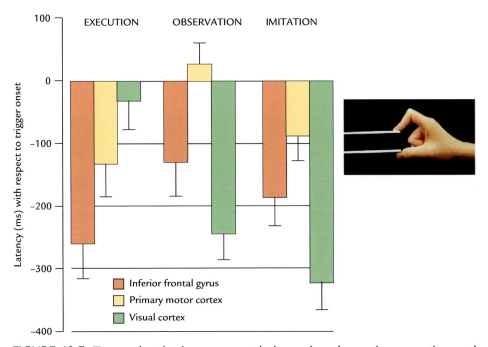

FIGURE 19.7. Temporal activation sequence during action observation, execution, and imitation. Mean (± SEM) peak latencies across seven subjects for MEG responses during execution, observation, and imitation of hand actions (stretching the hand to reach a manipulandum and then pinching it; see insert). Response latencies are shown for the inferior frontal gyrus, primary motor cortex, and visual cortex with respect to trigger onset, that is, the time when the subject either herself touched the manipulandum (during EXECUTION) or the experimenter himself touched the tip of his own manipulandum (OBSERVATION, IMITATION). In this study, the trigger for signal averaging was released when the experimenter touched a manipulandum. Adapted and reprinted from Nishitani N, Hari R: Temporal dynamics of cortical representation for action. *Proc Natl Acad Sci U S A* 2000, 97: 913–918. ©2000 National Academy of Sciences, USA.

Consistent cortical activation sequences have been also elicited by still pictures of facial gestures that the subjects had to imitate (Nishitani & Hari, 2002). The earliest activation was in the posterior visual cortex, followed within 350 ms by activation of the superior temporal sulcus, the inferior parietal cortex, the inferior frontal cortex, and finally the primary motor cortex. In a group of adult subjects with Asperger's syndrome, the latency at the inferior frontal cortex was delayed by about 50 ms, despite similar latencies *at earlier* stages of the neural response (Nishitani et al., 2004).

These results emphasize the large similarity (or overlap) of activations related to one's own and observed actions. It is then feasible to ask why healthy subjects do not automatically imitate other person's actions—a question that was studied in the experiments illustrated in Figure 19.8 (Hari et al., 2014). The subject (left panel) was viewing transient hand pinches made by the experimenter against a manipulandum (middle panels). The subject maintained a pinch against a similar manipulandum so that any movements could be detected, and the outflow from his motor cortex to the muscles was monitored by means of cortex–muscle coherence (cf. also Figures 17.4 and 17.5).

In agreement with previous studies, the experimenter's actions activated the viewer's primary motor cortex, phasically suppressing the 7- to 18-Hz MEG power in the motor cortex (right panel; sources at top and the time–frequency MEG power map in the middle). The right lowest panel, however, shows that, at the same time, the cortex–muscle coherence *increased* at slightly different frequencies (16–20 Hz). Because mu-rhythm power (and amplitude) and the level of cortex–muscle coherence typically covary, the opposite behavior

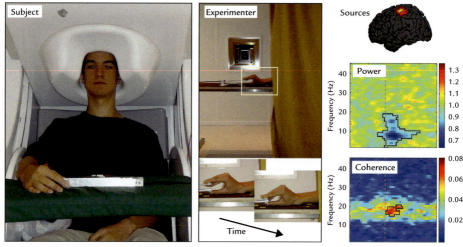

FIGURE 19.8. **Inhibition of unintentional imitation.** Left: Experimental setup. Subject is keeping a steady isometric contraction against a manipulandum containing force transducers while his brain activity is recorded with whole-scalp MEG. Middle: The experimenter, whose hand is visible to the subject, performs phasic pinches once every 3 to 6 s against a manipulandum. Right: Top panel shows group-level (N = 9) source map, implicating activation of the sensorimotor cortex. Middle panel represents a time–frequency plot of relative MEG power. Bottom panel displays a coherence map for the same time interval. Adapted and reprinted with permission from Hari R, Bourguignon M, Piitulainen H, Smeds E, De Tiège X, Jousmäki V: Human primary motor cortex is both activated and stabilized during observation of other person's phasic motor actions. *Philos Trans R Soc Lond B Biol Sci* 2014, 369: 20130171.

of these two measures in this case implies that whereas at least a part of the motor cortex was activated by the observed movement, another neuronal population in the motor cortex stabilized the cortex and likely prevented motor commands from passing from the cortex to the muscles.

These examples show *unidirectional* activation sequences from visual cortex in the occipital lobe to the motor areas in the Rolandic cortex; the sequence progresses via the STS, inferior parietal lobe, and inferior frontal cortex. On the basis of anatomical and functional monkey data, the connections between brain areas should, as a rule, be reciprocal and hierarchical (Friston, 2002), but due to the temporal overlap of such neural traffic in two directions it was not captured with the previous MEG recordings. Reciprocal connections are prerequisites of predictive-coding circuits (see Chapter 18), so that each processing stage of the action-observation system could generate predictions of the outcomes of the lower stages and thereby minimize prediction errors. We note that among all interactions that humans have with their environment, social encounters are the most complex and the most unpredictable ones, requiring constant adjustments of priors and predictions.

■ HYPERSCANNING

When we progress toward real-life interactional set-ups (corresponding to the lower right panel in Figure 19.1), we may consider "hyperscanning," or measuring brain signals simultaneously from two (or more) subjects. The term *hyperscanning* was first used to describe the yoking of two MRI scanners via an Internet connection to study behavior and brain activation in subjects playing an interactive game consisting of a deception task (Montague et al., 2002). However, since the game was not time-sensitive, the setup was more a proof of principle of the technical feasibility of hyperscanning than an absolutely necessary procedure for the study in question (see previous arguments in Figure 19.1 and the related text). Since then, hyperscanning has expanded by linking together two or multiple EEG devices or two MEG systems either in one laboratory or in two different locations, associated with an audio and video link either directly or via the Internet (Babiloni et al., 2006; Astolfi et al., 2010; Baess et al., 2012; Hirata et al., 2014; Zhdanov et al., 2015). Such links have to be made temporally accurate, which is relatively easy within the same laboratory space but may involve time-lags of the order of 100 to 150 ms if video must be transmitted via the Internet between two locations. In recent EEG hyperscanning setups, multiple subjects have been connected to a modular (high-density) EEG system, which has simplified synchronization between recordings of different individuals (e.g., Barraza et al., 2019). Interesting hyperscanning experiments are possible also with near-infrared spectroscopy (NIRS), and up to nine persons have been studied simultaneously in a NIRS "teamwork" hyperscanning study (Liu et al., 2021).

Interestingly, many decades ago two people were already connected to the same EEG system to study "extrasensory electroencephalographic induction" in identical twins and unrelated subjects. Subjects sat in separate rooms and modulation of their alpha rhythms were examined to verbal commands such as eye opening and closure (Duane & Behrendt, 1965). Technically speaking, this was the first-ever hyperscanning study. However, despite being published in a very prominent journal, the results were not properly controlled or replicated and thus made a negligible contribution to the scientific literature.

Figure 19.9 presents a 2PN MEG setup, where the MEG and other biological signals, including recordings of speech sounds, as well as all necessary triggers, are saved locally on files with accurate time stamps. As the audio signal in this older study was transmitted via the normal phone line ("landline"), the lags are minimal, corresponding to lags between

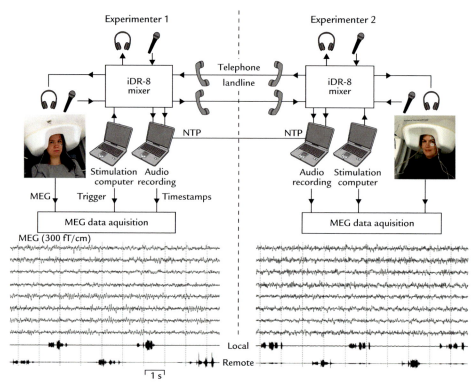

FIGURE 19.9. Hyperscanning setup for linking two MEG systems with one another. A schematic depicting the linking of two MEG systems located 5 km apart (left and right sides of the image). Subjects communicate via landline phone lines during MEG measurements. MEG and speech data, accurately time-locked with respect to each other, are saved locally at each site. A 10-s example of ongoing MEG is shown from both systems (from four temporal-lobe and four occipital-lobe gradiometers), with filter passband of 0.1 to 40 Hz. The lowest traces show audio recordings of speech while the subjects count numbers in alternation. Adapted and reprinted with permission from Baess P, Zhdanov A, Mandel A, Parkkonen L, Hirvenkari L, Mäkelä JP, Jousmäki V, Hari R: MEG dual scanning: a procedure to study real-time auditory interaction between two persons. *Front Hum Neurosci* 2012, 6: 83.

two people conversing in the same room at a distance of about 4 m. This kind of setting has been used for simultaneous recordings from dyads when one person was located far away from the other (e.g., in Espoo, Finland, and in Brussels, Belgium).

MEG/EEG hyperscanning studies have included tasks such as the prisoner's dilemma (Babiloni et al., 2006), a card game (played between four individuals) (Astolfi et al., 2010), playing music together (Lindenberger et al., 2009), initiating and imitating of movements (Dumas et al., 2010; Konvalinka et al., 2010; Zhou et al., 2016), verbal and nonverbal interaction between children and their caregivers (Hirata et al., 2014; Nguyen et al., 2020), social attention (Lachat et al., 2012), conversation (Mandel et al., 2016), and learning in educational settings (Bevilacqua et al., 2019). In general, any task requiring simultaneous actions (such as joint tasks or mutual adjustments during music playing) or rapid turn-taking (such as conversation) could be used in a hyperscanning setup. Whether that is the best option for data collection has to be carefully considered because hyperscanning setups tend to be much more time consuming and technically challenging for experimenters (for advice for implementing an EEG hyperscanning setup, see Barraza et al., 2019). A Python-based open-source code-processing pipeline is available for assessing interbrain connectivity between participants in MEG/EEG hyperscanning studies (Ayrolles et al., 2021).

We sound a word of caution for data interpretation for *any* MEG/EEG hyperscanning experiment. Some studies have concluded that certain brain rhythms (such as alpha or mu) of the two participants become synchronized during the interaction, so that they are sometimes "in phase" and at other times "out of phase." Here we would use astronomer Carl Sagan's "ECREE" principle saying that "extraordinary claims require extraordinary evidence." We consider this kind of synchronization between brain rhythms unlikely for a number of reasons. First, even in a single individual, brain rhythms have multiple sources with contributions that vary as a function of time. Second, the dominant brain rhythm frequencies in two individuals very likely differ, and third, free-running sinusoids of close frequencies synchronize at regular intervals determined by their frequency difference, so that, for example, sinusoids of 11 Hz and 12 Hz "beat" at 1 Hz. It is more likely to see interindividual synchronization in the envelopes of signal amplitudes or power than in the relative phases of certain brain rhythms.

There are also problematic claims regarding information flow during hyperscanning experiments. If subjects view the same movie (without interacting), then similar temporal behaviors in their brain signals do not reflect information flow *between* the two brains. Specifically, the confound of the externally driven activity in subjects facing similar conditions has to always be seriously considered.

Others have previously noted issues in analysis and interpretation that lead to spurious data and misinterpreted "hyperconnections" (see, e.g., Burgess, 2013; Holroyd, 2022). This shaky ground likely resulted from the lack of solid theory underlying most hyperscanning studies. Fortunately, conceptual frameworks emphasizing the centrality of social interaction for human brain function in terms of both "two-person neuroscience" (Hari & Kujala, 2009; Hari et al., 2015) and "second-person neuroscience" (Schilbach et al., 2013) are emerging. Moreover, theories are being developed regarding verbal communication (Kelsen et al., 2022) and how comforting touch affects tactile perception, shared distress, emotion regulation, and reward (Shamay-Tsoory & Eisenberger, 2021). So, it seems as though the hyperscanning field is indeed poised to start to set the theoretical contexts for future studies.

▪ VERBAL COMMUNICATION

Speech, a uniquely human means of communication, has attracted a large interest in neurophysiological and neuroimaging research. Until now, most language- and speech-related neuroimaging research has focused on either speech perception or speech production in *single individuals*, often studied with isolated fragments of language, and interactive studies with dialogues and turn-takings are rare.

On the perception side, speech sounds elicit very similar 100- to 200-ms onset and offset responses, as do any other sounds with similar acoustic features (see Chapter 13). Only later, at around 400 to 600 ms, do the responses start to depend on word meaning (see Chapter 18). On the basis of both EEG and MEG evoked-response latencies, the voice is recognized as voice by 170 ms, which is comparable to the latency of the face-sensitive N170, marking the time when a face is recognized as a face (Charest et al., 2009; Capilla et al., 2013).

One's own utterances also evoke responses in the supratemporal auditory cortex (Numminen et al., 1999), but these are dampened and delayed compared with responses to the same sounds replayed from tape. The likely reason, with acoustic dampening not able to account for the effect, is an internal control system that is necessary for automatic monitoring of the pitch, intensity, and phonemic quality of the speech. More convincing evidence of such an internal feed-forward ("efference copy") mechanism was obtained from a recording where subjects were asked to utter two vowels, a frequent /a/ (about 80% of the utterances) and rare /ae/ (about 20% of the utterances). When the sounds were recorded and played back to the subject, both of them elicited a 100-ms vertex response (N100m), and the rare sounds additionally elicited a clear mismatch field (MMF). In the recordings carried out *during* the utterances, transient 100-ms responses (now delayed by about 10 ms) were also elicited in auditory cortex, but the MMFs were absent (Curio et al., 2000). This result can be considered an indication of a prediction signal (efference copy) sent to the auditory cortex at the time of the utterance.

Speech elements typically comprise nonperiodic sounds of 2 to 10 kHz and periodic sounds of 50 to 500 Hz; the whole speech signal is amplitude-modulated at 2 to 50 Hz (Rosen, 1992). Thus the "temporal envelope" of speech overlaps with typical MEG/EEG frequencies, and, consequently, the MEG and EEG signals can be entrained by phase-locking to the speech envelope in the theta range (Peelle & Davis, 2012) or even in the delta range (Bourguignon et al., 2013; Gross et al., 2013; Doelling et al., 2014). Such a slow temporal envelope also carries prosody-related information. In human intracranial EEG recordings from Heschl's gyrus, gamma activity with spectral content up to 250 Hz actually tracks the speech envelope (Nourski et al., 2009; Kubanek et al., 2013).

One may criticize the ecological validity of studies that use language material in isolation, for example presenting single words to be memorized or learned. After all, children learn language in context and not as isolated utterances or words; moreover, the learning occurs during social interaction with other speakers. Thus some laboratories are already studying children's word learning in this context (Chen et al., 2021). The studies of brain activity during dialogues will likely be more prevalent in the future, it is hoped inspired by the idea that "humans are designed for dialogue rather than monologue" (Garrod & Pickering, 2004). Although the normal preparation time for one's own speaking is a few hundred milliseconds, during conversation the turn-takings occur extremely quickly, with lags of about 250 ms in all languages (Stivers et al., 2009), which means that the speakers cannot just react to the ends of each other's turns—rather they must multitask and prepare the content for their own turn while still listening to the other's voice. The preparation also involves prediction of the forthcoming speech. Importantly, conversation primes the participants so that the speakers do not need to start planning the next turn from scratch (Levinson, 2016), which considerably alleviates the burden of multitasking. The participants of a conversation are building together a sensible thread, and thus their interaction is like a joint task aiming at a common goal.

One benefit of studying conversation in hyperscanning settings is that subjects' behavior can be accurately monitored by recording the acoustic signals of the verbal utterances. One example is an MEG study that looked at how the speaker's versus listener's role would affect sensorimotor rhythms (Mandel et al., 2016). Unfortunately, the challenging analysis problem is the temporal overlap of the multiple processes that we mentioned above: the external speech stimulus itself, the reactions to the content of the partner's speech, anticipation of the partner's next utterance, and preparation for one's own turn to speak.

Very recently a literature has developed related to the perception and production of natural, continuous (connected) speech instead of isolated syllables, words, and phrases.

For example, when subjects attentively listened to a 1-hr audiobook, analysis of their MEG signals displayed signatures of word sequence predictability, with a main effect at multiple frequencies but peaking around 400 ms after word onsets. Before the main analysis, the effects of the acoustic waveform of the voice, as well as the frequency effects of each word, were removed from the MEG signals. Then the remaining signals were examined from the point of view of contextual word probabilities (local word probabilities in the context of neighboring words) obtained from a large text corpus (Koskinen et al., 2020). Thus, one important feature of this study was to introduce additional information into the analysis that aided the interpretation of the MEG results. A similar use of supplementary information might benefit the analysis of other complex signals related to social cognition and interaction.

■ REFERENCES

Adolphs R, Nummenmaa L, Todorov A, Haxby JV: Data-driven approaches in the investigation of social perception. *Philos Trans R Soc Lond B Biol Sci* 2016, 371: 20150367.

Astolfi L, Toppi J, De Vico Fallani F, Vecchiato G, Salinari S, Mattia D, Cincotti F, Babiloni F: Neuroelectrical hyperscanning measures simultaneous brain activity in humans. *Brain Topogr* 2010, 23: 243–256.

Ayrolles A, Brun F, Chen P, Djalovski A, Beauxis Y, Delorme R, Bourgeron T, Dikker S, Dumas G: HyPyP: a hyperscanning Python Pipeline for inter-brain connectivity analysis. *Soc Cogn Affect Neurosci* 2021, 16: 72–83.

Babiloni F, Cincotti F, Mattia D, Mattiocco M, De Vico Fallani F, Tocci A, Bianchi L, Marciani MG, Astolfi L: Hypermethods for EEG hyperscanning. *Conf Proc IEEE Eng Med Biol Soc* 2006, 1: 3666–3669.

Babo-Rebelo M, Puce A, Bullock D, Hugueville L, Pestilli F, Adam C, Lehongre K, Lambrecq V, Dinkelacker V, George N: Visual information routes in the posterior dorsal and ventral face network studied with intracranial neurophysiology and white matter tract endpoints. *Cereb Cortex* 2022, 32: 342–366.

Baess P, Zhdanov A, Mandel A, Parkkonen L, Hirvenkari L, Mäkelä JP, Jousmäki V, Hari R: MEG dual scanning: a procedure to study real-time auditory interaction between two persons. *Front Hum Neurosci* 2012, 6: 83.

Barraza P, Dumas G, Liu H, Blanco-Gomez G, van den Heuvel MI, Baart M, Pérez A: Implementing EEG hyperscanning setups. *MethodsX* 2019, 6: 428–436.

Bertenthal BI, Puce A: A look toward the future of social attention research. In: Puce A, Bertenthal BI, eds. *The Many Faces of Social Attention: Behavioral and Neural Measures.* London: Springer International, 2015: 221–245.

Bevilacqua D, Davidesco I, Wan L, Chaloner K, Rowland J, Ding M, Poeppel D, Dikker S: Brain-to-brain synchrony and learning outcomes vary by student-teacher dynamics: evidence from a real-world classroom electroencephalography study. *J Cogn Neurosci* 2019, 31: 401–411.

Bourguignon M, De Tiège X, Op de Beeck M, Ligot N, Paquier P, Van Bogaert P, Goldman S, Hari R, Jousmäki V: The pace of prosodic phrasing couples the reader's voice to the listener's cortex. *Hum Brain Mapp* 2013, 34: 314–326.

Brefczynski-Lewis JA, Berrebi ME, McNeely ME, Prostko AL, Puce A: In the blink of an eye: neural responses elicited to viewing the eye blinks of another individual. *Front Hum Neurosci* 2011, 5: 68.

Burgess AP: On the interpretation of synchronization in EEG hyperscanning studies: a cautionary note. *Front Hum Neurosci* 2013, 7: 881.

Caetano G, Jousmäki V, Hari R: Actor's and observer's primary motor cortices stabilize similarly after seen or heard motor actions. *Proc Natl Acad Sci U S A* 2007, 104: 9058–9062.

Capilla A, Belin P, Gross J: The early spatio-temporal correlates and task independence of cerebral voice processing studied with MEG. *Cereb Cortex* 2013, 23: 1388–1395.

Charest I, Pernet CR, Rousselet GA, Quinones I, Latinus M, Fillion-Bilodeau S, Chartrand JP, Belin P: Electrophysiological evidence for an early processing of human voices. *BMC Neurosci* 2009, 10: 127.

Chen C, Houston DM, Yu C: Parent–child joint behaviors in novel object play create high-quality data for word learning. *Child Development* 2021, 92: 1889–1905.

Curio G, Neuloh G, Numminen J, Jousmäki V, Hari R: Speaking modifies voice-evoked activity in the human auditory cortex. *Hum Brain Mapp* 2000, 9: 183–191.

daSilva EB, Crager K, Geisler D, Newbern P, Orem B, Puce A: Something to sink your teeth into: the presence of teeth augments ERPs to mouth expressions. *NeuroImage* 2016a, 127: 227–241.

daSilva EB, Crager K, Puce A: On dissociating the neural time course of the processing of positive emotions. *Neuropsychologia* 2016b, 83: 123–137.

de Gelder B: Towards the neurobiology of emotional body language. *Nat Rev Neurosci* 2006, 7: 242–249.

de Gelder B, Poyo Solanas M: A computational neuroethology perspective on body and expression perception. *Trends Cogn Sci* 2021, 25: 744–756.

Doelling KB, Arnal LH, Ghitza O, Poeppel D: Acoustic landmarks drive delta-theta oscillations to enable speech comprehension by facilitating perceptual parsing. *NeuroImage* 2014, 85 Pt 2: 761–768.

Duane TD, Behrendt T: Extrasensory electroencephalographic induction between identical twins. *Science* 1965, 150: 367.

Dumas G, Nadel J, Soussignan R, Martinerie J, Garnero L: Inter-brain synchronization during social interaction. *PLoS One* 2010, 5: e12166.

Dumas G, Lachat F, Martinerie J, Nadel J, George N: From social behaviour to brain synchronization: review and perspectives in hyperscanning. *IRBM* 2011, 32: 48–53.

Friston K: Beyond phrenology: what can neuroimaging tell us about distributed circuitry? *Annu Rev Neurosci* 2002, 25: 221–250.

Friston K, Frith C: A duet for one. *Consc Cogn* 2015, 35: 390–405.

Garrod S, Pickering MJ: Why is conversation so easy? *Trends Cogn Sci* 2004, 8: 8–11.

Gastaut H, Bert J: EEG changes during cinematographic presentation. *Electroencephalogr Clin Neurophysiol* 1954, 6: 433–444.

Gross J, Hoogenboom N, Thut G, Schyns P, Panzeri S, Belin P, Garrod S: Speech rhythms and multiplexed oscillatory sensory coding in the human brain. *PLoS Biol* 2013, 11: e1001752.

Hari R, Salmelin R: Human cortical oscillations: a neuromagnetic view through the skull. *Trends Neurosci* 1997, 20: 44–49.

Hari R, Forss N, Avikainen S, Kirveskari E, Salenius S, Rizzolatti G: Activation of human primary motor cortex during action observation: a neuromagnetic study. *Proc Natl Acad Sci U S A* 1998, 95: 15061–15065.

Hari R, Kujala MV: Brain basis of human social interaction: from concepts to brain imaging. *Physiol Rev* 2009, 89: 453–479.

Hari R, Bourguignon M, Piitulainen H, Smeds E, De Tiège X, Jousmäki V: Human primary motor cortex is both activated and stabilized during observation of other person's phasic motor actions. *Philos Trans R Soc Lond B Biol Sci* 2014, 369: 20130171.

Hari R: Magnetoencephalography studies of action observation. In: Ferrari PF, Rizzolatti G, eds. *New Frontiers in Mirror Neurons Research*. Oxford: Oxford University Press, 2015: 58–70.

Hari R, Henriksson L, Malinen S, Parkkonen L: Centrality of social interaction in human brain function. *Neuron* 2015, 88: 181–193.

Hari R, Sams M, Nummenmaa L: Attending to and neglecting people: bridging neuroscience, psychology and sociology. *Phil Trans Royal Soc B* 2016, 371: 1–9.

Hinojosa JA, Mercado F, Carretie L: N170 sensitivity to facial expression: a meta-analysis. *Neurosci Biobehav Rev* 2015, 55: 498–509.

Hirata M, Ikeda T, Kikuchi M, Kimura T, Hiraishi H, Yoshimura Y, Asada M: Hyperscanning MEG for understanding mother–child cerebral interactions. *Front Hum Neurosci* 2014, 8: 118.

Holroyd CB: Interbrain synchrony: on wavy ground. *Trends Neurosci* 2022, 45: 346–357.

Jonas J, Jacques C, Liu-Shuang J, Brissart H, Colnat-Coulbois S, Maillard L, Rossion B: A face-selective ventral occipito-temporal map of the human brain with intracerebral potentials. *Proc Natl Acad Sci U S A* 2016, 113: E4088–E4097.

Kelsen BA, Sumich A, Kasabov N, Liang SHY, Wang GY: What has social neuroscience learned from hyperscanning studies of spoken communication? A systematic review. *Neurosci Biobehav Rev* 2022, 132: 1249–1262.

Konvalinka I, Vuust P, Roepstorff A, Frith CD: Follow you, follow me: continuous mutual prediction and adaptation in joint tapping. *Q J Exp Psychol* 2010, 63: 2220–2230.

Koskinen M, Kurimo M, Gross J, Hyvärinen A, Hari R: Brain activity reflects the predictability of word sequences in listened continuous speech. *NeuroImage* 2020, 219: 116936.

Kubanek J, Brunner P, Gunduz A, Poeppel D, Schalk G: The tracking of speech envelope in the human cortex. *PLoS One* 2013, 8: e53398.

Lachat F, Hugueville L, Lemarechal JD, Conty L, George N: Oscillatory brain correlates of live joint attention: a dual-EEG study. *Front Hum Neurosci* 2012, 6: 156.

Lankinen K, Saari J, Hari R, Koskinen M: Intersubject consistency of cortical MEG signals during movie viewing. *NeuroImage* 2014, 92: 217–224.

Latinus M, Love SA, Rossi A, Parada FJ, Huang L, Conty L, George N, James K, Puce A: Social decisions affect neural activity to perceived dynamic gaze. *Soc Cogn Affect Neurosci* 2015, 10: 1557–1567.

Levinson SC: Turn-taking in human communication – Origins and implications for language processing. *Trends Cogn Sci* 2016, 20: 6–14.

Lindenberger U, Li SC, Gruber W, Müller V: Brains swinging in concert: cortical phase synchronization while playing guitar. *BMC Neurosci* 2009, 10: 22.

Liu T, Duan L, Dai R, Pelowski M, Zhu C: Team-work, Team-brain: exploring synchrony and team interdependence in a nine-person drumming task via multiparticipant hyperscanning and inter-brain network topology with fNIRS. *NeuroImage* 2021, 237: 118147.

Mandel A, Helokunnas S, Pihko E, Hari R: Neuromagnetic brain responses to other person's eye blinks seen on video. *Eur J Neurosci* 2014, 40: 2576–2580.

Mandel A, Helokunnas S, Pihko E, Hari R: Brain responds to another person's eye blinks in a natural setting—the more empathetic the viewer the stronger the responses. *Eur J Neurosci* 2015, 42: 2508–2514.

Mandel A, Bourguignon M, Parkkonen L, Hari R: Sensorimotor activation related to speaker vs. listener role during natural conversation. *Neurosci Lett* 2016, 614: 99–104.

Montague PR, Berns GS, Cohen JD, McClure SM, Pagnoni G, Dhamala M, Wiest MC, Karpov I, King RD, Apple N, Fisher RE: Hyperscanning: simultaneous fMRI during linked social interactions. *NeuroImage* 2002, 16: 1159–1164.

Nasiopoulos E, Risko EF, Kingstone A: Social attention, social presence, and the dual function of gaze. In: Puce A, Bertenthal BI, eds. *The Many Faces of Social Attention: Behavioral and Neural Measures.* London: Springer International, 2015: 221–245.

Nguyen T, Bánki A, Markova G, Hoehl S: Studying parent–child interaction with hyperscanning. *Prog Brain Res* 2020, 254: 1–24.

Nishitani N, Hari R: Temporal dynamics of cortical representation for action. *Proc Natl Acad Sci U S A* 2000, 97: 913–918.

Nishitani N, Hari R: Viewing lip forms: cortical dynamics. *Neuron* 2002, 36: 1211–1220.

Nishitani N, Avikainen S, Hari R: Abnormal imitation-related cortical activation sequences in Asperger's syndrome. *Ann Neurol* 2004, 55: 558–562.

Nourski KV, Reale RA, Oya H, Kawasaki H, Kovach CK, Chen H, Howard MA 3rd, Brugge JF: Temporal envelope of time-compressed speech represented in the human auditory cortex. *J Neurosci* 2009, 29: 15564–15574.

Numminen J, Salmelin R, Hari R: Subject's own speech reduces reactivity of the human auditory cortex. *Neurosci Lett* 1999, 265: 119–122.

Peelle JE, Davis MH: Neural oscillations carry speech rhythm through to comprehension. *Front Psychol* 2012, 3: 320.

Peräkylä A, Ruusuvuori J: Facial expression in an assessment. In: Knoblauch H, Schnettler B, Raab J, Soeffner H-G, eds. *Video-Analysis, Methodology and Methods: Qualitative Audiovisual Data Analysis in Sociology.* Frankfurt-am-Main: Peter Lang, 2006: 127–142.

Pitcher D, Dilks DD, Saxe RR, Triantafyllou C, Kanwisher N: Differential selectivity for dynamic versus static information in face-selective cortical regions. *NeuroImage* 2011, 56: 2356–2363.

Pitcher D, Ungerleider LG: Evidence for a third visual pathway specialized for social perception. *Trends Cogn Sci* 2021, 25: 100–110.

Ponkanen LM, Alhoniemi A, Leppänen JM, Hietanen JK: Does it make a difference if I have an eye contact with you or with your picture? An ERP study. *Soc Cogn Affect Neurosci* 2011, 6: 486–494.

Porter S, ten Brinke L: Reading between the lies: identifying concealed and falsified emotions in universal facial expressions. *Psychol Sci* 2008, 19: 508–514.

Puce A, Smith A, Allison T: ERPs evoked by viewing facial movements. *Cogn Neuropsychol* 2000, 17: 221–239.

Puce A: Perception of nonverbal cues. In: Ochsner K, Kosslyn S, eds. *The Oxford Handbook of Cognitive Neuroscience: Vol. 2: The Cutting Edges.* Oxford: Oxford University Press, 2013: 148–164.

Puce A, Latinus M, Rossi A, daSilva EB, Parada FJ, Love SA, Ashourvan A, Jayaraman S: Neural bases for social attention in healthy humans. In: Puce A, Bertenthal BI, eds. *The Many Faces of Social Attention: Behavioral and Neural Measures.* London: Springer International, 2016: 93–127.

Rellecke J, Sommer W, Schacht A: Does processing of emotional facial expressions depend on intention? Time-resolved evidence from event-related brain potentials. *Biol Psychol* 2012, 90: 23–32.

Retter TL, Jiang F, Webster MA, Rossion B: All-or-none face categorization in the human brain. *NeuroImage* 2020, 213: 116685.

Rizzolatti G, Craighero L: The mirror-neuron system. *Annu Rev Neurosci* 2004, 27: 169–192.

Rosen S: Temporal information in speech: acoustic, auditory and linguistic aspects. *Philos Trans R Soc Lond B Biol Sci* 1992, 336: 367–373.

Rossi A, Parada FJ, Kolchinsky A, Puce A: Neural correlates of apparent motion perception of impoverished facial stimuli: a comparison of ERP and ERSP activity. *NeuroImage* 2014, 98: 442–459.

Rossi A, Parada FJ, Latinus M, Puce A: Photographic but not line-drawn faces show early perceptual neural sensitivity to eye gaze direction. *Front Hum Neurosci* 2015, 9: 185.

Rossion B: Understanding face perception by means of human electrophysiology. *Trends Cogn Sci* 2014, 18: 310–318.

Schilbach L, Timmermans B, Reddy V, Costall A, Bente G, Schlicht T, Vogeley K: Toward a second-person neuroscience. *Behav Brain Sci* 2013, 36: 393–414.

Shamay-Tsoory SG, Eisenberger NI: Getting in touch: a neural model of comforting touch. *Neurosci Biobehav Rev* 2021, 130: 263–273.

Stivers T, Enfield NJ, Brown P, Englert C, Hayashi M, Heinemann T, Hoymann G, Rossano F, de Ruiter JP, Yoon K-E, Levinson SC: Universals and cultural variation in turn-taking in conversation. *Proc Nat Acad Sci U S A* 2009, 106: 10587–10592.

Wheaton KJ, Pipingas A, Silberstein RB, Puce A: Human neural responses elicited to observing the actions of others. *Vis Neurosci* 2001, 18: 401–406.

Zhdanov A, Nurminen J, Baess P, Hirvenkari L, Jousmäki V, Mäkelä JP, Mandel A, Meronen L, Hari R, Parkkonen L: An Internet-based real-time audiovisual link for dual MEG recordings. *PLoS One* 2015, 10: e0128485.

Zhou G, Bourguignon M, Parkkonen L, Hari R: Neural signatures of hand kinematics in leaders vs. followers: A dual-MEG study. *NeuroImage* 2016, 125: 731–738.

CHAPTER 20

BRAIN DISORDERS

Medicine is a science of uncertainty and an art of probability.

—WILLIAM OSLER

There is only one difference between a madman and me. The madman thinks he is sane. I know I am mad.

—SALVADOR DALI

■ INTRODUCTION

EEG and evoked potentials have been used in the clinical environment since their inception, and—as we have already mentioned—in-depth textbooks and best-practice guidelines exist relating to clinical applications. Until now, MEG's main clinical role has been in preoperative evaluation of tumor or epilepsy patients, especially in the identification of epileptic foci (see, e.g., Burgess et al., 2011; Hari et al., 2018; Schomer & Lopes da Silva, 2018).

It is important to make a distinction between studies of clinical populations for research purposes and the practice of clinical assessment. In the first type of study, data are typically reported *at a group level*, and the results are compared with a group of healthy individuals. In contrast, in clinical assessment the diagnostic process requires the evaluation, and sometimes monitoring, of *individuals* with a suspected abnormality. Clinically feasible findings in individual patients must not only be reliable but also differ statistically significantly from normative values of a healthy group of individuals with similar attributes, including sex and age. The normative values of healthy subjects will have typically been collected at the test site, using the same equipment and conditions as for the patients. Any test for assessing an individual patient must have high specificity and high sensitivity. Specificity is the true positive rate, that is, the chance of an individual showing a positive test result *and* having the disorder, whereas sensitivity is the true negative rate, meaning that the test is negative and the person has no disorder.

In this chapter we describe some clinical applications of MEG/EEG where patients can be assessed on an individual basis. An in-depth discussion of EEG's well-established clinical uses is available (Schomer & Lopes da Silva, 2018), and we recommend it highly to any clinically oriented EEG (or MEG) user.

■ EPILEPSY

An "epileptic seizure" is a paroxysmal alteration of brain function caused by excessive hypersynchronous discharge of neurons. This abnormal brain activity commonly causes visible convulsions (i.e., muscle contractions and jerks that can also be associated with speech arrest and loss of consciousness). The term *epilepsy* refers to a group of conditions that produce recurrent, typically unprovoked, seizures, although some seizure disorders can have certain triggers. About 0.6% of the general population suffers from some type of recurring seizure (GBD 2016 Epilepsy Collaborators, 2019), the most common of which are the febrile convulsions of childhood, occurring in about 2–4% of children in Europe and the USA and in 1–14% of children in the rest of the world (Hauser, 1994). Fortunately, febrile convulsions are benign in the majority of cases, meaning they do not recur or produce further health problems. However, 25% of these children do go on to have recurrent seizures (Fine & Wirrell, 2020).

Epilepsies are identified using an international classification system (for the latest revision, see Scheffer et al., 2017; and recent update for neonates, see Pressler et al., 2021), which involves three hierarchical tiers divided according to seizure type, epilepsy type, and syndrome type. Broadly speaking, these guidelines classify epilepsy in terms of *both* seizure semiology and onset of associated neurophysiological activity. Generalized seizures engage bilaterally distributed brain networks, whereas focal seizures begin in a limited brain area and thereafter may, or may not, spread and generalize to involve other brain regions or the whole brain. However, the borders between these classes are not rigid, and sometimes the onset type is unknown. The classical generalized tonic–clonic (previously known as grand mal) seizures start with tonic muscle contractions that then become clonic, and the seizures are associated with full loss of consciousness. Absence seizures (previously known as petit mal) also belong to the group of generalized seizures. They do not include convulsions but rather consist of short (10–15 s) lapses of awareness during which the individual loses contact with the environment; the eyes may roll upward with rhythmic eyelid movements. Other types of generalized seizure include myoclonic seizures that manifest as uncontrollable muscle jerking involving one or more limb or the body and atonic seizures that produce a complete loss of muscle tone, whereby the individual may fall to the ground and injure themselves (previously known as drop attacks). That all said, patients may have more than one seizure type, making definitive diagnosis without a detailed clinical investigation challenging. Fortunately, different seizure types can have different EEG/MEG signatures.

Figure 20.1 shows a clinical EEG recording from a 51-year-old woman who has had seizures for many years and recently began to have absences. This ambulatory EEG recording displays two generalized 3-Hz "spike-and-wave" discharges of 1 to 2 s duration. The discharges—typical for absence seizures—arise from an essentially normal EEG background where alpha rhythm over the posterior scalp waxes and wanes.

In focal seizures, discharges confined to a brain region may give rise to diverse and often complex behavioral manifestations, such as cognitive and/or motor aberrations or automatisms, or loss of consciousness during which the individual may not react to the external environment. These seizures can last for two to three minutes. Some focal seizures are drug-resistant and are treated surgically after a thorough presurgical assessment, sometimes involving continuous long-term intracranial EEG (ECoG and SEEG) recordings with associated video in a specialized monitoring room often sited in a neurosurgical intensive care unit.

EEG and MEG remain, due to their excellent temporal resolution, the methods *par excellence* for diagnosing and identifying epileptic syndromes. Some epileptic abnormalities

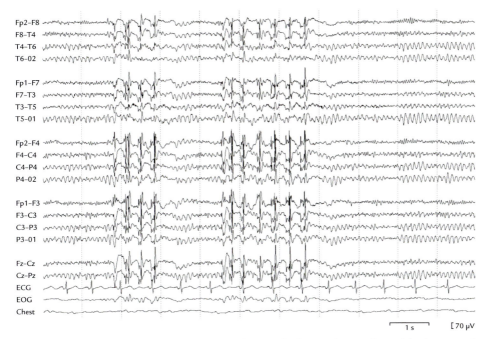

Fp2–F8
F8–T4
T4–T6
T6–02

Fp1–F7
F7–T3
T3–T5
T5–01

Fp2–F4
F4–C4
C4–P4
P4–02

Fp1–F3
F3–C3
C3–P3
P3–01

Fz–Cz
Cz–Pz
ECG
EOG
Chest

1 s   [70 µV

FIGURE 20.1. An example of 3-Hz spike-and-wave discharges in a patient with absence seizures. A double-banana EEG montage (see Figure 5.11) with 18 EEG channels shows spontaneous activity over an 11.5-s period, with regular rhythmic posterior alpha and frontal
oscillatory beta (due to benzodiazepine medication; see Chapter 11). This background activity is interrupted twice, for 1 to 2 s, with high-amplitude 3-Hz spike-and-wave discharges.
The bottom three traces depict ECG, EOG, and respiration (Chest). Note that the discharges
are seen to some extent also on the EOG channel, so that simultaneous eyeball or eyelid
movements cannot be discerned from this recording. Figure provided by Dr. Erika Kirveskari,
Department of Clinical Neurophysiology, Helsinki University Hospital, Finland.

can be seen in the MEG/EEG both interictally (between seizures) and ictally (during seizures). Note, however, that although ictal activity (especially seizure onset) typically has
accurate localizing value, interictal abnormalities can occur at the seizure focus or in other
regions, particularly when patients are withdrawn off their medications to elicit spontaneous seizures during monitoring.

The term *epileptic focus* refers to the cortical generator of epileptic discharges.
Sometimes, an epileptic focus, due to its frequent firing, can produce a "mirror focus" in a
homologous area in the other hemisphere. Figure 20.2 shows such a mirror focus in the left
hemisphere of an 18-year-old woman; the focus was driven by the primary focus in the right
hemisphere. Careful examination of the timing of the single traces from both hemispheres
indicated a transfer time of 17 to 20 ms from the primary focus in the right hemisphere
to the mirror focus on the left (Hari et al., 1993). The timing difference is a critical distinction between a primary and mirror focus and will directly affect any surgical resection
plan. Generalized seizure disorders, as their name suggests, produce generalized discharges
appearing at (about) the same time throughout the cortex.

Epileptic discharges can be provoked or exacerbated during a routine clinical EEG/
MEG recording by a number of activation procedures, including photic stimulation,

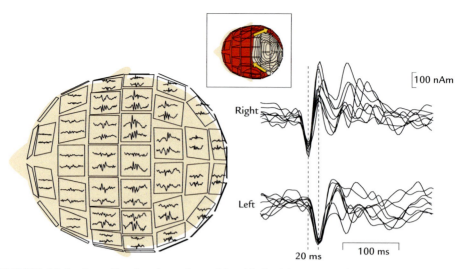

FIGURE 20.2. An epileptic mirror focus identified with MEG. Left: A 300-ms epoch of spontaneous MEG shown on a 122-channel array of planar gradiometers; in this view of the sensor helmet (with the eyes facing left), only about half of the signals are visible. The traces on each unit are from orthogonal gradiometers. An epileptic spike (or multispike) is largest in centroparietal sensors over both hemispheres. Inset at top: Field pattern during a single spike, with the red shading indicating flux leaving the head and the tan area showing flux entering the head. The isocontours depict steps of 400 fT/cm. Two equivalent current dipoles (yellow arrows), with opposite current directions in the right and the left hemispheres, can account for the observed field pattern. Right: Dipole moments as a function of time for eight single spikes for which the field pattern agrees with sources in the right and left parietal cortex (see the insert). Note the 20-ms time difference (broken vertical lines) between the hemispheres so that the right hemisphere leads the left. Adapted and reprinted from Hari R, Ahonen A, Forss N, Granström M-L, Hämäläinen M, Kajola M, Knuutila J, Mäkelä JP, Paetau R, Salmelin R, Simola J: Parietal epileptic mirror focus detected with a whole-head neuromagnetometer. *Neuroreport* 1993, 5: 45–48. With permission from Wolters Kluwer Health, Inc.

hyperventilation, or sleep deprivation, and sometimes pharmacological activation. Photic stimulation with a stroboscope typically uses a range of frequencies from 1 to 25 Hz, and it can provoke epileptiform discharges in light-sensitive individuals. Hyperventilation for a couple of minutes causes alkalosis (and, when sufficient, dizziness and paresthesia in the arms) and can also facilitate the appearance of epileptiform abnormalities in the EEG/MEG.

Status epilepticus (SE) is a potentially fatal state of continuous or repetitive seizures. In the United States, about 40,000 individuals die annually from SE, making it the most common neurological emergency (Stafstrom & Carmant, 2015). SE indicates a serious breakdown of the brain's natural inhibitory mechanisms. If SE progresses for a prolonged period, the visible convulsion in the patient can be suppressed, but SE is still typically recognizable from the ongoing seizure activity in the ambulatory EEG.

■ PREOPERATIVE MAPPING

MEG and EEG are particularly well suited for preoperative mapping that aims to ascertain the functional neuroanatomy of brain regions lying in the vicinity of the brain tissue to be removed due to a tumor, vascular abnormality, or epileptogenic cortex. To this end, invasive EEG recordings and direct electrical brain stimulation can be performed over several days using chronically implanted electrodes while the patient is being long-term EEG–video monitored in the hospital, or acutely during surgery with testing being performed in an awake patient. Depending on where the tissue to be resected is located, preoperative functional localization may include identification of the sensory and motor cortices posterior and anterior to the central sulcus (CS), mapping of language-sensitive areas, as well as visual (and face-sensitive) cortices. Such preoperative functional mapping may include scalp EEG, MEG, fMRI, NIRS, and TMS studies, as well as invasive EEG recordings.

Functional Identification of the Central Sulcus

Figure 20.3 shows an example of preoperative MEG mapping in a patient who had a large brain tumor in the region immediately posterior to the right CS. On the left image in the figure, the blue and red dots refer to the location of primary somatosensory cortex (SI) identified by means of electric stimulation of the foot (tibial nerve, red dot) and hand (median nerve, blue dot; for somatosensory responses, see Chapter 15). The yellow and green dots denote the location of precentral primary motor cortex (MI), identified by means of cortex–muscle coherence with respect to a foot muscle (yellow) and hand muscle (green; for cortex–muscle coherence, see Chapter 17). Good agreement has been demonstrated between the preoperative cortex–muscle coherence measures and intraoperative electrical stimulation in pinpointing the location of the primary motor cortex (Mäkelä et al., 2001).

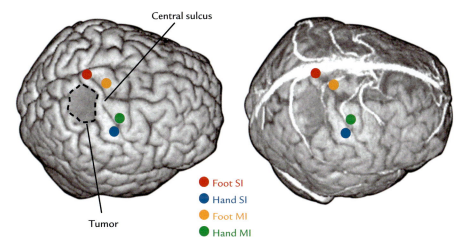

FIGURE 20.3. Preoperative identification of primary somatosensory and motor cortices in a tumor surgery patient. Left: A superolateral rendered view of the brain (based on 1.5-T structural images) showing the location of the right central sulcus relative to a brain tumor (surrounded by a dashed line). The locations of the hand and foot areas in the SI cortex posterior to the central sulcus (blue and red dots, respectively, as identified by means of somatosensory-evoked field recordings) and in the MI cortex anterior to the central sulcus (green and yellow dots, as identified by means of cortex–muscle coherence) are indicated. See main text for further explanation. Courtesy of CliniMEG, Brain Research Unit, Low Temperature Laboratory, Helsinki University of Technology (currently Aalto University), Finland.

Thus the CS can be preoperatively identified as the sulcus that delineates the SI from the MI cortices. In the image on the right, the surface rendering of the brain also shows the vasculature that is used by the surgeon to orient to the local anatomy during the operation.

Anatomical Identification of the Central Sulcus

To aid functional preoperative mapping, it is necessary to identify brain areas directly from the structural MRI scan. Although the CS is usually well seen in the structural MRIs and rendered brains of healthy subjects, it may be difficult to identify in patients whose brain structure is distorted by an abnormality. Additionally, even in MRI-guided intraoperative mapping, the CS can be difficult to identify from visual inspection of the craniotomy alone. Thus the following four partly redundant anatomical approaches can be applied to identify the CS preoperatively from structural MRI scans (Figure 20.4).

1. Identify the omega-shaped "hand knob" in axial slices as the motor-cortex hand representation (Figure 20.4, left image, yellow tracings) (Rumeau et al., 1994; Puce et al., 1995; Yousry et al., 1997). In sagittal slices this structure can be seen as a "hook" just anterior to the CS (Figure 20.4, middle image, yellow tracing) (Yousry et al., 1997).
2. Browse the axial MRI slices from top to bottom to find the superior frontal sulci, which run in an anterior-posterior direction and terminate at the precentral sulcus (Figure 20.4, left image, green tracings). The CS is the sulcus immediately posterior to the precentral sulcus.
3. Examine the mesial wall of the hemisphere in the sagittal MRI and search for the horizontally oriented cingulate sulcus and its posterior ramus, which runs dorsally (Figure 20.4, right image, green tracing). Where the posterior ramus terminates toward the dorsal aspect of the hemisphere, a tiny end of the CS is visible just anterior to it (Figure 20.4, right image, yellow tracing). The CS can then be followed to the lateral surface in other sagittal slices (Figure 20.4, middle image, yellow tracing), where the hand hook is visible.
4. The precentral gyrus (the MI) is typically broader than the postcentral gyrus (the SI), seen for example in axial MRI slices (Figure 20.4, left image).

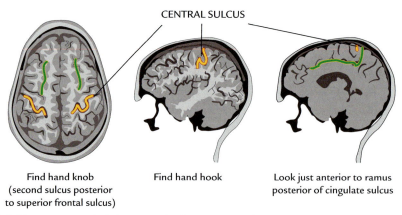

CENTRAL SULCUS

Find hand knob
(second sulcus posterior
to superior frontal sulcus)

Find hand hook

Look just anterior to ramus
posterior of cingulate sulcus

FIGURE 20.4. **How to find the central sulcus.** See text for details.

The noninvasive functional landmarks should converge with these findings. The sources of somatosensory-evoked fields and somatosensory-evoked potentials should be posterior to the CS and the sources of cortex–muscle coherence anterior to it, as demonstrated in Figure 20.3. Similarly, direct electrical cortical stimulation applied posterior to the CS should produce sensations of tingling. In contrast, stimuli applied anterior to the CS would elicit movements of the respective body part.

Hemispheric Dominance for Speech and Language

Drug-resistant epileptic foci that need to be surgically resected are most often located in the temporal lobe. To avoid associated speech and memory impairments, the temporal-lobe resection has to be less extensive in the language-dominant than in the language-nondominant hemisphere. Of course, although both clinical data and fMRI studies indicate, at the group level, a predominantly left-sided language network both in right-handed and left-handed subjects, right-hemisphere loci are also reliably activated both in fMRI (for a review, see Hickok, 2009) and MEG (Salmelin et al., 1994) recordings. Therefore, a very strict hemispheric lateralization for speech and language would not be expected with these assessment methods.

Classically, the Wada test has been used to map language dominance (Wada, 1949; Wada & Rasmussen, 1960) and lateralization of verbal memory (Milner et al., 1962). A bolus of sodium amytal is injected into internal carotid artery while the patient holds up both arms and performs a counting task. Amytal puts one brain hemisphere to sleep and produces a contralateral hemiplegia (arm drop). If the language-dominant hemisphere has been injected, a transient but profound speech arrest will follow as well. If the non-language-dominant hemisphere is injected, the patient can continue to count, albeit more slowly. EEG recorded during this test shows (ideally unilateral) slowing following amytal injection, and it can rule out behavioral changes that are the result of a simultaneous seizure. The Wada test is performed separately on the left and right hemispheres to ascertain language dominance. During the consequent resection of the temporal lobe, the language dominance is tested again by direct cortical stimulation. Typically, in most patients, the Wada test identifies one hemisphere as being dominant for language—somewhat at odds with results of human brain imaging.

Noninvasive tests, such as brain activations visible in, for example, fMRI and MEG, have been actively searched for to replace the invasive Wada test in the determination of language dominance but so far without definitive results at the single-individual level. For example, as noted, language tasks activate both hemispheres, although left-hemisphere activation is typically more extensive and can show stronger responses. Hence, a typical approach is to report "lateralization indices" for language dominance. A lateralization index (LI) is the difference of the left- and right-hemisphere activations (L – R) divided by their sum; thus LI = (L – R)/(L + R). LIs can be used equally well in the analysis of MEG/EEG and fMRI data.

In one preliminary MEG study, LIs were compared for two-sound vowels versus tones. Although the results pinpointed left-hemisphere language dominance in 11 out of 11 right-handed subjects (Gootjes et al., 1999), further work is needed to find out whether this pattern is consistent in a much larger number of individuals.

In an MEG language-lateralization study on 100 patients, lateralization indices were computed to quantify how long a current-dipole model explained long-latency auditory-evoked fields in each hemisphere (Papanicolaou et al., 2004). The results did not fully agree with those of the Wada test. However, one may also question the Wada test or direct cortical stimulation as the gold standards for language lateralization, as these tests themselves can yield data that are open to more than one interpretation.

A promising, although invasive, presurgical language mapping ("the Detroit Procedure") is based on intracranial recordings of focal high-gamma activity (70–110 Hz) to auditory verbal stimuli using ECoG or SEEG data obtained from 77 patients aged 4 to 56 years who underwent long-term video seizure monitoring (Kambara et al., 2018).

At the time of writing the second edition of this *Primer*, there was still an acute need for noninvasive studies with a large number of patients to nail down reliable language lateralization criteria that generalize across epilepsy centers (for a review, see Mégevand & Seeck, 2018).

Given the existing limitations of the current state of the field, the *combined use* of brain imaging (MEG/EEG and fMRI) and TMS has been suggested as a noninvasive future tool to replace the Wada test and invasive cortical stimulation (Papanicolaou et al., 2014). The most pragmatic approach currently would be to perform multiple assessments and look for converging evidence—preferably across multiple centers so that a large sample size could provide enough statistical power for a definitive assessment. One rarely considered variable that can potentially influence language dominance is the number of languages that the patient can speak and whether the tests are conducted in the first or second language or both. Another variable is the potential changeability or plasticity of the language network itself in response to a brain insult. The cortical language network is plastic and can be modified by an epileptic focus, by the presence of a lesion itself, or by ischemia that may be associated with a lesion (Bowyer et al., 2020; Pasquini et al., 2022).

■ STROKE

A stroke occurs when the blood supply to brain region(s) is impeded, usually due to an obstruction or rupture in the vasculature. Stroke can lead to various symptoms, such as impairments of motor function, inability to produce or understand speech, and sensory deficits. Stroke incidence varies by country, with reported incidences of about 30 to 240 individuals per 100,000 (Thrift et al., 2014). In stroke treatment, "time is brain," and it is urgent to resolve whether the patient has had an ischemic or a hemorrhagic stroke as their treatments are vastly different. In ischemic stroke, the occlusion or blood clot can be dissolved (with thrombolysis) or mechanically removed (via thrombectomy) up to a few hours after stroke onset, whereas in hemorrhagic stroke drugs dissolving blood clots are contraindicated. Unfortunately, the longest delays occur in getting patients to a hospital, which largely affects treatment success. Approximately one-third of stroke patients die soon after the incident, one-third recover fully, and one-third remain severely disabled. In addition to the individual suffering, stroke is also a heavy economic burden to society.

The main brain imaging methods for acute stroke are X-ray computerized tomography, structural and diffusion-weighted MRIs, and perfusion MRI. Importantly, the timing of brain scans with respect to stroke onset largely affects the findings and therefore also their interpretation.

After the acute phase of stroke, it is time to estimate the prognosis and rehabilitation possibilities of patients on the basis of their individual neurological injuries and affected functions. For the rehabilitation to be effective, it must commence very soon after the stroke.

Given that a stroke involves a breakdown in local neurovascular coupling that affects fMRI-based methods, MEG/EEG can provide essential information about the functional state of a stroke patient's brain (Rossini et al., 2004). A wider use of modern MEG/EEG analyses, beyond just eye-balling the spontaneous activity, would be welcome in the study of stroke patients, especially in the assessment of their prognoses. Useful information regarding the affected network and modified cortical excitability can be obtained from slow activity in the vicinity of the lesion (Laaksonen et al., 2013), the reactivity of sensorimotor cortex after voluntary and passive movements, and responses to TMS (Mäkelä et al., 2015) and to selective proprioceptive input (Piitulainen et al., 2013). Moreover, characterization of the functional state of the whole somatosensory system, including both primary and second somatosensory cortices (Forss et al., 1999; 2012) and the motor network, would guide neuroscientifically based and individualized rehabilitation. In stroke recovery, the relative functional roles of *both* hemispheres and the reorganization of the *contralesional* hemisphere have been flagged as playing important roles (Buetefisch et al., 2014; Buetefisch, 2015); an activity imbalance between nonlesioned and lesioned hemispheres is countered by compensatory activity in the nonlesioned hemisphere.

New rehabilitation methods, including real-time feedback of the level of action- or intention-related brain rhythms (Paggiaro et al., 2016), obtained from either MEG (Buch et al., 2012) or scalp EEG (Prasad et al., 2010) are still in the testing phase. In one study, the hand function of chronic stroke patients (mean duration ~2.5 y) improved when an orthotic device was taught—on the basis of the reactivity of the patient's magnetic 9–12-Hz mu rhythm—to assist the fingers of the affected hand into an open or closed grasping posture depending on which posture the patient had been imagining (Buch et al., 2012). Another promising method for stroke rehabilitation relies on action observation (see Chapter 19), presented either live or on video (e.g., Zhu et al., 2019).

Multimodal approaches, combining neurophysiological (MEG, EEG, TMS), neuropharmacological, and hemodynamic monitoring, have been used to develop biomarkers and standardized test protocols for purposes of rehabilitation (Buetefisch & Puce, 2012). Another approach, currently under development, is to use TMS–EEG (see Chapter 21) to assess both functional and effective connectivity in the affected hemisphere, as well as between the hemispheres (Keser et al., 2022).

Neurophysiological methods using brain–computer interfaces (BCIs) have an important role also in the rehabilitation of spinal-injury patients (see Chapter 22). The main BCI applications are geared toward either compensating for injuries at the spinal or even brain level (e.g., motor control to restore ambulation) or augmentation of sensory function when the peripheral sensory system does not function properly (one can, for example, provide visual or auditory signals to the subject).

The controlling signals that drive BCI hardware/software can come from many sensory modalities, or from the brain or body (for a comprehensive review, see Bockbrader et al., 2018). Noninvasive EEG signals can be used to control varied effectors and functions, for example, selecting individual letters on a screen for writing text, changing the position of a cursor on a computer screen, triggering electrical stimulation of a muscle, or starting the operation of an orthotic device, such as an exoskeleton, or prosthetic or robotic limb. The control commands for these last devices might even come via a mobile-phone application, and they vary, depending on the application, from digitized noninvasive EEG to invasive ECoG/SEEG signals; in both cases, attributes of frequency and/or amplitude can be used as the driving signal. Manipulation of objects with one's upper limb requires tactile and proprioceptive feedback; for a prosthetic hand that cannot provide tactile information, auditory feedback that arises from the contact between the object and the prosthetic hand can largely replace the effects of the tactile feedback (Lundborg et al., 1999). Whatever the ultimate, customized goal is for the BCI device, the most important thing is to consider the end users and their comfort and ability to use their new functions.

■ CRITICALLY ILL PATIENTS

Coma

Coma is a disorder of consciousness where the individual is unresponsive to the environment and cannot be awakened. The etiologies vary from toxic and metabolic insults (e.g., drug overdose or hepatic failure) to cerebral anoxia (following, e.g., cardiac arrest or ischemic stroke) and severe traumatic brain injury.

EEG is recommended (Claassen et al., 2013) for critically ill patients in neurointensive care for monitoring generalized convulsive SE, as well as for ruling out nonconvulsive epileptic disorders both in brain-injured patients and in comatose patients in whom the primary brain disorder is unknown. Other indications are the detection of ischemia in comatose patients who have suffered from subarachnoid hemorrhage as well as in patients who are comatose after cardiac arrest and in whom any prognostic information is badly needed.

The serious EEG abnormalities found in comatose and critically ill patients include, for example, slowing or flattening of the background activity, epileptiform discharges, and lateralization of pathological activity. More details of these abnormalities can be found in textbooks on clinical EEG (e.g., Schomer & Lopes da Silva, 2018).

Brain Death

Technically, *brain death* means that all brain functions have completely and irreversibly ceased. The presence of a flat (isoelectric) EEG (either invasively or noninvasively recorded) in addition to clinical signs at the bedside was originally proposed to signal brain death (Jouvet, 1959). However, EEG is not consistently included in brain-death determinations (Citerio et al., 2014), and the legal criteria for brain death and the required examinations vary from country to country (Wahlster et al., 2015).

A recent meta-analysis of 37 studies about the prognosis for recovery from a cardiac arrest concluded that, among a number of clinical criteria, the presence of the somatosensory N20 response with an amplitude of > 4 µV and a background EEG without discharges within 72 hours from the return of spontaneous circulation are positive signs for a good neurological outcome (Sandroni et al., 2022).

■ WHY HAVE THE CLINICAL APPLICATIONS FOR MEG DEVELOPED SO SLOWLY?

Since its naissance EEG has been used as a diagnostic tool on the basis of visual analysis of distinct "graphoelements," unique EEG waveforms (e.g., spikes, spike–slow-wave complexes, and slowing of activity) that have been correlated with different disease states (for an extensive survey of this field, see Schomer & Lopes da Silva, 2018). With the advent of accurate source analysis of MEG signals, the hopes were high that MEG would soon become clinically useful. Yet this direction of MEG development has been extremely slow, with only two well-established clinical applications so far: (1) diagnosis of epilepsy and localization of epileptic foci and (2) functional preoperative evaluation for focal epilepsy and brain tumors. The other clinical applications discussed in this chapter are still used only sporadically by specialized research teams; for example, magnetic auditory evoked responses can be very informative in hearing disorders and various neurological diseases (for a review, see Shvarts & Mäkelä, 2020).

A number of reasons may explain why the uptake of MEG in the clinic has been so slow. First, the MEG community is still missing evidence-based guidelines for clinical applications, although such guidelines have long existed in the EEG community via the International Federation for Clinical Neurophysiology. We note that MEG guidelines have been published previously (Burgess et al., 2011; Hari et al., 2018), but they are based—in addition to experience obtained in research and clinical environments—on existing small-*n* studies. Future MEG guidelines should be based on larger sample sizes. Perhaps an MEG initiative, similar to the #EEGManyLabs study (Pavlov et al., 2021), would help to achieve this goal?

Second, the number of MEG instruments worldwide has remained very small; for example, at present there are about 200 times as many MRI scanners than whole-scalp MEG devices (i.e., ~50,000 vs. 220!), and EEG devices are common in any midsize or large hospital, as well as private clinics.

Third, the human-powered analysis requirements for MEG data are very high. MEG measurements themselves require a good understanding of the basic principles of the recording instruments. Currently, there are still no fully automatic analysis tools. Therefore, the data analyzers and also interpreters of test results all need a solid background in understanding the physiological generation of the signals, the analysis pipelines, including statistical decision-making. Importantly, those who acquire and analyze data cannot succumb to basic pitfalls. They also must be able to connect the results to current basic and clinical neuroscience. Training of such scientist–clinicians is one aim of our *Primer*. All disciplines need to work together toward a common goal, using a "convergence research" approach (see Chapter 22).

A further aspect in the utility of clinical MEG (and EEG) results is that clinicians are used to evaluating numbers (e.g., in blood tests) and images (as in X-ray or MRI), whereas the clinical significance of temporal waveforms is more difficult to grasp. Perhaps the onus is on the MEG/EEG field itself to come up with better ways in which to present these sorts of data?

To understand why some brain responses are delayed beyond the lab's normative values one may also need to test peripheral sensory pathways, for example, by recording simultaneous ERG (for visual evoked responses), plexus compound action potentials (for somatosensory evoked responses), or the brainstem evoked responses (for cortical auditory evoked responses). Other sources of potential confounds include limb length and skin temperature (which can slow down peripheral sensory conduction), impaired visual acuity, and an elevated (often frequency-selective) hearing threshold (see Chapter 7).

Inadequate skills in sophisticated MEG/EEG data acquisition and analysis can easily lead to technically poor publications that do not push the field forward but rather can be misleading for clinical practice and thereby potentially harmful for individual patients. Only on the basis of a solid foundation can joint efforts of appropriately trained clinicians and clinical neurophysiology-trained scientists carry out the necessary sophisticated exams and data analysis to arrive at the correct conclusions for the benefit of their patients.

▪ REFERENCES

Bockbrader MA, Francisco G, Lee R, Olson J, Solinsky R, Boninger ML: Brain computer interfaces in rehabilitation medicine. *Phys Med Rehab* 2018, 10 (9 Suppl 2): S233–S243.

Bowyer SM, Zillgitt A, Greenwald M, Lajiness-O'Neill R: Language mapping with magnetoencephalography: an update on the current state of clinical research and practice with considerations for clinical practice guidelines. *J Clin Neurophysiol* 2020, 37: 554–563.

Buch ER, Modir Shanechi A, Fourkas AD, Weber C, Birbaumer N, Cohen LG: Parietofrontal integrity determines neural modulation associated with grasping imagery after stroke. *Brain* 2012, 135: 596–614.

Buetefisch C, Puce A: Multimodal investigations. In: Carey L, ed. *Stroke Rehabilitation: Insights from Neuroscience and Imaging*. Oxford: Oxford University Press, 2012: 54–72.

Buetefisch CM, Revill KP, Shuster L, Hines B, Parsons M: Motor demand-dependent activation of ipsilateral motor cortex. *J Neurophysiol* 2014, 112: 999–1009.

Buetefisch CM: Role of the contralesional hemisphere in post-stroke recovery of upper extremity motor function. *Front Neurol* 2015, 6: 214.

Burgess RC, Funke ME, Bowyer SM, Lewine JD, Kirsch HE, Bagić AI, Committee ACPG: American Clinical Magnetoencephalography Society clinical practice guideline 2: presurgical functional brain mapping using magnetic evoked fields. *J Clin Neurophysiol* 2011, 28: 355–361.

Citerio G, Crippa IA, Bronco A, Vargiolu A, Smith M: Variability in brain death determination in Europe: looking for a solution. *Neurocrit Care* 2014, 21: 376–382.

Claassen J, Taccone FS, Horn P, Holtkamp M, Stocchetti N, Oddo M, Neurointensive Care Section of the European Society of Intensive Care Medicine: Recommendations on the use of EEG monitoring in critically ill patients: consensus statement from the neurointensive care section of the ESICM. *Intensive Care Med* 2013, 39: 1337–1351.

Fine A, Wirrell EC: Seizures in children. *Pediatr Rev* 2020, 41: 321–347.

Forss N, Hietanen M, Salonen O, Hari R: Modified activation of somatosensory cortical network in patients with right-hemisphere stroke. *Brain* 1999, 122 1889–1899.

Forss N, Mustanoja S, Roiha K, Kirveskari E, Mäkelä JP, Salonen O, Tatlisumak T, Kaste M: Activation in parietal operculum parallels motor recovery in stroke. *Hum Brain Mapp* 2012, 33: 534–541.

GBD 2016 Epilepsy Collaborators: Global, regional, and national burden of epilepsy, 1990–2016: a systematic analysis for the Global Burden of Disease Study 2016. *Lancet Neurol* 2019, 18: 357–375.

Gootjes L, Raij T, Salmelin R, Hari R: Left-hemisphere dominance for processing of vowels: a whole-scalp neuromagnetic study. *Neuroreport* 1999, 10: 2987–2991.

Hauser WA: The prevalence and incidence of convulsive disorders in children. *Epilepsia* 1994, 35 (Suppl 2): S1–S6.

Hari R, Ahonen A, Forss N, Granström ML, Hämäläinen M, Kajola M, Knuutila J, Lounasmaa OV, Mäkelä JP, Paetau R, et al.: Parietal epileptic mirror focus detected with a whole-head neuromagnetometer. *Neuroreport* 1993, 5: 45–48.

Hari R, Baillet S, Barnes G, Burgess R, Forss N, Gross J, Hämäläinen M, Jensen O, Kakigi R, Mauguière F, Nakasato N, Puce A, Romani GL, Schnitzler A, Taulu S: IFCN-endorsed practical guidelines for clinical magnetoencephalography (MEG). *Clin Neurophysiol* 2018, 129: 1720–1747.

Hickok G: The functional neuroanatomy of language. *Phys Life Rev* 2009, 6: 121–143.

Jouvet M: Diagnostic électro-sous-corticographique de la mort du système nerveux central au cours de certains comas. [Electro-subcorticographic diagnosis of death of the central nervous system during various types of coma]. *Electroencephalogr Clin Neurophysiol* 1959, 11: 805–808.

Kambara T, Sood S, Alqatan Z, Klingert C, Ratnam D, Hayakawa A, Nakai Y, Luat AF Agarwal R, Rothermel R, Asano E: Presurgical language mapping using event-related high-gamma activity: the Detroit procedure. *Clin Neurophysiol* 2018, 129: 145–154.

Keser Z, Buchl SC, Seven NA, Markota M, Clark HM, Jones DT, Lanzino G, Brown RD Jr, Worrell GA, Lundstrom BN: Electroencephalogram (EEG) with or without transcranial magnetic stimulation (TMS) as biomarkers for post-stroke recovery: a narrative review. *Front Neurol* 2022, 13: 827866.

Laaksonen K, Helle L, Parkkonen L, Kirveskari E, Mäkelä JP, Mustanoja S, Tatlisumak T, Kaste M, Forss N: Alterations in spontaneous brain oscillations during stroke recovery. *PLoS One* 2013, 8: e61146.

Lundborg G, Rosen B, Lindberg S: Hearing as substitution for sensation: a new principle for artificial sensibility. *J Hand Surg [Am]* 1999, 24: 19–24.

Mäkelä J, Kirveskari E, Seppä M, Hämäläinen M, Forss N, Avikainen S, Salonen O, Salenius S, Kovala T, Randell T, Jääskeläinen J, Hari R: Three-dimensional integration of brain anatomy and function to facilitate intraoperative navigation around the sensorimotor strip. *Hum Brain Mapp* 2001, 12: 181–192.

Mäkelä JP, Lioumis P, Laaksonen K, Forss N, Tatlisumak T, Kaste M, Mustanoja S: Cortical excitability measured with nTMS and MEG during stroke recovery. *Neural Plast* 2015, 2015: 309546.

Mégevand P, Seeck M: Electroencephalography, magnetoencephalography and source localization: their value in epilepsy. *Curr Opin Neurol* 2018, 31: 176–183.

Milner B, Branch C, Rasmussen T: Intracarotid injection of sodium amytal for lateralization of cerebral speech dominance *Trans Am Neurol Assoc* 1962, 87: 224–226.

Paggiaro A, Birbaumer N, Cavinato M, Turco C, Formaggio E, Del Felice A, Masiero S, Piccione F: Magnetoencephalography in stroke recovery and rehabilitation. *Front Neurol* 2016, 7: 35.

Papanicolaou AC, Simos PG, Castillo EM, Breier JI, Sarkari S, Pataraia E, Billingsley RL, Buchanan S, Wheless J, Maggio V, Maggio WW: Magnetocephalography: a noninvasive alternative to the Wada procedure. *J Neurosurg* 2004, 100: 867–876.

Papanicolaou AC, Rezaie R, Narayana S, Choudhri AF, Wheless JW, Castillo EM, Baumgartner JE, Boop FA: Is it time to replace the Wada test and put awake craniotomy to sleep? *Epilepsia* 2014, 55: 629–632.

Pasquini L, Di Napoli A, Rossi-Espagnet MC, Visconti E, Napolitano A, Romano A, Bozzao A, Peck KK, Holodny AI: Understanding language reorganization with neuroimaging: how language adapts to different focal lesions and insights into clinical applications. *Front Hum Neurosci* 2022, 16: 747215.

Pavlov YG, Adamian N, Appelhoff S, Arvaneh M, Benwell CSY, Beste C, Bland AR, Bradford DE, Bublatzky F, Busch NA, Clayson PE, Cruse D, Czeszumski A, Dreber A, Dumas G, Ehinger B, Ganis G, He X, Hinojosa JA, . . . Mushtaq F: #EEGManyLabs: investigating the replicability of influential EEG experiments. *Cortex* 2021, 144: 213–229.

Piitulainen H, Bourguignon M, De Tiège X, Hari R, Jousmäki V: Corticokinematic coherence during active and passive finger movements. *Neuroscience* 2013, 238: 361–370.

Prasad G, Herman P, Coyle D, McDonough S, Crosbie J: Applying a brain–computer interface to support motor imagery practice in people with stroke for upper limb recovery: a feasibility study. *J Neuroeng Rehabil* 2010, 7: 60.

Pressler RM, Cilio MR, Mizrahi EM, Moshé SL, Nunes ML, Plouin P, Vanhatalo S, Yozawitz E, de Vries LS, Vinayan KP, Triki CC, Wilmshurst JM, Yamamoto H, Zuberi SM: The ILAE classification of seizures and the epilepsies: modification for seizures in the neonate. Position paper by the ILAE Task Force on Neonatal Seizures. *Epilepsia* 2021, 62: 615–628.

Puce A, Constable RT, Luby ML, McCarthy G, Nobre AC, Spencer DD, Gore JC, Allison T: Functional magnetic resonance imaging of sensory and motor cortex: comparison with electrophysiological localization. *J Neurosurg* 1995, 83: 262–270.

Rossini PM, Altamura C, Ferretti A, Vernieri F, Zappasodi F, Caulo M, Pizzella V, Del Gratta C, Romani GL, Tecchio F: Does cerebrovascular disease affect the coupling between neuronal activity and local haemodynamics? *Brain* 2004, 127: 99–110.

Rumeau C, Tzourio N, Murayama N, Peretti-Viton P, Levrier O, Joliot M, Mazoyer B, Salamon G: Location of hand function in the sensorimotor cortex: MR and functional correlation. *Am J Neuroradiol* 1994, 15: 567–572.

Salmelin R, Hari R, Lounasmaa OV, Sams M: Dynamics of brain activation during picture naming. *Nature* 1994, 368: 463–465.

Sandroni C, D'Arrigo S, Cacciola S, Hoedemaekers CWE, Westhall E, Kamps MJA, Taccone FS, Poole D, Meijer FJA, Antonelli M, Hirsch KG, Soar J, Nolan JP, Cronberg T: Prediction of good neurological outcome in comatose survivors of cardiac arrest: a systematic review. *Intensive Care Med* 2022, 48: 389–413.

Scheffer IE, Berkovic S, Capovilla G, Connolly MB, French J, Guilhoto L, Hirsch E, Jain S, Mathern GW, Moshé SL, Nordli DR, Perucca E, Tomson T, Wiebe S, Zhang YH, Zuberi SM: ILAE classification of the epilepsies: position paper of the ILAE Commission for Classification and Terminology. *Epilepsia* 2017, 58: 512–521.

Schomer DL, Lopes da Silva FH, eds. *Niedermeyer's Electroencephalography: Basic Principles, Clinical Applications, and Related Fields.* New York, NY: Oxford University Press, 2018.

Shvarts V, Mäkelä JP: Auditory mapping with MEG: an update on the current state of clinical research and practice with considerations for clinical practice guidelines. *J Clin Neurophysiol* 2020, 37: 574–584.

Stafstrom CE, Carmant L: Seizures and epilepsy: an overview for neuroscientists. *Cold Spring Harb Perspect Med* 2015: 5: a022426.

Thrift A, Cadilhac D, Thayabaranathan T, Howard G, Howard V, Rothwell P, Donnan G: Global stroke statistics. *Int J Stroke* 2014, 9: 6–18.

Wada J: A new method for the determination of the side of cerebral speech dominance: a preliminary report on the intra-carotid injection of sodium amytal in man (in Japanese). *Igaku to Seibutsugaki* 1949, 14: 221–222.

Wada J, Rasmussen T: Intracarotid injection of sodium amytal for lateralization of cerebral speech dominance *J Neurosurg* 1960, 17: 266–282.

Wahlster S, Wijdicks EF, Patel PV, Greer DM, Hemphill JC 3rd, Carone M, Mateen FJ: Brain death declaration: practices and perceptions worldwide. *Neurology* 2015, 84: 1870–1879.

Yousry TA, Schmid UD, Alkadhi H, Schmidt D, Peraud A, Buettner A, Winkler P: Localization of the motor hand area to a knob on the precentral gyrus: a new landmark. *Brain* 1997, 120 141–157.

Zhu JD, Cheng CH, Tseng YJ, Chou CC, Chen CC, Hsieh YW, Liao YH: Modulation of motor cortical activities by action observation and execution in patients with stroke: an MEG study. *Neural Plast* 2019, 2019: 8481371.

CHAPTER 21

MEG/EEG COMBINED WITH OTHER BRAIN IMAGING METHODS

You make different colors by combining those colors that already exist.

HERBIE HANCOCK

A good tool improves the way you work. A great tool improves the way you think.

JEFF DUNTEMANN

The main advantage of MEG and EEG for studying human brain function is their ability to noninvasively reveal millisecond-scale dynamics of neuronal populations. Figure 21.1 may be illustrative for comparing these neurophysiological methods with the hemodynamic response of functional magnetic resonance imaging (fMRI). The image is the now famous "daguerreotype" *Boulevard du Temple, Paris* taken on a spring morning in 1838 by Louis Daguerre when the street was typically at its busiest. However, the street looks totally empty, and the only visible people are a shoe-shiner and his client on the street corner. The extremely long exposure time of many minutes has completely eliminated the brief trajectories of pedestrians rushing about their morning chores. Similarly, with fMRI we will capture the relatively long time course of the hemodynamic response and not detect the faster, millisecond-range activity that we capture with MEG and EEG. Therefore, we again stress the complementarity of the various brain imaging methods. Below we discuss the advantages of combining the various methods to help fill in our knowledge gaps.

■ COMBINING MEG AND EEG

We have emphasized throughout this primer that MEG and EEG provide complementary information. An excellent recent case in point is the different sensitivities of the two methods to pick up neural signals emerging from the cerebellum (see Chapters 2 and 22). The complementary nature of MEG and EEG signals has a number of major consequences. First, the researcher applying either of these methods should be aware of *similar experiments carried out with the other method*. Second, in some cases one method might be clearly better than the other for studying a particular type of neural activity. Third, and ideally, MEG and EEG recordings would be carried out simultaneously and then the data analyzed and interpreted jointly. Such a combined approach has been long been advocated strongly also

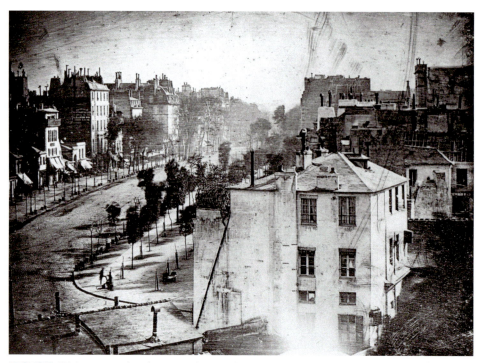

FIGURE 21.1. An early photograph, a "daguerreotype," with people, taken by Louis Daguerre in 1838. The image presents the Boulevard du Temple in Paris—a major road that separates the 3rd and 11th arrondissements. Image courtesy of Wikimedia commons: https://en.wikipedia.org/wiki/File:Boulevard_du_Temple_by_Daguerre.jpg.

for clinical investigations of epileptic activity (Ebersole & Ebersole, 2010), and it is more common today because of readily available hardware and software options.

Despite the theoretical benefits, combined MEG–EEG studies and their appropriate analyses continue to be rare for practical reasons. Possible solutions are to analyze both data sets separately and then compare the modeled sources and their behavior or to pool the data from multiple sensor types and generate models for the sources. Another approach, frequently applied in the interpretation of early evoked response studies (Hari, 1988), is to find, on the basis of MEG recordings, the *tangential* currents and then try to explain with them the measured EEG distribution. What cannot be explained must be generated by either *radial* or *deep* sources, which then should be identifiable on the basis of the EEG data. The main reason impeding this kind of straightforward workflow is that the conductivity structure of the tissues in the head considerably affects detailed modeling of the EEG signals, and such accurate information for building up a realistic head model has been laborious or impossible to obtain and requires, at minimum, a high-resolution structural MRI of the subject's head.

The skull is a particularly difficult tissue to model as it consists of three layers—two outer, harder layers with lower conductivity and an inner spongiform layer with higher conductivity (McCann et al., 2019)—and it also has large intra- and interindividual variations in thickness across the head (Antonakakis et al., 2020). This nonhomogeneous skull conductivity across the head has led to inaccurate estimates of source-current strengths based on EEG signals. Further inaccuracies in source-strength estimates can arise from thin skull bones and fontanelles (discontinuities between skull plates) in children (McCann & Beltrachini, 2022), as well as from burr holes and steel plates in neurosurgical patients.

In network-based (e.g., graph-theoretical) analyses, the interpretation of MEG/EEG source areas is complicated by two issues. First, for tractability of computation, sources must be put into a parcellated brain scheme, but, until very recently, the available brain parcellation schemes have included only the cerebral hemispheres (e.g., Glasser et al., 2016), omitting cerebellar, midline subcortical, and brainstem structures. Recent atlases, however, include the human midline structures (extension to the Human Connectome Project, HCPex; Huang et al., 2022) and the human brainstem (Coulombe et al., 2021). Anatomical atlases of the cerebellum are also available (Diedrichsen et al., 2009; Park et al., 2014).

Second, despite the accurate probabilistic atlases that parcellate cerebral cortex into cytoarchitectonically homogeneous regions (Amunts et al., 2020), it is not possible to associate a behavioral function to a specific brain "region" or "area" (see Genon et al., 2018), and specific brain functions do not necessarily respect anatomical borders. Fortunately, multilevel perspectives from the brain's micro- and macroscale organization are currently starting to be linked with cognitive functions using advanced computational tools and multiple research technologies (e.g., Amunts et al., 2022).

■ COMBINING MEG/EEG WITH MRI/FMRI

Since the 1990s, sources of MEG signals have been typically presented superimposed on individual images from structural brain MRI, with the same praxis more recently entering into the EEG community as well. Such a combination of functional and structural data requires careful alignment of the respective coordinate systems (discussed in Chapter 7). The match between the MEG/EEG and MRI/fMRI coordinate systems is improved by the currently widely applied practice to use MRI surface renderings for defining fiducial landmarks and sensor locations on the structural images and displaying the actual digitized scalp locations on the rendering.

Individual realistic conductor models for the head can be extracted from high-quality T1 and T2 anatomical MRI images. The methods that have been available for some time (Fujimoto et al., 2014) typically include segmentation of different head/brain tissues and their triangulation or voxelization, necessary for boundary- and finite-element models (BEM and FEM, respectively). An additional, extremely important procedure for this type of data analysis is to extract cortical geometry from the structural MRI images and use the cortical strip (and currents perpendicular to it) as a constraint in the source analysis (Dale & Sereno, 1993). As already noted, for EEG source analysis, a model is needed for the whole head rather than just for the brain alone, whereas for MEG analysis one needs only information about sensor locations with respect to the brain. The whole-head model is especially important for geodesic EEG electrode arrays, where electrodes cover the lower face and neck. This analysis also requires the accurate segmentation and modeling of additional tissues of the head (e.g., the eyes, muscles, fat, and skin) obtainable from high-resolution structural MRI of the *head* (Taberna et al., 2021). However, a number of neuroimaging data-analysis packages have typically used anatomical templates that were based on optimally sampled structural MRI *brain-only* images (e.g., the MNI [Montreal Neurological Institute] brain atlas and the Collins atlas). Consequently, experimenters often have had to generate their own custom-made whole-head templates or use other methods to produce a whole-head model (Cottereau et al., 2015; Huang & Parra, 2015).

Because MEG and EEG provide excellent temporal and fMRI accurate spatial information, it was initially proposed that brain areas activated in fMRI studies be used as "seeds" in MEG/EEG analysis to extract the time courses of the activated areas (A. K. Liu et al., 1998). However, it was soon evident that this procedure was not optimal, mainly because there is not necessarily a one-to-one correspondence of fMRI activation sites and the neurophysiological data, as has been demonstrated by comparing subdural recordings and fMRI data during face processing (Puce et al., 1997), as well as MEG and fMRI data during object and action naming (Liljeström et al., 2009) and during reading (Vartiainen et al., 2011). Still, individual fMRI-based retinotopic maps are used as seeds for the EEG source analysis of visual EEG responses (see, e.g., Cottereau et al., 2015; and Chapter 14).

Next, we compare in more detail activation sequences obtained from MEG and fMRI recordings in identical experimental conditions to learn how these two imaging modalities differ. Figure 21.2 shows schematics of possible time courses of MEG and fMRI signals: the beginning of the MEG response follows initial neuronal activation very closely, whereas the BOLD (blood-oxygen-dependent) response lags neural activity by several seconds and typically lasts longer than the neuronal activity.

In the left upper panel, we assume that brain is activated at equal time steps successively from regions 1 to 5. If the fMRI and MEG signals would reflect the same activation

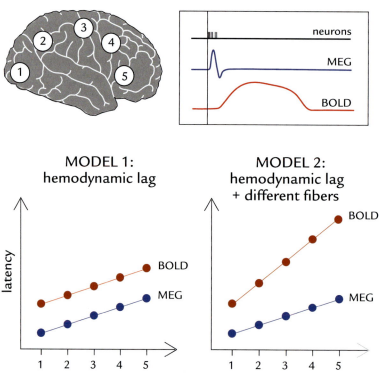

FIGURE 21.2. Two simple models for contrasting MEG and fMRI signals. Top left: An assumed activation sequence from areas 1 to 5. Top right: Schematic presentation of generalized time courses of neuronal activation, the MEG evoked response, and the BOLD response. Bottom panels: The latencies of MEG and BOLD responses could vary with respect to one another in two possible models. In MODEL1, the fMRI BOLD signals follow the time course of the MEG signals only with a hemodynamic lag. In MODEL2, the two signals differ, in addition to the hemodynamic lag, cumulating during the activation sequence because of the assumed weighing of slower transmission fibers by fMRI than MEG.

sequence (from the same brain regions), then their time courses should differ only by the hemodynamic lag, as is indicated in Model 1. Importantly, the interareal time differences—from, for example, area 1 to 5—should be the same in both recordings. However, if the fMRI and MEG signals would be transmitted via fibers of different conduction velocities, we could end up with a relationship that looks more like Model 2. Below we discuss some real results from three MEG–fMRI experiments, to further consider these two models.

Example 1. Figure 21.3 presents data from an experiment with separate fMRI and MEG sessions where the same subjects were presented with three types of stimuli: faces alone, houses alone, and double-exposure stimuli consisting of superimposed faces and houses. In the last case, subjects attended either to faces or to houses in separate runs. In the fMRI study, attending to faces activated roughly the same "face area" as for viewing single faces, and attending to houses activated the same "house area" as for viewing single houses. The MEG responses to faces (red traces in Figure 21.3) were similar to fMRI results in that they did not differ for superimposed faces versus faces alone. However, MEG responses to attended houses (blue dashed trace) were similar to those to *faces* during the first 190 ms, after which they were similar to the responses to houses alone (blue solid trace). The face-sensitive M170 response was considered to reflect rapid, feedforward processing, whereas the later and longer duration activity (which was more likely to be reflected in the fMRI signals) was likely affected by feedback connections (Furey et al., 2006). These findings do not fit with Model 1 because at latencies < 190 ms the source areas indicated by MEG differed from the fMRI-based activation locations but agreed with them at later latencies. Thus the relationship between the MEG and fMRI signals is likely complex, potentially consistent with Model 2.

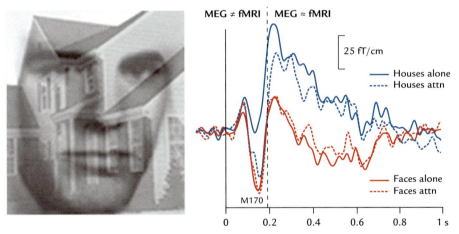

FIGURE 21.3. **MEG responses elicited by face and house images.** Left: An example of a double-exposure face–house stimulus. Right: MEG responses to faces and houses presented alone (solid lines) and attended (attn) in double-exposure images (dashed lines). Faces in both stimuli (red traces) and attended houses in double-exposure images (blue broken line) elicit a similar M170 response, which, however, is very small to single houses (blue solid line). For differences and similarities with respect to fMRI data (MEG ≠ fMRI and MEG ≈ fMRI, respectively), see the text. Generated from the dataset of Furey ML, Tanskanen T, Beauchamp MS, Avikainen S, Uutela K, Hari R, Haxby JV: Dissociation of face-selective cortical responses by attention. *Proc Natl Acad Sci USA* 2006, 103: 1065–1070.

Example 2. Early sensory areas tend to exhibit reasonably good convergence between neurophysiological and fMRI data sets, as far as activated brain areas are concerned. However, the dependence of somatosensory responses on stimulus repetition rate largely differs between methods: The MEG (and EEG) responses *decrease* when stimulation rate increases, whereas fMRI signals *increase* (Figure 21.4). This striking discrepancy, however, largely disappears when the rectified or squared MEG signals, or squared source strengths, are aggregated across the entire analysis period without focusing on any temporal aspects of the signal (Nangini et al., 2009). This aggregation of signals (to make the MEG signal resemble fMRI activity) contrasts the typical analysis of MEG/EEG rate effects that is based on the peaks of the most prominent responses (Figure 21.4, right panel). Hence, these results agree with the idea that the fMRI signal is closely related to the aggregated, time-integrated neural response, although lagging it due to the hemodynamic delay. This observation is more consistent with Model 1.

Example 3. A comparison of fMRI and MEG timing during a visuomotor task, recorded with 100-ms temporal resolution for BOLD (applying so-called inverse imaging), implied a linear relationship between latencies of the two signals across five brain regions from the visual to motor cortex (Lin et al., 2013). Similar linear relationships between the two imaging modalities were obtained, although with somewhat different slopes, for different timing indices. This finding nicely demonstrated that BOLD signals obtained with inverse imaging can be used to follow relatively quick time sequences in the brain, and that both fMRI and MEG might track the same activation sequence. However, the *interareal* time lags differed between methods in an interesting manner. For example, in the left hemisphere, the average lag from visual to motor cortex was around 250 ms for evoked MEG responses but 1,200 ms for the BOLD onset times,

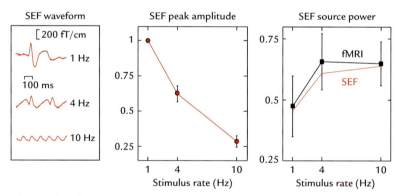

FIGURE 21.4. **The effect of interstimulus interval on MEG and fMRI responses in primary somatosensory cortex.** Left: Somatosensory evoked fields (SEFs) of a healthy subject to pneumotactile stimuli to fingertips at repetition rates of 1, 4, and 10 Hz. Middle: Mean ± SEM amplitudes across nine subjects of current dipole strengths for SEF peaks as a function of stimulus rate. Right: Mean ± SEM source power (the strength of the equivalent-current dipole squared, red line) over equal time periods (not only response peaks) for all stimulus rates for the same data, and mean ± SEM fMRI (BOLD) amplitudes (expressed as percentual signal change) of the same nine subjects as a function of stimulus rate (black line). Adapted and reprinted from Nangini C, Hlushchuk Y, Hari R: Predicting stimulus-rate sensitivity of human somatosensory fMRI signals with MEG. *Hum Brain Mapp* 2009, 30: 1824–1832. With permission from John Wiley & Sons.

implying that MODEL 1, with hemodynamic lag as the only explaining factor for timing differences, would not be valid. Yet, the induced MEG response (computed by means of temporal spectral evolution, TSE; see Chapter 10) does show closer temporal correspondence with the BOLD response (e.g., time-to-half BOLD signal)—more consistent perhaps with Model 1.

These three examples of combined MEG and fMRI recordings showcase obvious differences between the neurophysiological and hemodynamic data, with more support for Model 2 of Figure 21.2, meaning that prominent MEG/EEG deflections reflect the most synchronously activated neuronal populations, whereas fMRI tends to pick up all activity more evenly. Given that the long-distance thick fibers, likely supporting the synchrony-reflecting MEG/EEG responses, are sparse between brain areas (Wang et al., 2008; Buzsáki et al., 2013; Markov et al., 2013; Rosen & Halgren, 2022; see also Chapter 2), it is likely that fMRI signals mainly reflect gray matter activation transmitted via the dense and thin neuronal fibers (Hari & Parkkonen, 2015), which are far more abundant than the sparse fast-conducting thick fibers. It should be noted that here we have not considered responses of astrocytes or differences in hemodynamic response across different brain regions—factors that may well add further variation to the already complex relationship between measured neuronal and hemodynamic responses.

The observed differences between MEG and fMRI signals also emphasize the complementarity of hemodynamic and neurophysiological measures. A crucial difference to be considered is that fMRI responses are usually quantified as *differences between conditions*, whereas MEG/EEG analyses typically extract signals *with respect to individual conditions* in their own right. Further, identification of timing differences of less than 100 ms is feasible only in neurophysiological data.

A final important consideration relates to how multimodal data have been gathered. Two critical points bear noting. First, in the studies we have featured above, neurophysiological (MEG) and hemodynamic (fMRI) data were *not collected* within the same session. Therefore, potential differences may exist between the subject's mental state across the two sessions, and there may be task habituation effects.

Second, an important but rarely considered variable is the subject's physical position during the recording because body posture (e.g., standing, sitting, lying) has multiple effects on the subject's cognition, memory, and basic physiology, affecting, for example, cardiovascular, respiratory, and metabolic functions, as well as vigilance (Thibault & Raz, 2016). For example, performance is better in arithmetic tasks while sitting and words are recalled better while walking (Abou Khalil et al., 2020). Thus, the postures of the subjects matter while their brain activity is recorded during various tasks.

Based on structural MRI measurements, the cerebrospinal fluid (CSF) layer between the occipital brain and skull is thinner by ~30% when subjects are in a supine rather than prone position (Rice et al., 2013). Accordingly, sensor-space and source-space EEG signal power increased when subjects switched from a prone to supine position. These changes also have implications for EEG source modeling if the subject has been in a supine position during MRI data collection and sitting during EEG recording. In this context, Rice and colleagues (2013) also raised an additional concern related to brain atrophy due to normal aging and neurodegenerative diseases: the thickened CSF layer may dampen scalp potentials, although the cortical signals were unchanged. We want to emphasize that whereas the thickness of the CSF layer does not as such affect MEG signals, the associated change in the distance between the source currents and the sensors can affect the estimated source strengths. Moreover, the other mentioned position effects on cognition and bodily functions are relevant for MEG as well. Given all of above considerations, the merging and interpretation of MEG/EEG and fMRI data need careful attention even at the preliminary planning stages of a multimodal study.

■ EEG DURING NONINVASIVE BRAIN STIMULATION

When EEG is used concurrently with TMS, information may be potentially obtained about the connectivity between the stimulated area and other brain regions. Since TMS causes large artifacts in the EEG, some TMS-compatible EEG amplifiers have tradition-ally automatically been switched off for the duration of the TMS pulse. Hence, additional analysis methods need to be applied to either reduce and remove the artifacts or deal with data discontinuities (Ilmoniemi & Kicic, 2010; Rogasch et al., 2014; Mutanen et al., 2020; Hernandez-Pavon et al. 2022). After such precautions, both evoked and induced EEG ac-tivity can be examined.

Figure 21.5 illustrates an earlier study of TMS-evoked activity and its frequency content and scalp voltage topography after TMS stimulation of the left prefrontal cortex (Rogasch et al., 2014). Initially after stimulus delivery, higher-frequency (20–45 Hz) broadband activity is seen over the left frontal scalp, concurrently with lower-frequency (8–15 Hz) activity in the same scalp region. Activity over the posterior scalp is seen 80 to 200 ms after the TMS pulse and is suggestive of functional connections between anterior and posterior brain regions.

The TMS–EEG approach is a potentially powerful method. Combined with source lo-calization of timed neurophysiological activity, it could provide a good tool to study effec-tive connectivity and brain networks (Hallett et al., 2017). TMS–EEG might also be used in the future in the clinical environment to (a) assess local cortical excitability, (b) chart the spatiotemporal spread of induced activation, and (c) measure conduction times between the stimulated region and other cortical regions (Borich et al., 2015). Recent guidelines should be consulted regarding skills and competencies needed for safe use of noninvasive brain stimulation (Fried et al., 2021). Work is in progress to overcome technical problems in combining TMS and MEG in the same session.

The relevance and potential of TMS–EEG have been enthusiastically advertised for multiple clinical conditions, such as stroke recovery and other neurological and psychi-atric disorders (Tremblay et al., 2019; Keser et al., 2022). However, currently the clinical feasibility of the TMS–EEG method requires refinement from a technical point of view (application, artifact suppression, signal reliability, analysis, standardization). Additionally, meta-analyses are needed for assessing the sensitivity and specificity of the obtained results (Julkunen et al., 2022).

As we briefly mentioned in Chapter 9, EEG has also been used with transcranial direct-current stimulation (tDCS) in the study of synchronization of cortical activity (Roy et al., 2014). At the time of writing (2022), work examining the direct acute effects of tDCS and other transcranial electrical stimulation methods, such as transcranial alternating current stimulation (tACS), had started to enter the literature (A. Liu et al., 2018). However, the exact underlying neural mechanisms remain to be clarified, and it is still not certain at this stage how combined tDCS–EEG data will ultimately be used and interpreted.

An interesting new brain neuromodulation tool is low-intensity transcranial focused ultrasonic stimulation (FUS), which has a higher spatial selectivity than transcranial mag-netic and electric stimulation and that also penetrates much deeper, down to central brain structures (Bystritsky et al., 2011). Moreover, concomitant auditory or sensorimotor stim-ulation effects are small (although present) with FUS, in contrast to TMS, which produces loud clicks, tingling sensations, and muscle contractions (Darmani et al., 2022). Available FUS–EEG studies do not appear to have had issues with stimulus artifacts (Lee et al., 2015;

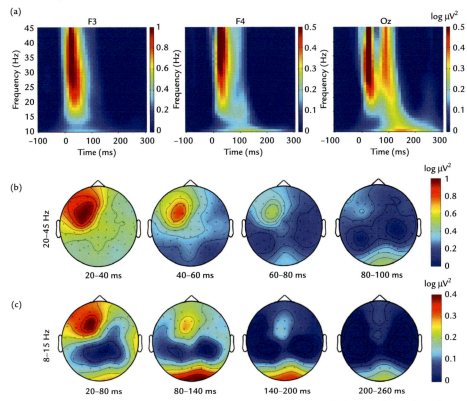

FIGURE 21.5. EEG recording during TMS stimulation of the left dorsolateral prefrontal cortex. (a) Grand-average (across 30 subjects) time–frequency plots of TMS-evoked oscillations at electrodes F3, F4, and Oz, showing a broadband response to the TMS pulse delivered at time zero and a second broadband response at Oz electrode about 100 ms later. Artifacts have been removed. Passband DC–3.5 kHz, sampling rate 20 kHz. (b) Topographies of TMS-evoked 20 to 45 Hz oscillations during 20-ms intervals from 20 to 100 ms. (c) Topographies of TMS-evoked 8 to 15 Hz oscillations during 60-ms intervals from 20 to 260 ms. Adapted and reprinted from Rogasch NC, Thomson RH, Farzan F et al: Removing artefacts from TMS–EEG recordings using independent component analysis: importance for assessing prefrontal and motor cortex network properties. *NeuroImage* 2014, 101: 425–439. With permission from Elsevier.

Darvas et al., 2016; Lee et al., 2016). In a 7-T fMRI study, FUS application to the thumb representation area in the primary motor cortex produced a larger activation volume relative to a standard finger-tapping task (Ai et al., 2018). Reliable somatosensory and visual evoked potentials have been elicited with FUS stimulation of primary somatosensory and visual cortices (Lee et al., 2015, 2016), but future work will have to compare these responses with conventional somatosensory evoked potentials (SEPs) and visual evoked potentials (VEPs) in the same subjects to understand how FUS affects the cortex. Safety of low-intensity FUS (e.g., Pasquinelli et al., 2019) has to be carefully considered because of potential tissue heating and injury; in fact, FUS at higher intensities is also used therapeutically, either to transiently open the blood-brain barrier for drug administration or to thermoablate a targeted tissue (Meng et al., 2021).

■ HYBRID MEG–MRI

An interesting technological development, intended specifically for the clinical environment, is the hybrid MEG–MRI method where ultra-low field (ULF) MRI and MEG are recorded with the same SQUIDs in the same device. In contrast to the conventional high-field (1.5, 3, or 7 T) MRI, the ULF MEG–MRI operates at very low fields of less than 200 mT but requires prepolarization of the proton spins (McDermott et al., 2004; Zotev et al., 2008; Vesanen et al., 2013). The ULF MRI has enhanced T1 contrast, which can be useful in detecting abnormal tissue, and critically *the device is silent during operation*. This technology allows accurate co-registration of the functional (MEG) and structural (MRI) data as both are measured at the same time. Consequently, the neural sources can be located accurately for purposes such as presurgical evaluation, and the connectivity analyses will be more reliable (Chella et al., 2019). One limitation of the MEG–MRI method is that, with this design, blood-oxygenation-level-based functional MRI signals cannot be recorded.

■ MULTIPLE METHODS AND THE "NEW NORMAL"

In this *Primer*, we have repeatedly championed the use of multiple assessment methods to provide converging evidence for studies in systems, social, and cognitive neuroscience. The literature using multiple methods in the same subjects continues to grow and is starting to provide valuable data that inform multiple branches of neuroscience. It is important that this trend continue so that our cutting-edge research methods can sooner become clinically feasible. In the next and final chapter of this *Primer*, we examine some exciting future developments in MEG/EEG research. It is our genuine belief that the future is particularly bright for these neurophysiological methods.

■ REFERENCES

Abou Khalil G, Doré-Mazars K, Senot P, Wang DP, Legrand A: Is it better to sit down, stand up or walk when performing memory and arithmetic activities? *Exp Brain Res* 2020, 238: 2487–2496.

Ai L, Bansal P, Mueller JK, Legon W: Effects of transcranial focused ultrasound on human primary motor cortex using 7T fMRI: a pilot study. *BMC Neurosci* 2018, 19: 56.

Amunts K, Mohlberg H, Bludau S, Zilles K: Julich-Brain: a 3D probabilistic atlas of the human brain's cyto-architecture. *Science* 2020, 369: 988–992.

Amunts K, DeFelipe J, Pennartz C, Destexhe A, Migliore M, Ryvlin P, Furber S, Knoll A, Bitsch L, Bjaalie JG, Ioannidis Y, Lippert T, Sanchez-Vives MV, Goebel R, Jirsa V: Linking brain structure, activity, and cognitive function through computation. *eNeuro* 2022, 9: ENEURO.0316-21.2022.

Antonakakis M, Schrader S, Aydin Ü, Khan A, Gross J, Zervakis M, Rampp S, Wolters CH: Inter-subject variability of skull conductivity and thickness in calibrated realistic head models. *NeuroImage* 2020, 223: 117353.

Borich MR, Brown KE, Lakhani B, Boyd LA: Applications of electroencephalography to characterize brain activity: perspectives in stroke. *J Neurol Phys Ther* 2015, 39: 43–51.

Buzsáki G, Logothetis N, Singer W: Scaling brain size, keeping timing: evolutionary preservation of brain rhythms. *Neuron* 2013, 80: 751–764.

Bystritsky A, Korb AS, Douglas PK, Cohen MS, Melega WP, Mulgaonkar AP, DeSalles A, Min BK, Yoo SS: A review of low-intensity focused ultrasound pulsation. *Brain Stimul* 2011, 4: 125–136.

Chella F, Marzetti L, Stenroos M, Parkkonen L, Ilmoniemi RJ, Romani GL, Pizzella V: The impact of improved MEG–MRI co-registration on MEG connectivity analysis. *NeuroImage* 2019, 197: 354–367.

Cottereau BR, Ales JM, Norcia AM: How to use fMRI functional localizers to improve EEG/MEG source estimation. *J Neurosci Meth* 2015, 250: 64–73.

Coulombe V, Saikali S, Goetz L, Takech MA, Philippe É, Parent A, Parent M: A topographic atlas of the human brainstem in the ponto-mesencephalic junction plane. *Front Neuroanat* 2021, 15: 627656.

Dale AM, Sereno MI: Improved localization of cortical activity by combining EEG and MEG with MRI cortical surface reconstruction: a linear approach. *J Cogn Neurosci* 1993, 5: 162–176.

Darmani G, Bergmann TO, Butts Pauly K, Caskey CF, de Lecea L, Fomenko A, Fouragnan E, Legon W, Murphy KR, Nandi T, Phipps MA, Pinton G, Ramezanpour H, Sallet J, Yaakub SN, Yoo SS, Chen R: Noninvasive transcranial ultrasound stimulation for neuromodulation. *Clin Neurophysiol* 2022, 135: 51–73.

Darvas F, Mehić E, Calerb CJ, Ojemann JG, Mourad PD: Towards deep brain monitoring with superficial EEG sensors plus neuromodulatory focused ultrasound. *Ultrasound Med Biol* 2016, 42: 1834–1847.

Diedrichsen J, Balsters JH, Flavell J, Cussans E, Ramnani N: A probabilistic MR atlas of the human cerebellum. *NeuroImage* 2009, 46: 39–46.

Ebersole JS, Ebersole SM: Combining MEG and EEG source modeling in epilepsy evaluations. *J Clin Neurophysiol* 2010, 27: 360–371.

Fried PJ, Santarnecchi E, Antal A, Bartres-Faz D, Bestmann S, Carpenter LL, Celnik P, Edwards D, Farzan F, Fecteau S, George MS, He B, Kim YH, Leocani L, Lisanby SH, Loo C, Luber B, Nitsche MA, Paulus W, . . . Pascual-Leone A: Training in the practice of noninvasive brain stimulation: recommendations from an IFCN committee. *Clin Neurophysiol* 2021, 132: 819–837.

Fujimoto K, Polimeni JR, van der Kouwe AJ, Reuter M, Kober T, Benner T, Fischl B, Wald LL: Quantitative comparison of cortical surface reconstructions from MP2RAGE and multi-echo MPRAGE data at 3 and 7 T. *NeuroImage* 2014, 90: 60–73.

Furey ML, Tanskanen T, Beauchamp MS, Avikainen S, Uutela K, Hari R, Haxby JV: Dissociation of face-selective cortical responses by attention. *Proc Natl Acad Sci U S A* 2006, 103: 1065–1070.

Genon S, Reid A, Langner R, Amunts K, Eickhoff SB: How to characterize the function of a brain region. *Trends Cogn Sci* 2018, 22: 350–364.

Glasser MF, Coalson TS, Robinson EC, Hacker CD, Harwell J, Yacoub E, Ugurbil K, Andersson J, Beckmann CF, Jenkinson M, Smith SM, Van Essen DC: A multi-modal parcellation of human cerebral cortex. *Nature* 2016, 536: 171–178.

Hallett M, Di Iorio R, Rossini PM, Park JE, Chen R, Celnik P, Strafella AP, Matsumoto H, Ugawa Y: Contribution of transcranial magnetic stimulation to assessment of brain connectivity and networks. *Clin Neurophysiol* 2017, 128: 2125–2139.

Hari R: Interpretation of cerebral magnetic fields elicited by somatosensory stimuli. In: Basar E, ed. *Springer Series of Brain Dynamics*, vol. 1. Berlin: Springer Verlag, 1988: 305–310.

Hari R, Parkkonen L: The brain timewise: how timing shapes and supports brain function. *Philos Trans R Soc Lond B Biol Sci* 2015, 370: 20140170.

Hernandez-Pavon JC, Kugiumtzis D, Zrenner C, Kimiskidis VK, Metsomaa J: Removing artifacts from TMS-evoked EEG: a methods review and a unifying theoretical framework. *J Neurosci Methods* 2022, 376: 109591.

Huang Y, Parra LC: Fully automated whole-head segmentation with improved smoothness and continuity, with theory reviewed. *PLoS One* 2015, 10: e0125477.

Huang CC, Rolls ET, Feng J, Lin CP: An extended Human Connectome Project multimodal parcellation atlas of the human cortex and subcortical areas. *Brain Struct Funct* 2022, 227: 763–778.

Ilmoniemi RJ, Kicic D: Methodology for combined TMS and EEG. *Brain Topogr* 2010, 22: 233–248.

Julkunen P, Kimiskidis VK, Belardinelli P: Bridging the gap: TMS-EEG from lab to clinic. *J Neurosci Methods* 2022, 369: 109482.

Keser Z, Buchl SC, Seven NA, Markota M, Clark HM, Jones DT, Lanzino G, Brown RD Jr, Worrell GA, Lundstrom BN: Electroencephalogram (EEG) with or without transcranial magnetic stimulation (TMS) as biomarkers for post-stroke recovery: a narrative review. *Front Neurol* 2022, 13: 827866.

Lee W, Kim H, Jung Y, Song IU, Chung YA, Yoo SS: Image-guided transcranial focused ultrasound stimulates human primary somatosensory cortex. *Sci Rep* 2015, 5: 8743.

Lee W, Kim H, Jung Y, Chung YA, Song IU, Lee JH, Yoo SS: Transcranial focused ultrasound stimulation of human primary visual cortex. *Sci Rep* 2016, 6: 34026.

Liljeström M, Hultén A, Parkkonen L, Salmelin R: Comparing MEG and fMRI views to naming actions and objects. *Hum Brain Mapp* 2009, 30: 1845–1856.

Lin FH, Witzel T, Raij T, Ahveninen J, Tsai KW, Chu YH, Chang WT, Nummenmaa A, Polimeni JR, Kuo WJ, Hsieh JC, Rosen BR, Belliveau JW: fMRI hemodynamics accurately reflects neuronal timing in the human brain measured by MEG. *NeuroImage* 2013, 78: 372–384.

Liu A, Vöröslakos M, Kronberg G, Henin S, Krause MR, Huang Y, Opitz A, Mehta A, Pack CC, Krekelberg B, Berényi A, Parra LC, Melloni L, Devinsky O, Buzsáki G: Immediate neurophysiological effects of transcranial electrical stimulation. *Nat Commun* 2018, 9: 5092.

Liu AK, Belliveau JW, Dale AM: Spatiotemporal imaging of human brain activity using functional MRI constrained magnetoencephalography data: Monte Carlo simulations. *Proc Nat Acad Sci U S A* 1998, 95: 8945–8950.

Markov NT, Ercsey-Ravasz M, Lamy C, Gomes ARR, Magrou L, Misery P, Giroud P, Barone P, Dehay C, Toroczkai Z, Knoblauch K, Van Essen DC, Kennedy H: The role of long-range connections on the specificity of the macaque interareal cortical network. *Proc Natl Acad Sci U S A* 2013, 110: 17161–17161.

McCann H, Pisano G, Beltrachini L: Variation in reported human head tissue electrical conductivity values. *Brain Topogr* 2019, 32: 825–858.

McCann H, Beltrachini L: Impact of skull sutures, spongiform bone distribution, and aging skull conductivities on the EEG forward and inverse problems. *J Neural Eng* 2022, 19: 016014.

McDermott R, Lee S, ten Haken B, Trabesinger AH, Pines A, Clarke J: Microtesla MRI with a superconducting quantum interference device. *Proc Natl Acad Sci U S A* 2004, 101: 7857–7861.

Meng Y, Jones RM, Davidson B, Huang Y, Pople CB, Surendrakumar S, Hamani C, Hynynen K, Lipsman N: Technical principles and clinical workflow of transcranial MR-guided focused ultrasound. *Stereotact Funct Neurosurg* 2021, 99: 329–342.

Mutanen TP, Biabani M, Sarvas J, Ilmoniemi RJ, Rogasch NC: Source-based artifact-rejection techniques available in TESA, an open-source TMS-EEG toolbox. *Brain Stimul* 2020, 13: 1349–1351.

Nangini C, Hlushchuk Y, Hari R: Predicting stimulus-rate sensitivity of human somatosensory fMRI signals with MEG. *Hum Brain Mapp* 2009, 30: 1824–1832.

Park MT, Pipitone J, Baer LH, Winterburn JL, Shah Y, Chavez S, Schira MM, Lobaugh NJ, Lerch JP, Voineskos AN, Chakravarty MM: Derivation of high-resolution MRI atlases of the human cerebellum at 3T and segmentation using multiple automatically generated templates. *NeuroImage* 2014, 95: 217–231.

Pasquinelli C, Hanson LG, Siebner HR, Lee HJ, Thielscher A: Safety of transcranial focused ultrasound stimulation: a systematic review of the state of knowledge from both human and animal studies. *Brain Stimul* 2019, 12: 1367–1380.

Puce A, Allison T, Spencer SS, Spencer DD, McCarthy G: Comparison of cortical activation evoked by faces measured by intracranial field potentials and functional MRI: two case studies. *Hum Brain Mapp* 1997, 5: 298–305.

Rice JK, Rorden C, Little JS, Parra LC: Subject position affects EEG magnitudes. *NeuroImage* 2013, 64: 476–484.

Rogasch NC, Thomson RH, Farzan F, Fitzgibbon BM, Bailey NW, Hernandez-Pavon JC, Daskalakis ZJ, Fitzgerald PB: Removing artefacts from TMS–EEG recordings using independent component analysis: importance for assessing prefrontal and motor cortex network properties. *NeuroImage* 2014, 101: 425–439.

Rosen BQ, Halgren E: An estimation of the absolute number of axons indicates that human cortical areas are sparsely connected. *PLoS Biol* 2022, 20: e3001575.

Roy A, Baxter B, He B: High-definition transcranial direct current stimulation induces both acute and persistent changes in broadband cortical synchronization: a simultaneous tDCS–EEG study. *IEEE Trans Biomed Eng* 2014, 61: 1967–1978.

Taberna GA, Samogin J, Mantini D: Automated head tissue modelling based on structural magnetic resonance images for electroencephalographic source reconstruction. *Neuroinformatics* 2021, 19: 585–596.

Thibault RT, Raz A: Imaging posture veils neural signals. *Front Hum Neurosci* 2016, 10: 520.

Tremblay S, Rogasch NC, Premoli I, Blumberger DM, Casarotto S, Chen R, Di Lazzaro V, Farzan F, Ferrarelli F, Fitzgerald PB, Hui J, Ilmoniemi RJ, Kimiskidis VK, Kugiumtzis D, Lioumis P, Pascual-Leone A, Pellicciari MC, Rajji T, Thut G, . . . Daskalakis ZJ: Clinical utility and prospective of TMS–EEG. *Clin Neurophysiol* 2019, 130: 802–844.

Vartiainen J, Liljeström M, Koskinen M, Renvall H, Salmelin R: Functional magnetic resonance imaging blood oxygenation level-dependent signal and magnetoencephalography evoked responses yield different neural functionality in reading. *J Neurosci* 2011, 31: 1048–1058.

Vesanen PT, Nieminen JO, Zevenhoven KC, Dabek J, Parkkonen LT, Zhdanov AV, Luomahaara J, Hassel J, Penttilä J, Simola J, Ahonen AI, Mäkelä JP, Ilmoniemi RJ: Hybrid ultra-low-field MRI and magnetoencephalography system based on a commercial whole-head neuromagnetometer. *Magn Reson Med* 2013, 69: 1795–1804.

Wang SS, Shultz JR, Burish MJ, Harrison KH, Hof PR, Towns LC, Wagers MW, Wyatt KD: Functional trade-offs in white matter axonal scaling. *J Neurosci* 2008, 28: 4047–4056.

Zotev VS, Matlashov AN, Volegov PL, Savukov IM, Espy MA, Mosher JC, Gomez JJ, Kraus RH Jr: Microtesla MRI of the human brain combined with MEG. *J Magn Reson* 2008, 194: 115–120.

CHAPTER 22

STEPPING BACK AND LOOKING FORWARD: TOWARD UNDERSTANDING THE HUMAN BRAIN

Knowledge comes by taking things apart.
But wisdom comes by putting things together.

JOHN A. MORRISON

We have inherited the past. We can create the future.

ANONYMOUS

In this chapter we take a step back to view the big picture in systems-level human neuroscience regarding the role of time-sensitive MEG and EEG recordings. The starting point for any solid experimental work is understanding the basics of one's methods and ensuring the quality and reproducibility of the results. One also needs to understand the limitations of the applied instrumentation and analysis tools. At the same time, one must be open to the multitude of new possibilities that the innovative use of these methods could provide. The starting point always is to collect data that are as clean and replicable as possible, so that the results are reliable and of interest to other scientists, thereby pushing the science forward.

To avoid incremental science, it is essential to carefully select the research questions among the unlimited number of unsolved issues in the world. In this final chapter, we therefore attempt to provide some food for thought by discussing the human brain as a multi-level dynamic system. We also remind the reader of the importance of converging multiple sources of information for building understanding of how the human brain works. But before addressing those more overarching points, we briefly examine some future developments of instrumentation and analysis tools, pinpoint some MEG/EEG research areas that could deserve more attention, and discuss some promises and challenges of the "big data" movement in science.

▪ FURTHER DEVELOPMENTS OF INSTRUMENTATION

In previous chapters we examined the recently rapidly expanding fields in MEG/EEG instrumentation, such as the increasing popularity of portable EEG devices that allow experiments to be carried out in real-life settings, although movement artifacts still remain an issue. Somewhat ironically, a very strong push for the development of light portable systems has come from the gaming industry.

We reiterate the importance of recording other physiological signals (e.g., heart rate, respiration, muscle activity, joint position, eye gaze, pupil dilation) and video of the body and surrounding environment to aid interpretation of EEG data (Pantelopoulos & Bourbakis 2010; Rehman et al. 2013). The physiological signals may be continuously monitored with, for example, capacitive micro-electro-mechanical (MEM) systems or textiles manufactured of conductive fibers (e.g., Patel et al. 2012; Babusiak et al. 2018). This kind of "smart clothing" also allows electrical signals from the brain and body to be recorded in naturalistic environments and in ambulatory patients. However, because of the small size of the EEG and some other physiological signals, considerable improvements in design will need to occur before these textile sensors can be used more widely (Tseghai et al. 2021).

Data from wearable sensors can be sampled and rapidly analyzed online and used, for example, for closed-loop *neurofeedback* to enhance the ongoing neural activity in certain frequency bands. Alternatively, the analyzed data could be used for a brain–computer interface (BCI) to control devices (e.g., a wheelchair or a prosthesis) using invasively or non-invasively recorded brain activity, especially of the motor cortex (Mojarradi et al. 2003; Aflalo et al. 2015; Murphy et al. 2015; for reviews, see Lebedev & Nicolelis 2006; Moxon & Foffani 2015). Latest developments are allowing mobile phone app control of these BCIs (Sun et al. 2020).

The brain signals could also be used to complement advanced spinal-cord stimulation via flexible electrode arrays implanted, somewhat unexpectedly, *beneath* the lesion site. These implants have already helped paraplegic people to stand up, walk, and initiate movements (Wagner et al. 2018; Rowald et al. 2022). This kind of targeted neurotechnology is a brilliant example of effective translational research arising from solid basic research, in this case assessing the physiological mechanisms of walking.

In MEG hardware, the largest change during the last 5 years has been the rapidly increasing popularity of optically pumped magnetometers (OPMs; see Chapter 5) that allow brain signals to be measured in flexible user-determined arrays with sensors positioned much closer to the scalp than traditional SQUID (superconducting quantum interference device) sensors. The improved OPM devices have the potential to significantly impact future clinical recordings as the adaptable sensor arrays can fit heads so closely that it is possible to obtain the maximum possible signal strength in each case *independent of the shape and size of the head*, infants included. Another very nice feature of OPMs is that they can be inserted into 3D-printed individualized scanner casts. Hence, extra sensors can be placed close to the eye to record noninvasive MRGs (magnetoretinograms) (Westner et al. 2021), on the cheeks or even in the mouth to improve signal detection from medial temporal lobes (Tierney et al. 2021). The versatility of the OPM sensor placements is also evident in recent work with concurrent recordings of brain *and* spinal signals with a customized head and spinal cast (Mardell et al. 2022). Moreover, combined OPM–EEG recordings can be made by inserting electrodes directly into the OPM helmet to prespecified locations.

Although OPM systems tolerate more subject movements than do SQUID-based MEG measurements, OPMs cannot (currently) operate in a patient ward or intensive-care unit because the measurements must remain restricted to the field-compensation region provided by sets of additional field-nulling coils, typically (but not necessarily) sited within a magnetically shielded room. For now, because of their low noise and fixed sensor positions, the SQUID-based neuromagnetometers continue to remain superior as far as the signal quality is considered and when high-frequency (> 200 Hz) activity is of interest. However, the recent helium-based technology, ^{4}He-OPMs, offers a wide band from direct current to 2 kHz, although the current noise levels exceed the SQUID-sensor noise by a factor of 10 (Zahran et al. 2022). Other room-temperature MEG sensors under development include cesium-based OPMs (Sheng et al. 2017) as an alternative to rubidium-based OPMs, solid-state yttrium–iron garnet magnetometers (Koshev et al. 2021), and tunnel magnetoresistive sensors (Kanno et al. 2022); with all these sensors, reliable brain signals have already been recorded.

Altogether, the ongoing extremely intensive development of OPMs that can be placed very close to the scalp (and skin of other body parts) will likely extensively increase the popularity of MEG recordings in both basic research and in clinical settings, thereby dramatically increasing the interest in applying time-sensitive methods in systems, cognitive, and social neuroscience.

■ WORKING WITH "BIG DATA"

With ever-increasing computational power and data storage capability, neuroscience has entered the epoch of "big data" (for standardization, see Chapter 8), associated with data-driven research in very large sample sizes of subjects to search for biomarkers, to decode brain states, and to classify disease states. Big data sets are also collected to study data *reproducibility* and *replicability*, as well as to promote *open science*. For all of these applications, the standardization, annotation, storage, processing, and curation of the data sets and the analysis pipelines need keen attention and scrutiny.

The *file size* of a state-of-the-art MEG/EEG from even one subject's recording can be large. Take for example a recording comprising 306-channel MEG, 74-channel EEG recording, 8 physiological signals, and say 4 stimulus/response channels. If all these signals are sampled at 1 kHz for 1 hour, and if they are digitized with 24-bit accuracy (with an additional 3 bits at the low signal level end, and final raw data storage options as either 16 or 32 bits), then the file size *could be as large as* $(306 + 74 + 8 + 4) * 1,000/s * 3,600\ s * 32$ = about 4.5 GB. Therefore, for a study with, for example, 25 subjects, one experiment would produce greater than 110 GB of data that, of course, could be compressed by down-sampling or by other means.

Mining Knowledge From Large Data Sets

"Data mining" with various machine learning (ML) tools can be used to identify or classify brain signatures at both the individual level and between subject populations, such as patients versus healthy subjects. In a typical classification problem, a training data set is used to train a set of classifiers (ML algorithms) equipped with a set of best-data separation parameters to predict the class to which data in a different (and independent) data set belong, for example, if someone has been viewing images of cats or dogs. A large data set can be split into two, with one half forming the training set and the other the set to be classified. Classifier accuracy can be calculated as a function of condition, and confusion matrices provide information about types of misclassifications occurring during analysis. The results can be used to understand underlying brain mechanisms or to generate new testable hypotheses in future experiments.

However, even if databases are really big, they are not equal to knowledge per se (Frégnac 2017). For example, classification of diseases or brain states can be inaccurate even though backed up by big data. Some humility and down-tuning of the hype around ML methods is called for, and the recent poor results in forecasting the spread and time courses of the COVID-19 pandemic (Ioannides et al. 2022) are an excellent case in point. Hundreds of AI (artificial intelligence) specialists rushed in to assist, but a critical appraisal of the results of 232 new AI-based algorithms showed that all, except two promising ones, were clinically useless for various reasons (Wynants et al. 2020). From these recent failures, we must learn many lessons (Roberts et al. 2021). First, caution should be exercised in selecting the training data sets themselves. In some cases, the data can be repackaged from other data sets that, in part, already exist in a public database, resulting in skewed training of ML algorithms. Biases may also arise from missing information or poor documentation, such as lacking demographic data for the included individuals. In the case of chest X-rays of COVID-19 patients, ML algorithms sometimes classified the individuals according to some secondary feature in the images, for example, imaging position (seriously ill patients were more often imaged supine) or text fonts in images acquired with different equipment. To remediate these irrelevant confounds, well-curated validation data sets are essential, as are collaborative efforts of the AI teams both to validate their algorithms and to work in close contact with clinicians.

Shared neuroinformatics tools help to integrate and analyze large data sets as, for example, brain-wide association studies that aim to understand the relationship between individual cognitive capabilities and brain size/structure. These studies are considered to require thousands of individuals for adequate statistical power (Marek et al. 2022). Another line of big data research goes toward large-scale simulations of the brain, aiming to explore mechanisms of different brain functions, behavior, and disease in silico (Frackowiak & Markram 2015). In general, we advocate moving from big data to *big science*, so that we can make real progress in accumulating *new knowledge*.

For data sharing to be effective, a number of requirements must be satisfied. First, the data must exist in common standardized formats (see Chapter 8). Second, data provenance must be thoroughly documented, together with adequate documentation of instrumentation, stimuli, and tasks, as well as descriptions and code used in all analyses with version control and unique digital object identifiers. National and international regulatory bodies also must agree on how, and where, data will be housed so that they can be accessed in perpetuity. These requirements currently differ between the European Union, the United Kingdom, and the United States, for example, related to research-subject privacy regulations. Thus it may be challenging for research groups to work on a particular scientific question using multiple data sets derived from, for example, the UK Biobank and Human Connectome Project. In our highly interactive and innovative neuroimaging community, many initiatives are currently being discussed at both grassroots and higher levels to overcome these regulatory challenges.

Biomarkers

In classical medicine, an experienced clinician makes a diagnosis on the basis of clinical signs and the patient's symptoms and anamnesis (history), combined with some laboratory tests. The efficiency of this set of diagnostic tools can, at least in principle, be significantly improved by accurate *biomarkers*, which can be combinations of measures, such as genotyping, brain imaging, and behavioral partitions. Biomarkers can aid clinical assessment, diagnosis, prognosis, and treatment of patients. Therefore, big data sets obtained with common experimental protocols in homogeneous patient populations have a tremendous potential to provide answers to clinical questions that would not otherwise be addressable in single medical centers.

In the data-mining analyses of large data sets, the privacy of sensitive healthcare information in individual subjects must be balanced with the benefits that the accumulating medical knowledge will provide for healthcare in society, as individual subjects usually do not benefit directly from these investigations (Fears et al. 2014). The public is typically very willing to share their *anonymized* and *deidentified* data to benefit others. Still, national legislation in many countries continues to prevent data sharing across international borders because of concerns related to private health information. The ethics issues arising in sharing the data must be considered *prior to data collection*, already at the stage of protocol submission to ethics committees, which play a critical role in balancing the risks and benefits of the proposed research. The consent forms that the subjects must sign need to contain complete information about current and future sharing plans of data with, or without, personal information.

■ NEW TARGETS IN MEG/EEG RESEARCH

Deep Sources

Over the years there has been continuing debate about the plausibility of recording MEG/ EEG responses from deep brain structures, such as thalamus, hippocampus, amygdala, insula, and cerebellum. Sampling activity from these structures is problematic as signal detectability rapidly decreases the deeper we go in the brain and the longer the distance from the sensors grows. For MEG, an additional strong effect arises from the spherical geometry because a source in the middle of an ideal sphere causes no magnetic field outside the sphere (see Chapter 1 and Figure 1.4). Thus, the conclusions that certain MEG/EEG signals come from these deep structures have typically been based on converging evidence from multiple methods (e.g., from intracranial human or animal data) and based on *more advanced analyses than just source localization* of MEG/EEG signals. We mention some these additional approaches below.

Neurophysiological signals can contain rich information about the spatial configuration of activity even when the source locations cannot be accurately identified (Stokes et al. 2015). Many deep structures, such as amygdala, hippocampus, and thalamus, likely contribute to EEG/MEG signals, as is evident from combined intracranial and MEG recordings in patients (Pizzo et al. 2019), from simulations using realistic anatomical and electrophysiological models for the deep activity (Attal & Schwartz 2013), and from MEG recordings in patients with altered cortical rhythms (e.g., in Parkinson's disease; [Salenius et al. 2002] or thalamic infarctions [Mäkelä et al. 1998]). However, these MEG/EEG findings speak only to the implied cortical consequences of activity in subcortical structures, but they do not indicate how likely it would be to identify activity in specific subcortical areas.

In Chapter 10 we discussed the probabilities of detecting with MEG recordings currents that are located at different parts of the cerebral cortex of individual subjects (Hillebrand & Barnes 2002) and the statistical power of detecting such cortical sources in a subject group as a function of the number of trials and the number of subjects (Chaumon et al. 2021). These studies, however, did not investigate the cerebellum or subcortical regions.

Figure 22.1 shows the calculated theoretical sensitivity maps of *cerebellar cortex* for measurements with MEG magnetometers and gradiometers and with EEG (Samuelsson

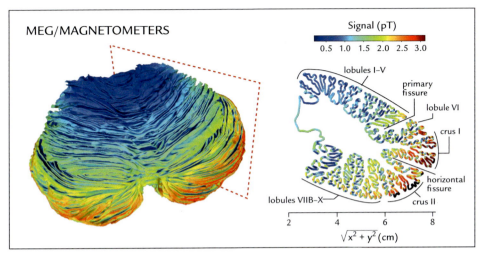

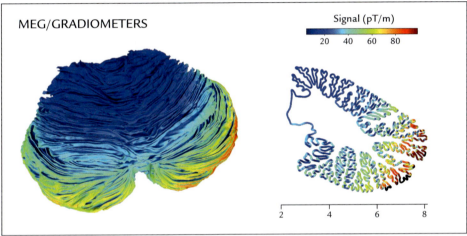

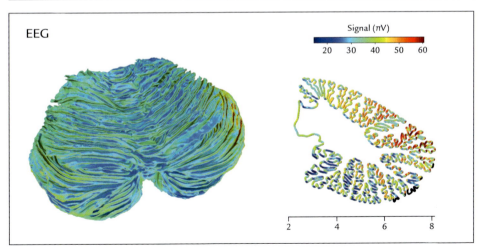

FIGURE 22.1. Cerebellar sensitivity maps showing different sensitivities for MEG and EEG recordings. The maps were calculated by inserting 100 nAm current dipoles at each source point in the cerebellar tissue, and the sensitivities are displayed separately for MEG

et al. 2020). These calculations were based on ultrahigh-resolution structural MRIs (magnetic resonance images) provided at 9.4 T of an ex vivo human cerebellum. One would expect that the highly convoluted thin folia of the cerebellar cortex would contribute to strong signal cancellation (see Chapter 2). Somewhat surprisingly, however, the simulations showed that cerebellar signals could be 40–70% of the size of signals from cerebral cortex if identical source currents are assumed (Samuelsson et al. 2020). Of course, the extent and distributions of cerebellar activation strongly depend on the stimuli and task, which leaves much space for insightful experimental design.

The few available intracranial recordings indicate that the cerebellum (see Chapter 2) can produce both low-frequency and high-frequency (up to 250 Hz) oscillations that exhibit task-related modulation (for a review, see Dalal et al. 2013). Such signals could, in principle, be picked up also with noninvasive MEG/EEG recordings. Multiple previous MEG studies have suggested sources in cerebellum in different experiments: during saccadic movements (Jousmäki et al. 1996); before and after somatosensory stimulation (Tesche & Karhu 1997, 2000); during slow repetitive finger movements (Gross et al. 2001); during a visuomotor tracking task (Jerbi et al. 2007); and during observation of other person's hand movements (Bourguignon et al. 2013); for a recent review, see Andersen et al. (2020).

Insular cortex would also be a very important target of MEG/EEG research for a number of reasons. First, it is among the least understood of brain regions (Uddin et al. 2017), possibly because it is cloaked by the opercula of the frontal, temporal, and parietal lobes. Additionally, its lengthy extent of finely folded tissue in the depths of the Sylvian fissure spans multiple cytoarchitectonic areas. Second, the insula is activated by information from multiple senses, such as olfaction, gustation, and interoception (Chapter 16), the latter of which includes pain, disgust, and bowel distension. Consequently, interoceptive awareness has been tied to the insular function. Direct stimulation of insular cortex in behaving monkeys (Jezzini et al. 2012) posits a major division between a caudal–dorsal sensorimotor field and anterior–ventral mosaic devoted to orofacial motor programs. The human insula also shows clear areal specialization with, for example, the parietal operculum preferentially encoding pain (Horing et al. 2019). In human intracranial recordings, responses with latencies ~500 ms occur to noxious heat stimuli in the posterior insula. However, these responses are not specific to nociception since responses of similar morphology and latency were also elicited by tactile, auditory, and visual stimuli (Liberati et al. 2016). Direct electrophysiological monitoring of the human insula is compromised by the rich and dense vasculature in that area (Türe et al. 2000). Moreover, even when clean electrocorticography/stereoencephalography (ECoG/SEEG) data are obtained, their interpretation is demanding as the insula is also active in various forms of disgust, with dissociable neural signaling in the somatic and parasympathetic systems (as measured with ECG [electrocardiogram] and EGG [electrogastrogram]) (Harrison et al. 2010). Accurate sensitivity maps

---

FIGURE 22.1. Continued
magnetometers (top panel), planar gradiometers (middle panel) and EEG (bottom panel). Note the large topographical differences in sensitivity (indicated by signal strength), particularly between MEG and EEG sensors. In the top panel, the cut level across the right cerebellar hemisphere is indicated by the dotted-lined rectangle, and major anatomical cerebellar features are labeled in the cerebellar slice. Adapted from Samuelsson JG, Sundaram P, Khan S, Sereno MI, Hämäläinen MS: Detectability of cerebellar activity with magnetoencephalography and electroencephalography. *Hum Brain Mapp* 2020, 41: 2357–2372. With permission from John Wiley & Sons.

based on individual anatomy would help interpretation of the MEG/EEG data suggesting activation of the insula.

What about other deep structures, such as brainstem, thalamus, amygdala, and hippocampus? All attempts to locate subcortical activity—be it in *brainstem, thalamus, amygdala,* or *hippocampus*—benefit from the anatomic and functional knowledge of subcortical pathways. Even if source locations cannot be identified by millimeter resolution, the results can still provide valuable information regarding the timing of brain activity. Validation of the results requires converging evidence from other methodologies. For example, studies of patients with circumscribed lesions in the areas of interest can provide additional evidence to support likely neuronal sources of MEG/EEG activity. In the early days of MEG when the generation of 100-ms AEFs (auditory evoked fields) in supratemporal auditory cortex was disputed, the abolition of these responses unilaterally in the affected hemisphere by a temporoparietal stroke (Mäkelä et al. 1991) was an important additional piece of evidence.

The detectability of subcortical evoked responses can be improved by increasing their signal-to-noise ratio by averaging. For example, averaging 16,000 trials helped to pinpoint multiple sources of auditory brainstem responses (see Figure 13.3; Parkkonen et al. 2009). Another strategy involves scanning interesting brain areas and their neighboring regions—selected on the basis of individual brain anatomy—as potential source areas; such a strategy has been used to detected thalamic activity to somatosensory median-nerve stimuli (Tesche 1996) and hippocampal activity to auditory oddball stimuli (Tesche et al. 1996).

Combination of a high number of averaged responses and anatomically determined regions of interest (ROIs) allowed Coffey et al. (2016, 2021; with $N = 14,000$ and $N = 11,000$, respectively) to pinpoint activity for speech-syllable-elicited frequency-following responses (FFRs) in the cochlear nucleus, inferior colliculus, and medial geniculate body, in addition to the cortical activity.

One interesting analysis strategy relies on the *sparsity* of stimulus-locked cortical activity (i.e., the activity is limited to a few cortical locations rather than being widely distributed), allowing a hierarchical algorithm to discriminate between *sparse cortical versus subcortical activity* (Krishnaswamy et al. 2017). Another promising possibility is to suppress—by computational means—the cortical signals and thereby improve the detectability of subcortical sources, a method that has been applied already to separation of cortical and subcortical auditory steady-state responses (Samuelsson et al. 2019).

We have learned in this *Primer* that both MEG and EEG studies have until now strongly focused on cortical activity, with the main subcortical EEG target in the auditory brainstem. However, the accumulating evidence about the detectability of signals from deep sources encourages the MEG/EEG community to pay increasing attention also to these less explored brain areas. Although the source localization accuracy is considerably worse for deep than superficial sources, complementary information obtained by other means can help considerably. For example, one can use anatomically defined ROIs and available anatomical and physiological information about the brain circuits of interest to test specific hypotheses and/or suppress the cortical activity by advanced computational means. After all, the most important contribution of MEG/EEG recordings for understanding human brain function derives from accurate timing, which is very valuable even when derived from source locations that contain some uncertainty.

Inhibition

Inhibition is a very important and energetically costly part of brain function (Buzsáki et al., 2007), sharpening and tuning neural processing and preventing the system from descending into disorder (e.g., an epileptic seizure). However, very little is known of inhibition's explicit hemodynamical (functional MRI [fMRI]) or gross neurophysiological (MEG/EEG) signatures. One reason for such sparsity of data might derive from the close coupling of inhibition to excitation. This coupling can take spatial form (e.g., Mexican-hat inhibition), temporal form (e.g., in-field inhibition), or a combination of both. In fMRI, tactile stimulation of one hand's fingers elicits a normal positive BOLD (blood-oxygen-dependent) response in the contralateral somatosensory cortex, but a negative BOLD in the ipsilateral side (Hlushchuk & Hari 2006). This finding is suggestive of neural inhibition because monkey recordings have shown similar negative BOLD responses that coincided with suppression of neuronal activity recorded directly from the visual cortex (Shmuel et al. 2006). In contrast, no such hemispheric distinction has been demonstrated in MEG/EEG recordings where ipsilateral SI responses are nonexistent. This interesting discrepancy in MEG and fMRI data raises many questions. For example, would the potential inhibition of the ipsilateral side be multisynaptic or be transmitted via slow fibers (see Chapter 21) and thus not be visible in the direct neurophysiological recordings that reflect the most synchronized activity?

Although detailed information is still missing regarding signs of inhibition in the temporospatial MEG/EEG time course, GABAergic drugs are known to enhance 20-Hz and 40- to 80-Hz rolandic rhythms (Jensen et al. 2005; Saxena et al. 2021). Quite striking is the suggestion, based on multielectrode recordings in monkey and human cortex (in two epilepsy patients), that local field potentials—which we assume to be the main contributors to MEG and EEG signals—are primarily associated with spiking of inhibitory neurons (Telenczuk et al. 2017). In this framework, the interpretation of many available MEG/EEG data apparently may need reconsideration.

More Focus on Developmental and Life-Span Studies

As totally noninvasive tools, MEG and EEG are extremely well suited for monitoring brain function throughout the life span. Recordings of spontaneous EEG are well established in the monitoring of newborn babies, including preterm infants, with known patterns varying according to the baby's vigilance (Pearl et al. 2018). Epileptic discharges are also easy to detect in the infant EEG (Pressler et al. 2021). An interesting research area centers on the relationship between developing brain function and nursing and care (see, e.g., Lehtonen et al. 2016). Therefore, hyperscanning studies (see Chapter 19), that is, simultaneous recordings from the infant and the caregiver, might more specifically assess some questions related to the development of brain mechanisms underlying social interaction.

MEG/EEG recordings have already been used to study, for example, the infant's sensitivity to speech sounds in their own and foreign languages, as well as the responses of the *fetal* brain to auditory and visual stimuli. Of course, questions similar to those studied in adults are also relevant, such as brain's responses to music, syllables, speech, and somatosensory stimuli; multisensory interactions; and motor function; for a recent review listing tens of infant MEG studies, see Kao and Zhang (2019).

Infant studies require careful subject preparation, such as feeding the newborn before the recording, letting the parent and infant experience the magnetically shielded room and even test the measurement chair or bed prior to the recording session, and letting older children choose a video for viewing during the measurement; see Clarke et al. (2022) for different aspects of infant MEG recordings. Fortunately, infants' EEG signals are large because of the discontinuities in their thin skull bones. Both EEG and OPM MEG can bring sensors very close to the brain, the latter even without touching the skin. For source modeling, however, ideally the infant's own structural MRI of brain should be used, as fontanelle closure has a wide temporal variation across individuals.

High-Resolution Assessment of Behavior

The combination of multiple physiological signals (discussed in Chapter 16) as part of MEG/EEG analyses will likely become a mainstay in cognitive, social, and systems neuroscience, as it allows the brain, the body, and the environment to be studied as an intimately interconnected system. Cognitive and social neuroscience methods provide rich measures of behavior. For example, infrared eye tracking provides both continuous measures of eye gaze and pupil diameter. As with ECG recordings of heart-rate variability, pupil diameter can also serve as an index of autonomic nervous system (ANS) activity during both resting-state and task-related EEG/MEG recordings.

At the same time, the importance of accurate assessment of motor actions cannot be overemphasized, and it is extraordinary how coarse our existing methods to measure behavior remain in the twenty-first century. In many neuroimaging experiments, motor actions have just two categories—pressing or not pressing a response button—whereas brain activity is measured with high temporal resolution in complex stimulus settings. A considerable improvement can be obtained by mouse tracking, which provides more nuanced responses, for example about emotional evaluation during a lengthy movie (Nummenmaa et al. 2012) or about the subject's change of mind during the response process (Stillman et al. 2018).

In an ML study where 3D poses of mice were video-monitored and then classified, the results indicated that the complex movements actually formed combinations of elementary movements and postures, very much like syllables in language, each lasting less than a second (typically 200–900 ms) (Wiltschko et al. 2015). Similar sequence analyses could be applied extensively to human actions, as seen in either high-temporal resolution video recordings or motion-capture data. Once again, the entertainment industry with its generous financial and technical resources leads the way; for example, "live" concerts with avatar performers based on human motion-capture data staged in specialized light and sound spaces have already been presented to audiences.

The latest developmental studies in human infants are an excellent example of what the potential gains can be from behavioral approaches. Video recordings from two cameras mounted on an infant's head (one to record the scene that the infant sees and the other facing the infant and recording their eye movements) can capture the image statistics that the infants experience in their first year of life. Not surprisingly, in the first 3 months human faces—caregivers' mainly as well as family members'—form the major input for infants lying on their back in the crib (Jayaraman & Smith 2019). During the first 2 years, however, the scenes viewed from the infant's perspective change from an earlier "face-dense" to a later "hands-dense" visual input as the social interactions start to transit to shared engagement with toys and other objects (Fausey et al. 2016). Various action monitoring devices, such as the wearable diaper cover containing accelerometer and gyroscope sensors to record the infant's respiration rate, body posture, and motor activity, can be added to the arsenal of behavioral monitoring (Ranta et al. 2021).

Multiple streams of behavioral measures, obtained from infants' and caregivers' head and eye cameras, have already been used examine how infants predict the actions of their caregivers (Monroy et al. 2021). Such behavioral infant studies have an impact on AI research, where AI is taught to learn in similar ways to young animals, including human infants (Prasad et al. 2019). The goal is to let the AI algorithms or devices learn better about the real world to avoid catastrophic failures, such as self-driving cars hitting pedestrians and cyclists or running into the back of buses or trucks.

Finally, the vestibular system, although behaviorally very relevant, remains ignored in both laboratory and naturalistic studies. The vestibular system provides an interface between the body and the environment, with direct control to musculature. Much more attention should be also devoted to proprioception, which is not only an important part of haptics (the combination of proprioception and touch), but a central component—with interoception—of bodily self-image.

■ TOWARD UNDERSTANDING THE HUMAN BRAIN

Systems-level neuroscience is a particularly appealing research field for multiple reasons. First, the brain is fundamental to human existence, with functions extending from not only basic physiological processes to thinking, acting, and caring, but also to violence, deception, and destruction. Second, because of the brain's immense complexity, interpretive challenges exist at multiple spatiotemporal scales, from molecules and single cells to brain networks and behaviors that include complex social interactions and the propagation of culture, requiring close interaction between multiple disciplines. Third, neurological and psychiatric disorders are extremely costly for society and emotionally damaging for patients and their loved ones. Finally, studies of brain structure and function can inspire development of "neuromorphic" devices for performing low-energy parallel computation.

Still, one of the most important goals of neuroscience is to understand the human mind and associated behavior. Obviously, these big problems cannot be adequately addressed without also considering the evolutionary, developmental, and aging trajectories of the human brain and without integrating results from many different sources across multiple analysis scales. For example, integration of human and animal data with computational modeling and theoretical neuroscience informs us about the generation mechanisms of brain rhythms (Sherman et al. 2016) and evoked responses (Neymotin et al. 2020; Kohl et al. 2022). Recent developments in ultrahigh-density chronic electrode arrays may help to bridge gaps between the microscopic cellular level and larger (meso)scale neural mechanisms. For example, at the time of writing (2022), silicon Neuropixels probes already allow chronic simultaneous recordings from up to 200 cortical single units with microelectrode contacts separated by 20 μm (Paulk et al. 2022).

From Micro- to Macrolevel and Back

As neuroscientists we may often forget that the human brain is not isolated in a vat but rather is situated in the body of its owner, who, by acting in, and on, the environment, receives continuous sensory feedback from the environment that, importantly, also includes other people. The brain is thus a part of an omnipresent action–perception loop where predicted action outcomes are compared with sensory feedback received during own actions (Chapter 17). During these processes, the highly plastic brain reorganizes itself on the basis of sensorimotor experiences.

Incredibly, the human nervous system's spatial scales vary by 9 decades: from nanometers (the scale of proteins) to about 2 m (the length of an adult human), and temporal scales vary by 19 decades from picoseconds (the scale of molecular dynamics) to about 100 years (the age of the oldest humans), as displayed in Figure 22.2. At each level of this multilayer system, different elements are connected as a complex network, forming "connectomes"

Spatial scales

Temporal scales

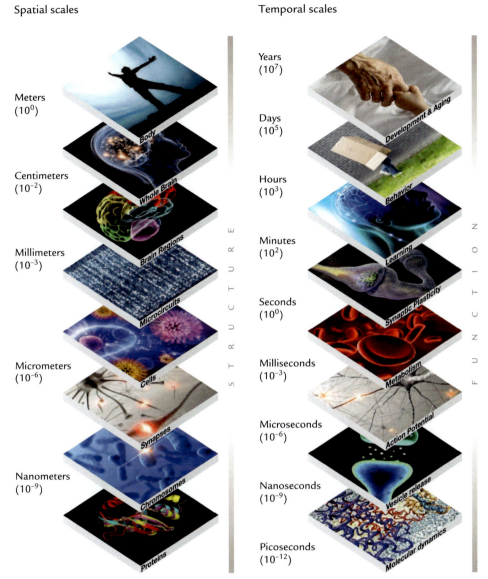

FIGURE 22.2. Multiple spatial (left column) and temporal (right column) scales of a human brain. For a more detailed explanation, see the main text. Reproduced from the HBP Report April 2002; Public Report to the European Commission.

of different spatial scales. When we move from lower to upper levels, qualitatively different new functions "emerge" from lower-level functions. The emerging higher-level functions (e.g., behavior) depend on lower levels (e.g., genotype), but cannot be reduced to them. For example, the contracting heart as a pulsating pump cannot, in an ontological sense, be reduced to the properties of the heart's muscle cells and neurons. In other words, groups of elements may have properties that do not exist in the elements themselves—or, in line with the words of the 1977 Nobel laureate in physics Philip W. Anderson: "More is different" (Anderson 1972). Even the most accurate understanding of the details of a single level does not permit us to understand how the human brain works, since we need to consider the brain as a *multilevel dynamical system*. Thus, it is evident that human brain imaging, working at temporal scales from milliseconds to seconds and spatial scales from millimeters to centimeters cannot tell us the whole story.

The brain also exhibits *downward causation* (or consequential properties) from upper to lower levels (Figure 22.2) so that, for example, genetic programming of proteins (and thereby plasticity) can be modified by the person's behavior, such as learning a manual skill. Moreover, even tiny differences in the environment can change these genetically coded outcomes—a phenomenon known as the "epigenetic landscape" (proposed by Conrad Waddington in 1940), meaning that the end results of two *identical* starting conditions can differ due to environmental influences.

The importance of the environment on behavior is nicely characterized by the famous "Herbert Simon's ant." Herbert Simon, the Nobel laureate of economics from 1978, was interested in decision processes and pointed out that the irregular path of an ant on a beach cannot be understood by studying (only) the ant (or its brain as we neuroscientists would do), but rather by considering the environment where various barriers block, or guide, the ant to choose a particular path. Similarly, the environment has a strong effect on human behavior and should be better scrutinized in human brain imaging research.

Living Matter Is Special

Sometimes brain states are considered to arise from atoms or molecules, similar to gas pressure that arises as the result of the thermokinetics of a large number of gas molecules. However, living matter is special in the sense that its smallest unit is a cell rather than a (sub) atomic particle or a molecule. Daniel E. Koshland characterized living systems by seven pillars supporting the "goddess of life, PICERAS" (Koshland 2002):

P stands for program (genetic programming via DNA);
I for improvisation (e.g., mutations allowing the organism to survive in changing environments);
C for compartmentalization (meaning that life takes place in limited volumes constrained by structural boundaries);
E for energy (life is always energetically an open system);
R for regeneration (e.g., this *Primer's* authors' hearts have already beaten about 2.5 billion times, requiring much cellular housekeeping and replacement of cardiac tissue, which would be impossible with other available natural or human-made materials);
A for adaptability (e.g., quick avoidance of a hot plate to prevent tissue lesion);
S for seclusion (e.g., specificity of enzymes to avoid unintended interactions as they operate in the same cytoplasm).

These pillars of PICERAS elaborate why brain function *cannot* be explained only in terms of the statistical mechanics of atoms and molecules. Indeed, we people consist of particles, but it is not their physical properties that determine who we are.

The Brain as a Nonlinear Timing System

In this *Primer* we have emphasized electric signaling of neurons, but the brain is also a chemically driven organ, with about 100 neurotransmitters that each have their specific time courses affecting postsynaptic neurons. Altogether this "wet timing machine" predicts the future on the basis of the past and present, being accurate or sluggish in its function, lagging or anticipating the triggering events for reasons that we do not yet fully understand.

MEG/EEG recordings have identified multiple activation sequences between human brain areas, but the situation is much more complicated than just feedforward progression of signals from one step to another with inter-step intervals caused by axonal conduction and synaptic delay times. In fact, the temporally overlapping activations in early visual cortices, revealed by intracranial recordings from monkey cortex (see Figure 14.6; Schmolesky et al. 1998) indicated that the activation sequences cannot be due only to simple feedforward connections. Therefore, we should strive to learn more about re-entrant connections that may be layer specific and operate in different canonical EEG frequency bands (Fries 2015) and thus potentially be distinguishable from each other. Lamina-specific OPM-MEG data have already been potentially differentiated in experiments where the subject's head movements were effectively constrained with individualized head casts (Meyer et al. 2017; Bonaiuto et al. 2018, 2021).

The brain as a complex dynamical system displays nonlinear behavior with, for example, phase transitions that can be evident also in overt behavior, such as falling asleep or suddenly becoming extremely alert because of a threatening event in the surrounding environment. A major cause of such transitions is the changed balance between excitatory and inhibitory signaling (Dehghani et al. 2016). Due to internal regulation, the healthy brain stays as excitable as possible without surging into disorder, such as an epileptic seizure.

Since the earliest *nonlinear analyses* of ictal EEG (Babloyantz & Destexhe 1986), hopes were placed on the analysis of nonlinear EEG dynamics to predict epileptic seizures, so that these might be prevented, or suppress epileptic activity by, for example, counter electrical stimulation (Kalizin & Lopes da Silva 2018). It has been assumed that the epileptic brain varies between different states—for example, seizures and normal interictal activity—due to noise or other internal fluctuations in the system, or due to external perturbations such as flickering light.

More recently, nonlinear MEG/EEG analyses assessing brain *criticality* have been similarly applied to (1) predict seizures, (2) forecast recovery from a persistent comatose state, (3) provide novel biomarkers for neurodegenerative disorders, and (4) imply signs of brain maturation from infancy to adolescence and adulthood (Zimmern 2020). Criticality refers to fluctuations of a system's state between order and disorder without any particularly preferred spatial or temporal scales (for reviews, see Beggs & Timme 2012; Cocchi et al. 2017; Palva & Palva 2018), acting as a set point between different states when a control parameter changes. For example, in water, a well-known physical system, increasing temperature results in a phase transition from solid to liquid, with another critical phase transition from liquid to gas. In a neural system, criticality could potentially underlie transitions between different resting-state networks, vigilance changes from wakefulness to sleep or anesthesia (Varley et al. 2020), or transition of normal brain activity to epileptiform discharges (Meisel & Loddenkemper 2020). The neurophysiological phenomena suggested to be linked to brain criticality include entrainment of brain rhythms, the nesting of frequencies associated with CFC (cross-frequency coupling), power-law scaling in time and space, and the scale-free temporal statistics of MEG/EEG/ECoG rhythms across a range of frequencies (Cocchi et al. 2017; Palva & Palva 2018).

Critical systems are of interest from brain function points of view because they are assumed to optimize information processing, allow a wider dynamical range for responses, and recall history better than noncritical systems. Although criticality phenomena have been demonstrated in the electric activity of neuronal cultures and in MEG/EEG signal patterns of human subjects, the interpretation of systems-level brain data still require much caution given the multilayer temporospatial organization of the human brain that we discussed above. In other words, the human brain forms a huge interconnected *system of systems*, where each subsystem—say, for example, the sensorimotor system—can have complex dynamic behavior of its own. Thus considering the moment-to-moment MEG/EEG nonlinear dynamics as reflecting a single "brain state" seems too coarse a simplification. It has also been questioned whether the brain operates at criticality at all (Destexhe & Touboul 2021). More robust methods, including statistical testing, are still being searched for to answer this question. One important task is to determine to what extent the criticality analyses are descriptive only or whether they can unravel underlying brain mechanisms.

Finally, an extremely important part of our research in the twenty-first century should also be devoted to attempting *to determine causality* and not being content with just studying correlation.

■ TOWARD CONVERGENCE RESEARCH

Teamwork and cooperation between researchers is required to share knowledge, and many research teams are justifiably proud of their multidisciplinary or interdisciplinary approaches. Yet, a more advanced collaborative approach is *convergence research* (National Research Council 2014), where the whole team has a common research goal that is approached with the concerted action of researchers with multiple backgrounds, all on equal footing. Only then can it be possible to completely share and integrate diverse perspectives, insights, knowledge and understanding, which is especially important when tackling really thorny (or "wicked") scientific problems that do not conveniently fit into the area of any single discipline or can be solved with the force of a single discipline. The wicked problems (Rittel & Webber 1973) typically include complex sociocultural and geopolitical issues with worldwide significance, such as the United Nations Sustainable Development Goals (United Nations 2021). Examples include climate action, health (e.g., the fight against pandemics), maintenance of peace and justice, and prevention of poverty and hunger. Understanding the human brain and mind is also a wicked problem in the sense that it needs the effort of many disciplines working in concert and that it does not have a set number of solutions.

Convergence scientists need deep roots that are anchored in their own specialty, complemented with a wide scope; for example, a strong foundation in mathematics/physics and coding is necessary for research in human brain imaging. It is essential to learn to work in a team (not only in a group that is typically a temporary collection of people) and to communicate effectively to *really interact* with other disciplines and to avoid ingroup–outgroup siloes. Passion for sincere science should be the reason to join convergence research, not grant money or possible high-impact publications.

Disciplinary borders are illusionary, with historical determinants. For example, neurology and psychiatry have historically diverged from neuropsychiatry to strengthen the identity and teaching of both branches. Today more and more people are trying to collaborate across these disciplinary borders, and in future these two disciplines may well be aligned more closely again.

■ LOOKING FORWARD

It is hoped that now you, our reader, are enthusiastically expecting to use your toolbox of new tools, gadgets, and gizmos to explore human brain function. Your goals may be in clinical diagnostics and follow-up or in researching a deeper understanding of the workings of the human brain.

Two decades ago, Paydarfar and Schwartz (2001) gave some timeless advice in their editorial in *Science* magazine that we wholeheartedly endorse: (1) slow down to explore; (2) read, but not too much; (3) pursue quality for its own sake; (4) look at the raw data; and (5) cultivate smart friends.

We would also add here the importance of forming a solid worldview, that is, making predictions of how the data might look. Only then can one be alerted to anomalies in the data and be prompted to totally new paths of scientific exploration; in fact, many advances in science have been serendipitous. It is also important to maintain common sense in data interpretation, as well as in statistical testing (Goodman et al. 2014).

Do not become enamored with a single tool. Rather, combine several methods and multiple views and you will take significant steps forward.

Now it's time to get out into the world and enjoy your new time-sensitive neurophysiological tools!

■ REFERENCES

Aflalo T, Kellis S, Klaes C, Lee B, Shi Y, Pejsa K, Shanfield K, Hayes-Jackson S, Aisen M, Heck C, Liu C, Andersen RA: Neurophysiology: decoding motor imagery from the posterior parietal cortex of a tetraplegic human. *Science* 2015, 348: 906–910.

Andersen LM, Jerbi K, Dalal SS: Can EEG and MEG detect signals from the human cerebellum? *NeuroImage* 2020, 215: 116817.

Anderson PW: More is different. *Science* 1972, 177: 393–396.

Attal Y, Schwartz D. 2013. Assessment of subcortical source localization using deep brain activity imaging model with minimum norm operators: a MEG Study. *PLoS One* 2013, 8: e59856.

Babloyantz A, Destexhe A: Low-dimensional chaos in an instance of epilepsy. *Proc Natl Acad Sci U S A* 1986, 83: 3513–3517.

Babusiak B, Borika S, Balogovab L: Textile electrodes in capacitive signal sensing applications. *Measurement* 2018, 114: 69–77.

Beggs JM, Timme T: Being critical of criticality in the brain. *Front Physiol* 2012, 3: 163.

Bonaiuto JJ, Meyer SS, Little S, Rossiter H, Callaghan MF, Dick F, Barnes GR, Bestmann S: Lamina-specific cortical dynamics in human visual and sensorimotor cortices. *eLife* 2018, 7: e33977.

Bonaiuto JJ, Little S, Neymotin SA, Jones SR, Barnes GR, Bestmann S: Laminar dynamics of high amplitude beta bursts in human motor cortex. *NeuroImage* 2021, 242: 118479.

Bourguignon M, De Tiège X, Op de Beeck M, Van Bogaert P, Goldman S, Jousmäki V, Hari R: Primary motor cortex and cerebellum are coupled with the kinematics of observed hand movements. *NeuroImage* 2013, 66: 500–507.

Buzsáki G, Kaila K, Raichle M: Inhibition and brain work. *Neuron* 2007, 56: 771–783.

Chaumon M, Puce A, George N: Statistical power: implications for planning MEG studies. *NeuroImage* 2021, 233: 117894.

Clarke MD, Bosseler AN, Mizrahi JC, Peterson ER, Larson E, Meltzoff AN, Kuhl PK, Taulu S: Infant brain imaging using magnetoencephalography: challenges, solutions, and best practices. *Hum Brain Mapp* 2022, 43: 3609–3619.

Cocchi L, Gollo LL, Zalesky A, Breakspear M: Criticality in the brain: a synthesis of neurobiology, models and cognition. *Prog Neurobiol* 2017, 158: 132–152.

Coffey EBJ, Herholz SC, Chepesiuk AMP, Baillet S, Zatorre RJ: Cortical contributions to the auditory frequency-following response revealed by MEG. *Nat Commun* 2016, 7: 11070.

Coffey EBJ, Arseneau-Bruneau I, Zhang X, Baillet S, Zatorre RJ: Oscillatory entrainment of the frequency-following response in auditory cortical and subcortical structures. *J Neurosci* 2021, 41: 4073–4087.

Dalal SS, Osipova D, Bertrand O, Jerbi K: Oscillatory activity of the human cerebellum: the intracranial electrocerebellogram revisited. *Neurosci Biobehav Rev* 2013, 37: 585–593.

Dehghani N, Peyrache A, Telenczuk B, Le Van Quyen M, Halgren E, Cash SS, Hatsopoulos NG, Destexhe A: Dynamic balance of excitation and inhibition in human and monkey neocortex. *Sci Rep* 2016, 6: 23176.

Destexhe A, Touboul JD: Is there sufficient evidence for criticality in cortical systems? *eNeuro* 2021, 8: ENEURO.0551-20.2021.

Fausey CM, Jayaraman S, Smith LB: From faces to hands: changing visual input in the first two years. *Cognition* 2016, 152: 101–107.

Fears R, Brand H, Frackowiak R, Pastoret PP, Souhami R, Thompson B: Data protection regulation and the promotion of health research: getting the balance right. *QJM* 2014, 107: 3–5.

Frackowiak R, Markram H: The future of human cerebral cartography: a novel approach. *Phil Trans R Soc Lond B Biol Sci* 2015, 370: 20140171.

Frégnac Y: Big data and the industrialization of neuroscience: a safe roadmap for understanding the brain? *Science* 2017, 358: 470–477.

Fries P: Rhythms for cognition: communication through coherence. *Neuron* 2015, 88: 220–235.

Goodman A, Pepe A, Blocker AW, Borgman CL, Cranmer K, Crosas M, Di Stefano R, Gil Y, Groth P, Hedstrom M, Hogg DW, Kashyap V, Mahabal A, Siemiginowska A, Slavkovic A: Ten simple rules for the care and feeding of scientific data. *PLoS Comput Biol* 2014, 10: e1003542.

Gross J, Kujala J, Hämäläinen M, Timmermann L, Schnitzler A, Salmelin R: Dynamic imaging of coherent sources: Studying neural interactions in the human brain. *Proc Natl Acad Sci U S A* 2001, 98: 694–699.

Harrison NA, Gray MA, Gianaros PJ, Critchley HD: The embodiment of emotional feelings in the brain. *J Neurosci* 2010, 30: 12878–12884.

Hillebrand A, Barnes GR: A quantitative assessment of the sensitivity of whole-head MEG to activity in the adult human cortex. *NeuroImage* 2002, 16: 638–650.

Hlushchuk Y, Hari R: Transient suppression of ipsilateral primary somatosensory cortex during tactile finger stimulation. *J Neurosci* 2006, 26: 5819–5824.

Horing B, Sprenger C, Buchel C: The parietal operculum preferentially encodes heat pain and not salience. *PLoS Biol* 2019, 17: e3000205.

Ioannidis JPA, Cripps S, Tanner MA: Forecasting for COVID-19 has failed. *Int J Forecast* 2022, 38: 423–438.

Jayaraman S, Smith LB: Faces in early visual environments are persistent not just frequent. *Vision Res* 2019, 57: 213–221.

Jensen O, Goel P, Kopell N, Pohja M, Hari R, Ermentrout B: On the human sensorimotor-cortex beta rhythm: sources and modeling. *NeuroImage* 2005, 26: 347–355.

Jerbi K, Lachaux J-P, N'Diaye K, Pantazis D, Leahy RM, Garnero L, Baillet S: Coherent neural representation of hand speed in humans revealed by MEG imaging. *Proc Natl Acad Sci U S A* 2007, 104: 7676–7681.

Jezzini A, Caruana F, Stoianov I, Gallese V, Rizzolatti G: Functional organization of the insula and inner perisylvian regions. *Proc Natl Acad Sci U S A* 2012, 109: 10077–10082.

Jousmäki V, Hämäläinen M, Hari R: Magnetic source imaging during a visually guided task. *Neuroreport* 1996, 7: 2961–2964.

Kalizin S, Lopes da Silva F: EEG-based anticipation and control of seizures. In: Schomer DL, Lopes da Silva F, eds. *Niedermeyer's Electroencephalography: Basic Principles, Clinical Applications, and Related Fields*. New York: Oxford University Press, 2018: 659–670.

Kanno A, Nakasato N, Oogane M, Fujiwara K, Nakano T, Arimoto T, Matsuzaki H, Ando Y: Scalp attached tangential magnetoencephalography using tunnel magneto-resistive sensors. *Sci Rep* 2022, 12: 6106.

Kao C, Zhang Y: Magnetic source imaging and infant MEG: current trends and technical advances. *Brain Sci* 2019, 9: 181.

Kohl C, Parviainen T, Jones SR: Neural mechanisms underlying human auditory evoked responses revealed by Human Neocortical Neurosolver. *Brain Topogr* 2022, 35: 19–35.

Koshev N, Butorina A, Skidchenko E, Kuzmichev A, Ossadtchi A, Ostras M, Fedorov M, Vetoshko P: Evolution of MEG: a first MEG-feasible fluxgate magnetometer. *Hum Brain Mapp* 2021, 42: 4844–4856.

Koshland DE Jr: The seven pillars of life. *Science* 2002, 295: 2215–2216.

Krishnaswamy P, Obregon-Henao G, Ahveninen J, Khan S, Babadi B, Iglesias JE, Hämäläinen MS, Purdon PL: Sparsity enables estimation of both subcortical and cortical activity from MEG and EEG. *Proc Natl Acad Sci U S A* 2017, 114: E10465–E10474.

Lebedev MA, Nicolelis MA: Brain–machine interfaces: past, present and future. *Trends Neurosci* 2006, 29: 536–546.

Lehtonen J, Valkonen-Korhonen M, Georgiadis S, Tarvainen MP, Lappi H, Niskanen JP, Pääkkönen A, Karjalainen PA: Nutritive sucking induces age-specific EEG-changes in 0–24 week-old infants. *Infant Behav Dev* 2016, 45: 98–108.

Liberati G, Klocker A, Safronova MM, Ferrao Santos S, Ribeiro Vaz JG, Raftopoulos C, Mouraux A: Nociceptive local field potentials recorded from the human insula are not specific for nociception. *PLoS Biol* 2016, 14: e1002345.

Mäkelä JP, Hari R, Valanne L, Ahonen A: Auditory evoked magnetic fields after ischemic brain lesions. *Ann Neurol* 1991, 30: 76–82.

Mäkelä JP, Salmelin R, Kotila M, Salonen O, Laaksonen R, Hokkanen L, Hari R: Modification of neuromagnetic cortical signals by thalamic infarctions. *Electroenceph Clin Neurophysiol* 1998, 106: 433–443.

Mardell LC, O'Neill GC, Tierney TM, Timms RC, Zich C, Barnes GR, Bestmann S: Concurrent spinal and brain imaging with optically pumped magnetometers. *bioRxiv* preprint 2022, May 13. https://doi.org/10.1101/2022.05.12.491623.

Marek S, Tervo-Clemmens B, Calabro FJ, Montez DF, Kay BP, Hatoum AS, Donohue MR, Foran W, Miller RL, Hendrickson TJ, Malone SM, Kandala S, Feczko E, Miranda-Dominguez O, Graham AM, Earl EA, Perrone AJ, Cordova M, Doyle O, . . . Dosenbach NUF: Reproducible brain-wide association studies require thousands of individuals. *Nature* 2022, 603: 654–660.

Meisel C, Loddenkemper T: Seizure prediction and intervention. *Neuropharmacology* 2020, 172: 107898.

Meyer SS, Bonaiuto J, Lim M, Rossiter H, Waters S, Bradbury D, Bestmann S, Brookes M, Callaghan MF, Weiskopf N, Barnes GR: Flexible head-casts for high spatial precision MEG. *J Neurosci Methods* 2017, 276: 38–45.

Mojarradi M, Binkley D, Blalock B, Andersen R, Ulshoefer N, Johnson T, Del Castillo L: A miniaturized neuroprosthesis suitable for implantation into the brain. *IEEE Trans Neural Syst Rehabil Eng* 2003, 11: 38–42.

Monroy C, Chen CH, Houston D, Yu C: Action prediction during real-time parent-infant interactions. *Dev Sci* 2021, 24: e13042.

Moxon KA, Foffani G: Brain–machine interfaces beyond neuroprosthetics. *Neuron* 2015, 86: 55–67.

Murphy MD, Guggenmos DJ, Bundy DT, Nudo RJ: Current challenges facing the translation of brain computer interfaces from preclinical trials to use in human patients. *Front Cell Neurosci* 2015, 9: 497.

National Research Council. 2014. *Convergence: Facilitating Transdisciplinary Integration of Life Sciences, Physical Sciences, Engineering, and Beyond*. Washington, DC: National Academies Press. https://doi.org/10.17226/18722.

Neymotin SA, Daniels DS, Caldwell B, McDougal RA, Carnevale NT, Jas M, Moore CI, Hines ML, Hämäläinen M, Jones SR: Human Neocortical Neurosolver (HNN), a new software tool for interpreting the cellular and network origin of human MEG/EEG data. *eLife* 2020, 9: e51214.

Nummenmaa L, Glerean E, Viinikainen M, Jääskeläinen IP, Hari R, Sams M: Emotions promote social interaction by synchronizing brain activity across individuals. *Proc Natl Acad Sci U S A* 2012, 109: 9599–9604.

Palva S, Palva JM: Roles of brain criticality and multiscale oscillations in temporal predictions for sensorimotor processing. *Trends Neurosci* 2018, 41: 729–743.

Pantelopoulos A, Bourbakis NG: A survey on wearable sensor-based systems for health monitoring and prognosis. *IEEE Trans Syst Man Cybern* 2010, 40: 1–12.

Parkkonen L, Fujiki N, Mäkelä JP: Sources of auditory brainstem responses revisited: contribution by magnetoencephalography. *Hum Brain Mapp* 2009, 30: 1772–1782.

Patel S, Park H, Bonato P, Chan L, Rodgers M: A review of wearable sensors and systems with application in rehabilitation. *J Neuroeng Rehabil* 2012, 9: 21.

Paulk AC, Kfir Y, Khanna AR, Mustroph ML, Trautmann EM, Soper DJ, Stavisky SD, Welkenhuysen M, Dutta B, Shenoy KV, Hochberg LR, Richardson RM, Williams ZM, Cash SS: Large-scale neural recordings with single neuron resolution using Neuropixels probes in human cortex. *Nat Neurosci* 2022, 25: 252–263.

Paydarfar D, Schwartz W: An algorithm for discovery. *Science* 2001, 292: 13.

Pearl PL, Beal JC, Eisermann M, Misra SN, Plouin P, Moshe SL, Riviello JJ, Nordli DR, Mizrahi EM: Normal EEG in wakefulness and sleep, preterm, term, infant, adolescent. In: Schomer DL, Lopes da Silva F, eds. *Niedermeyer's Electroencephalography: Basic Principles, Clinical Applications, and Related Fields*. New York, NY: Oxford University Press, 2018: 167–201.

Pizzo F, Roehri N, Villalon SM, Trebuchon A, Chen S, Lagarde S, Carron R, Gavaret M, Giusiano B, McGonigal A, Bartolomei F, Badier M, Benar CG: Deep brain activities can be detected with magneto-encephalography. *Nat Commun* 2019, 10: 971.

Prasad A, Wood SMW, Wood JN: Using automated controlled rearing to explore the origins of object permanence. *Dev Sci* 2019, 22: e12796.

Pressler RM, Cilio MR, Mizrahi EM, Moshe SL, Nunes ML, Plouin P, Vanhatalo S, Yozawitz E, de Vries LS, Puthenveettil Vinayan K, Triki CC, Wilmshurst JM, Yamamoto H, Zuberi SM: The ILAE classification of seizures and the epilepsies: Modification for seizures in the neonate. Position paper by the ILAE Task Force on Neonatal Seizures. *Epilepsia* 2021, 62: 615–628.

Ranta J, Ilen E, Palmu K, Salama J, Roienko O, Vanhatalo S: An openly available wearable, a diaper cover, monitors infant's respiration and position during rest and sleep. *Acta Paediatr* 2021, 110: 2766–2771.

Rehman A, Mustafa M, Israr I, Yaqoob M: Survey of wearable sensors with comparative study of noise reduction ECG filters. *Int J Comp Netw Technol* 2013, 1: 61–82.

Rittel HWJ, Webber MM: Dilemmas in a general theory of planning. *Policy Sci* 1973, 4: 155–169.

Roberts M, Driggs D, Thorpe M, Gilbey J, Yeung M, Ursprung S, Aviles-Rivero AI, Etmann C, McCague C, Beer L, Weir-McCall JR, Teng Z, Gkrania-Klotsas E, AIX-COVNET, Rudd JHF Sala E, Schönlieb C-B: Common pitfalls and recommendations for using machine learning to detect and prognosticate for COVID-19 using chest radiographs and CT scans. *Nat Mach Intell* 2021, 3: 199–217.

Rowald A, Komi S, Demesmaeker R, Baaklini E, Hernandez-Charpak SD, Paoles E, Montanaro H, Cassara A, Becce F, Lloyd B, Newton T, Ravier J, Kinany N, D'Ercole M, Paley A, Hankov N, Varescon C, McCracken L, Vat M, . . . Courtine G: Activity-dependent spinal cord neuromodulation rapidly restores trunk and leg motor functions after complete paralysis. *Nat Med* 2022, 28: 260–271.

Salenius S, Avikainen S, Kaakkola S, Hari R, and Brown P: Defective cortical drive to muscle in Parkinson's disease and its improvement with levodopa. *Brain* 2002, 125: 491–500.

Samuelsson JG, Khan S, Sundaram P, Peled N, Hämäläinen MS: Cortical signal suppression (CSS) for detection of subcortical activity using MEG and EEG. *Brain Topogr* 2019, 32: 215–228

Samuelsson JG, Sundaram P, Khan S, Sereno MI, Hämäläinen MS: Detectability of cerebellar activity with magnetoencephalography and electroencephalography. *Hum Brain Mapp* 2020, 41: 2357–2372.

Saxena N, Muthukumaraswamy SD, Richmond L, Babic A, Singh KD, Hall JE, Wise RG, Shaw AD: A comparison of GABA-ergic (propofol) and non-GABA-ergic (dexmedetomidine) sedation on visual and motor cortical oscillations, using magnetoencephalography. *NeuroImage* 2021, 245: 118659.

Schmolesky MT, Wang Y, Hanes DP, Thompson KG, Leutgeb S, Schall JD, Leventhal AG: Signal timing across the macaque visual system. *J Neurophysiol* 1998, 79: 3272–3278

Sheng J, Wan S, Sun Y, Dou R, Guo Y, Wei K, He K, Qin J, Gao JH: Magnetoencephalography with a Cs-based high-sensitivity compact atomic magnetometer. *Rev Sci Instrum* 2017, 88: 094304.

Sherman MA, Lee S, Law R, Haegens S, Thorn CA, Hämäläinen MS, Moore CI, Jones SR: Neural mechanisms of transient neocortical beta rhythms: converging evidence from humans, computational modeling, monkeys, and mice. *Proc Natl Acad Sci U S A* 2016, 113: E4885–E4894.

Shmuel A, Augath M, Oeltermann A, Logothetis NK: Negative functional MRI response correlates with decreases in neuronal activity in monkey visual area V1. *Nat Neurosci* 2006, 9: 569–577.

Stillman PE, Shen X, Ferguson MJ: How mouse-tracking can advance social cognitive theory. *Trends Cogn Sci* 2018, 22: 531–543.

Stokes MG, Wolff MJ, Spaak E: Decoding rich spatial information with high temporal resolution. *Trends Cogn Sci* 2015, 19: 636–638.

Sun KT, Hsieh KL, Syu SR: Towards an accessible use of a brain-computer interfaces-based home care system through a smartphone. *Comput Intell Neurosci* 2020, 2020: 1843269.

Telenczuk B, Dehghani N, Le Van Quyen M, Cash SS, Halgren E, Hatsopoulos NG, Destexhe A: Local field potentials primarily reflect inhibitory neuron activity in human and monkey cortex. *Sci Rep* 2017, 7: 40211.

Tesche CD: Non-invasive imaging of neuronal population dynamics in human thalamus. *Brain Res* 1996, 729: 253–258.

Tesche CD, Karhu J, Tissari SO: Non-invasive detection of neuronal population activity in human hippocampus. *Brain Res Cogn Brain Res* 1996, 4: 39–47.

Tesche CD, Karhu J: Somatosensory evoked magnetic fields arising from sources in the human cerebellum. *Brain Res* 1997, 744: 23–31.

Tesche CD, Karhu JJT: Anticipatory cerebellar responses during somatosensory omission in man. *Hum Brain Mapp* 2000, 9: 119–142.

Tierney TM, Levy A, Barry DN, Meyer SS, Shigihara Y, Everatt M, Mellor S, Lopez JD, Bestmann S, Holmes N, Roberts G, Hill RM, Boto E, Leggett J, Shah V, Brookes MJ, Bowtell R, Maguire EA, Barnes GR: Mouth magnetoencephalography: a unique perspective on the human hippocampus. *NeuroImage* 2021, 225: 117443.

Tseghai GB, Malengier B, Fante KA, Van Langenhove L: The status of textile-based dry EEG electrodes. *AUTEX Res J* 2021, 21: 63–70.

Türe U, Yaşargil MG, Al-Mefty O, Yaşargil DC: Arteries of the insula. *J Neurosurg* 2000, 92: 676–687.

Uddin LQ, Nomi JS, Hébert-Seropian B, Ghaziri J, Boucher O: Structure and function of the human insula. *J Clin Neurophysiol* 2017, 34: 300–306.

United Nations. 2021. UNSDG report: The Sustainable Developmental Goals report, United Nations. https://unstats.un.org/sdgs/report/2021/

Varley TF, Sporns O, Puce A, Beggs J: Differential effects of propofol and ketamine on critical brain dynamics. *PLoS Comput Biol* 2020, 16: e1008418.

Wagner FB, Mignardot JB, Le Goff-Mignardot CG, Demesmaeker R, Komi S, Capogrosso M, Rowald A, Seanez I, Caban M, Pirondini E, Vat M, McCracken LA, Heimgartner R, Fodor I, Watrin A, Seguin P, Paoles E, Van Den Keybus K, Eberle G, . . . Courtine G: Targeted neurotechnology restores walking in humans with spinal cord injury. *Nature* 2018, 563: 65–71.

Westner BU, Lubell JI, Jensen M, Hokland S, Dalal SS: Contactless measurements of retinal activity using optically pumped magnetometers. *NeuroImage* 2021, 243: 118528.

Wiltschko AB, Johnson MJ, Iurilli G, Peterson RE, Katon JM, Pashkovski SL, Abraira VE, Adams RP, Datta SR: Mapping sub-second structure in mouse behavior. *Neuron* 2015, 88: 1121–1135.

Wynants L, Van Calster B, Collins GS, Riley RD, Heinze G, Schuit E, Bonten MMJ, Dahly DL, Damen JAA, Debray TPA, de Jong VMT, De Vos M, Dhiman P, Haller MC, Harhay MO, Henckaerts L, Heus P, Kammer M, Kreuzberger N, . . . van Smeden M: Prediction models for diagnosis and prognosis of covid-19: systematic review and critical appraisal. *BMJ* 2020, 369: m1328.

Zahran S, Mahmoudzadeh M, Wallois F, Betrouni N, Derambure P, Le Prado M, Palacios-Laloy A, Labyt E: Performance analysis of optically pumped ^{4}He magnetometers vs. conventional SQUIDs: from adult to infant head models. *Sensors (Basel)* 2022, 22: 3093.

Zimmern V: Why brain criticality is clinically relevant: a scoping review. *Front Neural Circuits* 2020, 14: 54.

INDEX

For the benefit of digital users, indexed terms that span two pages (e.g., 52–53) may, on occasion, appear on only one of those pages.

Tables and figures are indicated by *t* and *f* following the page number